Clinical Cardiac Rehabilitation:
A Cardiologist's Guide

Second Edition

Clinical Cardiac Rehabilitation:

A Cardiologist's Guide

Second Edition

Edited by

Fredric J. Pashkow, MD

Associate-Director, Preventive Cardiology and Rehabilitation
Medical Director, Exercise Testing Laboratory
Department of Cardiology
The Cleveland Clinic Foundation
Cleveland, Ohio

William A. Dafoe, MD

Director, Prevention and Rehabilitation Centre
University of Ottawa Heart Institute
Ottawa, Ontario, Canada

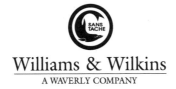

Williams & Wilkins

A WAVERLY COMPANY

BALTIMORE • PHILADELPHIA • LONDON • PARIS • BANGKOK
BUENOS AIRES • HONG KONG • MUNICH • SYDNEY • TOKYO • WROCLAW

Editor: Jonathan W. Pine, Jr.
Managing Editor: Leah Ann Kiehne Hayes
Marketing Manager: Daniell Griffin
Project Editor: Lisa J. Franko
Design Coordinator: Mario Fernandez

351 West Camden Street
Baltimore, Maryland 21201-2436 USA

Rose Tree Corporate Center
1400 North Providence Road
Building II, Suite 5025
Media, Pennsylvania 19063-2043 USA

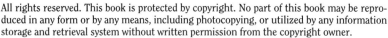

Printed in the United States of America

First Edition, 1993

Library of Congress Cataloging-in-Publication Data

Clinical cardiac rehabilitation: a cardiologist's guide / [edited by]
    Fredric J. Pashkow, William A. Dafoe. — 2nd ed.
        p.   cm.
    Includes bibliographical references and index.
    ISBN 0-683-30224-8
    1. Heart—Diseases—Exercise therapy.   2. Heart—Diseases—Patients—Rehabilita-
tion.   I. Pashkow, Fredric J., 1945– .   II. Dafoe, William A.
    [DNLM: 1. Heart Diseases—rehabilitation.   2. Exercise Therapy.   3. Heart Diseases—
prevention & control.   4. Heart Diseases—psychology.   WG 210 C641 1999]
    RC684.E9C55   1999
    616.1′ 203—dc21
    DNLM/DLC
    for Library of Congress   98-15106
                                                                                    CIP

To purchase additional copies of this book, call our customer service department at **(800)
638-0672** or fax orders to **(800) 447-8438.** For other book services, including chapter reprints
and large quantity sales, ask for the Special Sales department.

Canadian customers should call **(800) 665-1148,** or fax **(800) 665-0103.** For all other calls originating outside of the United States, please call **(410) 528-4223** or fax us at **(410) 528-8550.**

Visit Williams & Wilkins on the Internet: http://www.wwilkins.com or contact our customer service department at **custserv@wwilkins.com.** Williams & Wilkins customer service representatives are available from 8:30 am to 6:00 pm, EST, Monday through Friday, for telephone access.

98 99 00
1 2 3 4 5 6 7 8 9 10

This book is rededicated to our wives, Peg and Marie, and to our families, the people who truly sustain our day-to-day lives with meaningfulness.

Preface to the Second Edition

Seven years will have passed since we first conceived of the idea for such a book and the publication of this second edition. A lot has happened in this relatively short period of time in the world of cardiovascular disease. When we first approached the subject 7 years ago, physicians seemed mainly focused on the application of hard technologies for cardiac diagnosis and therapy—consisting of catheter intervention and bypass surgery for the most part. Cardiac rehabilitation and preventive cardiology were frankly neglected areas of specialization by our colleagues in our respective specialties of cardiology and physical medicine and rehabilitation. Our main purpose at the time of the creation of the first edition was to collect the most essential information under a single cover for the physician or other advanced professional involved in some way in cardiac rehabilitation programs—either as a medical director or supervising physician, or even as a referring doctor. We purposely included chapters rarely encountered in the cardiovascular literature covering the psychosocial aspects of heart disease, physical medicine issues relevant to the management of cardiac patients, and discourses on diverse areas—patient education, compliance, and applied technology.

Our first edition was well received and several strong reviews appeared in publications of general medical interest such as the *New England Journal of Medicine* and the *Lancet* in addition to the cardiac and cardiopulmonary rehabilitation literature. We embraced all of the constructive suggestions: six new chapters were added in an effort to expand coverage of the areas of growing interest, such as behavior and behavioral modification, the issue of gender, and the analysis of outcomes, in addition to expanded coverage on coronary disease risk factor management and preventive cardiology.

Our efforts are especially timely. It seems as if there is a real awakening regarding coronary disease risk factors with the growing realization that modification of these risks can slow or arrest the progression of the disease and, possibly more importantly, greatly impact the incidence of events such as myocardial infarction and unstable angina. This is spurred by the expanding understanding of how risk factors relate to the clinical manifestations of the disease, for example, how exercise alters the lipid profile and how those alterations may effect a patient's symptoms or the occurrence of an acute coronary event. This has led to a heightened interest in the practical aspects of program development and rehabilitation, and prevention programs seem to be popping up all over. Ironically, this comes at a time when the largest underwriter of health care, the U.S. government, in concert with some of the other influential policymakers and watchdogs of health care, would like to see any expansion of cardiovascular services contained.

Some other important things have happened in the interim as well. A Clinical Practice Guideline on Cardiac Rehabilitation was released in October 1995 by the U.S. Department of Health and Human Services. This effort looked exhaustively at cardiac rehabilitation and its components with regard to the scientific and clinical relevancy of the services. The results of this effort are incorporated into at least half of the chapters of this revised edition.

Lastly, we would like to emphasize another trend that we anticipated in our first edition and that has proven to be a major direction for this area of specialization. As a consequence of how cardiac rehabilitation evolved as a service historically, its development as a multidisciplinary field, and its orientation to outpatient and often extrainstitutional care, it is often the most appropriate "place" to implement newer models of long-term cardiovascular disease management, which inherently advances the concept of secondary prevention. Cardiac rehabilitation specialists have been doing this type of care for years now, and our experience and understanding of this paradigm are highly worthwhile for application to this evolving concept.

Preface to the First Edition

This book is intended for clinical cardiologists and for other physicians who need to extend their knowledge and involvement in the expanding area of cardiac rehabilitation. Furthermore, the mission of the book is to provide the clinician with a perspective about his or her pivotal role in this important field and an understanding that encompasses the contemporary and the controversial in a historical and clinical context.

By our current definition, cardiac rehabilitation consists of activities that include exercise, education, and reduction of modifiable heart disease risk factors, leading to a more normal state of cardiovascular health. In that sense, cardiac rehabilitation is maturing as a distinct modality of cardiac therapy. Historically, it began as a formalization of the concept of early ambulation postacute myocardial infarction, with risk stratification entering the process as predischarge or low-level exercise testing.

Cardiac rehabilitation has long been recognized for its subjective psychosocial value. Ironically, prospective studies have appeared in literature to confirm its efficacy for the reduction of morbidity and morality post acute ischemic coronary events just as quality of life issues are becoming increasingly important endpoints for medical intervention. Two major reviews, one by Oldridge and the other by O'Connor, demonstrate a 20% to 25% reduction in mortality for those patients who receive cardiac rehabilitation compared to those who receive "usual care." O'Connor's study notes a striking 45% reduction in the incidence of cardiac sudden death within the first year following myocardial infarction among those patients who receive rehabilitation. In this era of thrombolysis and more aggressive intervention—resulting in earlier and more appropriate revascularization—are we likely to observe further improvement in mortality? Are there other equally appropriate goals of therapy?

Studies that document regression of coronary atherosclerotic lesions in patients whose risk factors are favorably controlled are beginning to appear in the literature. As clinicians, we have been painfully aware of how difficult it is for patients to change behaviors critical to risk factor modification. Formalized cardiac rehabilitation programs can provide a forum for such a change. Can we influence our patients' compliance effectively and improve our results in making the required modifications of coronary risk? Studies suggest that, with appropriate program format, changes can be made and they make economic and financial sense.

The profile of patients who receive cardiac rehabilitation is changing and the population is growing. This reflects growth in both the absolute numbers of patients who have coronary disease, despite declining incidence, as well as the expanding population for whom rehabilitation is now felt appropriate. Patients who have poor left ventricular function or histories of malignant arrhythmia (perhaps with implanted defibrillator), for example, are being referred increasingly to cardiac rehabilitation programs. Exercise therapy for even these patients has now been demonstrated as safe, and there is a growing consensus as to which patients require continuous ECG monitoring versus intermittent ECG monitoring or exercise with staff supervision alone.

Those patients who are profiled at lower risk, however, have important needs. They require risk factor modification—especially smoking cessation, cholesterol and blood pressure lowering—and deserve attention from physicians and cardiac rehabilitation professionals despite their lower level of medical acuity and their greater level of medical stability. They need education and guidance and encouragement to comply.

How do we identify patients who are at greater risk for recurrence of coronary events or for untoward outcomes after a primary event? The exercise test remains a valuable tool for the process of assessing risk and prognosis and has been augmented greatly by newer, noninvasive techniques such as cardiac ultrasound and radionuclide imaging. Gas analysis during exercise testing is being used increasingly as an adjunct to combined cardiopulmonary assessment, especially for patients with complex problems who are being referred for cardiac rehabilitation with increasing frequency. New technologies also are available for risk factor diagnosis and patient monitoring, as well as patient education and the encouragement of compliance.

Patients and families all experience some psychological distress from their encounter with cardiovascular disease. Problems may arise from surgical or medical procedures. Such issues need to be addressed as part of the rehabilitation continuum. Returning to work may pose a concern if work demands appear excessive or the patient's medical condition has changed significantly. The clinician plays a significant role in the return-to-work process.

Patients and their families are also more aware of the existence of rehabilitation programs and are requesting referral to them more often, mainly because of expectations for improved functional capability and increased well-being. Cardiac rehabilitation has become an attractive ingredient in the services mix of many hospitals and has enhanced their self-image of excellence. A recent survey found that two-thirds of the hospitals in the United States with more than 500 beds offer outpatient cardiac rehabilitation now or will do so in the future. We estimate, however, that only 60,000 to 100,000 of the 2.5 million people with active coronary heart disease participate in cardiac rehabilitation.

Although cardiac rehabilitation has become increasingly popular among patients and hospital administrators, the truth is, few patients are enrolled relative to the large number of eligible persons. This is relative to the lack of consistent insurance reimbursement and to the costs related to the provision of the service. Although not nearly as expensive as other types of cardiovascular therapy, cardiac rehabilitation is sufficiently costly so that without insurance assistance it is prohibitive for most patients. There are low-cost alternative home and community-based programs that can be implemented successfully. Private corporations too have shown some interest in the development of rehabilitation programs to reduce the number of employees who require long-term disability and to reduce the expense of replacing employees prematurely. Physician involvement enhances the chances of success for these alternative strategies.

Improving participation in cardiac rehabilitation requires greater physician sensitivity to the rehabilitation needs of patients, an understanding of the suitable rehabilitation regimen for an individual patient, support for the development of multiple program options within a given patient-care area, and program referrals. This book outlines the important elements for implementing new programs, the medical-legal issues, and various program models that are presently effective. The goal of this book is to facilitate the use of this worthwhile therapy by cardiologists and other physicians who care for the cardiac patient.

Acknowledgments

We again thank our patients and staff for posing the questions that have challenged us to look for clinical and management solutions in cardiac rehabilitation and prevention from the clinicians' perspective. Special thanks go to our secretaries, Joann Kraynak and Jill Doane, who relayed hundreds of messages and packaged and repackaged manuscripts and never lost a chapter, and to Paula Schalling, Darrell Debowey, and their talented staff in the Cardiology Graphics and Design Section at the Cleveland Clinic who provided assistance with so many of the figures. We thank Jonathan Pine who steadfastly supported this book through its first edition and made possible a second expanded and embellished edition. We also thank the great staff at Williams & Wilkins, especially Leah Hayes, who handled our project with equanimity and patience, and all the other folks—our copy editors, production specialists, and the marketing and sales people—who worked and continue to work so hard on the book's behalf. We express special gratitude to our respective institutions, The Cleveland Clinic Foundation and the University of Ottawa Heart Institute, who continue to provide the vision, administrative support, and encouragement that allowed us to complete such an endeavor.

Contributors

Joseph A. Abate, MD
Clinical Assistant Professor of
Orthopedics and Rehabilitation
University of Vermont
College of Medicine
McClure Musculoskeletal
Research Center
Burlington, Vermont

Susan E. Abbey, MD
Associate Professor of Psychiatry
University of Toronto Faculty of Medicine
Director, Program in Medical Psychiatry
The Toronto Hospital
Toronto, Ontario, Canada

Philip A. Ades, MD
Professor of Medicine
Division of Cardiology
Director of Cardiac Rehabilitation
and Preventive Cardiology
University of Vermont
College of Medicine
Burlington, Vermont

John A. Bergfeld, MD
Head, Section of Sports Medicine
Department of Orthopedic Surgery
The Cleveland Clinic Foundation
Cleveland, Ohio

Kathy A. Berra, MSN, ANP
Clinical Trial Director
Stanford Center for
Research in Disease Prevention
Stanford Medical Center
Palo Alto, California

Gordon G. Blackburn, PhD
Program Director
Cardiac Health Improvement and
Rehabilitation Program
Department of Cardiology
The Cleveland Clinic Foundation
Cleveland, Ohio

Hank L. Brammell, MD
Cardiac Wellness Program Consultant
Leadville, Colorado

Laura Cupper, MSW
Vocational Rehabilitation Counselor
Prevention and Rehabilitation Centre
University of Ottawa Heart Institute
Ottawa Civic Hospital
Ottawa, Ontario, Canada

William A. Dafoe, MD
Director, Prevention and Rehabilitation Centre
University of Ottawa Heart Institute
Ottawa, Ontario, Canada

Pat Dunn, MS, MBA
Berkeley HeartLab, Inc.
San Mateo, California

JoAnne Micale Foody, MD
Department of Cardiology
Section of Preventive Cardiology
The Cleveland Clinic Foundation
Cleveland, Ohio

Barry A. Franklin, PhD
Professor of Physiology
Wayne State University School of Medicine
Detroit, Michigan
Director, Cardiac Rehabilitation and
Exercise Laboratories
Department of Cardiology
William Beaumont Hospital
Royal Oak, Michigan

Nancy Frasure-Smith, PhD
Associate Professor of Psychiatry and Nursing
McGill University Faculty of Medicine
Senior Research Associate
Montreal Heart Institute
Montreal, Quebec, Canada

Victor F. Froelicher, MD
Professor of Medicine
Stanford University School of Medicine
Stanford, California
Director, ECG and Exercise Laboratory
Division of Cardiovascular Medicine
Palo Alto Health Care System
Palo Alto, California

George O. Gey, MB, BCh
Clinical Assistant Professor of Cardiology
University of Washington School of Medicine
Chief, Preventive Medicine
Boeing Company
Seattle, Washington

Neil F. Gordon, MD, PhD
Director of Preventive
Cardiology and Rehabilitation
Savannah, Georgia

Sharon A. Harvey, MA
Manager, Stress Testing Laboratories
Section of Cardiovascular Imaging
Department of Cardiology
The Cleveland Clinic Foundation
Cleveland, Ohio

William L. Haskell, PhD
Professor of Medicine
Stanford University School of Medicine
Palo Alto, California

David L. Herbert, Esq.
Senior Partner
Herbert & Benson Attorneys at Law
Director, Professional Reports Corporation
Canton, Ohio

William G. Herbert, PhD
Professor and Director
Laboratory for Health and Exercise Sciences
Virginia Polytechnic Institute and
State University
Blacksburg, Virginia

William R. Hiatt, MD
Professor of Medicine
Section of Vascular Medicine
University of Colorado School of Medicine
Executive Director, Colorado Prevention Center
Denver, Colorado

Byron J. Hoogwerf, MD
Staff Physician
Department of Endocrinology
Director, Internal Medicine Residency Program
The Cleveland Clinic Foundation
Cleveland, Ohio

Robert F. Hunter, MA
Department of Cardiology
The Cleveland Clinic Foundation
Cleveland, Ohio

Arvind Koshal, MD
Clinical Professor and Director
Department of Cardiovascular and
Thoracic Surgery
University of Alberta Faculty of Medicine
Regional Clinical Director,
Cardiac Sciences Program
University of Alberta Hospital
Edmonton, Alberta, Canada

Michael S. Lauer, MD
Department of Cardiology
The Cleveland Clinic Foundation
Cleveland, Ohio

Sharon Lefroy, MEd, MHA
Business Manager
Prevention and Rehabilitation Centre
University of Ottawa Heart Institute
Ottawa, Ontario, Canada

François Lespérance, MD
Assistant Professor of Psychiatry
Université de Montréal Faculty of Medicine
Department of Psychosomatic Medicine
Montreal Heart Institute
Montreal, Quebec, Canada

Thomas H. Marwick, MD
Professor of Medicine
Unversity of Queensland
Princess Alexandra Hospital
Brisbane, QLD 4102, Australia

Louise Morrin, BSc, PT
Senior Physiotherapist
Prevention and Rehabilitation Centre
University of Ottawa Heart Institute
Ottawa, Ontario, Canada

James R. Nestor, PhD
Vice President
Cardium Health Services
Simsbury, Connecticut

Ira S. Ockene, MD
Professor of Medicine
Director, Preventive Cardiology Program
Division of Cardiovascular Medicine
University of Massachusetts Medical Center
Worcester, Massachusetts

Judith K. Ockene, PhD
Professor of Medicine
Director, Division of Preventive and
Behavioral Medicine
University of Massachusetts Medical School
Boston, Massachusetts

Neil B. Oldridge, PhD
Professor of Physical Therapy and Medicine
Indiana University
Center for Aging Research
Regenstrief Institute for Health Care
Indianapolis, Indiana

Jeffrey W. Olin, DO
Chairman, Department of Vascular Medicine
The Cleveland Clinic Foundation
Cleveland, Ohio

Fredric J. Pashkow, MD
Associate-Director Preventive Cardiology
and Rehabilitation
Medical Director, Exercise Testing Laboratory
Department of Cardiology
The Cleveland Clinic Foundation
Cleveland, Ohio

Peg L. Pashkow, PT, MEd
President
HeartWatchers International, Inc.
Solon, Ohio

Ileana L. Piña, MD
Professor of Medicine
Director, Cardiomyopathy and
Cardiac Rehabilitation
Cardiomyopathy and Transplant Center
Temple University School of Medicine
Philadelphia, Pennsylvania

Paul M. Ribisl, PhD
Professor and Chairman
Department of Health and Exercise Science
Bowman Gray School of Medicine of
Wake Forest University
Winston-Salem, North Carolina

Suzanne M. Rodkey, MD
Assistant Staff Cardiologist
Department of Cardiology
Section of Heart Failure and
Cardiac Transplant Medicine
The Cleveland Clinic Foundation
Cleveland, Ohio

Milagros C. Rosal, PhD
Assistant Professor of Medicine
Division of Preventive and Behavioral Medicine
Department of Medicine
University of Massachusetts Medical School
Worcester, Massachusetts
Instructor in Psychology
Department of Psychiatry
Massachusetts General Hospital/
Harvard Medical School
Boston, Massachusetts

Teresa M. Rudkin, MSc
Prevention and Rehabilitation Centre
University of Ottawa Heart Institute
Ottawa, Ontario, Canada

Robert A. Schweikert, MD
Department of Cardiology
The Cleveland Clinic Foundation
Cleveland, Ohio

Wayne M. Sotile, PhD
Director of Psychological Services
Cardiac Rehabilitation Program
Wake Forest University
Co-Director, Sotile Psychological Associates
Winston-Salem, North Carolina

Dennis L. Sprecher, MD
Head, Section of Preventive Cardiology
Department of Cardiology
The Cleveland Clinic Foundation
Cleveland, Ohio

Ray W. Squires, PhD
Associate Professor of Medicine
Mayo Medical School
Director, Cardiovascular Health Clinic
Division of Cardiovascular Diseases and
Internal Medicine
Mayo Clinic and Foundation
Rochester, Minnesota

H. Robert Superko, MD
Cholesterol, Genetics, and
Heart Research Institute
San Mateo, California

J. Robert Swenson, MD
Associate Professor of Psychiatry
University of Ottawa Faculty of Medicine
Director, Medical-Psychiatric Unit
Ottawa General Hospital
Ottawa, Ontario, Canada

Nanette Kass Wenger, MD
Professor of Medicine
Division of Cardiology
Emory University School of Medicine
Consultant, Emory Heart Center
Director, Cardiac Clinics
Grady Memorial Hospital
Atlanta, Georgia

Bruce L. Wilkoff, MD
Director, Cardiac Pacing and
Tachyrhythmia Devices
Department of Cardiology
The Cleveland Clinic Foundation
Cleveland, Ohio

James B. Young, MD
Head, Section of Heart Failure and
Cardiac Transplant Medicine
Department of Cardiology
Medical Director
Kaufman Center for Heart Failure
The Cleveland Clinic Foundation
Cleveland, Ohio

Contents

SECTION I. Current Perspectives in Cardiac Rehabilitation

SECTION II. Functional Assessment and Prescription of Exercise

SECTION III. Medical Considerations in Cardiovascular Rehabilitation

SECTION IV. Psychosocial Considerations in Cardiovascular Rehabilitation

SECTION I.

Current Perspectives in Cardiac Rehabilitation

Cardiac Rehabilitation as a Model for Integrated Cardiovascular Care

Fredric J. Pashkow and William A. Dafoe

HISTORICAL CONTEXT OF CARDIAC REHABILITATION

Early Ambulation Postmyocardial Infarction

Following the clinical description of myocardial infarction (MI) by Herrick in 1912, patients generally were confined to bed rest for 2 months. The fear was that physical activity would lead to the formation of ventricular aneurysm, heart failure, cardiac rupture, and sudden death (1).

In the late 1930s, Mallory and associates (2) described the pathologic evolution of MI as a process maturing during 6 weeks from the initial ischemic necrosis to the formation of a stable scar. This time characterization of infarct evolution reinforced the prevailing clinical practice of strict bed rest for 6 to 8 weeks after acute MI. Any activity defined as strenuous, such as stair climbing, was restricted for protracted periods, sometimes indefinitely. Needless to say, return to normalcy, including gainful employment, was rare.

The modern correlate of this concern is the concept of myocardial remodeling after an infarct. With expansion of the infarcted and noninfarcted tissue, there is concern that inappropriate physical activity may lead to aneurysmal formation. Indeed, Jugdutt et al. (3), in a retrospective analysis, observed such a phenomenon in cardiac patients with large anterior wall infarcts who followed a high-intensity exercise program. Increased aneurysmal formation in patients with large anterior wall myocardial infarcts was reported after early, recurrent high-level exercise, suggesting that adverse ventricular remodeling may occur (3).

More recently, a multicenter trial has demonstrated that patients with poor left ventricular (LV) function 1 to 2 months after anterior MI are prone to develop further global and regional dilatation. Exercise training does not appear to influence this spontaneous deterioration. Thus, postinfarction patients without clinical complications, even those with a large anterior MI, may benefit from long-term physical training without any additional negative effect on ventricular size and topography (4).

By the late 1940s, papers that questioned the efficacy of prolonged bed rest appeared (5, 6). Levine and Lown (7, 8) advocated the use of chair therapy as an alternative to prolonged bed confinement. The proposed physiologic rationale was that the dependency of the lower extremities led to reduced venous return, a decreased stroke volume, and a resultant lessening of the amount of expended cardiac work. Today, we realize that their interpretation of decreased cardiac work in a sitting position is slightly erroneous, because this position, in fact, results in a smaller increase in oxygen consumption than the supine position. This added energy requirement is minimal, however, and is more than offset by the advantages of early mobilization. Nevertheless, Levine and Lown's change in clinical practice represented one of the first liberalizations of the strict bed rest practice.

Newman and coworkers (9) characterized as "early ambulation" 3 to 5 minutes of walking twice daily during the fourth week of postinfarction convalescence. Brummer and colleagues (in 1956) appear to be among the first to report on the use of early ambulation—that is, within 14 days of the acute event (10). Cain and associates (11) also reported on the efficacy and safety of an early graded activity program in 1961. Thereafter, an awareness grew among clinicians that early mobilization after MI might not be harmful and, in fact, might avoid some of the complications of bed rest, such as pulmonary emboli and significant deconditioning (12). Subsequent studies have shown that the adverse hemodynamic effects of bed rest are related to the disorganization of the normal upright response to gravity (13) and are not related to alterations in sympathetic or pressor responses (14) or to muscular deconditioning per se. The physiologic effects of bed rest and restricted activity have recently been extensively reviewed (15).

By the late 1960s, 3 weeks' hospitalization after MI was considered clinically routine in the United States. The early 1970s saw a flurry of research activity related to early mobilization, particularly in the United Kingdom and in other countries in which the cost of hospitalization had already become a major social welfare issue. Studies by Groden and others (12, 16, 17) demonstrated the similarity in outcome and safety of early ambulation after MI but were not prospective or randomized. Controlled studies by Boyle, Hutter, Bloch, Abraham, and their associates (18–21) confirmed no significant difference in the occurrence of angina, reinfarction, heart failure, or death. Bloch and associates (20) showed significantly greater disability up to 1 year later in the patients who had not performed early mobilization.

Abraham and colleagues (21) found that early ambulation is beneficial regardless of the occurrence of complications such as angina or congestive heart failure (CHF) during the early infarction period, but in general, morbidity and mortality in postinfarction patients who have complicated courses (Table 1.1) are much higher than in those who have uncomplicated courses (22, 23). The most important clinical predictors are prior MI and the presence of CHF, or cardiogenic shock (1). Ambulation should be deferred in these patients until they have been stabilized medically and then performed gradually under close observation (24).

As early ambulation was applied increasingly, the process became more formalized and evolved into what we currently define as phase I, or inpatient cardiac rehabilitation (25). Wenger and coworkers (25) have done much to systemize the technique and to promote it for clinical use. Activities performed in the coronary intensive care unit were limited to 2 METs (1 MET = 3.5 mL O_2 consumed per kilogram body weight per minute). It should be noted that the MET formulation is a de-

Table 1.1.   Criteria for Classification of a Complicated Myocardial Infarction[a]

Continued cardiac ischemia (pain, late enzyme rise)
Left ventricular failure (congestive heart failure, new murmurs, roentgenographic changes)
Shock (change in mentation, oliguria, metabolic acidosis)
Important cardiac dysrhythmias (sustained atrial or ventricular)
Conduction disturbances (LBBB, >mobitz type 1–2nd degree AV block)
Severe pericarditis
Concurrent illness (severe respiratory disease, renal insufficiency, etc.)
Marked CK rise without a noncardiac explanation or after thrombolysis

AV = atrioventricular; CK = creatine kinase; LBBB = left bundle branch block.
[a]One or more criteria classify a myocardial infarction as complicated. (Adapted from Froelicher V: Cardiac rehabilitation. In: Parmley W, Chatterjeek, eds. Cardiology. Philadelphia: JB Lippincott Co., 1988;1:1–17.)

scription of *total* oxygen requirements by the body. In general, there is a correlation between METs and myocardial oxygen demands, but the relationship varies according to the type of activity. Upper extremity activities or isometric activities, for instance, may invoke higher myocardial oxygen demands than lower extremity activities. Activities that require fewer than 2 METs include self-care activities such as bed-bathing, use of a bedside commode, chair sitting, and passive and active range of motion. This portion of the experience usually is supervised by the unit nursing staff but sometimes involves a specialized rehabilitation team (26).

Once transferred from the coronary care to a regular nursing unit, patients commonly find that "specialists" supervise their rehabilitation. These specialists may be nurses, physical or occupational therapists, or exercise physiologists with special training and experience (26). Surveillance of the response to early ambulation is facilitated by the use of telemetered electrocardiographic monitoring (25). Untoward responses to activity include dyspnea, ischemic chest pain, dysrhythmia, or a disproportional heart rate (HR) response to exercise. ST-segment abnormalities during ambulation by noncalibrated telemetry monitoring may be misleading and require confirmation by 12-lead recording. The postexercise HR should remain within 20 beats per minute, and blood pressure (BP) should be within 20 mm Hg of the resting level (1). A fall in systolic blood pressure (SBP) of 15 mm Hg or greater below resting baseline is a worrisome sign. The inability to maintain or increase SBP with low workload suggests a significant compromise in pump function that may reflect either extensive intrinsic damage or large amounts of myocardium under ischemic stress. Any one of these adverse findings warrants clinical reassessment. An appropriate response to a given level of activity indicates that the patient can be advanced safely to activities of greater intensity (25).

The major goal for the physical activity portion of the phase I program is to condition the patient for the exertional demands required after discharge (27). This is a reasonably easy task because most activities of daily living (ADLs) in the home environment are less than 3 to 4 METs. If stairs are involved, this activity should be performed under monitoring and supervision until competency is achieved. Initially the tendency was to prescribe activity in rather rigid steps, and the MET level of each step was tied closely to the time elapsed after the event. Numerous early ambulation protocols that define from 7 to 14 steps have been made available (1, 28). The exercises prescribed correlated with various ADLs as well as with many educational and recreational activities.

We advocate the individualizing of exercise therapy by supervising progress closely with appropriate alterations in exercise frequency, time, and distance. Given that progress occurs in fractions of a MET and that patients may be fatigued related to concurrent medical procedures or other activities, this individualization seems suitable. Predefined activity formats continue to be useful in environments in which cardiac rehabilitation is not performed by specialists. It provides medical and nursing staff with an activities template and dispenses with the tedious requirement of writing specific daily activity orders for each patient (28).

With time, the limits of activity have been extended safely, and from the mid-1970s to the mid-1980s, length of hospital stay was shortened from 14 to approximately 10 days (29, 30). Length of stay for uncomplicated MI in the United States at the time of this writing may be as short as 4 to 5 days. This has significant implications both for goals and realistic expectations for inpatient programs as well as for the development of appropriately designed outpatient programs. In fact, the time has come for us to rethink the traditional concept of the three or four distinct phases of cardiac rehabilitation and to perhaps merge our experience in clinical exercise therapy with those providing home nursing and chronic disease management.

Expansion of the Rehabilitation Concept

Education about cardiovascular disease and informational transfer intended for reassurance and psychosocial support also are key elements in the cardiac rehabilitative process (23, 31). Historically, this patient education in the form of one-on-one counseling was added to the structured exercise and began during the course of routine hospitalization. Ideally, it should begin at the moment of the patient's initial encounter with the medical care system. Although hospitalization for an acute coronary event usually "gets the attention" of coronary patients, they often are so overwhelmed by the pain, confusion, fear, and anxiety of the experience that not much didactic information is retained. We suggest straightforward responses to patients' questions in the early hours or days of the acute event, followed by a more formal, structured educational process when the patient is further along in the physical and psychological recovery. Repetition of key parts of the material is essential to overcome emotional obstacles and is consistent with generally accepted learning theory. Studies suggest that such education can affect quality of life positively (32, 33).

With continuing shortening of length of stay, we see greater need for structured outpatient rehabilitation programs in the home, hospital, or the community environment. As we alluded to above, the amount of time spent in hospital is no longer adequate to acquire the skills required to monitor exercise activity or to cover the educational material adequately (34).

Outpatient programs began to appear in the mid-1960s. To some degree, they represented a direct extension of phase I. Several alternative models were available essentially from the beginning. Hellerstein and colleagues (35, 36) advocated that exercise be performed under close medical monitoring and supervision, and this established a precedent that is followed today in many phase II formats, in which both continuous electrocardiogram (ECG) monitoring and exercise supervision are provided.

Alternatively, gymnasium-based programs also

became popular (26, 37, 38). Physicians frequently volunteered their time for supervision, and the programs often received community support (39). Drug boxes, bottled oxygen, and a cardioverter/defibrillator were available on site. The defibrillator often was equipped with "quick-look" paddles, and patients were taught to monitor their own blood pressures and pulse rates (26). This degree of caution was believed to be appropriate, given the estimated safety of the therapy (40). Data have accumulated that demonstrate the significant safety of outpatient exercise rehabilitation, regardless of the model followed (41, 42). The gymnasium- or community-based programs were identified as "phase III" and were thought to be ideal for those persons who had graduated from phase II programs. By the late 1970s, however, patients with uncomplicated courses who were thought to be at "low risk" were being referred directly (39).

The concept of risk stratification became more widely applied and was extended further in the mid-1980s by DeBusk, Haskell, and others (43–45), who advocated home exercise programs. (This is discussed in more detail later in this chapter and in chapter 24.)

The relative time-course relationship of phases I through III rehabilitation is illustrated in Figure 1.1.

Cardiac Rehabilitation Perspectives

The World Health Organization (WHO) has defined cardiac rehabilitation as the "sum of activity required to ensure cardiac patients the best possible physical, mental, and social conditions so that they may by their own efforts, regain as normal as possible a place in the community and lead an active life" (46).

Implicit in this definition is the concept of *secondary prevention,* which can be defined as the effort toward risk factor reduction designed to lessen the chance of a subsequent cardiac event and to slow and perhaps stop the progression of the disease process. A conceptual model of cardiac rehabilitation is depicted in Figure 1.2.

This Venn-type diagram shows that secondary prevention goals are embedded in the overall goal of cardiac rehabilitation. Each component of a cardiac rehabilitation program is shown by the rectangles. For example, a formal exercise program has approximately equal benefits for secondary prevention and rehabilitation alike. Rehabilitation "end points" from the exercise program might be less depression, greater confidence for resumption of normal activities, and so forth. Secondary prevention "end points" from this same modality could be the effects that exercise has on risk factors (increased high-density lipoprotein [HDL] cholesterol, improved weight control). Another program component, such as smoking cessation, would have most of its benefits directed toward secondary prevention.

The history of cardiac rehabilitation from the WHO perspective is outlined by Lamm (47). The WHO became interested in the problem of cardiovascular disease in the late 1950s with the recognition of the high rate of coronary heart disease

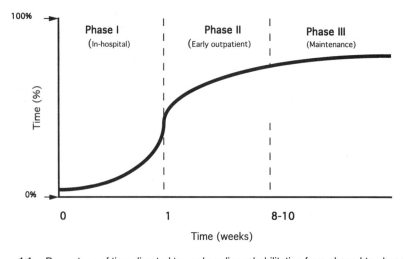

Figure 1.1.   Percentage of time directed toward cardiac rehabilitation from phase I to phase III.

Rehabilitation goals

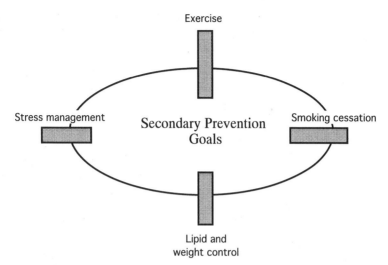

Figure 1.2. Components of cardiac rehabilitation. Relative contribution to rehabilitation versus secondary prevention goals.

(CHD) in the western world and rheumatic fever and Chagas disease in developing countries. A cardiovascular disease unit was established at the WHO headquarters in Geneva in 1958. An expert committee on rehabilitation was established in 1964 and reviewed the acute and long-term facilities for treatment, the prevailing medical attitudes, and the available health care facilities (46).

After this meeting, two major philosophical directions emerged and persisted for many years. One group believed that cardiac rehabilitation was synonymous with physical training. This group looked at the role of exercise testing and training for cardiac patients. Further efforts led to the publication of two WHO monographs, *Fundamentals of Exercise Testing* and *Assessment of Habitual Activity*.

The other group concentrated on the following areas: the cardiovascular situation in Europe, the formulation of practical recommendations that used existing knowledge, and the issues that required more research. In the early 1970s, an increasing number of working groups evaluated different components of rehabilitation. Some of the emerging concepts included the following:

1. Physical exercise should be only one part of rehabilitation.
2. Rehabilitation is only one part of secondary prevention.

3. Noncardiologic aspects—psychological, social, and vocational—play an important role in the success or failure of rehabilitation.
4. Nearly all existing attempts to assess sustained regular physical exercise in MI patients have failed because of the high drop-out rates of initial participants.

Presently, the role of the WHO is to bring together experts who work in the fields of epidemiology, primary prevention, clinical cardiology, and rehabilitation for the conceptualization and implementation of practical secondary prevention strategies. The institutions in Europe that promoted and performed cardiac rehabilitation were fostered by these WHO principles.

By its very nature, cardiac rehabilitation is heterogeneous and involves health care practitioners from various disciplines. The American Heart Association (AHA) and the American College of Cardiology (ACC) have recurrently developed and published standards and guidelines that will be discussed throughout the book.

The American College of Sports Medicine (ACSM) has supported cardiac rehabilitation by offering certification procedures for personnel involved with the exercise training of cardiac patients (48). The first 20 candidates were certified in 1975 from a workshop held in Aspen, Colorado. Presently, more than 200 exercise specialists are certified each year in the United States. Other countries, including Japan and Canada, have similar certifications that involve ACSM procedures. The ACSM has two references pertinent to cardiac rehabilitation: *The Guidelines for Exercise Testing and Prescription* (49) and *The Resource Manual for Exercise Testing and Prescription* (50).

The American Association of Cardiovascular and Pulmonary Rehabilitation (AACVPR) was founded in 1986 and serves as the national association for cardiac rehabilitation specialists. The *Journal of Cardiopulmonary Rehabilitation* is the AACVPR official publication. Other national associations of cardiac rehabilitation are emerging. The Canadian Association of Cardiac Rehabilitation (CACR) was officially incorporated in 1991 and has a similar mandate as the AACVPR.

Policy Statements on Cardiac Rehabilitation

The WHO formed an expert committee on prevention of CHD in 1981. Their general statement regarding the prevention of the recurrence and progression of CHD is as follows (51):

A substantial proportion of CHD deaths occur in people already known to have the disease; measures to influence the course of already recognized CHD might help significantly to reduce the total attributable mortality. The long-term prognosis after a heart attack is influenced by many of the same risk factors that provoked the first attack, suggesting that atherosclerosis continues to progress, and hence that preventive measures are still relevant.

The Expert Committee recommended that, for every CHD patient, planned preventive measures should be part of the usual care. The expectation of long-term benefit is unlikely to be less, and could well be more, than in primary prevention.

The American Heart Association and American College of Cardiology in 1996 published guidelines for the management of patients with acute MI (52). These guidelines for long-term management stated:

The patient should be instructed to achieve an ideal weight and educated about a diet low in saturated fat and cholesterol. The patient with a low-density lipoprotein cholesterol measurement greater than 130 mg/dL (3.36 mmol/L) despite diet should be given drug therapy with the goal of reducing LDL to less than 100 mg/dL (2.59 mmol/L). Smoking cessation is essential. Finally, the patient should be encouraged to participate in a formal rehabilitation program.

The Canadian Cardiovascular Society in 1995 issued the following recommendations for cardiac rehabilitation after a consensus conference for the management of the post-MI patient (53):

The aim of rehabilitation is to relieve symptoms and to improve both cardiovascular performance and quality of life. Rehabilitation strategies should include services to help control weight, smoking, blood pressure, and lipid disorders; to help manage emotional stress and facilitate social support; and an exercise prescription to help increase exercise tolerance. The immediate and long-term aims of rehabilitation are to relieve symptoms and to improve both cardiovascular performance and quality of life.

In 1995, The Clinical Practice Guideline Panel applied the U.S. Public Health Service definition for cardiac rehabilitation (54):

Cardiac rehabilitation services are comprehensive, long-term programs involving medical evaluation, prescribed exercise, cardiac risk factor modification, education, and counseling. These programs are designed to limit the physiologic and psychological effects of cardiac illness, reduce the risk for sudden death or reinfarction, control cardiac symptoms, stabilize or reverse the atherosclerotic process, and enhance the psychosocial and vocational status of selected patients.

Predischarge Exercise Testing

Exercise ECG ("stress") testing has proved to be an important tool in the assessment of the status of patients who recover from acute MI (55). It is extremely useful for assessing and reassuring patients of their capability for returning to work and normal recreational activities (27). Early studies demonstrated its feasibility and safety

(56, 57), as well as its ability to predict the risk of occurrence of angina, recurrent MI, and death after infarction (58–60). Early exercise testing contributed to the developing concept of risk stratification and the recognition of the need for further intervention. As outpatient rehabilitation programs have come into being, the graded exercise test, even when performed before discharge, has become a prerequisite first step.

Originally, the studies were performed to a level that approximated the degree of physical activity achieved during the latter days of hospitalization and was stopped on the basis of fixed end points, usually HR or MET-level limited (57). Even early on, studies showed that selected patients can be tested safely to symptom- or sign-limited end points (58–61). Currently, a HR limit of 130 beats per minute and 5 METs is used for patients older than 40 years of age, and 140 beats per minute and 7 METs for patients younger than 40. A perceived exertion level in the range of 15 to 16 on the Borg scale can also be used to end the test (see chapter 5).

Evolution of Risk Stratification

During the 1980s, various designated therapies for particular subsets of patients were shown to improve survival after acute MI (62). Studies have confirmed that predischarge exercise ECG testing may help identify patients who are likely to experience ischemically mediated events, such as subsequent infarction, and who are candidates for more aggressive interventions, such as surgical revascularization (63). As we know, the process by which these various subsets of patients are identified emerged as *risk stratification*.

Topol and associates (64) established that submitting patients who are recovering from an infarction to exercise testing actually may expedite and optimize discharge from the hospital. Early submaximal exercise testing also has been shown to be useful in evaluating unstable angina patients for the presence of multivessel CHD after stabilization (65).

Low-level exercise testing before discharge predicted subsequent events better than a submaximal test performed at 6 weeks after MI. Almost 20% of patients tested early were unable to undergo testing 6 weeks later because they had destabilized as a result of recurrent ischemia, in-

farction, or death (66). Krone and colleagues confirm that just performing a predischarge study is associated with a 10% lower mortality and a lower incidence of subsequent coronary events, but they imply that low-level exercise testing is most useful in patients who show other clinical markers of higher risk (66).

A trend toward earlier higher level testing is at odds with our understanding of the pathophysiology of the MI process. As already stated, the duration of the healing phase after MI is about 6 weeks. Traditionally, we have assumed that if the heart is subjected to a major increase in HR or BP during this period, deleterious effects could result. The hypothetical hazards of exertion in MI patients are cardiac rupture, aneurysm formation, extension of infarction, CHF, and serious dysrhythmias (27). In actual experience, these problems rarely are reported in patients who perform moderately intense exercise after the first or second week after infarction. For purposes of risk stratification the point, however, is that abnormal responses at higher workloads are not as predictive as those at lower workloads (67).

As alluded to previously, it appears that clinical judgment can be used effectively to identify high-risk patients (68), and that ST-segment shifts are not as predictive of high risk as an abnormal SBP response or poor exercise capacity (67). When Froelicher and his colleagues (67) subgrouped the studies by time of testing, that is, predischarge or postdischarge, a high proportion of predischarge test results were accurate predictors of poor outcome. Risk predictors from exercise testing best identify the patients who die early after MI—before later testing can be done. This coincides with the observation that one-third of first-year mortality occurs within the first 6 weeks after acute infarction (63).

The process of risk stratification has become an integral part of the management of patients during and after an acute myocardial event. The results of the process serve as signposts for patient management (Fig. 1.3). In addition, the results of risk stratification define the management of the patient throughout the rehabilitative process. The designations of low-, intermediate-, or high-risk patients are then applied for purposes of guidelines and standards used for program planning (e.g., staffing and resource allocation or reimbursement of program services).

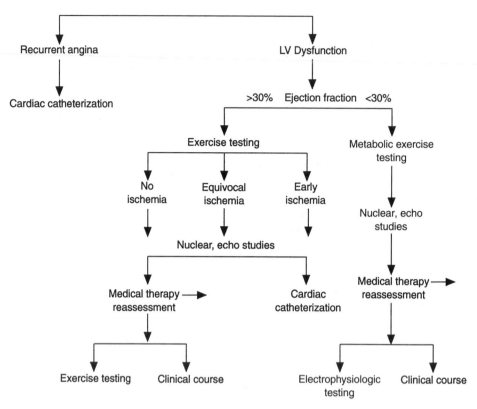

Figure 1.3. Risk stratification of patients after myocardial infarction. (Adapted from Wenger NK. Risk stratification after myocardial infarction. Myocardium 1988;1:5.)

On behalf of the Health and Public Policy Committee of the American College of Physicians (ACP), Greenland and Chu (69) have recommended that intermediate-risk patients be defined as those who experience shock or CHF during a recent (less than 6 months) MI, those who demonstrate less than 2 mm of ischemic ST-segment depression, or those who are unable to self-monitor or comply with the exercise prescription. For these patients, a time-limited program has been recommended, but not the full 8- to 12-week program that has been commonly prescribed.

High-risk patients are defined as those who have severe depression of LV function (ejection fraction less than 30%); resting complex ventricular dysrhythmias; ventricular arrhythmia that increases during exercise; a decrease in SBP of 15 mm Hg with exercise; recent MI (less than 6 months) complicated by serious arrhythmias; or survival of sudden cardiac arrest or marked, exercise-induced ischemia indicated by angina of 2

mm or more of ST-segment depression on ECG (69). Patients who demonstrate these clinical features are believed to be appropriate candidates for telemetry ECG monitoring during exercise.

Guidelines for risk stratification have been produced by other organizations as well. The AACVPR published its guidelines in 1991 (70, 71), with the major focus of this risk stratification scheme to provide guidance for the extent of patient supervision and to establish appropriate levels for reimbursement. The AACVPR guidelines are outlined in chapter 23 (see Table 23.2). Major differences between ACP and AACVPR risk stratification schemes include in-hospital heart failure as intermediate (ACP) rather than high risk (AACVPR); less than (ACP) versus more than (AACVPR) 2 mm ST-segment depression as intermediate; and changing pattern angina as intermediate (AACVPR), not specifically covered (ACP). The AACVPR guidelines also list combinations of ischemic markers thought to be associated with increased risk: functional capacity less than or equal to 5 with hypotensive blood pressure response or more than or equal to 1 mm ST-segment depression; and more than or equal to 2 mm ST-segment depression at peak HR less than or equal to 135 beats per minute.

Three factors determine the prognosis of any patient who has CHD: the amount of myocardium at risk, the extent of LV dysfunction, and the arrhythmic potential of the cardiac substrate (Table 1.2). Regardless of how the various schemas are defined, the responses that reflect ischemia include not just ST-segment (ECG) changes but also global exercise capacity and the presence or absence of angina. Ventricular function is best reflected by the ability to maintain an appropriate SBP response and the accomplishment of adequate aggregate of work. Arrhythmic potential can be highly deceptive, but it clearly is a risk when sustained ventricular arrhythmia is present spontaneously or can be induced. Patients who demonstrate single or multiple elements of these factors we identify as high risk. It is this kind of patient whom we are seeing with greater frequency in our programs.

Changing Demographics and the Impact of Aging

The 20th century has seen prodigious growth in the number of people we identify as elderly, and projections indicate that there will be increases in both the absolute and relative proportions of the population who are older (72, 73). This phenomenon is related to the current birthrate and the decline in age-specific mortality. Because of the increasing population and its high component of elderly, we can expect an increase in the absolute numbers of patients who have CHD (74). These demographic changes related to the aging population will inevitably have a huge impact on health care utilization and expenditures (75).

Levy and others (76, 77) have observed that since the late 1960s, there has been an unprecedented decline in mortality from cardiovascular disease in the United States, especially from CHD and stroke. The decline has been observed in all age groups, especially in the elderly (76). The fall in CHD mortality is attributable to the development of specialized acute coronary care, potent cardiovascular drugs for the treatment of heart failure *and* ischemia, surgical techniques for coronary revascularization, accurate noninvasive diagnostic methods such as echocardiography, and the identification of specific cardiovascular risk factors (including the major modifiable ones of cigarette smoking, hypertension, and blood lipids). The decline in mortality correlates with the development of increasing risk factor awareness and modification. Not only improved treatment regimens but also risk factor modification through lifestyle changes have played important roles in the reduction of cardiovascular mortality (76). Because of the demographics of the growing population, however, we must not misinterpret the decline in cardiovascular mortality to imply a lower future prevalence of disease, at least not in the next decade or two. If anything, we should expect the prevalence of CHD to increase by about 30% by the year 2015, even with 20% to 25% decreases in case fatality and incidence rates (74).

The demographics of those patients undergoing surgical coronary revascularization are changing rapidly as well (78). The population of patients who undergo coronary artery bypass graft (CABG) surgery is characteristically older, more commonly female, advanced in age, and likely to have three-vessel disease or abnormal LV function (Table 1.3). At the Cleveland Clinic, the percentage of patients who undergo CABG surgery and who are older than 70 years of age has risen from 0.2% in the period 1967–1970 to more than 35% in 1996. More than 65% of procedures are now done for three-vessel disease, whereas only 13% were performed in the previ-

Table 1.2. Characteristics of Low-, Intermediate-, and High-Risk Disease During Exercise ECG Testing

Low-risk
   ≥8 METs 3 weeks after cardiac event
   No symptoms
Intermediate-risk
   ≤8 METs 3 weeks after cardiac event
   Angina with moderate or intense exercise
   History of congestive heart failure
High-risk
   ≤5 METs 3 weeks after cardiac event
   Exercise-induced hypotension
   Ischemia induced at low levels of exercise
   Persistence of ischemia after exercise
   Sustained arrhythmia

METs = metabolic equivalents.

Table 1.3.   Characteristics of Patients Who Undergo Primary Coronary Revascularization: The Cleveland Clinic Foundation[a]

	1967–1970	1976	1982	1988	1994	1996
Preoperative Clinical Characteristics						
Age (median)	50	55	59	64	65	66
% ≥ 70 years	0.2	3	10	30	32	35
Men (%)	85	89	84	78	75	70
Angiographic Findings[b]						
One vessel	56	15	8	3	7	7
Two vessel	31	28	25	19	26	26
Three vessel	13	57	67	78	66	67
Left main	9	12	12	16	19	19
LV dysfunction[c]	41	45	55	57	57	56

[a]Adapted from Lytle B, Cosgrove D, Loop F. Future implications of current trends in bypass surgery. Cardiovasc Clin 1991;21:265–278.
[b]Percent prevalence of critical stenoses (≥50%).
[c]Left ventricular (LV) regional asynergy.

ously mentioned base period. Nearly 50% show some evidence of LV dysfunction, whereas only 41% previously did (78).

Acinapura and colleagues (79) suggest that because of the increasing number of elderly patients (defined as older than 70 years of age), the growing number of reoperative CABG cases, and acute MI patients with unstable angina pectoris who present for surgery, the operative mortality is likely to rise. To a significant degree, the advent of percutaneous transluminal coronary angioplasty (PTCA) is changing the patient population who undergo CABG surgery. Patients who undergo PTCA were considerably younger (55 years on average for those undergoing PTCA versus 68.5 years undergoing CABG surgery, with 38% being 70 years of age or older), and most had only one- or two-vessel disease. The left ventricular ejection fraction (LVEF) in patients who undergo CABG surgeries averaged 38% and was 55% for PTCA. The hospital mortality for elective CABG surgery in patients older than 70 years was 8% versus 1.8% for patients younger, for reoperative procedures, 3.6%, and for postinfarction or unstable angina pectoris, 4%, for a combined operative mortality of 4.8% (79). Patients who undergo CABG surgery today are thus older, more complex, and have intrinsically poorer pump function (80).

Urberg and associates (81) documented striking changes in the demographics and incidence of comorbid conditions among patients admitted for acute MI. Although the population is clearly becoming older and sicker, the prevalence of serious comorbid conditions such as diabetes mellitus is striking. Lavie and associates (82, 83) have collected data that document beneficial effects of cardiac rehabilitation and exercise training in the elderly, including modest improvements in lipids, obesity indexes, behavioral characteristics, and quality-of-life parameters, and marked improvements in exercise capacity. Their data suggest that elderly patients with CHD should be routinely referred to, and encouraged to participate in, formal outpatient cardiac rehabilitation and exercise training programs after major CHD events. A recent review by Hellman and Williams (84) corroborates this.

In 1990, Thompson (85) observed that "the future of aging persons in an aging society will depend equally upon the exogenous factors of the society and upon our attitudes and behaviors." He points out that the increase in the number and proportion of elderly will create "constraints and pressures upon resources and services" (85). These considerations for decision making will be reflected in our actions and attitudes about aging and the elderly. Thompson observes further that the role of the aging person is evolving from our stereotype of "retired," or "grandparent," to a more active and participatory role. The changing demographic profile compels us to anticipate newer approaches to health care for an older constituency. Although the primary concern to be addressed is the development and administration of a system of services for the chronically ill, these health services must be coordinated to meet a wide range of needs (85).

REDEFINING CARDIAC REHABILITATION

Role of Efficacy Studies

As health care dollars become more scarce, there will be more requests for "proof" of various rehabilitation modalities and programs. Cardiac rehabilitation is one of the areas that faces this issue. The close association with cardiology, an internal medicine discipline that scrutinizes most new medical advances rigorously, influences the evaluation of rehabilitation. The large potential population that requires rehabilitation deters third-party payers and prompts requests for "proof of efficacy."

The concept of proof is a difficult construct. In the context of cardiac rehabilitation, "proof of efficacy" implies that convincing evidence exists to show that cardiac rehabilitation can affect positively the so-called hard end points, such as an MI or death attributable to cardiovascular disease. It should be recognized from the outset that it is unrealistic to expect 100% absolute proof for any medical intervention. We are always left, therefore, with suboptimal proof for any condition. The question then becomes, "Does sufficient proof exist to recommend a certain therapeutic modality or program given the potential benefits and risks?"

The traditional guidelines for acceptance of the results of a clinical trial are generally well accepted with specific parameters given for an alpha level (usually less than .05) and a beta level (usually less than .1). There are no such fixed guidelines when summarizing the results of numerous trials. In general, one hopes only to satisfy Hill's postulates to accept proof (86):

1. Strength
2. Graded relationship
3. Consistency
4. Independence
5. Temporality
6. Congruence

For clinical trials, the pooling of data in the form of a meta-analysis has emerged as an accepted method of summarizing results from various studies. Recently, the guidelines panel applied a strength-of-evidence rating scale to designate the strength of the scientific evidence for each of the guideline recommendations. In this method the ratings were intended to reflect both the quality of the studies included (study design and methods), and the consistency of the results of the scientific evidence. To be designated an "A" a guideline recommendation required that scientific evidence be provided by "well-designed, well-conducted, controlled trials (randomized and nonrandomized) with statistically significant results," i.e., with adequate power and analytical methods. A "B" recommendation was indicated when the evidence provided was by observational studies or when controlled trials showed less consistent results. Finally, a guideline recommendation was designated a "C" when expert opinion supported it but controlled studies or consistent scientific evidence were lacking. The expert panel having reviewed the scientific literature concluded "that cardiac rehabilitation services are an essential component of the contemporary management of patients with multiple presentations of CHD and heart failure" (54). The Clinical Practice Guideline that resulted from the methodology is discussed in greater detail in chapter 23.

In 1992, the First International Heart Health Conference (Victoria Declaration on Heart Health, 1992) stressed that sufficient proof existed and efforts should be directed toward implementation (87). In a similar manner, given the Clinical Practice Guideline review and recommendations, sufficient proof exists for widespread implementation of cardiac rehabilitation.

End Points of Rehabilitation Outcome

With the establishment of successful earlier ambulation after MI, the belief emerged that exercise would improve prognosis. Exercise represents the fundamental element of cardiac rehabilitation programs, with the major focus on improvement of functional capacity and the contingent achievement of other important secondary goals. Major end points of rehabilitation outcome thus include functional capacity, changes in psychosocial function, health education after acute ischemic event, morbidity and mortality, ventricular function, cardiac perfusion or collateral circulation, and secondary risk factor modification (88).

Traditional End Points—Death, Recurrent MI, Exercise Improvement

Meta-analyses that reviewed randomized, prospective studies of cardiac rehabilitation versus usual care have confirmed its efficacy for the reduction of death after heart attack (89, 90). Oldridge and coworkers (89) demonstrated a 20% to 25% reduction in overall mortality in integrated programs of rehabilitation after MI. Furthermore, the effects on mortality were influenced markedly by continuation of the program beyond the usual 8 to 12 weeks of therapy. In a meta-analysis of randomized trials of rehabilitation that incorporated exercise after MI, O'Connor and associates (90) found reductions in cardiovascular mortality to be consistent with the findings of Oldridge et al., but also demonstrated a 37% reduction in the incidence of sudden cardiac death during the first year after an acute cardiac event. We believe this reduction in sudden death rate is mostly related to the presence of skilled supervision and the early recognition of clinical destabilization during the rehabilitation sessions, but the possibility that intrinsic changes may occur in the cardiac substrate or catechol-mediated responses to exercise, although unlikely, has not, in fact, been ruled out entirely. The latter speculation is discussed in the next section in some detail.

A comprehensive cardiac rehabilitation program can reduce the incidence of subsequent infarction. This was demonstrated in a study that reviewed the 5-year follow-up experience of a nonselected intervention group of patients who survived acute MIs and were randomized to a rehabilitation program that included follow-up at a special post-MI clinic, exercise training, the provision of information on smoking cessation and diet, and psychological support to patients and their families. During the 5-year follow-up, no difference appeared in cardiac mortality between the groups, but the recurrence rate of nonfatal MI (17.3% versus 33.3%; $P = .02$) and the rate of total cardiac events (39.5% versus 53.2%; $P = .05$) were lower in the intervention group. This may reflect an alteration of risk factors, because there were fewer smokers and uncontrolled hypertensives in the intervention group. The program proved to be particularly effective in those patients younger than 55 years of age, in whom a significantly lower rate of total cardiac events was observed, and more patients returned to

work than in the reference group (91). Again, the issue here may, at least in part, be related to the increased supervision inherent in a rehabilitation program and the ability to appreciate early clinical destabilization.

Large numbers of studies have documented improvement in exercise capacity with training by an average of 15% to 25% (54, 88). Others have suggested, however, that patients self-condition to adequate levels without formalized exercise training (92), but the time course of conditioning may be improved considerably. Other studies suggest that a phase I rehabilitation experience in uncomplicated, low-risk patients obviates the need for phase II (93). Although the 15% to 25% improvement in patients who have normal exercise capacity has little practical impact, patients who are the most debilitated are likely to derive the largest benefit to their functional capacity with exercise training (94). Such observations have significant implications for the design of future cardiac rehabilitation programs (22, 34).

CONTEMPORARY ISSUES IN CARDIAC REHABILITATION

Surveillance in Cardiac Rehabilitation

A more recent use for rehabilitation programs is the concept of surveillance. Patients who are at high risk because of high-grade ectopy or congestive failure are being referred increasingly to rehabilitation programs for monitoring over a period of time. Even the traditional lock-step progression of hospitalization to rehabilitation has been relaxed. Occasionally, a patient awaiting CABG surgery will attend a "rehabilitation program" to lose weight or to stop smoking to lessen the surgical risk. In some cases, the decision is equivocal with regard to the need for surgery. Such patients sometimes are sent to "rehabilitation" to assess the maximum improvement achieved with lifestyle measures. Finally, some patients who have atypical chest pain and inconsistent physical findings have been evaluated further in rehabilitation programs.

Surveillance in Patients After Angioplasty and After MI

The mortality associated with acute MI has improved significantly during the last 25 years, but the 1980s were especially significant for the management of acute MI because of the introduction of intravascular thrombolysis (95). The message from more than 50,000 patients included in five key trials is clear: thrombolysis is now the cornerstone of acute MI treatment, producing a favorable epidemiologic picture. In the Gruppo Italiano per lo Studio della Sopravvivenza nell' Infarto Miocardico (GISSI-2) trial, the nationwide adoption of a package of recommended thrombolytic and adjunctive therapies for patients with acute MIs produced a significant modification of the natural history of the disease, reducing in-hospital mortality from 13% to 8.8% (about 40%) in just a few years (96). In the majority of cases (patients with a first infarction, less than 70 years of age, with normal LV function), the mortality has gone down to 3%, making a further reduction in acute mortality hard to obtain with new drugs or strategies. Will this have an impact on subsequent mortality and the likelihood that rehabilitation can reduce mortality even more?

Patients with failure of infarct-related artery recanalization after thrombolytic therapy have a poor clinical outcome (97). Interventions are being performed increasingly to establish patency of large infarct-related vessels. Moreover, any objective evidence of persistence of ischemia in areas identified as potentially significant after MI is likely to call for revascularization by interventional techniques or CABG surgery. On this basis, we should expect to see fewer patients in rehabilitation who are apt to experience improved mortality on the basis of reduced myocardium at ischemic risk. Angioplasty is associated with a high incidence of failure (98), however, and, if anything, phase II rehabilitation provides the kind of close supervision in which such failures can be detected early.

Although low-level exercise thallium testing is useful in identifying the high-risk patient after acute MI, it does not apply as well to patients who receive thrombolytic treatment during the course of their infarction, according to Tilkemeier and associates (99). The ability of ECG and thallium tests to predict future cardiac events was compared in patients who received thrombolysis and in those who did not receive the intervention. The only significant predictors of outcome were LV cavity dilatation in the intervention group and ST-segment depression and increased lung uptake in the non-intervention group. The sensitivity of exercise thallium was only 55% in the intervention group and 81% in the nonintervention group ($P < .05$). Nearly half the events after discharge are not predicted by predischarge, low-level exercise thallium testing in patients who receive thrombolytic therapy for acute MI (99).

The detection of restenosis after successful coronary angioplasty can be improved with the use of a logistic model that combines procedural and follow-up variables (100). Using logistic discriminant analysis, a model for the prediction of restenosis was developed by Renkin and colleagues (100). Multivariate analysis revealed four factors independently related to increased risk of restenosis: recurrence of angina ($P < .0001$), perfusion defects on exercise thallium Tl 201 scintigram ($P < .001$), absolute postangioplasty stenosis diameter ($P < .02$), and exercise ST-segment depression ($P < .01$). These predictors can be used to stratify patients into high-risk and low-risk probability groups with predictive values of 100% and 94%, respectively. This approach may be superior to the usual clinical practice of performing repeat coronary angiography in patients who have recurrent angina or ST-segment changes during exercise (100).

Beyond Risk Stratification

Some additional contingencies have been identified that serve as markers of risk for future cardiac events subsequent to acute MI. These factors are relevant to the rehabilitative process, because they appear to be time dependent and may be modifiable by exercise conditioning. They could account for at least some of the improvement in mortality related to sudden death reported by O'Connor and colleagues (90).

The presence of high-frequency late potentials in the terminal portion of the QRS complex (a principal deflection in an ECG) detected by signal-averaging technique has been shown to be a sensitive and powerful predictor of subsequent, sustained ventricular tachycardia and sudden cardiac death. In one large series (101), late potentials occurred in about one-third of patients studied, yielded a sensitivity of 94%, and produced a negative predictive value in 97% of cases.

Patients with late potentials in the signal-averaged ECG are more at risk for lethal arrhythmias in the period after acute MI. Eldar and associates (102) tested the effects of thrombolysis on the incidence and evolution of late potentials during the first 10 days after acute MI. The incidence of late potentials in the first 2 days after infarction was not significantly different between the thrombolytic and control groups (14% versus 11.8%). By 7 to 10 days, the occurrence of late potentials among patients who underwent thrombolysis remained unchanged (14%); however, it increased significantly in the control group (11.8% to 22.5%). Thrombolysis thus seems to reduce the evolution of late potentials within 10 days of infarction. Because the risk of fatal arrhythmias is higher in patients with late potentials, this study may partly explain the reduced mortality after thrombolysis (102).

A relationship has been established between patency of the infarct-related artery and the presence of late potentials on the signal-averaged ECG. Vatterott and colleagues (103) documented that in patients who had no prior MI and who underwent early reperfusion therapy, a patent artery was associated with a decreased incidence of late potentials (20% versus 71%) and that this finding was independent of LVEF as an index of infarct size. In the patients who received thrombolytic agents within 4 hours of symptom onset, the incidence of late potentials was slightly higher (24% versus 83%; $P < .04$). Vatterott suggests that these data imply that reperfusion of an infarct-related artery has a beneficial effect on the electrophysiologic substrate for serious ventricular arrhythmias that is independent of change in LVEF. These findings might explain, in part, the low late-mortality rate in survivors of MI with documented reperfusion of the infarct-related artery (103).

Heart rate variability has proved to be a sensitive indicator of risk for sudden cardiac death after MI as well (104). Reduced HR variability proved to be the single most powerful predictor of sudden cardiac death and sustained ventricular tachycardia among several variables studied by Cripps and associates (105). The effects of sympathetic stimulation on the occurrence of malignant arrhythmia, particularly in the setting of ischemic heart disease, have been described. Specifically, it has been shown that, although sympathetic hyperactivity is arrhythmogenic, increased vagal activity often exerts a beneficial effect (106). Vanoli and Schwartz have shown that MI and ischemia can interact synergistically to reduce HR variability, and that this interaction is associated with an increased risk for ventricular fibrillation. The protective effect of vagal activity was confirmed further in experimental studies in which muscarinic stimulation, induced electrically and pharmacologically, was able to prevent ventricular fibrillation during acute myocardial ischemia (106). There is also an established diurnal distribution to the loss of HR variability that tends to coincide with the recognized distribution of acute cardiac events (107).

Results from the Exercise Training in Anterior Myocardial Infarction (EAMI) study provided little corroboration of the hypothesis that exercise training after MI improves HR variability and thus contributes to the reduced incidence of sudden death observed in rehabilitated patients. Multiple measures of HR variability reflecting neuroregulatory activity were inconsistent and too small to reach any firm conclusions (108). However, a more recent study does in fact suggest that increased HR variability and enhanced parasympathetic tone occurred in patients who received cardiac rehabilitation after acute MI (109). Further, the effects appeared to persist after 1 year. In untrained patients, the autonomic control of HR variability did not change 8 weeks after MI and was only slightly modified by time. Thus, exercise training, performed for 8 weeks after an MI, modified the sympathovagal control of HR variability toward a persistent increase in parasympathetic tone. This may explain the decreased incidence of sudden death observed in patients who undergo rehabilitation.

Secondary Risk Modification (Vein Graft Atherosclerosis, Postangioplasty)

The available interventional therapies for CHD are not curative but are only temporizing (110–114). The percentage of patients who return for second and even third CABG operations continues to increase (115, 116). The implication for future health care planning is extremely serious.

The traditional approach to secondary prevention of CHD is based on one-to-one professional counseling to help patients modify risk factors that promote the progression of the disorder (117). A collective recognition of the need for prevention is occurring at a time when impending economic scarcity impels us to anticipate the enormous financial burden of providing one-to-one counseling and supervision to the huge population that requires guidance to alter lifestyle in a serious and meaningful way (118).

Recognition of the factors that increase the risk of developing CHD dates to the 1960s, from the Framingham Study (119, 120). The effectiveness of cholesterol lowering for primary prevention of CHD has been suggested (113, 118, 121, 122). Secondary prevention of atherosclerosis involves amelioration of the same risk factors (but after an acute event such as a heart attack or CABG surgery).

Evidence indicates that aggressive treatment of hypercholesterolemia can reduce effectively the rate of progression and probably can cause regression of atherosclerotic lesions (123–125). Data suggest that lifestyle intervention alone, including exercise, diet, and meditation without cholesterol-lowering drugs, can arrest or reverse coronary atherosclerosis (126). Most importantly, such lifestyle approaches can be targeted successfully toward patients who already have demonstrated major manifestations of the disease (127).

Sahni and associates (128) recently documented that cholesterol-lowering therapy reduces the incidence of angioplasty failure. Patients who had undergone successful angioplasty were randomized prospectively to treatment with lovastatin, a drug effective for lowering low-density lipoprotein cholesterol. There was a statistical difference in the incidence of angioplasty failure in patients treated with the drug (20 to 40 mg/day) compared with those who received no drug.

Although Greenland and Chu (88) expressed doubt about whether cardiac rehabilitation can reduce coronary risk factors, we believe that the study by Kallio and coworkers (129) has demonstrated the efficacy of comprehensive rehabilitation for the post-MI patient; Hedback et al. (130) have shown its efficacy for the reduction of multiple risks after CABG surgery, and Ornish and colleagues (126), as mentioned above, have shown its potential for patients who have obstructive atherosclerotic disease. The Clinical Practice Guidelines concluded that cardiac rehabilitation services have the following benefits: "improvement in blood lipid levels, reduction in cigarette smoking, improvement in exercise tolerance, improvement in psychosocial well-being and reduction of stress" (54).

Expanded Indications: Arrhythmia, Valve Replacement, Heart Failure

The incidence of CHF is about 500,000 cases per year in the United States, and the prevalence is about 2.5 million (127, 131). With improved therapy such as angiotensin-converting enzyme (ACE) inhibitors, home dobutamine therapy, and so on, we can expect that mortality from cardiac failure will continue to decrease and that more patients afflicted with this problem will enroll in group programs and be appropriate candidates for home therapy (132). Although the number of patients who receive transplants is small (about 2,000 per year), because of the severe level of deconditioning by the time of transplant, virtually all these patients are rehabilitation candidates. Similarly, the newer procedures such as the use of a left ventricular assist device (LVAD) are likely to be performed in significant numbers in the future and these patients derive tangible benefits from exercise training whether the device is used as a bridge to transplant or as a singular intervention (133).

Implantable devices that use direct-current shocks for the management of lethal arrhythmia, implantable cardioverter/defibrillators (ICDs), have had significant success, particularly since publication of the finding that drugs used for the suppression of lethal or potentially lethal arrhythmias may cause greater mortality than they prevent (134). These ICD devices, although limited initially to patients with histories of sudden death and those in whom sustained ventricular tachycardia can be induced in the electrophysiologic (EPS) laboratory (135), now are being placed increasingly in patients identified as having susceptible cardiac substrate and LV dysfunction (136, 137). More than 300,000 people per year sustain sudden cardiac death; a significant number of them will be identified and have one of these devices implanted. These patients can benefit from exercise (22) and psychosocial support (138).

On the one hand, the incidence of rheumatic heart disease has been on the decline; on the other, mitral repair for myxomatous valve degeneration is being performed increasingly more often, and aortic valvular stenosis as an age-correlated problem therefore is also on the increase (139). Although valvular heart disease accounts for a small number of patients compared with those who undergo CABG surgery, combined coronary-valve procedures are becoming increasingly common (140).

Although the majority of patients who enroll in cardiac rehabilitation have CHD, as the emphasis shifts toward higher risk patients in monitored programs, patients with heart failure, cardiac transplants, ventricular remodeling, serious arrhythmia, and implanted devices will come to represent an increasing number of the participants (22).

Modern End Points—Quality of Life, Cost-Effectiveness

Quality of life has become an increasingly prominent issue in cardiology and cardiovascular surgery during the last decade (141). Although interest has been focused on major "big-ticket" modalities of therapy (CABG surgery versus medical management) (142), almost every intervention now is regarded in the same way. Cardiac rehabilitation is no exception, and as measures of quality become better understood and more standardized, it will be more closely scrutinized (143).

Our impression, based on the positive feedback that we receive in an anecdotal way from our patients, is that cardiac rehabilitation makes a significant difference in their perceived quality of life. "I wouldn't have gotten back to normal as soon without the program," is a frequent response. There is no question that many participants enjoy and derive subjective improvement from rehabilitation, but does it make a measurable difference? Although Oldridge and associates (144) expressed doubt about regarding this in a study in which parameters on disease-specific and generic health-related quality of life, exercise tolerance, and return to work after acute MI were examined in low-risk patients who underwent brief rehabilitation, in most cases no differences were observed between those patients who participated in rehabilitation and those who received usual care. However, when the Guideline Panel reviewed the issue, their conclusion was "that cardiac rehabilitation exercise training—with and without other cardiac rehabilitation services—generally results in improvement in measures of psychological status and functioning. Exercise training as a sole intervention does not consistently result in improvement in measures of anxiety and depression" (54).

Wenger (141) pointed out that the goal of therapy in patients with severe symptomatic heart failure is improvement of symptoms and maintenance of functional abilities and comfort, and that generally a poor correlation exists between hemodynamic features of heart failure (such as ejection fraction) and quality of life attributes. In low-risk patients, it is likely that they will achieve normalcy in the performance of routine ADLs regardless of whether they participate in an exercise rehabilitation program. Rehabilitation is less likely to impact on their perception of quality of life. For a person who is severely limited, however, even modest improvement is likely to have a noticeable impact on functional capacity (145). Exercise training appears quite beneficial in patients with the most impaired exercise capacity (146) and those with compensated heart failure (147). It seems ironic that we previously excluded patients with severely reduced exercise tolerance on the assumption that they would derive little tangible benefit, defined as large, expected incremental measures in exercise function.

Oldridge and Rogowski (148) also looked at the efficacy of ward ambulation versus exercise in specialized centers for patients in phase I rehabilitation. Self-efficacy variables were measured at various intervals after the event (baseline, discharge, and 7 and 28 days after discharge). For the majority of self-efficacy variables considered, either approach appeared to be equally effective. As discussed earlier in this chapter, historically, and for many institutions today, ward ambulation serves as the exercise mode of choice during the inpatient experience.

Oldridge and Rogowski's study does raise the question, however, of cost-effectiveness relative to benefit for rehabilitation services. The issue of the economic impact of cardiac rehabilitation has been studied infrequently (149) until the early 1990s, when more research focused on this important aspect of care began to appear (150). As Dennis has pointed out in one of the first publications that specifically focused on this issue, consideration of cost-effectiveness and cost-benefit ratio seems especially important in cardiac rehabilitation, where there appears to be little short-term impact on morbidity and mortality, but important potential long-term benefits on mortality, disability, and psychological well-being (150).

Coors Industries was quoted that they save

$6.00 for every $1.00 expended in their comprehensive wellness program, which includes mandatory cardiac rehabilitation for those workers who experience an acute coronary event (151), although this policy has been changed given the changing realities of health care financing (see section on Coors Industries in chapter 23). Picard and associates (152) examined the impact of rehabilitation on earned income and medical care costs and found that those persons who receive rehabilitation have higher earned incomes in the 6 months after an acute coronary event and generate $500 less in medical care costs. Much more research, however, is needed in this area. The issues of rehabilitation economics are discussed further in the next section and in subsequent chapters.

ECONOMIC EVALUATION OF CARDIAC REHABILITATION SERVICES

Approximately 1 million people in the United States survive acute MIs annually (127), and it is estimated that approximately 10% to 15% of these patients subsequently are observed in supervised outpatient cardiac rehabilitation (153). Assuming that supervised rehabilitation costs about $1800 per patient, then the annual cost of supervised cardiac rehabilitation is estimated at approximately $200 million. To make informed decisions about the allocation of limited resources to health care services such as cardiac rehabilitation, it is important to apply some type of economic evaluation (154, 155).

Economic evaluation may be defined as "the comparative analysis of alternative courses of action in terms of both costs and consequences" (156–158). The term "costs" usually refers to the direct costs borne by health care providers and by the patient, whereas "consequences" include effects of the intervention, such as changes to the physical, social, and emotional functioning of patients (23). Economic evaluations are classified according to the way in which consequences are measured in the analysis—in cost-benefit analysis, consequences are measured in terms of dollars; in cost-effectiveness analysis, consequences are measured in terms of natural units such as life-years gained; and in cost-utility analysis, consequences are measured in quality-adjusted life-years (QALYs), which can be estimated (157, 159).

Oldridge and coinvestigators (144) included an economic evaluation in the design of a randomized clinical trial of 8 weeks of comprehensive cardiac rehabilitation initiated after acute MI. Patients who showed mild to moderate in-hospital anxiety or depression after acute MI were randomized to rehabilitation ($n = 99$) or to usual care ($n = 102$). Outcomes, including health-related quality of life measured by time trade-off scores (159), were determined before and after the 8-week comprehensive cardiac rehabilitation intervention and 4, 8, and 12 months later. By the end of the trial, the cardiac rehabilitation patients had gained 20 quality-adjusted "life-days" (0.052 QALYs) per patient over usual-care patients and used fewer ($P < .0001$) "other rehabilitation visits" during the follow-up period of the trial (160).

The investigators then performed cost-utility and cost-effectiveness analyses for the 1 year using life-years gained (LYG) estimates from previously published meta-analyses of cardiac rehabilitation (89, 90). The best estimate of net direct 12-month costs ($1990) for patients randomized to cardiac rehabilitation after acute MI was $480 per patient with a cost utility per QALY gained of $9200 during the year of follow-up. Using the reduced 3-year mortality from the meta-analyses of cardiac rehabilitation, and quality-of-life data from the prior study (144), the cost-effectiveness of cardiac rehabilitation after acute MI was $5615 per LYG, with a cost-utility estimate of $3293 per QALY gained, making it a considerably more efficient use of resources than most treatments for CHD for which we have cost-utility estimates.

We came to a similar conclusion after the application of a model for determining cost-effectiveness of cardiac rehabilitation in dollars per year of life saved ($/YLS) by combining published mortality rates from selected randomized trials of cardiac rehabilitation, as well as from epidemiologic studies of long-term survival in the overall postinfarction population, and studies of patient charges for rehabilitation services and averted medical expenses for hospitalizations after rehabilitation (161).

Cardiac rehabilitation participants experienced an incremental life expectancy of 0.202 years during a 15-year period. In 1988, we estimated the average cost of rehabilitation and exercise testing to be $1485, partially offset by averted cardiac rehospitalization costs of $850 per patient. A cost-effectiveness value of $2130/LYS was determined for the late 1980s, and projected to a value of

$4950/LYS for 1995. A sensitivity analysis strongly supported the study results (161).

Compared with other post-MI treatment interventions, cardiac rehabilitation is more cost-effective than single-vessel bypass (162–164), CABG surgery (163, 165), and cholesterol-lowering drugs (166–168), and is similar to that of β-adrenergic antagonist therapy in a 55-year-old man (169), though less cost-effective than smoking cessation programs (162, 170). However it is considerably more cost-effective than the brief office visit for smoking cessation if there is a 50% relapse at 1 year (171), or for the long-term drug therapy of diastolic hypertension of more than 94 mm Hg (172), something considered standard care by most cardiologists.

These economic data provide important preliminary evidence that cardiac rehabilitation after acute MI is an efficient use of health care resources and can be justified economically.

A FINAL WORD

Historically, we have witnessed an evolution in the field of cardiology in the appreciation of an intervention's value from reduction in morbidity and mortality, to quality-of-life issues, to economic valuation. For a therapeutic modality to maintain support in today's competitive and volatile environment, it must be demonstrably successful with respect to all these criteria. Cardiac rehabilitation can succeed in each of these ways, but to do so, it requires the appropriate understanding, support, participation, and use by physicians. With this in mind, we move on to discuss more specifically the physician and cardiac rehabilitation.

References

1. Froelicher V. Cardiac rehabilitation. In: Parmley W, Chatterjee K, eds. Cardiology. Philadelphia: JB Lippincott, 1988;1:1–17.
2. Mallory G, White P, Salcedo-Salgar J. The speed of healing of myocardial infarction: a study of the pathological anatomy in seventy-two cases. Am Heart J 1939;18:647–671.
3. Jugdutt B, Michorowski B, Kappagoda C. Exercise training after anterior Q wave myocardial infarction: importance of regional left ventricular function and topography [see comments]. J Am Coll Cardiol 1988; 12:362–372.
4. Giannuzzi P, Tavazzi L, Temporelli P, et al. Long-term physical training and left ventricular remodeling after anterior myocardial infarction: results of the Exercise in Anterior Myocardial Infarction (EAMI) trial. EAMI Study Group. J Am Coll Cardiol 1993;22:1821–1829.
5. Taylor H, Henschel A, Brozek J. Effects of bed rest on cardiovascular function and work performance. J Appl Physiol 1949;2:223–224.
6. Levine S. Some harmful effects of recumbency in the treatment of heart disease. JAMA 1944;126:80–84.
7. Levine S, Lown B. The "chair" treatment of acute coronary thrombosis. Trans Assoc Am Physicians 1951;64:316–327.
8. Levine S, Lown B. "Armchair" treatment of acute coronary thrombosis. JAMA 1952;148:1365–1369.
9. Newman L, Andrews M, Koblish M. Physical medicine and rehabilitation in acute myocardial infarction. Arch Intern Med 1952;89:552–561.
10. Brummer P, Linko E, Kasanen A. Myocardial infarction treated by early ambulation. Am Heart J 1956;52:269–272.
11. Cain H, Frasher W, Stivelman R. Graded activity program for safe return to self-care after myocardial infarction. JAMA 1961;177:111–115.
12. Groden B, Allison A, Shaw G. Management of myocardial infarction. The effect of early mobilisation. Scott Med J 1967;12:435–439.
13. Convertino V. Effect of orthostatic stress on exercise performance after bed rest: relation to inhospital rehabilitation. J Cardiac Rehabil 1983;3:660–663.
14. Chobanian A, Lille R, Tercyak A, et al. The metabolic and hemodynamic effects of prolonged bed rest in normal subjects. Circulation 1974;49:551–559.
15. Convertino V, Bloomfield S, Greenleaf J. An overview of the issues: physiological effects of bed rest and restricted physical activity. Med Sci Sports Exerc 1997;29:187–190.
16. Harpur J, Conner W, Hamilton M, et al. Controlled trial of early mobilisation and discharge from hospital in uncomplicated myocardial infarction. Lancet 1971;2:1331–1334.
17. Lamers H, Drost W, Kroon B, et al. Early mobilisation after myocardial infarction: a controlled study. Br Med J 1973;1:257–259.
18. Boyle J, Lorimer A. Early mobilisation after uncomplicated myocardial infarction. Lancet 1973;2:346–349.
19. Hutter A, Sidell V, Shine K, et al. Early hospital discharge after myocardial infarction. N Engl J Med 1973;288:1141–1144.
20. Bloch A, Maeder J, Haissly J, et al. Early mobilization after myocardial infarction. Am J Cardiol 1974; 34:152–157.
21. Abraham A, Sever Y, Weinstein M, et al. Value of early ambulation in patients with and without complications after acute myocardial infarction. N Engl J Med 1975;292:719–722.
22. Pashkow F. Rehabilitation strategies for the complex cardiac patient. Cleve Clin J Med 1991;58:70–75.
23. Pashkow F. Issues in contemporary cardiac rehabilitation: an historical perspective. J Am Coll Cardiol 1993;21:822–834.
24. Hurst J. "Ambulation" after myocardial infarction. N Engl J Med 1975;292:746–748.

25. Wenger N, Gilbert C, Skoropa M. Cardiac conditioning after myocardial infarction. An early intervention program. Cardiac Rehabil 1971;2:17–22.
26. Pashkow F, Schafer M, Pashkow P. HeartWatchers—low cost, community centered cardiac rehabilitation in Loveland, Colorado. J Cardpulm Rehabil 1986;6: 469–473.
27. Froelicher V. Exercise testing and training: clinical applications. J Am Coll Cardiol 1983;1:114–125.
28. Wenger N, Hellerstein H, Blackburn H, et al. Uncomplicated myocardial infarction: current physician practice in patient management. JAMA 1973;224: 511–514.
29. Swan H, Blackburn H, DeSanctis R, et al. Duration of hospitalization in "uncomplicated completed acute myocardial infarction." Am J Cardiol 1976;37:413–419.
30. Hlatky M, Cotugno H, Mark D, et al. Trends in physician management of uncomplicated acute myocardial infarction, 1970 to 1987. Am J Cardiol 1988;61:515–518.
31. Pashkow FJ. Cardiac rehabilitation: not just exercise anymore. Cleve Clin J Med 1996;63:116–123.
32. Pozen M, Stechmiller J, Harris W, et al. A nurse rehabilitator's impact on patients with myocardial infarction. Med Care 1977;15:830–837.
33. Ott C, Sivarajan E, Newton K, et al. A controlled randomized study of early cardiac rehabilitation: the Sickness Impact Profile as an assessment tool. Heart Lung 1983;12:162–170.
34. Wenger N. Future directions in cardiovascular rehabilitation. J Cardpulm Rehabil 1987;7:168–174.
35. Hellerstein H, Ford A. Rehabilitation of the cardiac patient. JAMA 1957;164:225–231.
36. Naughton J, Hellerstein H, Mohler I. Exercise testing and exercise training in coronary heart disease. 1st ed. New York: Academic Press, 1973.
37. Hartwig R. Cardiopulmonary research institute—CAPRI. J Cardiac Rehabil 1982;2:481–483.
38. Miller H, Ribisl P. Cardiac rehabilitation program at Wake Forest University. J Cardiac Rehabil 1982;2: 503–505.
39. Pashkow FJ, Pashkow PS, Schafer MN. Successful cardiac rehabilitation: the complete guide for building cardiac rehab programs. 1st ed. Loveland, CO: The HeartWatchers Press, 1988.
40. Haskell W. Cardiovascular complications during exercise training of cardiac patients. Circulation 1978;57: 920–924.
41. VanCamp S, Peterson R. Cardiovascular complications of outpatient cardiac rehabilitation programs. JAMA 1986;256:1160–1163.
42. Haskell W. The efficacy and safety of exercise programs in cardiac rehabilitation. Med Sci Sports Exerc 1994; 26:815–823.
43. Fletcher G, Chiaramida A, LeMay M, et al. Telephonically-monitored home exercise early after coronary artery bypass surgery. Chest 1984;86:198–202.
44. DeBusk R, Haskell W, Miller N, et al. Medically directed at-home rehabilitation soon after clinically uncomplicated acute myocardial infarction: a new model for patient care. Am J Cardiol 1985;55:251–257.
45. DeBusk RF, Blomqvist CG, Kouchoukos NT, et al. Identification and treatment of low-risk patients after acute myocardial infarction and coronary-artery bypass graft surgery. N Engl J Med 1986;314:161–166.
46. Report of the World Health Organization Expert Committee on Disability Prevention and Rehabilitation: Rehabilitation of patients with cardiovascular disease. Geneva, Switzerland: World Health Organization, 1964.
47. Lamm G. The World Health Organization's contributions to the advancement of rehabilitation. Bibl Cardiol 1986;40:8–19.
48. American College of Sports Medicine programs. In: Oldridge NB, Foster C, Schmidt DH, eds. Cardiac rehabilitation and clinical exercise programs: theory and practice. Ithaca, NY: Movement Publications, 1988: 351–356.
49. American College of Sports Medicine. Guidelines for exercise testing and prescription. 5th ed. Philadelphia: Lea & Febiger, 1995:314.
50. Blair S, Painter P, Pate RR, et al., eds. Resource manual for guidelines for exercise testing and prescription. 1st ed. Philadelphia: Lea & Febiger, 1988:436.
51. World Health Organization. Prevention of coronary heart disease: report of a WHO Expert Committee. Geneva, Switzerland: World Health Organization, 1982.
52. Ryan TJ, Anderson JL, Antman EM, et al. ACC/AHA guidelines for the management of patients with acute myocardial infarction: executive summary. A report of the American College of Cardiology/American Heart Association Task Force on Practice Guidelines (Committee on Management of Acute Myocardial Infarction). Circulation 1996;94:2341–2350.
53. Fallen EL, Cairns J, Dafoe W, et al. Management of the postmyocardial infarction patient: a consensus report—revision of 1991 CCS guidelines. Can J Cardiol 1995;11:477–486.
54. Wenger NK, Froelicher ES, Smith LK, et al. Cardiac rehabilitation. Rockville, MD: Department of Health and Human Services, Public Health Service, Agency for Health Care Policy and Research and National Heart, Lung, and Blood Institute, 1995:3.
55. DeBusk R, Dennis C. "Submaximal" predischarge exercise testing after acute myocardial infarction: who needs it? Am J Cardiol 1985;55:499–500.
56. Erricson M, Granath A, Ohlsen P, et al. Arrhythmias and symptoms during treadmill testing three weeks after myocardial infarction in 100 patients. Br Heart J 1973;35:787–790.
57. Sivarajan E, Lerman J, Mansfield L. Progressive ambulation and treadmill testing of patients with acute myocardial infarction during hospitalization: a feasibility study. Arch Phys Med Rehabil 1977;58:241–244.
58. Markiewitz W, Houston N, DeBusk R. Exercise testing soon after myocardial infarction. Circulation 1977; 56:26–31.
59. Sami M, Kraemer H, DeBusk R. The prognostic significance of serial exercise testing after myocardial infarction. Circulation 1979;60:1238–1241.
60. Theroux P, Waters D, Halphen C. Prognostic value of exercise testing soon after myocardial infarction. N Engl J Med 1979;301:341–344.
61. Wohl A, Lewis H, Campbell W, et al. Cardiovascular

function during early recovery from acute myocardial infarction. Circulation 1977;56:931–937.

62. Dwyer E, McMaster P, Greenberg H. Nonfatal cardiac events and recurrent infarction in the year after acute myocardial infarction. J Am Coll Cardiol 1984;4:695–702.

63. Krone R, Gillespie J, Weld F, et al. Low-level exercise testing after myocardial infarction: usefulness in enhancing clinical risk stratification. Circulation 1985;71:80–89.

64. Topol E, Juni J, O'Neill W, et al. Exercise testing three days after onset of acute myocardial infarction. Am J Cardiol 1987;60:958–962.

65. Butman S, Olson H, Butman L. Early exercise testing after stabilization of unstable angina: correlation with coronary angiographic findings and subsequent cardiac events. Am Heart J 1986;111:11–18.

66. Starling MR, Crawford MH, Kennedy GT, et al. Treadmill exercise tests predischarge and six weeks postmyocardial infarction to detect abnormalities of known prognostic value. Ann Intern Med 1981;94:721–727.

67. Froelicher V, Perdue S, Pewen W, et al. Application of meta-analysis using an electronic spread sheet to exercise testing in patients after myocardial infarction. Am J Med 1987;83:1045–1054.

68. Froelicher V, Duarte G, Oakes D, et al. The prognostic value of the exercise test. Dis Mon 1988;34:677–735.

69. Greenland P, Chu J. Cardiac rehabilitation services: position paper from the Health and Public Policy Committee, American College of Physicians. Ann Int Med 1988;109:671–673.

70. American Association of Cardiovascular and Pulmonary Rehabilitation. Guidelines for cardiac rehabilitation programs. 1st ed. Champaign, IL: Human Kinetics Books, 1991.

71. American Association of Cardiovascular and Pulmonary Rehabilitation. Guidelines for cardiac rehabilitation programs. 2nd ed. Champaign, IL: Human Kinetics Books, 1995.

72. Siegel J, Davidson M. Demographic and socioeconomic aspects of aging in the United States. Washington, DC: United States Department of Commerce, Bureau of the Census, 1984.

73. Keller N, Feit F. Atherosclerotic heart disease in the elderly. Curr Opin Cardiol 1995;10:427–433.

74. Frye R, Higgins M, Beller G, et al. Major demographic and epidemiologic trends affecting adult cardiology. J Am Coll Cardiol 1988;12:840–846.

75. Guralnik J, FitzSimmons S. Aging in America: a demographic perspective. Cardiol Clin 1986;4:175–183.

76. Levy R. Declining mortality in coronary heart disease. Arteriosclerosis 1981;1:312–325.

77. Goldman L, Cook E. The decline in ischemic heart disease mortality rates. An analysis of the comparative effects of medical interventions and changes in lifestyle. Ann Intern Med 1984;101:825–836.

78. Lytle B, Cosgrove D, Loop F. Future implications of current trends in bypass surgery. Cardiovasc Clin 1991;21:265–278.

79. Acinapura A, Jacobowitz I, Kramer M, et al. Demographic changes in coronary artery bypass surgery and

its effect on mortality and morbidity. Eur J Cardiothorac Surg 1990;4:175–181.

80. Katz N, Hannan R, Hopkins R, et al. Cardiac operations in patients aged 70 years and over: mortality, length of stay, and hospital charge. Ann Thorac Surg 1995;60:96–100.

81. Urberg M, Cano M, Yuzon D. Changes in the characteristics of myocardial infarction patients: 1980 vs 1988. Fam Pract Res J 1991;11:99–106.

82. Lavie C, Milani R, Littman A. Benefits of cardiac rehabilitation and exercise training in secondary coronary prevention in the elderly. J Am Coll Cardiol 1993;22:678–683.

83. Lavie C, Milani R. Effects of cardiac rehabilitation programs on exercise capacity, coronary risk factors, behavioral characteristics, and quality of life in a large elderly cohort. Am J Cardiol 1995;76:177–179.

84. Hellman E, Williams M. Outpatient cardiac rehabilitation in elderly patients. Heart Lung 1994;23:506–512.

85. Thompson P. Aging in the 1990s and beyond. Occup Med 1990;5:807–816.

86. Blackburn H. Epidemiologic evidence for the causes and prevention of atherosclerosis. In: Steinberg D, Olefsky J, eds. Hypercholesterolemia and atherosclerosis. New York: Churchill Livingstone, 1987:53–99.

87. Victoria declaration on heart health. Victoria, Canada: Health and Welfare Canada, 1992.

88. Greenland P, Chu J. Efficacy of cardiac rehabilitation services: with emphasis on patients after myocardial infarction. Ann Intern Med 1988;109:650–653.

89. Oldridge N, Guyatt G, Fischer M, et al. Cardiac rehabilitation after myocardial infarction. Combined experience of randomized clinical trials. JAMA 1988;260:945–950.

90. O'Connor G, Buring J, Yusuf S, et al. An overview of randomized trials of rehabilitation with exercise after myocardial infarction. Circulation 1989;80:234–244.

91. Hedback B, Perk J. 5-Year results of a comprehensive rehabilitation programme after myocardial infarction. Eur Heart J 1987;8:234–242.

92. Mayou R, MacMahon D, Sleight P, et al. Early rehabilitation after myocardial infarction. Lancet 1981;2:1399–1402.

93. Gulanick M. Is phase 2 cardiac rehabilitation necessary for early recovery of patients with cardiac disease? A randomized, controlled study. Heart Lung 1991;20:9–15.

94. Hammond H, Kelly T, Froelicher V, et al. Use of clinical data in predicting improvement in exercise capacity after cardiac rehabilitation. J Am Coll Cardiol 1985;6:19–26.

95. Muller D, Topol E. Selection of patients with acute myocardial infarction for thrombolytic therapy. Ann Intern Med 1990;113:949–960.

96. Tognoni G, Fresco C, Franzosi M, et al. Thrombolysis in acute myocardial infarction. Chest 1991;99:S121–S127.

97. Abbottsmith C, Topol E, George B, et al. Fate of patients with acute myocardial infarction with patency of the infarct-related vessel achieved with successful thrombolysis versus rescue angioplasty. J Am Coll Cardiol 1990;16:770–778.

98. Kahn J, Hartzler G. Frequency and causes of failure

with contemporary balloon coronary angioplasty and implications for new technologies. Am J Cardiol 1990;66:858–860.

99. Tilkemeier P, Guiney T, LaRaia P, et al. Prognostic value of predischarge low-level exercise thallium testing after thrombolytic treatment of acute myocardial infarction. Am J Cardiol 1990;66:1203–1207.

100. Renkin J, Melin J, Robert A, et al. Detection of restenosis after successful coronary angioplasty: improved clinical decision making with use of a logistic model combining procedural and follow-up variables. J Am Coll Cardiol 1990;16:1333–1340.

101. Ozawa Y, Yakubo S, Hatano M. Prospective study of late potentials to predict cardiac sudden death and ventricular tachycardias in patients with myocardial infarction surviving over 4 weeks. Jpn Circ J 1990;54:1304–1314.

102. Eldar M, Leor J, Hod H, et al. Effect of thrombolysis on the evolution of late potentials within 10 days of infarction. Br Heart J 1990;63:273–276.

103. Vatterott P, Hammill S, Bailey K, et al. Late potentials on signal-averaged electrocardiograms and patency of the infarct-related artery in survivors of acute myocardial infarction. J Am Coll Cardiol 1991;17:330–337.

104. Pipilis A, Flather M, Ormerod O, et al. Heart rate variability in acute myocardial infarction and its association with infarct site and clinical course. Am J Cardiol 1991;67:1137–1139.

105. Cripps T, Malik M, Farrell T, et al. Prognostic value of reduced heart rate variability after myocardial infarction: clinical evaluation of a new analysis method. Br Heart J 1991;65:14–19.

106. Vanoli E, Schwartz P. Sympathetic–parasympathetic interaction and sudden death. Basic Res Cardiol 1990;85:305–321.

107. Malik M, Farrell T, Camm A. Circadian rhythm of heart rate variability after acute myocardial infarction and its influence on the prognostic value of heart rate variability. Am J Cardiol 1990;66:1049–1054.

108. Mazzuero G, Lanfranchi P, Colombo R, et al. Long-term adaptation of 24-h heart rate variability after myocardial infarction. The EAMI Study Group. Exercise Training in Anterior Myocardial Infarction. Chest 1992;101:304S–308S.

109. Malfatto G, Facchini M, Bragato R, et al. Short and long term effects of exercise training on the tonic autonomic modulation of heart rate variability after myocardial infarction. Eur Heart J 1996;17:532–538.

110. Kouchoukos N, Kirklin J, Oberman A. An appraisal of coronary bypass grafting. Circulation 1974;50:11–16.

111. Campeau L, Lesperance J, Hermann J, et al. Loss of improvement of angina between 1 and 7 years after aortocoronary bypass surgery: correlations with changes in vein grafts and in coronary arteries. Circulation 1979;60(Part 2):1–5.

112. Campeau L, Enjalbert M, Lesperance J, et al. The relation of risk factors to the development of atherosclerosis in saphenous-vein bypass grafts and the progression of disease in the native circulation. A study 10 years after aortocoronary bypass surgery. N Engl J Med 1984;311:1329–1332.

113. The Lipid Research Clinics Coronary Primary Prevention Trial results. I. Reduction in incidence of coronary heart disease. JAMA 1984;251:351–364.

114. Alderman E, Bourassa M, Cohen L, et al. Ten-year follow-up of survival and myocardial infarction in the randomized Coronary Artery Surgery Study [see comments]. Circulation 1990;82:1629–1646.

115. Bourassa MG. Fate of venous grafts: the past, the present and the future. J Am Coll Cardiol 1991;17:1081–1083.

116. Lytle B, Loop F, Taylor P, et al. Vein graft disease: the clinical impact of stenoses in saphenous vein bypass grafts to coronary arteries. J Thorac Cardiovasc Surg 1992;103:831–840.

117. Squyres WD. Anticipating the "bottom line" in patient education in the twenty-first century. In: Wenger NK, ed. The education of the patient with cardiac disease in the twenty-first century. New York: LeJacq Publishing, 1986:30–44.

118. Stamler J, Wentworth D, Neaton JD. Is relationship between serum cholesterol and risk of premature death from coronary heart disease continuous and graded? Findings in 356,222 primary screenees of the Multiple Risk Factor Intervention Trial (MRFIT). JAMA 1986;256:2823–2828.

119. Kannel W, Castelli W, Gordon T, et al. Serum cholesterol, lipoproteins, and the risk of coronary heart disease. The Framingham Study. Ann Intern Med 1971;74:1–12.

120. Castelli W, Garrison R, Wilson P, et al. Incidence of coronary heart disease and lipoprotein cholesterol levels. The Framingham Study. JAMA 1986;256:2835–2838.

121. The Lipid Research Clinics Coronary Primary Prevention Trial results. II. The relationship of reduction in incidence of coronary heart disease to cholesterol lowering. JAMA 1984;251:365–374.

122. Frick M, Elo O, Haapa K, et al. Helsinki Heart Study: primary-prevention trial with gemfibrozil in middle-aged men with dyslipidemia. Safety of treatment, changes in risk factors, and incidence of coronary heart disease. N Engl J Med 1987;317:1237–1245.

123. Blackburn H, Taylor H, Keys A. Prognostic significance of the post-exercise electrocardiogram: risk factors held constant. Am J Cardiol 1970;25:85.

124. Blankenhorn D, Nessim S, Johnson R, et al. Beneficial effects of combined colestipol-niacin therapy on coronary atherosclerosis and coronary venous bypass grafts (published erratum appears in JAMA 1988; 259:2698). JAMA 1987;257:3233–3240.

125. Brown G, Albers J, Fisher L, et al. Regression of coronary artery disease as a result of intensive lipid-lowering therapy in men with high levels of apolipoprotein B [see comments]. N Engl J Med 1990;323:1289–1298.

126. Ornish D, Brown S, Scherwitz L, et al. Can lifestyle changes reverse coronary heart disease? The Lifestyle Heart Trial. Lancet 1990;336:129–133.

127. 1997 Heart and Stroke Statistics. Dallas, TX: American Heart Association, 1996.

128. Sahni R, Maniet A, Voci G, et al. Prevention of restenosis by lovastatin after successful coronary angioplasty. Am Heart J 1991;121:1600–1608.

129. Kallio V, Hämäläinen H, Hakkila J, et al. Reduction of

sudden deaths by a multifactorial intervention program after acute myocardial infarction. Lancet 1979; 2:1091–1094.

130. Hedback B, Perk J, Engvall J, et al. Cardiac rehabilitation after coronary artery bypass grafting: effects on exercise performance and risk factors. Arch Phys Med Rehabil 1990;71:1069–1073.

131. Smith W. Epidemiology of congestive heart failure. Am J Cardiol 1985;55:3A–8A.

132. Dubach P, Froelicher V. Cardiac rehabilitation for heart failure patients. Cardiology 1989;76:368–373.

133. McCarthy P, James K, Savage R, et al. Implantable left ventricular assist device. Approaching an alternative for end-stage heart failure. Implantable LVAD Study Group. Circulation 1994;90:II83–II86.

134. Investigators CASTC. Preliminary report: effect of encainide and flecainide on mortality in a randomized trial of arrhythmia suppression after myocardial infarction. N Engl J Med 1989;321:406–412.

135. Mirowski M. The automatic implantable cardioverter-defibrillator: an overview. J Am Coll Cardiol 1985; 6:461–466.

136. Tchou P, Kadri N, Anderson J, et al. Automatic implantable cardioverter defibrillators and survival of patients with left ventricular dysfunction and malignant ventricular arrhythmias. Ann Intern Med 1988; 109: 529–534.

137. Saksena S, Madan N, Lewis C. Implanted cardioverter-defibrillators are preferable to drugs as primary therapy in sustained ventricular tachyarrhythmias. Prog Cardiovasc Dis 1996;38:445–454.

138. Badger J, Morris P. Observations of a support group for automatic implantable cardioverter-defibrillator recipients and their spouses. Heart Lung 1989;18: 238–243.

139. Rahimtoola S, Cheitlin M, Hutter A. Cardiovascular disease in the elderly. Valvular and congenital heart disease. J Am Coll Cardiol 1987;10:60A–62A.

140. Lytle B. Impact of coronary artery disease on valvular heart surgery. Cardiol Clin 1991;9:301–314.

141. Wenger N. Quality of life: can it and should it be assessed in patients with heart failure? Cardiology 1989;76:391–398.

142. Booth D, Deupree R, Hultgren H, et al. Quality of life after bypass surgery for unstable angina. 5-Year follow-up results of a Veterans Affairs Cooperative Study [see comments]. Circulation 1991;83:87–95.

143. Katz S. The science of quality of life. J Chronic Dis 1987;40:459–463.

144. Oldridge N, Guyatt G, Jones N, et al. Effects on quality of life with comprehensive rehabilitation after acute myocardial infarction. Am J Cardiol 1991;67: 1084–1089.

145. Sullivan M, Higginbotham M, Cobb F. Exercise training in patients with chronic heart failure delays ventilatory anaerobic threshold and improves submaximal exercise performance. Circulation 1989;79:324–329.

146. Sjoland H, Wiklund I, Caidahl K, et al. Improvement in quality of life and exercise capacity after coronary bypass surgery. Arch Intern Med 1996;156:265–271.

147. Kavanagh T, Myers M, Baigrie R, et al. Quality of life and cardiorespiratory function in chronic heart failure: effects of 12 months' aerobic training. Heart 1996;76:42–49.

148. Oldridge N, Rogowski B. Self-efficacy and in-patient cardiac rehabilitation. Am J Cardiol 1990;66:362–365.

149. Luginbuhl W, Forsyth B, Hirsch G, et al. Prevention and rehabilitation as a means of cost containment: the example of myocardial infarction. J Public Health Policy 1981;2:103–115.

150. Dennis C. Cost-effectiveness in cardiac rehabilitation. J Cardpulm Rehabil 1991;11:128–131.

151. Cordtz D. For our own good. Financial World 1991; 160:50.

152. Picard M, Dennis C, Schwartz R, et al. Cost-benefit analysis of early return to work after uncomplicated acute myocardial infarction. Am J Cardiol 1989;63: 1308–1314.

153. Wittels E, Hay J, Gotto A. Medical costs of coronary artery disease in the United States. Am J Cardiol 1990; 65:432–440.

154. Eisenberg JM. Clinical economics. A guide to the economic analysis of clinical practices. JAMA 1989;262: 2879–2886.

155. Kupersmith J, Holmes-Rovner M, Hogan A, et al. Cost-effectiveness analysis in heart disease, part I: general principles. Prog Cardiovasc Dis 1994;37:161–184.

156. Weinstein M, Stason WB. Foundations of cost-effectiveness analysis for health and medical practices. New Engl J Med 1977;296:716–721.

157. Torrance G. Utility, decision, and quality of life. J Chron Dis 1987;40:593–600.

158. Drummond M, Stoddart G, Torrance G. Methods for the economic evaluation of health care programmes. Oxford: Oxford University Press, 1987:29.

159. Torrance G, Feeny D. Utilities and quality-adjusted life years. Intern J Tech Assess Health Care 1989;5: 559–575.

160. Oldridge N, Furlong W, Feeny D, et al. Economic evaluation of cardiac rehabilitation soon after acute myocardial infarction. Am J Cardiol 1993;72:154–161.

161. Ades P, Pashkow F, Nestor J. Cost-effectiveness of cardiac rehabilitation after myocardial infarction. J Cardpulm Rehabil 1997;17:222–231.

162. Kupersmith J, Holmes-Rovner M, Hogan A, et al. Cost-effectiveness analysis in heart disease, part II: preventive therapies. Prog Cardiovasc Dis 1995;37:243–271.

163. Kupersmith J, Holmes-Rovner M, Hogan A, et al. Cost-effectiveness analysis in heart disease, part III: ischemia, congestive heart failure, and arrhythmia. Prog Cardiovasc Dis 1995;37:307–346.

164. Wong J, Sonnenberg F, Salem D, et al. Myocardial revascularization for chronic stable angina. Analysis of the role of percutaneous transluminal coronary angioplasty based on data available in 1989. Ann Intern Med 1990;113:852–871.

165. Weinstein M, Statson W. Cost-effectiveness of coronary artery bypass surgery. Circulation 1982;66(Suppl 3):56–66.

166. Kinosian B, Eisenberg J. Cutting into cholesterol. Cost-effective alternatives for treating hypercholesterolemia. JAMA 1988;259:2249–2254.

167. Hay J, Wittels E, Gotto A. An economic evaluation of

lovastatin for cholesterol lowering and coronary artery disease reduction. Am J Cardiol 1991;67:789–796.

168. Goldman L, Weinstein M, Goldman P, et al. Cost-effectiveness of HMG-CoA reductase inhibition for primary and secondary prevention of coronary heart disease. JAMA 1991;265:1145–1151.

169. Goldman L, Sia S, Cook E, et al. Costs and effectiveness of routine therapy with long-term beta-adrenergic antagonists after acute myocardial infarction. N Engl J Med 1988;319:152–157.

170. Krumholz H, Cohen B, Tsevat J, et al. Cost-effectiveness of a smoking cessation program after myocardial infarction. J Am Coll Cardiol 1993;22:1697–1702.

171. Cummings S, Rubin S, Oster G. The cost-effectiveness of counseling smokers to quit. JAMA 1989;261:75–79.

172. Edelson J, Weinstein M, Tosteson A, et al. Long-term cost-effectiveness of various initial monotherapies for mild to moderate hypertension [see comments]. JAMA 1990;263:407–413.

The Physician and Cardiac Rehabilitation

Fredric J. Pashkow and William A. Dafoe

REFOCUSING UPSTREAM

Dr. Irving Zola once related the story of a physician that nicely illustrates the dilemma of modern cardiologic practice (1):

You know, sometimes it feels like this. There I am standing by the shore of a swiftly flowing river and I hear the cry of a drowning man. So I jump into the river, put my arms around him, pull him to shore, and apply artificial respiration. Just when he begins to breathe, there is another cry for help. So I jump into the river, reach him, pull him to shore, apply artificial respiration, and then just as he begins to breathe, another cry for help. So back in the river again, reaching, pulling, applying, breathing, and then another yell. Again and again, without end, goes the sequence. You know, I am so busy jumping in, pulling them to shore, applying artificial respiration, that I have no time to see who the hell is upstream pushing them all in.

Despite our earnest efforts, cardiovascular disease (CVD) is the leading cause of death in North America today (2). The available interventional therapies for CVD are not curative but temporizing (3). The percentage of patients who return for second, and even third, coronary artery bypass graft (CABG) operations continues to increase (4, 5). The implication for the cost of future health care is quite sobering. The time has come for us to address the fundamental causes of atherosclerotic heart disease and to develop effective, affordable, long-term strategies for primary and secondary prevention.

Recognition of factors that increase the risk of developing CVD dates to the 1960s from epidemiologic studies such as Framingham (6, 7). The effectiveness of lowering cholesterol for primary prevention of coronary heart disease has been experimentally demonstrated (8–13). Secondary prevention of atherosclerosis involves amelioration of the same risk factors, but after an acute event such as a heart attack or CABG surgery. The traditional risk factors assume prognostic importance for postmyocardial infarction after taking into account the mortality associated with the acute event (14–16). Despite this, physicians have been slow to adopt more aggressive treatment of hypercholesterolemia (17, 18), and even cardiologists have only recently embraced a more assertive treatment approach for hypercholesterolemia in patients with identified coronary heart disease (CHD) (19). The problem is that such intervention requires therapy (such as diet and exercise) that demands time for motivation, education, and a long-term commitment. Low adherence rates further frustrate these long-term efforts (20–23).

As we have stated earlier, cardiac rehabilitation has evolved to consist of exercise, psychosocial support, and education. Its major objectives are to reduce secondary risk factors for CVD through lasting modification of behavior and to facilitate readaptation to normal life through the realization of maximal functional capability (24–27). More than ever, rehabilitation appears to be an appropriate and needed modality of cardiovascular care. In addition to the scientific urgency, there are other serious, compelling reasons to attain these goals that touch on the individual practitioner's role and future in cardiovascular health care delivery.

EFFECT OF SUPERSPECIALIZATION IN CARDIOLOGY AND THE CHANGING ROLE OF PHYSICIANS IN HEALTH CARE

Until recently, in the United States at least, cardiologists have had total freedom with respect to decisions concerning subspecialization and allocation of time. More recently, significant internal and external trends have occurred that will affect the role of the cardiologist for the future. Externally, we are witnessing a significant aging of the population (28). This will have a major impact on cardiologists, because, on average, their patients are considerably older. Government and insurance carriers are becoming more involved in the standardization of the delivery of care in an effort to control costs (29). Some of these changes are already well under way in Canada, the United Kingdom, and western Europe. Business, which has been "footing the bill" for cost-shifting in the United States for indigent and underreimbursed care, is looking to prepaid health plans and other forms of capitation to control costs. Whether there is increasing interest by business in rehabilitation and prevention services has a lot to do with the documentation of cost savings and benefits from such programs. With the need to cut health care costs, all outpatient services are under scrutiny. If physicians and administrators inappropriately deem cardiac rehabilitation as an unnecessary service, it will be difficult to overcome such an obstacle, and a real danger continues to exist that physicians and administrators will come to such a point (30).

Within the discipline of cardiology, we see important trends as well. Overall, there is an increasing supply of doctors. Close to 20,000 cardiologists will be practicing in the United States by the year 2000, which will represent a 100% increase from the number practicing in 1980 (31, 32). There is likely to be a shift toward group and salaried practice, with more competition among physicians, increased monitoring, and application of practice norms, distinct changes in the style of practice—for instance, more outpatient procedures, greater use of physician extenders, and an expanding role of cardiologists as directors of programs and rehabilitation centers (31,

33). With these anticipated changes, no doubt a shift in reimbursement motive will occur, and cardiologists are likely to dedicate more of their efforts to preventive medicine (31). Currently, little personal incentive exists to emphasize prevention in a system that mainly compensates practitioners on the basis of procedures performed (34)—but this is, in fact, in the process of change (35–37).

In addition to the reimbursement issues, there are compelling reasons that our practices have had a procedural versus a more lifestyle-enhancing or behavior-modifying approach. The system has attributed greater prestige to the performance of invasive or other complex technical procedures (38); patients have demanded as instant a "fix" as possible for their coronary problems; and no prevalent infrastructure has arisen for the provision of alternative services. The tiny medical–industrial complex for rehabilitation (mainly a spin-off from the exercise equipment market) is dwarfed by the massive complexes that exist for medical imaging, interventional cardiology, and drug therapy.

At the same time, cardiologists are obliged to provide additional services and functions that seriously impinge on their available time. They are spending more hours producing ever-increasing medical documentation, serving on more quality assurance and utilization surveillance committees, and responding to the increasing demands of patients and their families for more personalized attention (39). A survey of internists (40) was undertaken to ascertain the perceived problems with counseling for prevention (in particular for exercise training). The findings of this survey gave the following barriers to counseling:

Lack of time	55%
Belief of inefficacy of counseling	35%
Need more counseling skills	33%
Patients not interested	31%
Unsure about content for counseling	28%
Lack of reimbursement	22%
Not convinced exercise helpful	11%
Lifestyle matter of personal choice	7%

Thus, lack of time was the major deterrent for initiating such preventive efforts.

CONSTRAINTS—CARDIAC REHABILITATION AS AN OPTIMAL USE OF PHYSICIAN RESOURCES

As the contemporary cardiologist is faced with the escalating internal and external changes described, cardiac rehabilitation appears increasingly attractive as a means of physician extension. Up to this point, we have focused mainly on aspects of education and secondary risk factor modification. A survey of physicians' reasons for referral several years ago indicated that education was cited as a rationale for referral only 25% of the time, whereas secondary risk factor modification per se was not even mentioned. The majority of referrals, nearly 75%, were motivated by the issue of patient surveillance during exercise (30). In chapter 1, we discussed in some detail the issue of surveillance with respect to patient destabilization after a coronary event (such as angioplasty). We discuss other aspects of the surveillance issue, namely electrocardiogram (ECG) monitoring, later in this chapter, as an extension of the physician's traditional role in rehabilitation. Before going on, however, we must discuss the important issue of how cardiac rehabilitation embodies more contemporary thinking about the medical practice model.

Conflict with the Traditional Medical Model

Until recently, medicine has been practiced in western culture mostly according to the principles of beneficence—the physician performs acts in the best interest of patients, producing benefits, good outcomes, and relief from problems and pain (41). Paternalism, usually justified by rationalizations that refer to the welfare, good, needs, and interests of the patient, is the extreme form of beneficence. The consequence of paternalistic practice, however, usually is interference with personal autonomy (42). Even the benefits of prevention need to be scrutinized with respect to potential benefit versus potential harm (43).

One of the few constructive aspects of the recent "malpractice" turmoil in American medicine was the realization (by physicians especially) that practice strictly according to the principle of beneficence transfers all the responsibility of outcome to the provider and leaves little responsibility for outcome to the patient. The principle of

beneficence has been yielding more to one of autonomy—respecting patients' rights to self-determination with the expectation of their greater acceptance of self-responsibility (41). We suspect that the growing numbers of successful rehabilitation programs over the last 25 years reflect this changing philosophy of practice. The evolution of the principle of autonomy has resulted in a greater acceptance of rehabilitation programs that exemplify self-responsibility.

Traditionally, the primary role of the physician in the rehabilitation program was to ensure patient safety. This was inherent in the appropriate selection of patients and supervision of the most advanced ("safest") monitoring methods available. With patients' growing acceptance of self-responsibility, the physician's role has evolved: in addition to appropriate patient selection, there is the prescription of medically compatible activity, the integration of the prescribed regimen with other means of therapy, and the cultivation of the rehabilitation concept with the patient, the primary physician, and the public. The cardiac rehabilitation physician often is viewed as an objective medical voice that provides a reasoned perspective among the various approaches and points of view.

Role of the Physician in Patient Selection

Patient assessment should be a process of individualized appraisal. As Froelicher has pointed out (44), "For every clinical situation there are exceptions: there is the high-risk patient who outlives his physician, the patient with barely any myocardium remaining who can run a marathon, and the low-risk patient who dies. Biological systems are complex, and we all continue to learn with each patient we treat."

The current consensus is that cardiac rehabilitation is appropriate for patients who have active CHD (angina pectoris, recent myocardial infarction [MI], CABG, or angioplasty), after congenital or valvular heart surgery, for patients who have cardiomyopathy, left ventricular (LV) dysfunction, or after cardiac transplantation or the insertion of specialized devices that may improve function in relation to exercise performance.

Once the candidate for rehabilitation has been identified, the initial step is to determine patient stability. Although this process of clinical evaluation is routine for any practicing cardiologist and essential to any initial assessment, it is so fundamental to the contemporary rehabilitation process that an overview is appropriate. At the time of assessment for rehabilitation, records may be "in the mail" and not at hand. As we have indicated previously, three things determine the prognosis for any patient who has CHD: the amount of myocardium at ischemic risk, the extent of LV dysfunction, and the arrhythmic potential of the cardiac substrate. Emerging strategies will assess the stability of the coronary plaque with intracoronary ultrasound and possibly nuclear tracers. How do we assess the relative status of these parameters?

We begin with the history and physical examination. The history should concentrate on the characterization of pain, quantification of physical capacity, recognition of serious markers of cardiac dysfunction, and assessment of arrhythmic potential (Table 2.1). With respect to pain, question carefully for precipitating factors, loca-

Table 2.1.   Characterization of Coronary Disease by History After Myocardial Infarction

Pain
   Ischemic[a]—classically exertional, squeezing, tight, pressure-like, substernal radiates to jaw or left arm, relieved by sublingual nitroglycerin
   Nonischemic—generally nonexertional, sharp, fleeting, not relieved by nitroglycerin
Physical capacity
   ≥2 METs—showers, descends stairs, desk work; walks 30-minute mile
   ≥4 METs—climbs stairs (1 flight) without carrying, runs power mower, walk/jogs (16-minute mile, no grade), golf (walking)
   ≥6 METS—climbs stairs (1 flight) carrying 20 lbs, heavier yard work, jogs (14-minute mile), tennis, downhill skiing
Heart failure
   Weight gain ≥½ pound/day, cough
   Dyspnea—on exertion, at rest, orthopnea, nocturnal
   Therapy—on Lasix, Bumex, or ACE inhibitor[b]
Arrhythmia
   Palpitation—fluttering, thumping, central chest fullness
   Sensorium—lightheadedness, syncope, near-syncope
   Therapy—on antidysrhythmic drugs, internal cardioverter defibrillator

ACE = angiotension-converting enzyme.
[a]**Warning**—pain may be absent in the presence of ischemia. Rest pain of ischemic quality may represent unstable angina, and may not respond to nitroglycerin.
[b]Also used for the treatment of hypertension.

tion, quality, response to sublingual nitrates, frequency, radiation, and associated symptoms. Try to characterize by history the extent of physical capability. Can the patient descend (2 METs) or climb stairs (4 METs)? Can the patient carry a grocery bag up a flight of stairs (5 METs) or a suitcase (7 METs)?

Has the patient had an MI? How extensive? Has the patient been hospitalized for heart failure or for taking prescribed drugs that are an indicator for heart failure? For the history of ventricular function, the characterization of dyspnea is probably most helpful because it may be titrated historically by how much effort elicits breathlessness. Does it occur with one flight, a few steps, at rest? Is orthopnea present? The history of low cardiac output is difficult because symptoms such as early fatigue, lassitude, and cool extremities may be associated with other systemic conditions.

Has the patient had symptomatic arrhythmia or a history of cardiac sudden death? Is there a history of antidysrhythmic therapy that is a clear marker for serious arrhythmic problems, or is there any history to suggest a proarrhythmic effect of these medications? Examples of such therapy currently are sotalol or amiodarone. In the current cardiologic climate, antidysrhythmic drugs for ventricular arrhythmia are being applied mainly in patients who have significant indications, such as documented or inducible ventricular tachycardia or fibrillation. The characterization of disease by use of the history is summarized in Table 2.1.

On the physical examination, we look for findings that predicate the historic data. Does the patient have findings that confirm noncardiac chest pain, for example? As Froelicher has pointed out (44), after a patient has had an acute coronary event, every subsequent chest pain is thought to be cardiac until proved otherwise. Cardiac patients can also have nonischemic chest pains. Findings that suggest noncardiac causes include chest wall tenderness, abnormal cervical precordial maneuvers, and characteristic symptoms with hyperventilation.

For the evaluation of ventricular function, signs of pump failure include the presence of a clearly abnormal precordial impulse, a ventricular gallop (S_3), and rales, although the latter may be found in chronic lung disease, particularly in chronic fibrosis or bronchitis. Neck vein distension, a positive hepatojugular reflux, and lower extremity edema are consistent with some element of right-sided failure, which may be secondary to decompensation of the left ventricle or indicate serious other concurrent disease.

Simple examination of the peripheral pulse can be revealing. The irregularly irregular pattern of atrial fibrillation is distinctive. The frequency of ventricular ectopic beats may be hemodynamically significant. A patient who has a sinus rate of 80 beats per minute with ventricular bigeminy may have only an effective peripheral pulse of 40 beats per minute. What is the ratio of awareness of the ectopy? Can the patient feel some of the ectopic beats, all of them, or none of them? This can be determined only by questioning during simultaneous palpation.

Once the history and physical examination are performed, the astute clinician has a good estimation of the stability and relative risk of this patient for participation in the exercise component of rehabilitation. The next step is to review studies, beginning with the simplest and progressing to the more complex and increasingly invasive.

The chest radiograph and resting 12-lead ECG are so routine that we take them for granted and their value sometimes is underappreciated. The extent of Q waves and the magnitude of R waves correlate reliably with the patient's long-term prognosis (44). Intraventricular conduction delay, usually of left bundle branch block (LBBB) type is almost invariably observed in patients with severely compromised LV function. The chest radiograph can be helpful in the determination of ventricular decompensation, including the overall heart size, large and small vessel vascularity, presence of infiltrates, or effusion, which, along with heart shape and configuration, contributes to this impression.

The physician then should survey the additional noninvasive studies that accompany the patient. Echocardiography provides a wealth of information concerning the structural condition of the heart: how extensive is the regional postinfarction damage, are the valves working properly, how is the global ventricular function? Radionuclide images can provide specific information about myocardial perfusion and function using isotopes such as thallium, rubidium, and labeled glucose. These techniques are improving regularly because of advancements in the radiophar-

maceuticals and the acquisition and processing of higher resolution images. (These techniques are reviewed in detail in chapter 7 on noninvasive diagnostic imaging.)

Ambulatory ECG monitoring of various types is useful for the assessment of the extent and severity of arrhythmia. The classic Holter monitor usually involves 24-hour ambulatory monitoring, which is useful to quantify the amount of dysrhythmia, document sustained and nonsustained runs, and correlate symptoms with dysrhythmic events. For symptoms that occur infrequently but are of sufficient duration, say 3 minutes or longer, a home arrhythmia monitor (basically, a small ECG recorder with a telephone transmitter) is more ideal. It can be maintained in the patient's possession for periods of time sufficient enough to document the problem. It is important to know the natural history of arrhythmias to properly interpret their significance. For example, it is common to observe ectopy after CABG surgery (45, 46).

Another important use of ambulatory monitoring is for the assessment of possible ischemic symptomatology. Most telemetry units are used for arrhythmia detection, and the practitioner needs to be sure the system has appropriate frequency response to assess for ischemic ST-segment changes. Similar caveats exist for Holter monitoring and ischemic changes.

Often, in the face of continuing problems or on the basis of abnormal findings in noninvasive studies, the patient will undergo cardiac catheterization. Angiographic imaging provides the "gold-standard" definition of coronary anatomy and, to some clinicians, ventricular function. The newer technique of intravascular ultrasound adds insight previously unavailable regarding the structure and distribution of the atherosclerotic plaque. Once the status of the coronary circulation is established, decisions concerning management usually are forthcoming. If the determination is to forego revascularization, some parameter, such as a change in the pattern of pain or progression in perfusion defects by thallium, serves as an indicator for the modification of the patient's therapeutic regimen by the managing clinicians. (A summary and the relative value of findings of various diagnostic techniques appear in Table 2.2, modified from Froelicher [44].)

Although the selection of adjunctive studies

Table 2.2.   Comparison of Various Risk Assessment Techniques Postmyocardial Infarction

	History	PE	CXR	ECG	ExT	Echo	Thal	PET	RNV	Holter	Cath
Ischemia	+ + + +[a]	+ +	+	+ +	+ + +	+/+ + +[b]	+ + +	+ + + +	+ +	+ +	+ + + +
LV Dys	+ + + +[a]	+ + +	+ +	+	+ + +	+ + + +	+	+ +	+ + + +	+	+ + +
Arrhythmia	+ + +[a]	+ +	+	+ + +	+ + +	+	+	+	+	+ + + +	+/+ + + +[c]
Cost[d]	Low	Low	Low	Low	Low	Low	Inter	Inter	Low	Low	High

Pe = physical examination; CXR = chest x-ray; ECG = electrocardiogram; ExT = exercise test; Thal = thallium myocardial scintigram; PET = positron emission tomogram; RNV = radionuclide ventriculogram; Holter = ambulatory electrocardiogram; Cath = coronary arteriogram with left ventriculogram; LV Dys = left ventricular dysfunction.
[a]+ indicates least helpful; + + = somewhat helpful; + + + = definitely helpful; + + + + = very helpful.
[b]Echocardiogram with exercise.
[c]Catheterization with electrophysiologic testing.
[d]Relates to range of costs and is not a judgment as to its economic value. Low = relatively lower cost; Inter = intermediate cost; High = relatively higher cost.

is, in part, individualized, it is our contention that the great majority of patients who enter cardiac rehabilitation exercise programs require exercise testing (47). Even though the primary purpose of such a study is to assign safe exercise limits, reassurance of the patient and spouse, establishment of ischemic and dysrhythmic markers, and management of medical therapy are other important indications for the entry study. Table 2.3 summarizes the common indications for exercise testing after MI. Patients who may not be appropriate for an exercise test include those who have considerable fear of the procedure (perhaps from a previous cardiac arrest), those who are starting at extremely low activity levels, those who are at very high risk (e.g., patients awaiting surgery), or those who refuse to have a test and only wish to follow a low-level program. Such patients should be kept at a low to moderate intensity of exercise and assessed frequently on telemetry.

The physician's preentry history, physical assessment, the exercise ECG, and other studies are then used to place the patient in one of several activity classifications. These classifications provide a blueprint for the activity guidelines, the need and extent for ECG and blood pressure (BP) monitoring, and the intensity of medical and nonmedical supervision. The activity classifications recommended by the American Heart Association (AHA) in the Exercise Standards (47) are summarized in Table 2.4.

A principal issue in activity classification has to do with the use of ECG monitoring. The medical concerns related to this have been satisfied by multiple studies that imply that risk of sudden cardiac arrest during exercise activity averages about one per 60,000 patient-hours of activity (47). The activity guidelines outlined in the AHA

Table 2.3.   Purposes of Exercise Testing After Acute Myocardial Infarction

Risk stratification for intensity of monitoring
Reassurance of patient, spouse, and employers
Identify exercise-induced ischemia
Selection and evaluation of medical therapy
Evaluation of ventricular function
Evaluation of dysrhythmias
Evaluation of functional capacity
   Establish safe exercise limits
   Exercise prescription
   Disability determination

Exercise Standards stipulate that continuous ECG monitoring during rehabilitation sessions is recommended until "safety" is established in those patients at moderate to high risk for cardiac complications during exercise (class D patients). The clinical characteristics of such patients include two or more MIs, New York Health Association (NYHA) functional class 3 or greater, exercise capacity less than 6 METs, ischemic (horizontal) or downsloping ST depression of 4.0 mm or more, angina during exercise, fall in systolic pressure during exercise, prior incident of cardiac sudden death, ventricular tachycardia during exercise, or a life-threatening concurrent medical condition.

This recommendation overlaps to only a small degree the criteria listed for ECG monitoring in the Position Report on Cardiac Rehabilitation by the American College of Cardiology (ACC) (48). The characteristics of patients most likely to benefit from continuous ECG monitoring according to the ACC criteria are listed in Table 2.5. The major implication is for program reimbursement, because it is the ECG monitoring for which many third-party payers are indemnified in reimbursement claims for cardiac rehabilita-

Table 2.4. Criteria for Activity Classification After Risk Stratification[a]

	Stable	Risk	NYHA[b]	METs[c]	CHF[d]	Ischemia	BP (Ex)[e]	VEA[f]	Activity[g]	Monitor[h]	Supervise[i]
Class A	Yes	Low	1	>7	No	No	⇑	No	Ad lib	NR	None
Class B	Yes	Low	1–2	>6	No	±	⇑	PVCs	Walk	6–12	NM
Class C	Yes	Low	1–2	>6	No	±	⇑	PVCs	Walk	6–12	M, NM
Class D	Yes	Mod	≥3	≤6	Yes	4 mm ⇓	⇓	VT-NS	by R$_x$	6–12	M, NM
Class E	No	High	≥4	<3	Yes	Unstable	⇓	VF, VT-S	None	NA	NA

[a]Class A = apparently healthy; B = known stable coronary artery disease (CAD)—low risk; C = known stable CAD—low risk, unable to self-regulate; D = moderate to high risk for complications during exercise; E = unstable disease requiring activity restriction.
[b]NYHA = New York Heart Association functional class.
[c]METs = Metabolic equivalents = 3.5 mL O$_2$ consumed/kg body weight per minute.
[d]CHF = Congestive heart failure.
[e]BP (Ex) = blood pressure response to exercise (normal = ⇑).
[f]VEA = ventricular ectopic activity; PVCs = premature ventricular complexes; VT-NS = ventricular tachycardia (nonsustained); VT-S = ventricular tachycardia (sustained); VF = ventricular fibrillation.
[g]Activity = exercise activity; Ad lib = no restrictions; Walk = walking by exercise prescription; by R$_x$ = by exercise prescription.
[h]Monitor = ECG and BP monitoring; NR = not required; NA = not applicable.
[i]Supervise = supervision required; NM = nonmedical staff (with CPR certification); M = medical supervision.

Table 2.5. Characteristics of Patients Most Likely to Benefit from Continuous ECG Monitor During Cardiac Rehabilitation

Severely depressed left ventricular function (ejection fraction <30%)
Resting complex ventricular arrhythmia
Ventricular arrhythmias appearing or increasing with exercise
Decrease in systolic blood pressure with exercise
Survivors of sudden cardiac death
Patients after MI complicated by CHF, cardiogenic shock, or serious ventricular arrhythmias
Patients with severe CAD and marked exercise-induced ischemia
Inability to self-monitor heart rate because of physical or intellectual impairment

CAD = coronary artery disease; CHF = congestive heart failure; MI = myocardial infarction.

tion. The financial and organizational implications of this matter are discussed in more detail in chapter 23.

Although for many physicians, the referral or the intake and enrollment of the patient into the rehabilitation program may be their primary involvement, we encourage physicians to be actively present for patient review sessions with the cardiac rehabilitation team and to provide medical leadership with regard to quality assurance and program development. During the course of rehabilitation, questions frequently arise concerning concurrent medical therapy, such as the management of angina during exercise or accelerating hypertension. These questions are referred to the patient's physician of record or to the medical adviser of the program in the absence or nonavailability of the primary physician.

Sometimes, the medical adviser is consulted when inconsistencies arise with written policy and procedures.

Medical supervision, meaning the presence of a physician during the course of exercise therapy, is not consistent in all programs but is probably adequate for current practice. A regional Medicare fiduciary attempted to rule several years ago that a doctor must be literally in the presence of patients who are exercising. This seems extreme given the low incidence of complications during exercise sessions and the fact that similar requirements do not exist even for coronary intensive care units. The AHA Exercise Standards state that for moderate- to high-risk patients, a "physician should be immediately available (in the facility) for these classes, although the presence of a properly trained nurse in the exercise room is acceptable if the physician is not available" (47).

A medical director is an essential person for the staff of a cardiac rehabilitation program, and the role of this physician has been defined (49). Table 2.6 summarizes the required and preferred qualifications for physicians who serve in the role of medical director or supervising physician. The definition of the physician's role, however, was deleted from the second edition of the American Association of Cardiovascular and Pulmonary Guidelines (50). We believe this is a serious omission and implies that physician input for program design and operations is unessential.

As a medical resource or spokesperson, the physician can be instrumental in achieving the mission and goals of the cardiac rehabilitation

Table 2.6.   Qualifications of Physicians Serving as Medical Directors or Supervising Physicians of Cardiac Rehabilitation Programs

Required qualifications
  Cardiologist, internist, or other physician with interest and experience in cardiac rehabilitation licensed to practice in the jurisdiction and with special competence in rehabilitative care
  Experienced in exercise testing, prescription, and counseling
  Certified in advanced cardiac life support (ACLS) or experienced and knowledgeable in emergency procedures

Preferred qualifications
  Board-certified or board-eligible cardiologist
  Experienced in medical supervision of cardiovascular rehabilitation services

Desirable qualifications
  Interested and knowledgeable in risk factor reduction techniques
  Able to lead a multidisciplinary team
  Able to represent cardiac rehabilitation in the medical hierarchy

program. Often, physicians who refer to or are involved in the program as medical advisers are willing to lead educational sessions with participants, particularly if they are given license to cover topics of their own special interests. This participation tends to be reinforcing and to intensify their own awareness of the program's potential.

COPING WITH INCREASING PATIENT EXPECTATIONS AND GROWING SELF-EFFICACY

We live in an era in which the latest findings from the *New England Journal of Medicine* are discussed in the media before practicing physicians receive the journal itself. Our patients receive this information and more through magazines, newsletters, the Internet, radio, and television. Special interest groups for various diseases network across the continent and invite expert speakers for presentations. Patients feel empowered with this information and evolve to become the "informed consumer." The image of a dependent patient who prefers to be sheltered from harsh truths is not supported according to Deber in a paper on the patient–physician partnership (51). It appears that most patients wish to have information, although there is an identifiable minority who prefer not.

The late Norman Cousins became a hero of

self-efficacy with his determination to "rehabilitate himself" from ankylosing spondylitis and a complicated MI (52). He developed a collaborative working relationship with his physician to augment the traditional medical treatment. He was an active partner in his treatment and was involved with all decision making. In addition, he used techniques such as humor and imagery to enhance his own therapeutic efforts. In a similar way, a number of patients wish to play an active role in their rehabilitative process. Such patients provide unique challenges to cardiac rehabilitation programs and physicians.

As with most complex issues, elements of controversy exist about the various risk factors (for example, minimal levels for cholesterol). Patients regard their cardiac rehabilitation physician as an expert resource and, in some cases, as an arbitrator for the mass of confusing information. This situation leads to increased patient expectations for health care staff. For the physician, it is difficult, if not impossible, to be conversant with all studies germane to a particular issue. In addition, it is difficult to spend the time to discuss the various perspectives and the merits of relevant studies with each patient. It is unrealistic to think that we will revert back to "simpler times" when patients just "did as they were told." We have found that the provision of patient discussion groups that outline the various aspects of risk factors (including a dialogue about sources of conflict), providing access to well-researched health newsletters (e.g., *The Berkeley Wellness Newsletter* or *The Cleveland Clinic Heart Advisor*), or suggested authoritative web sites such as the American Heart Association (http://www.amhrt.org/newhome.html) can help patients to become their own best advocate.

Physician Beliefs and Actions Concerning Cardiac Rehabilitation and Risk Factor Modification

Despite the continuing accumulation of evidence that links cholesterol and coronary disease, physicians have demonstrated a reluctance to diagnose and treat lipid abnormalities, even in patients with proven CHD. Cohen and coworkers (19) have demonstrated that patients who have coronary disease and hyperlipidemia were treated no more aggressively than other patients, and that cardiologists do not intervene any more than physicians in general, though this appears to be changing. A Canadian survey showed that only about 30% of family physicians are treating according to published guidelines (Fodor J, McPherson R, Dafoe W, et al. unpublished observations). Several plausible explanations for this reluctance to treat have been suggested. Physicians may not have been convinced of the cost-effectiveness of lipid management (38, 53, 54). Until recently, the therapy for hyperlipidemia was complex and the diets and drugs unpleasant to the extent that treatment of this problem was difficult and time-consuming. The perceived lack of time and lack of nutritional background and training required to perform the counseling task satisfactorily most likely accounts for the reluctance (55). Schectman and Hiatt's data suggest that physicians are now paying more attention to this important risk factor (23).

A survey of physicians done almost 20 years ago by Frances (56), long before the publication of findings on atherosclerotic regression, revealed that 50% of the physicians studied already believed that cardiac rehabilitation decreases the progression of coronary disease. In addition, approximately 50% of the respondents also thought that rehabilitation decreased mortality and reinfarction, and improved physician control; 75% felt that rehabilitation improved morbidity and return-to-work (56).

The potential positive influence of the physician in the reduction of other important risk factors has been demonstrated (57). Many techniques for smoking cessation are now available (58, 59), and a significant majority of physicians recommend smoking cessation to their patients (60). Demers and coworkers (61) examined the effect of a 3- to 5-minute unstructured physician discussion encouraging smoking cessation; the differences in quit rates, although not statistically significant, did suggest that physicians can affect patient smoking cessation positively. Even brief counseling by a physician may be extremely cost-effective (62). Another investigation suggests that a positive association is found between perceived physician humanism and patient satisfaction and that greater success in patients' attempts to quit smoking is associated with higher perceived physician interest and understanding (63).

Once the importance of risk factor modification is endorsed by the physician, what are the most effective practical methods of achieving change in patients (64)? How can we enhance the patient's motivation for change? What is the optimal focus for counseling, so that the patient can be made to feel that the activity of exploring or modifying their risk behavior is meaningfully connected with their personal goals and life priorities? Nolan (64) goes on to promote fostering a patient-centered clinical method. We currently are seeing the availability of a profusion of patient-focused educational materials (handouts, brochures, audiotape and videotape, and the like). Recent strategies help to guide the physician into different strategies for counseling depending on the readiness for change by the patient as described by the transtheoretical model of Prochaska and DiClimente (as cited by Nolan [64]). A coordinated effort with the rest of the office staff or cardiac rehabilitation team is integral to these approaches (65). Despite this material, it appears that the substance per se is not as important as doctor validation and serious, personal communication between doctor and patient (66).

In our experience, pure didactic programs—lectures—on risk factor modification are not as successful for the transfer of information to patients and spouses as more participatory experiences. We have found that informal discussions ("firesides"), although more challenging to perform to encompass the educational material, produce more personal participation and a more effective learning experience. These question-and-answer sessions led to our use of "field trips" for nutritional counseling. We found that a nutritionist with a small group in a supermarket was substantially more engaging than a classroom lecture. Another persuasive approach is a cooking class, in which the "students" (patients and spouses) actually participate in preparing heart-healthy dishes after a culinary arts demonstration. The nutritional content is woven into the demonstration and the transfer of information is painless. "Teach culinary arts and not nutrition," advises Dr. William Castelli of Framingham fame. One sobering note is the reality that risk factor modification is a lifelong process, and the challenge for cardiac rehabilitation patients and programs is the long-term maintenance of these changes.

Earlier in this chapter we discussed physician motivation for cardiac rehabilitation referral. Perhaps this is an appropriate time to discuss physicians' reasons for nonreferral. About two-thirds of the physicians surveyed indicated that cost was a consideration; 50% cited satisfaction with their own approach to patient management, and about 40% indicated that they disliked losing control over the patient or they "just did not believe" in exercise conditioning and rehabilitation (30).

It is important that the medical director of a cardiac rehabilitation program be aware of these perceptions. Because change takes place over an extended period of time, it is important to acknowledge the existence of such views. A thoughtful and reasoned response to these concerns can often lead to their amelioration. First, the concern about cost needs to be addressed and put into perspective. The cost for a complete course of cardiac rehabilitation is equivalent to approximately 1 day in the coronary care unit (CCU). The direct costs often are covered by third-party payers who already have certified the service as reimbursable. Next, a referral to cardiac rehabilitation does not lessen the effective job of an individual clinician. If anything, involvement in a structured program can act in a synergistic way to allow an enhanced effect. Patients often give credit to their own physicians for arranging their referral to a formal cardiac rehabilitation program. The concern about "loss of control" is a sensitive issue and needs to be addressed directly. It should be made clear in the program literature and in all staff pronouncements that the referring physician is in control of the patient's medical management. If there is a serious concern regarding a medical issue, resolution can be achieved by a discussion between the medical director and the referring physician. Finally, the more difficult issues of disbelief in the efficacy of exercise or risk factor reduction require time and frequent discussion. In our experience, a small, residual number of physicians have decided that cardiac rehabilitation is not appropriate despite the increasing amount of evidence to the contrary. Nevertheless, many of their patients are now requesting referrals to cardiac rehabilitation programs. Our favored approach is to respect these differing points of view when addressing program participants but to present our perspective with the appropriate evidence.

Although the referral of patients into formal cardiac rehabilitation remains physician controlled, we do find that increasing numbers of patients and their families are requesting the service. At the Cleveland Clinic, it was found that 78% of those patients eligible were interested in phase II participation, although the actual rate of participation is far lower (about 20%), mainly related to medical instability, geographic distance, or lack of reimbursement.

CHALLENGING ISSUES: HANDLING ANGER AND POTENTIAL LIABILITY, REFERRAL BIAS, AND CARDIAC ENTITIES BEYOND CORONARY ARTERY DISEASE

A difficult role for the cardiac rehabilitation physician is to address effectively, but not necessarily manage, all patient issues that may affect the success of the rehabilitation program. As previously mentioned, the referring physician continues to treat active medical issues and others, should they arise. But what should be done if a nonmedical problem involves the referring physician or other medical personnel?

A difficult scenario involves the patient who is angry at one of the treating physicians. Perhaps the anger results from a perceived delay in the diagnosis of the infarct, or because the treatment in hospital was "cold and callous." Whatever the cause, in today's litigious society, such anger may be a prelude to a lawsuit (see also chapter 24 on Medical–Legal Liability).

Anger is an issue that needs to be addressed if the patient is to have an effective experience. From a physiologic perspective, psychological distress (anger being a classic example) has been seen as a harbinger of ventricular arrhythmias (67, 68). From a rehabilitation perspective, it is difficult for the patient or the family to progress through the rehabilitation continuum when considerable energies are directed toward "past injustices." Furthermore, it is difficult for a trusting therapeutic relationship to flourish with the rehabilitation staff.

We have found that this particular issue of "patient anger" needs to be addressed early in the rehabilitation experience. It is not the role of the cardiac rehabilitation physician to take sides and attempt to defend other physicians or attitudes experienced in some other medical setting. In some cases, the cardiac rehabilitation physician may wish to provide some background information that may clarify the aggrieved situation. Patients need to work through this anger as part of the overall therapy. The process may involve the patient's being encouraged to have a meeting with the physician, to write a letter to record the issues of concern, or in some cases, to proceed with legal consultation. Whatever the selected course, patients should feel that such actions will not affect their rehabilitation course adversely. In some cases, it is appropriate to arrange a referral to a psychologist, social worker, or psychiatrist affiliated with the program to deal further with this anger.

Patients may ask the cardiac rehabilitation physician to become the treating physician or to facilitate the transfer to another cardiologist. Because either course of action is fraught with potential problems, a suggested approach is to discuss strategies to improve the therapeutic relationship with the original treating physician, and if this fails, to suggest that such a transfer should be arranged independently or through the primary or family physician.

An important issue for clinical studies involves referral bias to either an institution or to a particular physician. For example, the descriptive characteristics of the patient population at the Cleveland Clinic is markedly different from hospitals of vastly different size in nearby cities. Because formal cardiac rehabilitation programs can manage only a fraction of all potential referrals, the referring physician may select what are considered to be the most appropriate patients. This process forms the selection bias for the program. The knowledge of limited cardiac rehabilitation resources becomes known in the medical community. This may lead to the perception that uncomplicated patients or those who express few complaints have no need of rehabilitation services. The often touted phrase "this patient is too good for rehabilitation" is increasingly heard. Thus, patients who have only complex medical problems in addition to their cardiac difficulties are perceived as appropriate for referral. In some cases, an opposite bias—a hangover from the past—occurs in that complicated patients are not referred to cardiac rehabilitation.

Referral bias creates numerous problems. First, a proportion of eligible patients (uncomplicated ones in this instance, or the complex patients in another), fails to derive the benefits of any cardiac rehabilitation or preventive intervention. Second, in the case of complex patients, some have overwhelming problems that are unlikely to improve with exercise training. Third, the positive group atmosphere and confidence-enhancing effect of a cardiac rehabilitation program become jeopardized with too many complex patients. Thus, the cardiac rehabilitation physician needs to be aware of these perceptions in the community that form the referral bias. Patients who have overwhelming medical or psychosocial problems may tax the limited rehabilitation resources unduly and, thus, may have to be considered on a quota basis.

The traditional referrals to cardiac rehabilitation programs have been CHD patients. Patients with other cardiac disorders, however, have similar concerns as CHD patients (for example, a safe level of activity, coping with the disease process, and attempts to prevent recurrence). A growing cadre of patients exists who have cardiomyopathy or who have undergone heart failure surgery, including cardiac transplantation or implantation of defibrillators or left ventricular assist devices, and who form an appropriate patient referral pool. The cardiac rehabilitation physician needs to be knowledgeable about this patient group and must assume responsibility for the development of safe guidelines for the program. Each patient needs to be assessed individually for unique problems. For example, a transplantation patient may have muscle weakness and osteoporosis as a result of steroid therapy and months of bed rest. Or, a patient with an implantable defibrillator may be depressed and anxious because of the fear of the defibrillator firing. The cardiac rehabilitation team may need to alter the emergency procedures for such a patient when acute arrhythmia management is required to accommodate this patient's unique circumstance (the presence of the cardioverter/defibrillator).

RELATING TO THE POWER STRUCTURE: WITHIN THE INSTITUTION, THE MEDICAL COMMUNITY, AND THE GOVERNMENT

Inherent in the successful application of cardiac rehabilitation as a therapeutic mode is the acceptance of the concept of collaborative practice. Cardiac rehabilitation programs are most successful when they use a program management structure. This allows the required autonomy for cardiac rehabilitation programs including control over the budgeting process and staffing issues. This means that a significant amount of the responsibility for the program is shared by allied health and nonmedical professionals. A substantial amount of patient care and supervision may be performed distant from the hospital and clinical environment, often with the use of protocols. How comfortable the physician is with these collaborative relationships may contribute substantially to referrals to such programs (30).

Miller (30) has pointed out that enhancing physician involvement in cardiac rehabilitation programs requires a detailed understanding of the physician and the practice environment. Is the hospital a large teaching or tertiary referral institution in which specialty consultation is the norm and physician assistants and allied health professionals are routinely available? In addition to the primary physician, many persons may be important in the rehabilitation referral process, including consulting physicians, physician extenders involved in the day-to-day clinical care, specialists who perform inpatient rehabilitation, and so on. This does not necessarily mean that the road to patient referral is smooth, however. Sometimes, with so much fragmentation of care, the patient is never referred. Someone assumes that someone else has taken care of the outpatient rehabilitation referral. Large institutions require thorough procedures for the recruitment and enrollment of patients into the program. These standardized routines for referral can cause disagreement among medical staff. There will be physicians, usually vocal traditionalists, who will object vehemently to the use of routine referral procedures or, for that matter, to the standardized format of the educational materials or even the exercise components of the program. They will insist that only they know what is "good" for a particular patient and demand that their patients be excluded or handled in some unique way. In our experience, these issues need to be addressed at a departmental level. Such persons should be encouraged to express their views in committees or specific task forces. In the end, a consensus needs to be reached on a departmental or institutional basis. Similar problems sometimes are seen in smaller hospital environments in which there are few if any physician

extenders and the concept of collaborative practice is unknown. The development of a patient care map for different medical conditions requires the input of all concerned physicians. Disagreements about treatment algorithms can be addressed in the development of the map. An automatic referral to cardiac rehabilitation can be an integral component of the patient care map.

As noted previously, physicians are facing an increasingly competitive environment in medicine today and many are developing new attitudes about the importance of practice expansion and development. They understandably are protective of their patients but recognize the need to offer services that keep patients coming back (69). At the same time, physicians are aware of the issue of escalating cost in health care.

The hospital environment is one in which drastic changes are occurring. The length of stay is shortening radically to the point at which hospitalization for an uncomplicated MI or CABG operation is now, on average, less than 5 days. A major consequence of this marked abbreviation in length of stay is the time in which patients and families must absorb important information and process the psychological changes associated with the illness. This enhances the appeal of outpatient rehabilitation and, with greater participation likely, increases the interest of hospital administrators who see the programs as potential new revenue sources and enhancements to their hospital's image of excellence. The program may also have "marketing value" in the increasingly competitive health care environment. This increases the likelihood that the hospital administration will make the investment in facility, equipment, and staff to maximize the chances of program success. It is important, however, that the hospital administration have realistic expectations for what these programs can generate in direct and indirect income to offset the investment needed to establish them.

It is useful to remind ourselves of the prescient findings from a Task Force Report in 1974 from the National Heart and Lung Institute. This report represented the first significant involvement of a federal institution in cardiac rehabilitation. The report categorized knowledge in the area of cardiovascular rehabilitation, assessed techniques, and the importance of the discipline, and provided recommendations for future research and clinical practice (70). Although the role of the physician is discussed mainly in relation to the issues of medical practice and supervision, it does address the issue of the physician–patient relationship and some of the problems specifically extant at that time. These included problems in communication, especially related to cultural differences, insufficient information for clinical and vocational decisions, and physician reticence in returning patients to full activity, resulting in delay of rehabilitation and dealing with physician–patient discrepancies in degree of impairment (70).

In 1995, the United States Department of Health and Human Services released a Clinical Practice Guideline for Cardiac Rehabilitation from the Agency of Health Care Policy and Research (71). Although this represents the most detailed analysis of the efficacy and indications for cardiac rehabilitation as an intervention, little regarding the specific role of the physician is included. Coverage of role of intake assessment and risk stratification for exercise surveillance, usually the responsibility of the doctor, is deferred to the other practice guidelines. Other than these reports, the most tangible relationship currently between the physician involved in cardiac rehabilitation and the federal establishment is in the reimbursement milieu.

Changing attitudes provide timely opportunities. Cardiac rehabilitation is a valuable service at a relatively low price. It provides frequent contact with the patient and a bonding of the patient with the staff. If the physician is identified as part of the rehabilitation team, the patient–physician relationship will be enhanced, and the physician is correctly perceived as being interested in providing a full spectrum of services to ensure the attainment of the patient's better cardiovascular health (69).

CARDIAC REHABILITATION IN A TEAM SETTING, RELATING TO OTHER HEALTH CARE PROFESSIONALS

Rehabilitation requires a comprehensive approach for an effective treatment outcome. Traditional rehabilitation services for neurologic and musculoskeletal problems (cardiovascular accident [CVA], amputations) have used a team approach to bring together the expertise required for the patient. In a similar way, many cardiac rehabilitation programs have used the team approach. A "health care team" is defined by Halstead (72) as "a group of health care professionals from different disciplines who share common values and work toward common objectives." Halstead concluded that a coordinated team care appears to be more effective than fragmented care for patients who have long-term illness (72).

The rehabilitation team can use a multidisciplinary or interdisciplinary approach, or a combination of both (73). The multidisciplinary approach has each discipline treating the patient with unique activities. Each staff member only needs to know the skills inherent to his or her own discipline. An example of this approach would be a cardiac patient who sees an exercise physiologist on Monday, a dietitian on Tuesday, and a health educator on Wednesday. These three health care professionals may not be aware of the content and approach of the other expert resources. They might be able to interchange information on a particular patient at a team meeting. The interdisciplinary approach is somewhat more complex. In this model, each discipline provides input according to its expertise but also contributes to a group effort on behalf of the patient. An example using this approach would be a team in which a treatment strategy is discussed with the whole team at patient intake. Although most if not all cardiac patients would be following an exercise program and receiving education, other issues could be addressed on an individual basis. Perhaps one patient might find it easier to lose weight before smoking cessation. The interdisciplinary team then can work together in a synergistic manner to develop a treatment strategy. Whatever team approach is used, communication among team members is paramount. The cardiac rehabilitation physician may function as the head of this team, or if there is a program director (other than the physician who would be the medical director), the physician can provide input and assume responsibility for the medical issues. In either scenario, it is important for the physician to be fully conversant with the team model and the dynamics for optimal team functioning.

The assignment of responsibilities in a cardiac rehabilitation team is determined by a number of factors (historic, legal, discipline-specific responsibilities, site-specific needs, interests, and so forth). It is important at the outset to set guidelines and boundaries for different team members. A review of other cardiac rehabilitation programs may be helpful. The resolution of these needs helps to avoid "turf issues." The process of establishing discipline boundaries is dynamic because staff interests may change and the personnel in the various disciplines may change. Areas of overlap need to be acknowledged. For example, a psychologist and social worker may work with patients who have family problems. The cardiac rehabilitation physician may be called on to help establish staff responsibilities because medical and safety issues and previously established institutional guidelines will play a role.

A cardiac rehabilitation team is composed of personnel who have varied backgrounds, interests, and temperaments. An effective team does not just happen on its own. It is useful for the cardiac rehabilitation physician to become familiar with the literature and dynamics of team building. Expert facilitators may be well worth the investment for effective team functioning (74). To function effectively, it is important that the cardiac rehabilitation physician, as a senior member of the team, be aware of process issues. In some cases, the physician is called on to arbitrate a decision. If this situation is part of a more complex problem related to team dynamics, then the full issue needs to be explored. Conflict and complacency are important issues that each team has to address.

The characteristics of an effective working team have been outlined by McGregor as follows (75):

1. Atmosphere: tends to be informal, comfortable, and relaxed.
2. Discussion: there is considerable discussion in which virtually everyone participates, but it remains pertinent to the task of the group. The members listen to each other. There is disagreement. The group is comfortable with this and shows no sign of having to avoid conflict.
3. Objective of the group: the task or objective of the group is well understood and accepted by the members.
4. Decision making of the group: most decisions are reached by consensus in which it is clear

that everybody is in general agreement and willing to go along.
5. Criticism: frank, frequent, and relatively comfortable. There is little evidence of personal attack, either openly or in a hidden fashion.
6. Chairman or leader: does not dominate, or, on the contrary, the group does not defer unduly to the leader. As one observes the activity, it is clear that the leadership shifts from time to time, depending on the circumstances.
7. Conflict and disagreement: a normal and necessary part of team development. How it is handled determines its effect on team objectives and on the group process.
8. Mutual respect: important for the role and function of each discipline. Team members should feel comfortable in the role of "teacher" and "learner" alike with regard to various components of a patient's care.

Finally, it should be mentioned that the team approach is not sacrosanct. Keith (76) reviewed the concept of the rehabilitation team (primarily in general rehabilitation) and notes that there has been a paucity of research regarding its efficacy. He observes that the "evolution of the comprehensive rehabilitation team in its current form has been the product of a combination of technologic competencies, professional territoriality, and external economic and regulatory forces." It is important, therefore, for the cardiac rehabilitation physician to be aware of the historic evolution of rehabilitation teams and to know that future delivery of care, given the present economic climate, may change the team as we know it.

THE PHYSICIAN AND ISSUES OF REIMBURSEMENT

Reimbursement for cardiac rehabilitation remains the Achilles' heel of the discipline (77). The reason for this is complex, and the relationship of the physician to the implementation of successful reimbursement strategies is crucial. The first consideration is that because cardiac rehabilitation consists of several identifiable elements, including exercise therapy, counseling, patient education, ECG monitoring, and so on, the way in which therapy is identified and billed to insurers and third-party payers is inconsistent. Most often, the reimbursement procedure and coding vary from state to state or by region. Meyer (78) did a survey and found that 16 different codes were used for billing essentially the same phase II cardiac rehabilitation services. The second consideration is that, because of its heterogeneity, payers have difficulty recognizing cardiac rehabilitation as a specific therapy or as a well-defined service unlike the way that cardiac catheterization or a CABG operation is perceived. Despite demonstrations of its efficacy and endorsement of its appropriateness as an alternative model by the Clinical Practice Guideline (25), at-home rehabilitation is not likely to be reimbursable in the near future. First and foremost, no specific procedure code has been defined and assigned for at-home cardiac rehabilitation; in addition, there appears to be concern about the economic implications of greatly expanding the availability of this service.

Reimbursement for inpatient services is even more fragmented than for outpatient, but it is a less serious issue for patients with Medicare coverage in the United States because the cost of rehabilitation is included in the capitated fee paid for the hospitalization under the Diagnosis Related Group (DRG) system. Our main concern currently is that projected cutbacks in Medicare reimbursement under DRGs may result in the curtailing or elimination of inpatient rehabilitation programs. Physician involvement remains essential, however, to see that administrators continue to recognize the value of inpatient programs and to continue to secure reimbursement for phase II outpatient programs. The reimbursement standards have been defined effectively by Medicare, which covers a significant number of claims for these phase II services.

Coverage for individually prescribed exercise training and telemetered ECG monitoring in the United States is reimbursed under part B of Medicare. It has provided coverage for hospital-based outpatient cardiac rehabilitation programs since 1980, and for outpatient physician-directed programs since 1982 (78). Guidelines have been published that specify the role of the physician and define the extent of medical supervision required. They are summarized in Table 2.7.

Physician involvement in the supervision of the cardiac rehabilitation program provides more than just the expertise needed for the medical management and safety of patients. The physician's active participation justifies the con-

Table 2.7. Guidelines Concerning Physician Involvement for Medicare Reimbursement

A physician must be present on the premises during patient activity.

Each patient must be under the care of the hospital or clinic physician.

Cardiopulmonary emergency equipment, such as a defibrillator and a crash cart, must be immediately available.

Programs must be staffed by personnel trained in basic life support and cardiac exercise therapy.

A physician must supervise the nonphysician personnel.

cept of rehabilitation and imparts to the team members who perform the yeoman's portion of the day-to-day work the psychological fortitude needed to overcome the resistance of backsliding patients and skeptical critics. As secondary prevention is incorporated as an integral component of cardiac rehabilitation, physician input and development is essential.

References

1. McKinlay JB. A case for refocusing upstream: the political economy of illness. In: Conrad P, Kern R, eds. The sociology of health and illness. New York: St. Martin's Press, 1981:613.
2. 1997 Heart and stroke statistics. Dallas, TX: American Heart Association, 1996.
3. Alderman E, Bourassa M, Cohen L, et al. Ten-year follow-up of survival and myocardial infarction in the randomized Coronary Artery Surgery Study. Circulation 1990;82:1629–1646.
4. Bourassa MG. Fate of venous grafts: the past, the present and the future. J Am Coll Cardiol 1991; 17: 1081–1083.
5. Vanbrussel BL, Plokker HWT, Voors AA, et al. Progression of atherosclerosis after venous coronary artery bypass graft surgery—a 15-year follow-up study. Cathet Cardiovasc Diagn 1997;41:141–150.
6. Kannel W, Castelli W, Gordon T, et al. Serum cholesterol, lipoproteins, and the risk of coronary heart disease. The Framingham Study. Ann Intern Med 1971;74:1–12.
7. Castelli W, Garrison R, Wilson P, et al. Incidence of coronary heart disease and lipoprotein cholesterol levels. The Framingham Study. JAMA 1986;256:2835–2838.
8. The Lipid Research Clinics Coronary Primary Prevention Trial results. I. Reduction in incidence of coronary heart disease. JAMA 1984;251:351–364.
9. The Lipid Research Clinics Coronary Primary Prevention Trial results. II. The relationship of reduction in incidence of coronary heart disease to cholesterol lowering. JAMA 1984;251:365–374.
10. Stamler J, Wentworth D, Neaton J. Is relationship between serum cholesterol and risk of premature death

from coronary heart disease continuous and graded? Findings in 356,222 primary screenees of the Multiple Risk Factor Intervention Trial (MRFIT). JAMA 1986; 256:2823–2828.

11. Frick M, Elo O, Haapa K, et al. Helsinki Heart Study: primary-prevention trial with gemfibrozil in middle-aged men with dyslipidemia. Safety of treatment, changes in risk factors, and incidence of coronary heart disease. N Engl J Med 1987;317:1237–1245.

12. Gotto AJ. Lipid-lowering trials: what have they taught us about morbidity and mortality? [review]. Cardiology 1996;87:453–437.

13. LaRosa JC. Cholesterol lowering, low cholesterol, and mortality [review]. Am J Cardiol 1993;72:776–786.

14. Kannel W. Prospects for risk factor modification to reduce risk of reinfarction and premature death. J Cardpulm Rehabil 1981;1:64–71.

15. Tervahauta M, Pekkanen J, Nissinen A. Risk factors of coronary heart disease and total mortality among elderly men with and without preexisting coronary heart disease. Finnish cohorts of the Seven Countries Study. J Am Coll Cardiol 1995;26:1623–1629.

16. Assman G. Lipid metabolism disorders and coronary heart disease—primary prevention, diagnosis and therapy guidelines for general practice. Munich: Bertelsmann Publishing Group, 1989.

17. Superko H, Desmond D, de Santos V, et al. Blood cholesterol treatment attitudes of community physicians: a major problem. Am Heart J 1988;116:849–855.

18. Danielsson B, Aberg H. Hyperlipidaemia—management and views amongst physicians in general practice, in occupational health care and in internal medicine. J Intern Med 1993;234:411–416.

19. Cohen M, Byrne M, Levine B, et al. Low rate of treatment of hypercholesterolemia by cardiologists in patients with suspected and proven coronary artery disease. Circulation 1991;83:1294–1304.

20. Eraker S, Kirscht J, Becker M. Understanding and improving patient compliance. Ann Intern Med 1984; 100:258–268.

21. Fishman T. The 90-second intervention: a patient compliance mediated technique to improve and control hypertension. Public Health Rep 1995;110:173–178.

22. Urquhart J. Partial compliance in cardiovascular disease: risk implications [review]. Br J Clin Pract Symp Suppl 1994;73:2–12.

23. Schectman G, Hiatt J. Drug therapy for hypercholesterolemia in patients with cardiovascular disease: factors limiting achievement of lipid goals. Am J Med 1996;100:197–204.

24. Wenger NK. Future directions in cardiovascular rehabilitation. J Cardpulm Rehabil 1987;7:168–174.

25. Wenger NK, Froelicher ES, Smith LK, et al. Cardiac rehabilitation. Clinical practice guideline No. 17. Rockville, MD: Department of Health and Human Services, Public Health Service, Agency for Health Care Policy and Research and National Heart, Lung, and Blood Institute. AHCPR Publication No. 96–0672, 1995.

26. Dafoe W, Huston P. Current trends in cardiac rehabilitation. Can Med Assoc J 1997;156:527–532.

27. Merz CN, Rozanski A. Remodeling cardiac rehabilitation into secondary prevention programs [review]. Am Heart J 1996;132(2 Pt 1):418–427.

28. Guralnik J, FitzSimmons S. Aging in America: a demographic perspective. Cardiol Clin 1986;4:175–183.

29. Ginzberg E. What lies ahead for American physicians: one economist's views. JAMA 1985;253:2878–2879.

30. Miller M. A framework for enhancing physician involvement in the rehabilitation continuum. In: Hall L, Meyer G, eds. Cardiac rehabilitation: exercise testing and prescription. Champaign, IL: Human Kinetics, 1988:43–66.

31. Russell R, Beahrs M, Davis J, et al. Economic trends affecting adult cardiology. J Am Coll Cardiol 1988;12: 847–853.

32. Health, United States, 1996–97 and Injury Chartbook. Hyattsville, MD: National Center for Health Statistics, 1997.

33. Goldsmith JC. The US health care system in the year 2000. JAMA 1986;256:3371–3375.

34. Glanz K, Fiel S, Walker L, et al. Preventive health behaviors of physicians. J Med Educ 1982;57:637–639.

35. DeMaria A, Rodgers J, Carmichael D, et al. The impact of current health policy trends on adult cardiology. J Am Coll Cardiol 1988;12:853–858.

36. Feldman AM, Greenhouse PK, Reis SE, et al. Academic cardiology division in the era of managed care. A paradigm for survival [see comments]. Circulation 1997; 95:740–744.

37. Weingarten S, Stone E, Hayward R, et al. The adoption of preventive care practice guidelines by primary care physicians: do actions match intentions? J Gen Intern Med 1995;10:138–144.

38. Ginzberg E. High-tech medicine and rising health care costs. JAMA 1990;263:1820–1822.

39. Ginzberg E. US health policy–expectations and realities. JAMA 1988;260:3647–3650.

40. Sherman S, Hershman W. Exercise counseling: how do general internists do? J Gen Intern Med 1993;8: 243–248.

41. Gorovitz S. Dilemmas: moral conflict and medical care. New York: MacMillan, 1982:36–37, 41–54.

42. Zembaty JS. A limited defense of paternalism in medicine. In: Mappes T, Zembaty J, eds. Biomedical ethics. New York: McGraw-Hill, 1981:57–58.

43. Marshall KG. Prevention. How much harm? How much benefit? Influence of reporting methods on perception of benefits. Can Med Assoc J 1996;154:1493–1499.

44. Froelicher V. Cardiac rehabilitation. In: Parmley W, Chatterjee K, eds. Cardiology. Philadelphia: JB Lippincott, 1988;1:1–17.

45. Dolatowski R, Squires R, Pollock M. Dysrhythmia detection in myocardial revascularization surgery patients. Med Sci Sports Exerc 1983;15:281–286.

46. Kirdar JA, Sharma GV, Khuri SF, et al. Pathogenesis and prognostic significance of conduction abnormalities after coronary bypass surgery. Cardiovasc Surg 1996;4:832–836.

47. Fletcher GF, Balady G, Blair SN, et al. Statement on exercise: benefits and recommendations for physical activity programs for all Americans. A statement for health professionals by the Committee on Exercise

and Cardiac Rehabilitation of the Council on Clinical Cardiology, American Heart Association. Circulation 1996;94: 857–862.

48. Parmley W. Position report on cardiac rehabilitation. J Am Coll Cardiol 1986;7:451–453.

49. American Association of Cardiovascular and Pulmonary Rehabilitation. Guidelines for cardiac rehabilitation programs. 1st ed. Champaign, IL: Human Kinetics, 1991:35.

50. American Association of Cardiovascular and Pulmonary Rehabilitation. Guidelines for cardiac rehabilitation programs. 2nd ed. Champaign, IL: Human Kinetics, 1995:92.

51. Deber RB. Physicians in health care management: 7. The patient-physician partnership: changing roles and the desire for information. Can Med Assoc J 1994; 151:171–176.

52. Cousins N. Head first. New York: Penguin Books, 1989.

53. Jacobson TA. Cost-effectiveness of 3-hydroxy-3-methylglutaryl-coenzyme A (HMG-COA) reductase inhibitor therapy in the managed care era. Am J Cardiol 1996;78(Suppl 6A):32–41.

54. Oldridge NB. Cardiac rehabilitation and risk factor management after myocardial infarction—clinical and economic evaluation. Wien Klin Wochenschr 1997; 109(Suppl 2):6–16.

55. O'Keefe C, Hahn D, Betts N. Physicians' perspectives on cholesterol and heart disease. J Am Diet Assoc 1991;91:189–192.

56. Frances C. Cardiac rehabilitation: current physician attitudes. In: Cohen L, Mock M, Ringquist I, eds. Physical conditioning and cardiovascular rehabilitation. New York: John Wiley & Sons, 1981:239–246.

57. Schwartz J, Lewis C, Clancy C. Internists' practices in health promotion and disease prevention. Ann Intern Med 1991;114:46–53.

58. Silagy C, Mant D, Fowler G, et al. Meta-analysis on efficacy of nicotine replacement therapies in smoking cessation. Lancet 1994;343:139–142.

59. Schwartz JL. Methods of smoking cessation. Med Clin North Am 1992;76:451–476.

60. Nett LM. The physician's role in smoking cessation. A present and future agenda. Chest 1990;97(2 Suppl): 28S–32S.

61. Demers R, Neale A, Adams R, et al. The impact of physicians' brief smoking cessation counseling: a MIRNET study. J Fam Pract 1990;31:625–629.

62. Cummings S, Rubin S, Oster G. The cost-effectiveness of counseling smokers to quit. JAMA 1989;261:75–79.

63. Hauck F, Zyzanski S, Alemagno S, et al. Patient perceptions of humanism in physicians: effects on positive health behaviors. Fam Med 1990;22:447–452.

64. Nolan RP. How can we help patients to initiate change? Can J Cardiol 1995;11:16A–19A.

65. Calfas KJ, Long BJ, Sallis JF, et al. A controlled trial of physician counselling to promote the adoption of physical activity. Prev Med 1996; 25:225–233.

66. Campbell J, Tierney W. Information management in clinical prevention. Prim Care 1989;16:251–253.

67. Follick M, Gorkin L, Capone R, et al. Psychological distress as a predictor of ventricular arrhythmias in a post-myocardial infarction population. Am Heart J 1988;16:32–36.

68. Verrier RL, Mittleman MA. Life-threatening cardiovascular consequences of anger in patients with coronary heart disease [review]. Cardiol Clin 1996;14:289–307.

69. Pashkow FJ, Pashkow PS, Schafer MN. Successful cardiac rehabilitation: the complete guide for building cardiac rehab programs. Loveland, CO: The Heart-Watchers Press, 1988:329.

70. Task Force on Cardiovascular Rehabilitation. Needs and opportunities for rehabilitating the coronary heart disease patient. Bethesda, MD: The National Heart and Lung Institute, 1974: DHEW Publication No. 76–750.

71. American Association of Cardiovascular and Pulmonary Rehabilitation. Guidelines for cardiac rehabilitation programs. 2nd ed. Champaign, IL: Human Kinetics, 1995.

72. Halstead LS. Team care in chronic illness: critical review of literature of past 25 years. Arch Phys Med Rehabil 1976;57:507–511.

73. Melvin JL. Interdisciplinary and multidisciplinary activities and ACRM. Arch Phys Med Rehabil 1980;61: 379–380.

74. Francis D, Young D. Improving work groups. A practical manual for team building (revised). San Diego: Pfeiffer & Company, 1992.

75. McGregor D. The human side of enterprise. New York: McGraw-Hill, 1960:232–235.

76. Keith R. The comprehensive treatment team in rehabilitation. Arch Phys Med Rehabil 1991;72:269–274.

77. Wenger NK. Reimbursement for cardiac rehabilitation services. J Am Coll Cardiol 1997;29:473.

78. Meyer GC. Overview of insurance—obtaining and maintaining coverage in cardiovascular rehabilitation. In: Hall L, Meyer G, eds. Cardiac rehabilitation: exercise testing and prescription. Champaign, IL: Human Kinetics, 1988:67–102.

Improvement of Quality of Life in the Framework of Cardiac Rehabilitation

Nanette Kass Wenger

EMERGENCE OF QUALITY-OF-LIFE CONSIDERATIONS IN CLINICAL ASSESSMENTS

Among the influences reinforcing the validity of quality-of-life assessment as an outcome of clinical care are the increased prevalence of chronic cardiovascular (coronary) illness, the informed-consumer movement in health care, the escalating emphasis on preventive care, the emergence of a number of comparably effective therapeutic options for many cardiac problems, and the inclusion of quality-of-life data in the assessments of cost-effectiveness. Each will be addressed in turn. In chronic illness, therapies are not curative, but are designed to ameliorate symptoms and improve functional abilities, i.e., to limit the disabling consequences of the disease, such that the patients' perceptions about their resultant health status have clinical relevance. Particularly as regards chronic illness, patients as enlightened consumers of health care increasingly seek information about their disease, the therapeutic alternatives available to them for its management, and the anticipated outcome. Patient satisfaction with medical care appears predominantly related to whether, as a result of a treatment, they feel better and can function better; essentially, the treatment undertaken has improved the quality of their life. The increased emphasis on preventive therapies often relates to medical problems that are essentially asymptomatic. For patients with coronary heart disease, complicating hypertension, and hypercholesterolemia, as examples, typically entail long-term care including lifestyle modifications or pharmacotherapy or both. Adherence to these aspects of risk modification influences outcome; therefore, to achieve benefit from preventive interventions it must be realized that perceptions influence adherence and that the patients' perceptions thereby influence outcomes. Because, as Hoerr has stated, "it's hard to make an asymptomatic patient feel better," preventive therapies must be delivered in the context of an acceptable lifestyle for the patient. Although long-term benefits can be anticipated, the patient must not be hampered by short-term impedances to life quality. A further driving force for quality-of-life assessment relates to a variety of comparably effective therapeutic options—for the coronary patient, medical versus surgical therapies, and in the rehabilitation setting, a variety of approaches to exercise training and to education and counseling. The impact of these rehabilitative therapies may differ depending on patient characteristics, needs, and preferences; effect on work status; and requirements for surveillance. In the use of quality-of-life attributes in evaluating the cost-effectiveness of coronary care, determining features include the resultant functional independence of the patient, productivity, return to remunerative work, and level of life satisfaction.

QUALITY OF LIFE IN THE MEDICAL CARE CONTEXT

Aspects of outcome that require assessment in chronic cardiovascular illness include the total consequences of both the illness and its management. Quality of life, in the medical care context, is a measurable and quantifiable concept that encompasses the ways in which a patient's life is affected both by an illness and by the varied components of its care. Quality of life thus addresses the patient's resultant comfort, sense of well-being, and life satisfaction; his or her maintenance of physical, emotional, and intellectual function; and the ability to participate in valued activities in the family, in the workplace, and in the community (1). Spitzer (2) has characterized these multifactorial domains of quality of life applicable to medical care as "clinically relevant human attributes." Favorable alterations in these clinically relevant human attributes characteristically are the parameters that determine the patient's satisfaction with and perception of the effectiveness of the outcomes of medical care. The goals of cardiac rehabilitation address these valued outcomes.

Assessment of quality of life differs from a categorization of the symptomatic manifestations of an illness or the objective benefits and complications of a therapy or intervention. Quality-of-life attributes are subjective and personal; they reflect and incorporate a patient's personal value systems and judgments about general health status, well-being, and life satisfaction. In this approach to assessment, the focus is the individual patient. Quality-of-life assessment also reflects the patient's (and family's) expectations of the outcomes of therapy and the resultant improvements in functioning. These expectations can encompass a spectrum from simple survival and recovery, to feeling better or feeling completely well, to the resumption of an independent and active lifestyle, or, at times, to a return to remunerative employment. Given this great variability, it is important to ascertain the expectations of a specific coronary patient (and his or her family) about the benefits of undertaking a rehabilitation regimen. For symptomatic coronary patients whose activities are likely to have been restricted by long-term coronary illness, anticipation about the extent of functional improvement is likely to have lessened, thereby curtailing the potential benefits of rehabilitative interventions. The advent of newer therapies, as in coronary patients whose illness is complicated by heart failure, may require education and counseling about greater anticipated benefits than previously obtained. Further, evidence that the most impaired patients are more likely to benefit from exercise rehabilitation (3) should change patient expectations. With the advances in contemporary medical and surgical care, now included in the tasks of counseling patients recovering from a coronary event should thus be a

review of the reasonable functional improvement that can be anticipated and the approaches recommended for achieving them. As well, the escalating documentation of the value of secondary preventive interventions in limiting both coronary morbidity and mortality (4) can, with appropriate education and counseling, favorably alter patient expectations about outcomes.

The role of perceived health status (5, 6) has received increasing attention in recent years in that it correlates, in some studies (and particularly for older patients), with the risk of mortality. Further, perceived health status often correlates better with work resumption (7) and work performance than does the objectively measured functional capacity, as determined at exercise testing. Of particular importance is that the perception of health status can be altered favorably by education and counseling.

In many recent studies that encompassed considerations of the resultant quality of life of coronary patients, there has been a disproportionate focus on return to work as an outcome measure, with some investigators using work resumption virtually as a surrogate for quality-of-life assessment. Despite the importance of return to work for many coronary patients, it is only one component of life quality. Also, as commonly ascertained, return to work typically fails to address diverse life quality domains within the workplace (job satisfaction, job performance, opportunity for advancement, adequacy of income, and the like), which often are affected adversely by a cardiac, and particularly a coronary, illness. Finally, return to work is an inappropriate goal for many coronary patients, prominent among whom are elderly or retired patients or those medically complex, severely impaired patients with advanced coronary heart disease and its complications. For these patients, attainment and maintenance of an independent lifestyle is likely their most valued outcome and should, indeed, be the goal of their rehabilitative care. More recent studies assessing health-related quality of life have broadened the concept of work to include a range of productive activities, both paid and unpaid. Such measures include volunteer and community activities, household tasks, and caregiving activities, as well as paid employment. These instruments provide a more comprehensive view of the individual's functional status, with respect to productive activities, than focusing solely on return to work (8).

QUALITY OF LIFE: PATIENTS WITH CORONARY HEART DISEASE

Evaluation of quality of life assumes particular importance in patients with chronic illness (9, 10), typified by coronary heart disease, wherein the therapies for the illness are not designed to be curative, but, rather, to alleviate or limit the symptoms of the illness, to restore or improve the patient's functional capabilities to permit relative self-sufficiency and independence, to retard or limit progression of the underlying disease, to maintain a sense of well-being, and to decrease the adverse psychological consequences of the illness that may lead to unwarranted invalidism. The effects of coronary illness, coronary disability, and therapeutic interventions for coronary heart disease often extend beyond the patient and exert an impact on family members and significant others. Quality-of-life assessment addresses the ways in which the patients' (and families') lives are affected by the manifestations of coronary heart disease and the components of its management. Because a cure is not anticipated, it addresses the ways in which a patient must learn to live with and cope with the coronary illness.

As new therapies for coronary heart disease have lessened substantially the risks both of morbidity and of mortality, there may be less effective end points in the comparative evaluation of therapies. As an example, in the thrombolytic era, a majority of patients discharged from the hospital after an episode of myocardial infarction (MI) who are younger than 70 years of age are considered at low-risk status for a proximate coronary event; this is the case for many patients after myocardial revascularization procedures as well (11). Increased attention in assessing the outcome of interventions in these low-risk coronary patients likely will be directed to the life satisfaction that can be derived from a sense of well-being and from improved physical status, emotional state, and intellectual functioning, as well as from work performance when appropriate. These multiple variables that characterize a patient's overall function assume added importance in comparing interventions for symptomatic coronary disease that have comparable morbidity and mortality benefits, e.g., medical versus surgical therapies, different approaches to myocardial revascularization, structured or supervised versus unsupervised rehabilitative care, and the like.

Application of vasodilator therapies, particularly the use of angiotensin-converting enzyme inhibitor drugs, for coronary patients with complicating heart failure has prominently decreased their symptoms and improved their functional capacity. Nonetheless, a combination of pharmacotherapy and exercise training can decrease symptoms and improve functional capacity in such patients beyond the results achieved with angiotensin-converting enzyme inhibitor therapy alone (12). The addition of low-dose β-blockade may provide further benefit.

REHABILITATIVE GOALS IN THE CARE OF CORONARY PATIENTS: RELATIONSHIP TO QUALITY OF LIFE

The overall goals of the rehabilitative care of coronary patients are to enable the resumption of a normal or preillness lifestyle and to return the patient to a productive, active, and satisfying role in society. Because the results sought from rehabilitative care concern quality-of-life attributes, the evaluation of the outcomes of coronary rehabilitation should include, and possibly emphasize, assessment of the quality of the patient's life (see below).

Goals of Exercise Rehabilitation

Exercise training for coronary patients currently is prescribed predominantly to lessen activity-induced or activity-related symptoms and to improve physical functional capacity. The desired outcome is an improvement in these quality-of-life attributes.

In the early years of exercise rehabilitation, as well as in most of the clinical trials of exercise training efficacy, disproportionate attention was focused on the potential improvement in survival and decrease in reinfarction in coronary patients as a consequence of exercise training. Although no individual clinical trial of rehabilitative exercise training has demonstrated such advantage, meta-analyses of pooled data from a number of exercise trials in patients with coronary heart disease (13, 14) documented a 25% survival advantage among exercising patients (15). Less emphasis is currently directed to morbidity and mortality outcomes of exercise rehabilitation, likely reflecting the substantial reduction in postinfarction mortality and early reinfarction related to coronary thrombolysis or acute angioplasty in the early hours of MI, improved catheter-based and surgical myocardial revascularization techniques, and the burgeoning of effective pharmacotherapies for these coronary patients. Among the relatively low-risk coronary patients just described, there is less likelihood of significant additional improvement in survival resulting from any additional intervention, including exercise training (15). Stated another way, for the sizable number of low-risk postinfarction patients, morbidity and mortality data typically are not helpful in characterizing the outcome of any treatment; other outcome measures may assess better the efficacy of an added intervention and address the patient's main goal in seeking or undertaking medical care.

Exercise Rehabilitation of High-risk, Medically Complex, and Elderly Coronary Patients

A subgroup of seriously ill, medically complex coronary patients still remains, many of whom have had recurrent coronary events, are often elderly, many of whom have heart failure, and typically are not candidates for myocardial revascularization procedures. Among these patients, many of whom have significant residual myocardial ischemia, severe ventricular dysfunction, or potentially life-threatening arrhythmias, the risk of mortality or reinfarction is so high and their prognosis is generally so poor that any intervention is unlikely to alter substantially morbidity and mortality outcomes. Again, other outcome measures may assess better the efficacy of an intervention, for example, its ability to improve the patient's functional capabilities and comfort, even to a modest extent; its ability to enable the patient to perform self-care; its ability to enable the patient to remain in a reasonably independent living status or to participate in valued family or other social interactions. These all are measurable quality-of-life attributes that may be enhanced by even small improvements in physical work capacity.

A lower intensity, more gradually progressive, and more protracted course of exercise training, at times with ECG monitoring, is characteristic of the exercise rehabilitation recommended for many of these high-risk, medically complex, and often elderly coronary patients. In prior years, most of these categories of coronary patients were arbitrarily excluded from exercise rehabilitation. Despite the impairment caused by their coronary illness or because of their advanced age or comorbidity, a substantial improvement in exercise capacity has been demonstrated by many of these coronary patients, albeit requiring a longer time than for their younger counterparts (16–19).

The training-induced improvement in exercise capacity among these patients should not be surprising, given the predominant or exclusively peripheral (noncardiac) adaptations to low-intensity exercise training. These effects include an improved extraction of oxygen by trained skeletal muscle from the perfusing blood, and autonomic nervous system and peripheral blood flow changes that result in a decrease in myocardial oxygen demand (lower heart rate and lower systolic blood pressure) at any submaximal exercise intensity. Exercise training thereby increases the anginal threshold, with a resultant lessening of exercise-induced angina and a reduced curtailment of the performance of activities of daily living (ADL) and self-care. This improvement in exercise tolerance can reverse prior limitations of activity, particularly those related to the occurrence of angina pectoris.

These benefits of exercise training enhance the patient's ability to maintain an independent lifestyle, a valued goal of most seriously ill or elderly coronary patients, a goal that is measurable, and one that, in the medical care setting, is cost-saving as well. Long-term institutional care for elderly coronary patients or for those with end-stage coronary illness constitutes an expensive component of total cardiac care. The concomitant teaching of work simplification techniques can additionally enhance the physically impaired coronary patient's ability to maintain an independent living status.

Features of Exercise Rehabilitation That May Affect Life Quality Favorably

Among the substantial benefits anticipated from the exercise rehabilitation of the coronary patient, coupled with education and counseling, are a number of favorable changes that may lessen coronary risk (15): an improvement in blood lipid levels, reduction in cigarette smoking, and reduction in stress. Also, there is an improvement in joint mobility, musculoskeletal stability, and neuromuscular coordination, all of which may increase functional capability. A prominent improvement occurs in psychological well-being, with a decrease in fear, depression, and dependency; renouncing of the sick role; and improvements in self-confidence and in self-esteem. Both depression (20) and lack of emotional support (21) are independent risk factors for unfavorable outcomes after a coronary event.

The component of these benefits related to the exercise training per se and that related to education and counseling and to peer reinforcement and professional support in a group exercise setting remains uncertain. This, in part, addresses the role of the peer group setting in coronary rehabilitation as a social support system; social isolation in coronary patients is associated with increased mortality (22, 23). Exercise training also has been associated with an improvement in work attendance and an increase in leisure time activities; it also may lessen the need for the number or dosage of medications designed to control myocardial ischemia and hypertension.

Characteristics of Contemporary Coronary Patients

As previously cited, contemporary medical and surgical therapies for patients with coronary heart diseases often result in less residual myocardial ischemia and less myocardial dysfunction after a coronary event. In part, this relates to acute interventions used to maintain myocardial perfusion (for example coronary thrombolysis or acute angioplasty in the setting of MI) and in part is related to the wide application of myocardial revascularization techniques (coronary angioplasty or coronary artery bypass surgery).

For patients with initial coronary events, there is a low risk of proximate recurrence of such events. This favorable prognosis warrants intensive efforts at multifactorial coronary risk reduction, designed to enhance atherosclerotic plaque stability, prevent progression, and potentially induce regression of the underlying coronary atherosclerosis, and, thereby to maintain a favorable coronary risk status.

Unfortunately, particularly with the brief hospitalization for an initial episode of chest pain, as when coronary angioplasty is undertaken for myocardial revascularization and MI is averted, the patient often perceives the illness as minor and nondisruptive of the usual patterns of living. This feature is inappropriately translated into the consideration of the coronary illness as not potentially serious or life-threatening. As a result, adherence to recommendations for coronary risk modifications has been less than optimal among this patient subgroup and may have an unfavorable impact on the long-term course of the coronary illness.

Goals of Rehabilitative Education and Counseling for Coronary Patients

Coronary risk reduction is designed to arrest or retard the progression of coronary atherosclerosis, to stabilize atherosclerotic plaques, and potentially to induce regression of the obstructive coronary atherosclerotic lesions (4). Because these interventions predominantly involve behavioral modifications, the patient must be provided not only with the requisite cognitive information but also must be taught the skills required for the adoption of health-related behaviors, encouraged to practice these skills, and receive reinforcement for maintenance of successful coronary risk reduction (24).

Psychosocial counseling (including vocational counseling) has as its goal an improved perception of health status and resultant changes in behaviors in these spheres. The perception of health status often can be influenced favorably by interpreting clinical data to the patient, such as those related to exercise performance (as determined at exercise testing), as well as the benefits that can be anticipated from reduction of coronary risk (25). Whereas the satisfactory accomplishments of 7 or 8 METs of exercise on an exercise test protocol identifies the patient's favorable risk status for the treating physician, the patient can overcome the perception of serious illness and disability only when this value is translated into the performance of daily living or occupational and recreational activities (25, 26), and when this information is used to dispel the fears of resuming prior activities. Improvement in perceived health status characteristically may have favorable effects on many other variables, including return to sexual activity, return to remunerative employment (7), and resumption of preillness family, community, and social roles. These anticipated and measurable outcomes of successful rehabilitative education and counseling directly address enhancement of quality-of-life attributes.

Features of Education and Counseling That May Affect Life Quality Favorably

Patients who attain an improvement in their coronary risk status, showing themselves able to cope with the problems of illness, concomitantly improve their self-confidence and self-esteem. There is family and community approval for weight loss when indicated, for resumption of recommended levels of physical activity, and for return to work when it is reasonable to do so. Resumption of sexual activity, of leisure time pursuits, and return to preillness roles in the family and the community further enhance the life quality of the coronary patient.

Assessment of Quality of Life as an Outcome Measure of Coronary Rehabilitation

As discussed, the low-risk status for recurrent coronary events after an initial coronary episode of many patients who have received contemporary therapies is such that additional interventions are unlikely to alter morbidity and mortality substantially. In the context of evaluation of components of care for a chronic illness, coronary rehabilitation is one model in which quality-of-life variables can serve appropriately as outcome measures of the efficacy of this intervention. Quality-of-life assessments are singularly appropriate for evaluating the outcomes of coronary rehabilitation, given that most of the goals of coronary rehabilitation address quality-of-life domains.

Several well-validated quality-of-life assessment instruments have been documented as capable of assessing life quality attributes both in general and in the setting of acute and chronic coronary illness. Global or generic measures of quality of life are advantageous in that various functional domains can be anticipated to be affected by an exercise training regimen and by the educational and counseling components of coronary rehabilitation. Among these generic measures are the Nottingham Health Profile (27), the Quality of Well-Being Scale (28), the Sickness Impact Profile (29), and the Rand-36 Health Status Profile (30).

Although these global measures explore a wide variety of quality-of-life concerns, prominent among them being physical function, social and emotional function, intellectual function, symptoms and their consequences, occupational activities and job satisfaction, leisure activities, sexual adjustment, perceived health status, life satisfaction, and interpersonal relationships, it is of added value to use selected measures appropriate for those components of quality of life specifically related to coronary heart disease in the assessment of coronary rehabilitative interventions. These disease-specific measures better characterize detailed aspects of benefits or adverse effects of treatments for specific symptoms or functions related to a disease. For coronary heart disease, relevant test measures include the New York Heart Association (NYHA) functional classification that grades the limitations of ability to perform physical activity (31); the Specific Activity Scale (SAS), to be discussed later; and the Rose Chest Pain Questionnaire (32) and the Canadian Cardiovascular Society (CCS) Classification (33) for judging the severity of angina pectoris. For more impaired patients, the SAS, developed by Goldman et al. (34) is thought to define more precisely the ability to perform physical activity, in that the "usual" levels of activity, as addressed by the NYHA functional classification, may decrease with time and with progression of the severity of illness. The SAS grades the magnitude of tasks by metabolic indices of oxygen consumption (METs) to define the level of function that can be attained by the patient without stopping. For patients with heart failure complicating the coronary illness, measures of dyspnea may be of value (35, 36).

Virtually all life quality attributes can be addressed by comprehensive coronary rehabilitative care: physical and emotional function, cognitive function, social participation, general well-being, economic status, and the like. If only disease-specific measures are used, it becomes difficult to disentangle the complex interrelationships among quality-of-life dimensions. For example, has the increased intensity of physical symptoms (e.g., angina) resulted in a decrease in physical capabilities, with resultant anxiety and depression? Or has depression or other emotional dysfunction engendered a limitation in physical function? The quality-of-life global measures described previously can determine the impact of rehabilitative interventions and their interrelationships and can supplement the disease-specific outcome measures. Particularly for seriously ill patients, virtually all components of life quality may be influenced by cardiac rehabilitation, hence the value of using a broadly based assessment instrument with multivariant measures. Effects may be evident on self-care skills, ambulation ability, home management, ability to engage in pleasurable activities, performance of social roles with family and friends, intellectual and cognitive function, the need for and use of health resources, sense of control and self-reliance, autonomy, coping behavior, degree of denial, and other features of emotional status such as expectations, mood, life satisfaction, and optimism about the future (37). Mosteller and associates (38) summarized these issues in their delineation that

public impression to the contrary, the bulk of medical and surgical treatment is not life saving, but is aimed at improving the state or quality of life. Most diseases are not dramatically fatal, but chip away at comfort and happiness. At the same time, treatments for life-threatening diseases often have different impacts on patient comfort. To the extent that we are unable to measure and compare the effects of treatments on the quality of the patient's life, we are unable to document advantages of treatments as well as their defects.

Assessment of improvements in life quality domains may thus be an excellent technique for evaluating the efficacy of coronary rehabilitative care. Although this measurement is undertaken increasingly in the research setting (39), an unmet need is the development of a brief questionnaire for use in office practice to ascertain reliably life quality in coronary patients.

INDIVIDUALIZATION OF CORONARY REHABILITATION: RELATIONSHIP TO QUALITY OF LIFE

The trend for the delivery of coronary rehabilitative services in the next millennium increasingly will emphasize individualization of care (i.e.,

a patient-oriented rather than a program-oriented approach to rehabilitative care) (40). In prior years, many structured and supervised coronary rehabilitation programs were characterized by a relatively inflexible and indiscriminate multifactorial intervention approach, with the varied components of care delivered to all participating patients without particular regard for their timeliness, relevance, or interest to the patient.

The contemporary trend is for the selection of relevant rehabilitation services, tailored to the individual patient's needs and preferences and based on medical recommendations derived from the patient's clinical status, from among those available in a coronary rehabilitation setting (supervised or unsupervised). In addition, desired outcomes should be defined for each of these services or program components, and preferably these outcomes should be targeted as time-based goals. For example, the exercise training goal may be for the patient to improve exercise capacity from a 4-MET level to an 8-MET level within 3 months; or to lower LDL cholesterol level by dietary modification, weight loss, and pharmacotherapy from 170 mg/dL to 100 mg/dL within 4 to 6 months. In this way, acceleration of recovery with rehabilitative techniques, as compared with usual care, can be ascertained (39). Next, the selection of the specific rehabilitative services and the modes of their implementation should be based on medical care recommendations and on patient preference. Patient preferences may dictate, for example, whether a group exercise program or home exercise regimen is chosen for the low-risk coronary patient who does not require supervision of exercise; or whether the skills for implementing a cholesterol-lowering diet are to be learned in group discussions, using videotapes at home that can be shared with the family, using interactive television or computer-based learning, by participatory cooking and food shopping demonstrations—or by a combination of these techniques.

Individualization of coronary rehabilitation is likely to affect favorably the patient's functional capabilities, perceptions of personal health status, and coping skills and, thereby, to improve the quality of the coronary patient's life.

With appreciation to Julia Wright for help in the preparation of the manuscript.

References

1. Patrick DL, Erickson P. What constitutes quality of life? Concepts and dimensions. Qual Life Cardiovasc Care 1998;4:103–127.

2. Spitzer WO. Keynote address: state of science for 1986: quality of life and functional status as target variables for research. J Chron Dis 1987;40:465–471.

3. Balady GJ, Jette D, Scheer J, et al. Changes in exercise capacity following cardiac rehabilitation in patients stratified according to age and gender. Results of the Massachusetts Association of Cardiovascular and Pulmonary Rehabilitation Multicenter Database. J Cardpulm Rehabil 1996;16:38–46.

4. Fuster V, Pearson TA. 27th Bethesda conference: matching the intensity of risk factor management with the hazard for coronary disease events. J Am Coll Cardiol 1996;27:957–1047.

5. Kaplan GA, Camacho TC. Perceived health and mortality: a 9 year follow up of the human population laboratory cohort. Am J Epidemiol 1983;117:292–295.

6. Mossey JM, Shapiro E. Self-rated health: a predictor of mortality among the elderly. Am J Public Health 1982;72:800–808.

7. Fitzgerald ST, Becker DM, Celentano DD, et al. Return to work after percutaneous transluminal coronary angioplasty. Am J Cardiol 1989;64:1108–1112.

8. Wenger NK, Naughton MJ, Furberg CD. Cardiovascular disorders. In: Spilker B, ed. Quality of life and pharmacoeconomics in clinical trials. 2nd ed. New York: Raven Press, 1996:883–891.

9. Luginbuhl WH, Forsyth BR, Hirsch GB, et al. Prevention and rehabilitation as a means of cost containment: the example of myocardial infarction. J Public Health Policy 1981;2:103–115.

10. Parmley WW. President's page: position report on cardiac rehabilitation. J Am Coll Cardiol 1986;7:451–453.

11. Ryan TJ, Anderson JL, Antman EM, et al. ACC/AHA guidelines for the management of patients with acute myocardial infarction: executive summary. A report of the American College of Cardiology/American Heart Association Task Force on Practice Guidelines (Committee on Management of Acute Myocardial Infarction). Circulation 1996;94:2341–2350.

12. Meyer TR, Casadei B, Coats AJ, et al. Angiotensin-converting enzyme inhibition and physical training in heart failure. J Intern Med 1991;230:407–413.

13. Oldridge NB, Guyatt GH, Fischer ME, et al. Cardiac rehabilitation after myocardial infarction. Combined experience of randomized clinical trials. JAMA 1988; 260:945–950.

14. O'Connor GT, Buring JE, Yusuf S, et al. An overview of randomized trials of rehabilitation with exercise after myocardial infarction. Circulation 1989;80:234–244.

15. Wenger NK, Froelicher ES, Smith LK, et al. Cardiac rehabilitation. Clinical practice guidelines No. 17. Rockville, MD: U.S. Department of Health and Human Services, Public Health Service, Agency for Health Care Policy and Research and the National Heart, Lung, and Blood Institute. AHCPR Publication No. 96-0672. October 1995.

16. Wenger NK. Overview. Exercise and cardiac rehabilitation in the elderly. Geriatr Cardiovasc Med 1988;1: 87–88.

17. Wenger NK. Exercise for the elderly: highlights of preventive and therapeutic aspects. J Cardpulm Rehabil 1989;9:9–11.

18. Lavie CJ, Milani RV, Littman AB. Benefits of cardiac rehabilitation and exercise training in secondary coronary prevention in the elderly. J Am Coll Cardiol 1993;22:678–683.

19. Ades PA, Waldmann ML, Gillespie C. A controlled trial of exercise training in older coronary patients. J Gerontol 1995;50A:M7–M11.

20. Frasure-Smith N, Lesperance F, Talajic M. Depression and 18-month prognosis after myocardial infarction. Circulation 1995;91:999–1005.

21. Berkman LF, Leo-Summers L, Horwitz RI. Emotional support and survival after myocardial infarction. A prospective, population-based study of the elderly. Ann Intern Med 1992:117:1003–1009.

22. Appels A. Mental precursors of myocardial infarction. Br J Psychiatry 1990;156:465–471.

23. Orth-Gomer K, Unden A-L, Edwards M-E. Social isolation and mortality in ischemic heart disease. A 10-year follow-up study of 150 middle-aged men. Acta Med Scand 1988;224:205–215.

24. Zafari AM, Wenger NK. Secondary prevention of coronary heart disease. Arch Phys Med Rehabil 1998;Aug: in press.

25. Taylor CB, Bandura A, Ewart CK, et al. Exercise testing to enhance wives' confidence in their husbands' cardiac capability soon after clinically uncomplicated acute myocardial infarction. Am J Cardiol 1985;55: 635–638.

26. Ott C, Bergner M. The effect of rehabilitation after myocardial infarction on quality of life. Qual Life Cardiovasc Care 1985;1:176–190.

27. Hunt SM, McKenna SP, McEwen J. A quantitative approach to perceived health. J Epidemiol Community Health 1985;34:281–295.

28. Bush JW. General health policy model/Quality of Well-Being (QWB). In: Wenger NK, Mattson ME, Furberg CE, et al., eds. Assessment of quality of life in clinical trials of cardiovascular therapies. New York: Le Jacq Publishing, 1984:189–190.

29. Bergner M, Bobbitt RA, Carter WB, et al. The sickness impact profile: development and final revision of a health status measure. Med Care 1981;19:787–805.

30. Hays RD, Sherbourne CD, Mazel RM. The Rand 36-item health status survey 1.0. Health Econ 1993;2:217–227.

31. Harvey RM, Doyle EF, Ellis K, et al. Major changes made by the Criteria Committee of the New York Heart Association. Circulation 1974;49:390.

32. Rose GA, Blackburn H. Cardiovascular survey methods. Geneva: World Health Organization 1986;56:1–188.

33. Campeau L. Grading of angina pectoris. Circulation 1976;54:522–523.

34. Goldman L, Hashimoto B, Cook EF, et al. Comparative reproducibility and validity of systems for assessing cardiovascular functional class: advantages of a new Specific Activity Scale. Circulation 1981;64:1227–1234.

35. Foxman B, Lohr KN, Brook RH, et al. Conceptualization and measurement of physiological health in

adults, v. congestive heart failure. Santa Monica, CA: Rand Corp., September 1982.

36. Mahler DA, Weinberg DM, Wells CK, et al. The measurement of dyspnoea. Content, interobserver agreement and physiologic correlates of two new clinical indexes. Chest 1984;85:751–758.

37. Wenger NK. Quality of life: can it and should it be assessed in patients with heart failure? Cardiology 1989;76:391–398.

38. Mosteller F, Gilbert JP, McPeek B. Reporting standards and research strategies for controlled trials. Controlled Clin Trials 1980;1:37–58.

39. Oldridge N, Guyatt G, Jones N, et al. Effects on quality of life with comprehensive rehabilitation after acute myocardial infarction. Am J Cardiol 1991; 67:1084–1089.

40. Wenger NK. Future directions in cardiovascular rehabilitation. J Cardpulm Rehabil 1987;7:168–174.

Evaluation of Outcomes

Philip A. Ades, Peg L. Pashkow, James R. Nestor, and Fredric J. Pashkow

The current perspective of cardiac rehabilitation is of a structured "secondary prevention center" with on-site and home exercise programs, lipid clinics, and other risk factor modification components aimed at preventing second coronary events and cardiac rehospitalizations in patients with established coronary artery disease. Cardiac rehabilitation services include medical evaluation, prescribed exercise, and cardiac risk factor modification. Services are tied to a series of measurable short-term and longer-term outcomes such as measures of physical functioning, cardiac risk factors, cardiac symptoms, return to work, psychological well-being, progression of coronary atherosclerosis, recurrence of cardiac events, and cardiac rehospitalizations.

Objective and systematic measurement of specific cardiac rehabilitation outcomes serves multiple purposes.

1. It demonstrates the continuing integrity of a profession already deeply steeped in evidence-based demonstration of efficacy (1).
2. It provides a tool by which individual programs can measure results of their component interventions and continually improve delivery patterns.
3. It provides a tool by which case-managers can individualize therapy for cardiac rehabilitation participants to attain individualized goals.
4. It provides a framework to calculate cost-effectiveness of cardiac rehabilitation and its components. These data can be used to improve program efficiency and to calculate contracts with managed care and third-party payers.
5. It stimulates research into improved models of preventive care delivery.

Outcomes of cardiac rehabilitation can be classified as follows:

1. Clinical outcomes (primary and intermediate).
2. Quality-of-life outcomes.
3. Cost or economic outcomes.

Primary clinical outcomes are outcomes that can be sensed or appreciated by the patient, such as the presence of symptoms, measures of physical functioning, and recurrent cardiac events. Intermediate clinical outcomes are those that require the taking of a measurement and include factors that may modify the clinical or atherosclerotic process, such as lipid levels or blood pressure measures, but which are not of themselves symptomatic.

Quality-of-life measures are generally defined from the patient's point of view and form a major component of the patient's satisfaction with the health care process. Quality-of-life measures generally do not confer prognostic significance, although recent studies demonstrate that measures of social isolation and depression, in fact, predict an altered prognosis (2, 3).

Finally cost or economic outcomes are a crucial component of evaluating the efficacy of cardiac rehabilitation services. As economic pressures continually force health care personnel to maximize efficiency and minimize costs, the demonstration of cost-effectiveness for specific interventions will be required to maintain high quality care and availability of rehabilitative services.

CLINICAL OUTCOMES

Primary Clinical Outcomes

Primary clinical outcomes include measures of survival, recurrent cardiac events, symptomatic status, and physical functioning.

On the basis of meta-analytical data that includes patients from 21 randomized, controlled trials of cardiac rehabilitation, a reduction in cardiac and overall mortality of about 25% has been established for a 3-year follow-up period (4, 5). These studies included more than 4000 patients. It is notable that the beneficial mortality outcomes were greater in trials that used multifactorial cardiac rehabilitation versus exercise training alone (4, 5). These studies unfortunately involved principally male patients younger than 65 years of age, with less than 20% of patients being female.

Although it is beyond the scope of individual programs to provide statistically meaningful mortality data, it is important to track mortality rates both in short- and long-term rehabilitation. As programs see an influx of older patients and patients with chronic heart failure, mortality rates may be expected to increase. The occurrence of exercise-related mortality and morbidity rates should be closely observed, and in many cases this tracking will be required for hospital or program accreditation. Furthermore, the occurrence of cardiac events should trigger a review of the emergency care system of individual programs. The occurrence of non–exercise-related outpatient morbidities such as myocardial infarction, cardiac rehospitalizations, and intracoronary interventions should also be closely monitored. Several studies have documented a favorable effect of cardiac rehabilitation on requirements for subsequent cardiac rehospitalizations (6–8). Whether cardiac rehabilitation alters the rate of recurrent coronary events is less clear. Data from the above-mentioned meta-analyses of cardiac rehabilitation, performed in the 1970s and early 1980s, failed to show a decrease in recurrent myocardial infarction rates (4, 5). On the other hand, a more recent controlled trial of exercise rehabilitation from Sweden did show a significant decrease in recurrent myocardial infarction during a 5-year follow-up period (7). With the recent documentation of the value of lipid lowering (9, 10) and multifactorial rehabilitation (10) on coronary event rates and need for rehospitalizations and revascularization procedures, it is academic whether exercise alone has such effects. If cardiac rehabilitation programs could duplicate the multifactorial intervention described by Haskell et al. (10), which involves case-managed nutritional counseling (for weight loss or lipid lowering), behavioral treatment for smoking, exercise, and lipid-lowering drugs, similar reductions in total coronary event rates should be attained (Fig. 4.1).

At the intake assessment the symptomatic status of patients should be assessed such that response to the rehabilitation intervention can be determined. The presence and severity of angina and dyspnea can be categorized using the Canadian Cardiovascular Functional Classification, the New York Heart Association Functional Classification scale (11), or the Rose Questionnaire (12). The performance of an exercise tolerance test with electrocardiographic monitoring may demonstrate angina and dyspnea and provides an objective measure of exercise tolerance before training. The measurement of peak aerobic capacity, often termed $\dot{V}O_2$max, is of great value in studies of the physiologic benefits of exercise-based rehabilitation but is, in general, not required in a clinically oriented program.

Patient-described questionnaires of physical functioning and physical activity, describing the ability to perform daily activities such as climbing stairs, carrying groceries, and walking, are an important component of several QOL questionnaires (13). The supplementation of physical function questionnaires with physical performance testing, which includes an observed measure of the ability of patients to perform specific physical activities, gives the caregiver a sensitive measure of improvements in specific activities after rehabilitation. Commonly used physical performance tests, developed primarily for geriatric patients, include the Physical Performance Test (14), the Continuous Scale Physical Functional Performance Test (15), and the 6-minute walk.

Intermediate Clinical Outcomes

Intermediate clinical outcomes include measures of cardiac risk factors that are not of themselves symptomatic, but which modulate progression of the atherosclerotic process. These include measures of serum lipid levels, blood pressure, smoking status, measures of glucose tolerance and insulin resistance, body weight, body fat distribution, and exercise capacity.

At the intake evaluation, programs should systematically document baseline measures for fasting lipid profiles, serum glucose, body weight, body fat distribution (waist/hip ratio), smoking status, and a measure of fitness. These should be entered on a flow sheet with short-

FIGURE 1

CARDIAC REHABILITATION - PATIENT FLOWSHEET
PATIENT NAME:
CASE MANAGER:
INDEX EVENT:

PATIENT GOALS	SHORT TERM (6 WEEKS)	REALISTIC TERM (3 MONTHS)	GOALS LONG TERM (1 YEAR)	IDEAL FINAL GOALS
Cigarettes smoked/day				0
Total Cholesterol				<180 mg/dL
LDL — Chol				<100 mg/dL
HDL — Chol				>50 mg/dL
Triglycerides				<150 mg/dL
Body Weight				100%
Systolic Blood Pressure				<120 mm Hg
Diastolic Blood Pressure				<80 mm Hg
Fasting Glucose				<100 mg/dL
Exercise (sessions/week)				4–5
Return to Work				
ADDITIONAL GOALS				

Figure 4.1.   Patient flow sheet. (Adapted from Haskell WL Alderman EL, Fair JM, et al. Effects of intensive multiple risk factor reduction on coronary atherosclerosis and clinical cardiac events in men and women with coronary artery disease: the Stanford Coronary Risk Intervention Project (SCRIP). Circulation 1994;89:975–990.)

term and long-term goals that should be discussed with the patient and the primary physician (Fig. 4.1). Interventions to alter risk factors are developed and long-term follow-up is defined, again in coordination with the primary physician. Progress toward risk factor goals should be reassessed periodically in a systematic fashion. Authoritative guideline documents have defined goals of risk factor treatment in coronary patients (1, 16, 17).

QUALITY OF LIFE

Quality of life (QOL) is a multidimensional concept, which has gained prominence in the outcome arena as valid and reliable methods for its evaluation have become easier to quantify. Quality of life is generally measured by questionnaire with instruments that are both generic, or non–disease-specific, and those that are disease-specific. They include domains that are directly affected by the presence of disease, such as the presence of symptoms, and domains that are less directly linked to disease, such as emotional and social function. An important characteristic of QOL data is that it views life quality from the patient's point of view.

Definitions and Domains

Strictly speaking, QOL is the value assigned to duration of life as modified by impairments, functional states, perceptions, and social opportunities that are influenced by disease, injury, treatment, or policy (18). Health-related QOL is the component of life quality related to health, which the World Health Organization (WHO) defines as "a state of complete physical, mental and social well-being and not merely the absence of disease or infirmity" (19). Therefore, when measuring health-related QOL, one must include such issues as an individual's overall satisfaction with life and one's general sense of personal well-being.

There are a number of dimensions to QOL. The domains of QOL most commonly described are physical function, psychological well-being, and social function (20). Physical function includes the patient's abilities in self-care, mobility, physical activity, and communication. Self esteem, thoughts of the future, and feelings about critical life events are important components of psychological well-being. Social functioning, which includes work and social performance, material welfare, and support from and participation of family and friends, has been highly associated with economic status (21).

Quality of life, which is subjective by definition, must be evaluated by the patient, rather than by clinicians, who tend to focus on clinical conditions rather than QOL (22). The patient's perception of well-being is highly influenced by their values and beliefs, which is in turn influenced by their culture (23) and their life experiences.

Reasons for Measuring Quality of Life

When selecting an instrument for measuring QOL, objectives for the measurement must be identified to assure that the instrument selected meets predetermined needs. Most want an instrument that can measure change in patients or groups of patients with time (evaluative instrument). Also of interest is the ability to discriminate between patients or groups of patients at a given point in time (discriminative instrument). In outcome studies, preferred instruments are both evaluative and discriminative (24). The instruments described in Tables 4.1 and 4.2 are both evaluative and discriminative.

Selection of Measurement Instrument

Although in QOL trials the consensus is generally to use generic measures supplemented with disease-specific measures, in clinical cardiac rehabilitation programs time and financial constraints have dictated the need for a simple, quick, and effective measure (39). When determining which QOL instrument to use one must address whether a generic tool, a disease-specific tool, or both are needed for the patient population to be studied (Tables 4.3 and 4.4). Most generic instruments (Table 4.1) are designed for use in all illnesses and

Table 4.1.   Examples of Generic Quality-of-Life Instruments

General Quality of Life Measures
Medical Outcomes Study Short Form (SF-36) (25)
Nottingham Health Profile (26)
Sickness Impact Profile (27)
Quality of Well-Being Scale (28)
Illness Effects Questionnaire (29)
Dartmouth Primary Care Cooperative Information (30)
DUKE Health Profile (31)
Multidimensional Health Locus of Control Inventory (32)
Quality of Life Systemic Inventory (33)
Symptom Questionnaire (34)

to allow supplementation by additional measures (Table 4.2).

EXAMPLES OF CARDIAC-SPECIFIC QUALITY-OF-LIFE INSTRUMENTS

Historically, the gold standard for measuring the physical functioning domain of QOL in cardiac rehabilitation has been the New York Heart Association functional classification (11). This tool is used by the clinician to evaluate the patient's physical functioning. Though clinicians generally have the information and expertise to evaluate their patients' clinical outcome, consensus directs us to ask patients to evaluate their own QOL.

Instruments can be used alone or to supplement generic QOL measures. Disease-specific measures are of greatest interest to the patients themselves and to the clinicians who treat them. Generic measures, because they permit comparisons across conditions and populations, may be of greatest interest to the policy or decision maker. The use of both categories of measures will be most appropriate when the results could be of interest to both audiences (42). Generic measures may be of interest in clinical practice, providing clinicians with information they might not otherwise obtain.

A survey of outcome studies by individual rehabilitation programs and regional and state

outcome projects indicates the most commonly used instrument for measuring QOL is the Medical Outcome Trust SF-36 (25). In many cases, the SF-36 is used hospital-wide with computerized scoring and tracking mechanisms. Regional preferences in instrument selection exist as regional and state associations attempt to compare their outcomes.

Quality-of-Life Trials in Cardiac Rehabilitation

Although a number of studies have been published about QOL in cardiac patients (40, 43), they have focused on patients with hypertension (44, 45), chronic heart failure (36, 46), angina (47, 48), myocardial infarction (49, 50), and after coronary revascularization (51–53). Few studies have assessed the effects of cardiac rehabilitation.

An improvement in QOL has been demonstrated in patients who are referred after comprehensive cardiac rehabilitation that includes education, counseling, and exercise training after coronary artery bypass graft surgery (7, 54), after acute myocardial infarction (37, 55), and after coronary angioplasty. Lavie, Milani and associates have studied cohorts of coronary patients after cardiac rehabilitation and have shown improved QOL among the elderly (56, 57), those with diabetes (58), elderly women (59), the obese (60), and those depressed (61), as well as among general populations with coronary artery disease (62). It should be noted, however, that none of these studies included an untreated control group, and therefore a component of the measured improvement may have been the natural recovery after a coronary event.

Conclusions

The measurement of QOL provides the indispensable point of view of the patient in evaluat-

Table 4.2. Examples of Cardiac-specific Quality-of-Life Instruments

Cardiac-specific Quality-of-Life Measures

Minnesota Living with Heart Failure Questionnaire (35)
Outcomes Institute Angina type Specification (36)
Quality of Life after Myocardial Infarction (37)
Ferrans and Powers Quality of Life Index—Cardiac Version (24)
Seattle Angina Questionnaire (38)

Table 4.3. Qualities of Generic Quality-of-Life Instruments

Benefits of Generic QOL Instruments	Limitations of Generic QOL Instruments
Apply to heterogeneous population, regardless of existing conditions	Some items are not relevant to all populations
Allows cross-population comparisons (i.e., compare with other chronic diseases)	Large numbers of respondents needed to compare across populations
Address multiple issues related to limitations in health status (i.e., comorbibities, age)	Less responsive to disease-specific issues
Useful in cost-utility analysis for economic evaluation of health care service	Conceal individual variation in reaction to illness and its treatment (40)

Table 4.4.   Qualities of Disease-specific Quality-of-Life Instruments

Benefits of Disease-specific QOL Instruments	Limitations of Disease-specific QOL Instruments
Responsive to a specific population with same disease or condition	Does not allow comparison between populations with different conditions
Able to focus on relevant, problematic areas for a given population	Some items are not relevant to all within a specific population because of differences in severity, age, intervention, or comorbidity (41)
Addresses issues related to clinical manifestations of a disorder; able to measure small changes in specific conditions	The multidimensionality of QOL may not be addressed as focus is narrowed to specific areas
Allows comparison of a small cohort of respondents with same disease	

ing the value of medical interventions such as cardiac rehabilitation (63). These data complement physiologic, morbidity, and mortality outcome measures.

COST-EFFECTIVENESS ANALYSIS

Cost-effectiveness analysis measures address the cost of delivering care qualified by an outcome effect. Costs need to be distinguished from "charges," and direct costs for medical care need to be contrasted with indirect costs such as time lost from work or disability payments.

Several therapies commonly used in the treatment of coronary heart disease (CHD) have been the subject of extensive economic analysis undertaken to rank various procedures and treatment strategies according to their relative economic and social worth (Table 4.5). Cardiac rehabilitation (CR), as a stand-alone intervention in the post–myocardial infarction population, has been favorably evaluated within this relatively comprehensive volume of cost-effectiveness analysis (CEA), which has also considered major invasive and diagnostic procedures, use of acute care, drug therapies, and risk factor alteration efforts (64). Cardiac rehabilitation ranks among the most cost-effective. Only smoking cessation programs within the general CHD population and some drug therapies within specific subgroups are superior.

The objective of CEA is straightforward: to determine the cost of providing a specific quantity of health benefit to a specific patient group. The quantity of health benefit may be stated in various ways. The benefit can be stated in units of (average) incremental life expectancy when the measure results in avoidance or delay of early death.

For measures that provide benefit principally by enhancing life quality rather than life expectancy, units of (average) quality-adjusted life-years (QALYs) are used instead (termed cost-utility analysis). Measures that affect both the duration and QOL may be legitimately subjected to both analyses. Cost-effectiveness analysis is often expressed in dollars per years of life saved, which may be "quality adjusted." A cost measure may be expressed in several ways: the total value of goods and services consumed (raw cost), the price issued by the provider (charges), the actual monetary quantity exchanged (payment), or the value of the best possible alternate use of the goods and services consumed (opportunity cost).

Cost-effectiveness analysis has a useful role in several genuine clinical circumstances exemplified by the following situations:

1. Multiple self-exclusive strategies are available and are distinguishable according to cost and efficacy. The clinician must choose one strategy and reject the alternatives. A cost-effectiveness comparison can inform the decision-making process. The choice of streptokinase versus tissue plasminogen activator for acute thrombolytic reperfusion is a proper cardiovascular example.
2. A particular measure of health or safety has been found by CEA to have an extraordinarily high (low) level of economic and social worth and its use (disuse) without further consideration is to be generally promoted.
3. A specific disease state, identified with the consumption of a large and complex set of medical and social resources, is isolated for a comparative evaluation of its several components. A workable framework for such comparison is

Table 4.5.   Comparative Cost-Effectiveness Analysis for the Treatment of Coronary Heart Disease

Intervention	Patient Group	Cost-Effectiveness ($/YLS)	Cost Utility ($/QALY)	Time Period	Source
Cardiac rehabilitation					
Versus usual care	Mostly male, age 25–65 y	2,130		1985	64
		4,950		1995	
			9,200	1991	65
Smoking cessation					
Nurse counseling	Post-MI smoker, average age 58 y	220		1993	66
Physician counseling	Male smoker, age 55–59 y	728		1984	67
Nicotine patch	Male smoker, age 55–59 y		6,320	1995	68
Cholesterol-lowering drugs					
Simvastatin, 20 mg/day	Mostly male, secondary prevention	9,630		1996	69
Lovastatin, 20 mg/day	Age 55–64, baseline <250 mg/dL*	17,000		1989	70
	Age 35–44, baseline <250 mg/dL	38,000			
	Age 55–64, baseline >250 mg/dL	1,600			
	Age 35–44, baseline >250 mg/dL	0			
Antihypertension/antiangina drug therapy					
β-blocker	Post-MI, high risk of CV death	3,600		1993	71,72
	Post-MI, low risk	20,200			
Thrombolytic reperfusion					
Streptokinase	Anterior MI	12,300		1991	73
versus usual care	Inferior MI	69,500			
t-PA versus	Anterior MI, age 41–60	49,900		1993	74
streptokinase	Inferior MI, age 41–60	74,800			
		74,800			
Coronary artery bypass surgery					
Versus medical care	Left main, male, age 55	8,500		1993	72,75
	3 vessels	18,700			
	2 vessels	114,000			
	Left main, severe angina		9,200		
	3 vessels, severe angina		17,500		
	2 vessels, severe angina		42,500		
Coronary artery angioplasty					
Versus medical care	One vessel, severe angina		8,700	1993	76
	One vessel, mild angina		126,400		
Coronary artery stenting					
Versus Conventional angioplasty	Single vessel, symptomatic		23,600	1991	77
Autologous blood donation before bypass surgery					
Versus banked blood	2 units donated	305,000		1992	78
	5 units donated	588,000			

$/YLS = dollars per year of life saved; $/QALY = dollars per quality-adjusted life-year; MI = myocardial infarction; CV = cardiovascular; t-PA = tissue plasminogen activator
*250 mg/dL = 6.44 mmol/L

provided by CEA. Coronary heart disease, and CR as a component, is a notable example. The profusion of recent CEA efforts targeting CHD is consistent with the magnitude of expenditure for direct medical care (1997) for this disease: $47.5 billion per year in the United States, distributed among 13.7 million individuals with CHD, for an average of $3500 per individual (79). Direct medical expenditure includes professional services, out-patient care, hospitalization, nursing home, in-home care, drugs, and diagnostic tests. The total direct expenditure constitutes a significant fraction (~6%) of the nation's entire outlay for health care. Indirect expenditure, mostly disability and lost income, amounts to an additional $43.4 billion. Scrutiny of the pattern of allocation of the CHD budget is a rational activity for which CEA is intended to add guidance and to complement considerations of individual preferences, compassion, and availability of resources.

Cost-Effectiveness of Cardiac Rehabilitation

The cost-effectiveness of CR has been computed by using data from the meta-analysis of randomized studies of survival in the 3 years after rehabilitation in post-MI patients (64). The results are shown in Table 4.5. Monetary data, hospital and outpatient charges in this particular case, were taken from a comprehensive survey of CR providers in the United States and from a study of rehospitalization events after CR in the geographic region around Burlington, Vermont. The survival-based cost-effectiveness of CR was found to be $2100/year of life saved ($/YLS), with costs referenced to the year 1986. The figure is the computed result of a quotient in which the numerator contains the net cost of CR (the direct cost of the rehabilitation minus the total of rehospitalization costs averted as a consequence of the rehabilitation) and the denominator contains the gain in life expectancy (YLS) attributable to the rehabilitation for the average patient. The YLS value was determined by projecting 3-year survival data for rehabilitation and control groups over the nominal 15-year life expectancy of the study subjects. The primary finding was extrapolated forward in time by one decade to capture the impact of vigorous inflation of medical costs and modern survival rates during the period of time in question. The

1995 CEA value was $4900/YLS. The core data used in the development of these cost-effectiveness figures were as follows: direct 1986 cost (charges) for CR = $1280; net 1986 cost (charges) for cardiac rehabilitation = $430, 1986 YLS = 0.20 years. The corresponding figures for 1995 were $2810, $940, and 0.19 years.

In an earlier study by different investigators, cost-utility (as opposed to cost-effectiveness) was determined by direct measurement of the impact of CR on the QOL of MI survivors (65). Quality-of-life changes were gauged by a time trade-off test, and monetary value was expressed as raw costs for rehabilitation delivery in 1991 dollars. A cost-utility value of $9200/QALY was reported. In view of differing methodologies this value should not be quantitatively compared with the non-QALY-adjusted cost-effectiveness value described above, but rather, should lend further support to the finding that CEAs for CR fall well within the acceptable range for medical interventions after myocardial infarction. As a pair, these two CEAs of CR demonstrate some of the noncomparability alluded to above. It would not be correct to infer from these two results that, of the benefits available from CR, QALYs come at a higher price than YLS. The proper inference, as illustrated by the comparisons drawn in Table 4.5, is that CR is a rational measure of secondary prevention for most of the CHD population.

From the point of view of the individual program the collection of comprehensive cost-effectiveness data is impractical. To maximize cost-effectiveness, programs should focus on combining an efficient exercise intervention with a risk factor intervention program aimed at attaining specific risk factor goals (Table 4.3). Cost and charges of intervention components should be tabulated and specific cost-related outcome data, such as cardiac interventions, rehospitalizations, and incident-free event-years, should be kept.

Conclusions

The systematic collection of outcomes data in cardiac rehabilitation will provide program staff, patient participants, and referring physicians with information valuable for evaluating and perfecting the CR intervention. As CR programs evolve to become secondary prevention centers they will necessarily collect data upon which they will base therapy and follow-up. The collection of

QOL data and economic data broadens the ability of the CR program to integrate its intervention into the mainstream of therapy for CHD. In the long run, CR may have its most favorable impact on QOL in patients with CHD, and its effect on these measures warrants further attention.

References

1. Wenger NK, Froelicher ES, Smith LK, et al. Cardiac rehabilitation. Clinical practice guideline No. 17. Rockville, MD: US Department of Health and Human Services, Public Health Service, Agency for Health Care Policy and Research and the National Heart, Lung and Blood Institute. AHCPR Publication No. 96-0672, October 1995.
2. Ruberman W, Weinblatt E, Goldberg ID, et al. Psychosocial influences on mortality after myocardial infarction. N Engl J Med 1984;311:552–559.
3. Frasure-Smith N, Lesperance F, Talajic M. Depression following myocardial infarction impact on 6-month survival. JAMA 1993;270:1819–1825.
4. O'Connor GT, Buring JE, Yusuf S, et al. An overview of randomized trials of rehabilitation with exercise after myocardial infarction. Circulation 1989;80:234–244.
5. Oldridge NB, Guyatt GH, Fischer ME, et al. Cardiac rehabilitation after myocardial infarction. JAMA 1988; 260:945–950.
6. Ades PA, Huang D, Weaver SD. Cardiac rehabilitation participation predicts lower rehospitalization costs. Am Heart J 1992;123:916–921.
7. Perk J, Hedback B, Jutterdal S. Cardiac rehabilitation: evaluation of a long-term program of physical training for outpatients. Scand J Med 1989;21:13–17.
8. Bondestam E, Breikss A, Hartford M. Effects of early rehabilitation on consumption of medicare during the first year after acute myocardial infarction in patients >65 years of age. Am J Cardiol 1995:75;767–771.
9. Scandinavian Simvastatin Survival Study Group. Randomised trial of cholesterol lowering in 4444 patients with coronary heart disease: the Scandinavian Simvastatin Survival Study (4S). Lancet 1994;344:1383–1389.
10. Haskell WL, Alderman EL, Fair JM, et al. Effects of intensive multiple risk factor reduction on coronary atherosclerosis and clinical cardiac events in men and women with coronary artery disease: the Stanford Coronary Risk Intervention Project (SCRIP). Circulation 1994; 89:975–990.
11. Harvey R, Doyle E, Ellis K, et al. Major changes made by the Criteria Committee of the New York Heart Association. Circulation 1974; 49:390.
12. Rose G, McCartney P, Reid DD. Self-administration of a questionnaire on chest pain and intermittent claudication. Br J Prev Soc Med 1977;31:42–48.
13. Kriska DM, Casperson CJ, eds. A collection of physical activity questionnaires for health-related research. Med Sci Sports Exerc 1997;29:S1–S205.
14. Reuben DB, Siv AL. An objective measure of physical function of elderly outpatient. The Physical Performance Test. J Am Geriatr Soc 1992;38:1105–1111.
15. Cress ME, Buchner DM, Questad KA, et al. Continuous scale physical functional performance in broad range of older adults: a validation study. Arch Phys Med Rehabil 1996;7:1243–1250.
16. National Cholesterol Education Program Detection, Evaluation and Treatment of high blood cholesterol in adults (Adult Treatment Panel II). Bethesda, MD: National Institutes of Health (NHLBI), NIH Publication No. 93-3095, September 1993.
17. National High Blood Pressure Education Program. The Fifth Report of the Joint National Committee on Detection, Evaluation and Treatment of High Blood Pressure. Bethesda, MD: National Institutes of Health (NHLBI), NIH Publication No. 93-1088, January 1993.
18. Patrick D, Erickson P. Health status and health policy. Quality of life in health care evaluation and resource allocation. New York: Oxford University Press, 1993.
19. World Health Organization. Constitution of the World Health Organization. Basic documents. Geneva: World Health Organization, 1948.
20. Rubenstein L, Catkin D, Grundlund S, et al. Health status assessment for elderly patients. Report of the Society of General Internal Medicine Task Force on Health Assessment. J Am Geriatr Soc 1988; 37:562–569.
21. Calman K. Quality of life in cancer patients—an hypothesis. J Med Ethics 1984; 10:124–127.
22. Campbell A. Subjective measurement of well-being. Am Psychol 1976; 31:117–124.
23. Spilker B. Introduction. In: Spilker B, ed. Quality of life assessments in clinical trials. New York: Raven Press, 1990:3–9.
24. Ferrans C, Powers M. Psychometric assessment of the Quality of Life Index. Res Nurs Health 1992;15:29–38.
25. Stewart A, Hays R, Ware JJ. The MOS short-form general health survey. Reliability and validity in a patient population. Med Care 1988;26:724–735.
26. Hunt S, McEwen J, McKenna S. A quantitative approach to perceived health. J Epidemiol Community Health 1980;34:281–295.
27. Gibson B, Gibson J, Bergner M, et al. The sickness impact profile—development of an outcome measure of health care. Ann Intern Med 1975;65:1304–1310.
28. Kaplan R, Atkins C, Timms R. Validity of a quality of well-being scale as an outcome measure in chronic obstructive pulmonary disease. J Chron Dis 1984;37:85–95.
29. Greenberg G, Peterson R, Heilbronner R. Illness effects questionnaire (unpublished). Philadelphia: Psychology Department, Children's Rehabilitation Hospital, Thomas Jefferson University Hospital, 1989.
30. Wasson J, Keller A, Rubenstein L, et al. Benefits and obstacles of health status assessment in ambulatory settings. Med Care 1992;30:42–49.
31. Parkerson G, Gehlbach S, Wagner E, et al. The Duke-UNC Health Profile: an adult health status measure. Med Care 1981;10:806–828.
32. Wallston K, Wallston B. Health locus of control scales. In: Lefcourt H, ed. Research with the locus of control construct. New York: Academic Press, 1981:36–42.
33. Dupuis G, Perrault J, Lambany M, et al. A new tool to as-

sess quality of life: the Quality of Life Systemic Inventory. Qual Life Cardiovasc Care 1989;Spring:36–40.

34. Kellner R. Manual of the symptom questionnaire (unpublished). Albuquerque, NM: Dept of Psychiatry, School of Medicine, 1987.

35. Rector T, Kubo S, Cohn J. Patients' self-assessment of their congestive heart failure. Heart Failure 1987; Oct/Nov:198–209.

36. Rogers W, Johnstone D, Yusuf S, et al. Quality of life among 5025 patients with left ventricular dysfunction randomized between placebo and enalapril: the study of left ventricular dysfunction. J Am Coll Cardiol 1994;23:393–400.

37. Oldridge N, Guyatt G, Jones N, et al. Effects on quality of life with comprehensive rehabilitation after acute myocardial infarction. Am J Cardiol 1991;67:1084–1089.

38. Spertus J, Winder J, Dewhurst T, et al. Development and evaluation of the Seattle Angina Questionnaire: a new functional status measure for coronary artery disease. J Am Coll Cardiol 1995;25:333–341.

39. Spilker B. Introduction. In: Spilker B, ed. Quality of life and pharmacoeconomics in clinical trials. Philadelphia: Lippincott-Raven, 1996:9–14.

40. Mayou R, Bryant B. Quality of life in cardiovascular disease. Br Heart J 1993;69:460–466.

41. Wenger N, Naughton M, Furgerg C. Cardiovascular disorders. In: Spilker B, ed. Quality of life and pharmacoeconomics in clinical trials. Philadelphia: Lippincott-Raven, 1996:883–891.

42. Guyatt G, Jaeschke R, Feeny D, et al. Measurements in clinical trials: choosing the right approach. In: Spilker B, ed. Quality of life and pharmacoeconomics in clinical trials. Philadelphia: Lippincott-Raven, 1996:41–48.

43. Kinney M, Burfitt S, Stullenbarger E, et al. Quality of life in cardiac patient research: a meta-analysis. Nurs Res 1996;45:173–180.

44. Dahlof C. Well-being (quality of life) in connection with hypertensive treatment. Clin Cardiol 1991;14:97–103.

45. Turner R. Role of quality of life in hypertension therapy: implications for patient compliance. Cardiology 1992;80S:11–22.

46. Guyatt G. Measurement of health-related quality of life in heart failure. J Am Coll Cardiol 1993;22:185A–191A.

47. Chen A, Daley J, Thibault G. Angina patients' ratings of current health and health without angina: associations with severity of angina and comorbidity. Med Decis Making 1996;16:169–177.

48. Visser M, Fletcher A, Parr G, et al. A comparison of three quality of life instruments in subject with angina pectoris: the Sickness Impact Profile, the Nottingham Health Profile, and the Quality of Well-being Scale. J Clin Epidemiol 1994;47:157–163.

49. O'Brien B, Buxton M, Patterson D. Relationship between functional status and health-related quality of life after myocardial infarction. Med Care 1993;31:950–955.

50. Wiklund I, Herlitz J, Hjalmarson A. Quality of life five years after myocardial infarction. Eur Heart J 1989; 10:464–472.

51. Krumholz H, McHorney C, Clark L, et al. Changes in health after elective percutaneous coronary revascu-

larization. A comparison of generic and specific measures. Med Care 1996;34:754–759.

52. McKenna K, McEniery P, Mass F, et al. Clinical results and quality of life after percutaneous transluminal coronary angioplasty: a preliminary report. Cathet Cardiovasc Diagn 1992;27:89–94.

53. Bliley A, Ferrans C. Quality of life after coronary angioplasty. Heart Lung 1993;22:193–199.

54. Engblom E, Korpilahti K, Hamalainen H, et al. Quality of life and return to work 5 years after coronary artery bypass surgery. Long-term results of cardiac rehabilitation. J Cardpulm Rehabil 1997;17:29–36.

55. Conn V, Taylor S, Casey B. Cardiac rehabilitation program participation and outcomes after myocardial infarction. Rehabil Nurs 1992;17:58–62.

56. Lavie C, Milani R. Effects of cardiac rehabilitation programs on exercise capacity, coronary risk factors, behavioral characteristics, and quality of life in a large elderly cohort. Am J Cardiol 1995;76:117–179.

57. Lavie C, Milani R. Effects of cardiac rehabilitation and exercise training programs in patients > or = 75 years of age. Am J Cardiol 1996;78:675–677.

58. Milani R, Lavie C. Behavioral differences and effects of cardiac rehabilitation in diabetic patients following cardiac rehabilitation. Am J Med 1996;100:517–523.

59. Lavie C, Milani C. Benefits of cardiac rehabilitation and exercise training in elderly women. Am J Cardiol 1997;79:664–666.

60. Lavie C, Milani R. Effects of cardiac rehabilitation, exercise training, and weight reduction on exercise capacity, coronary risk factors, behavioral characteristics, and quality of life in obese coronary patients. Am J Cardiol 1997;79:397–401.

61. Milani R, Lavie C, Cassidy M. Effects of cardiac rehabilitation and exercise training programs on depression in patients after major coronary events. Am Heart J 1996;132:726–732.

62. Maines T, Lavie C, Milani R, et al. Effects of cardiac rehabilitation and exercise programs on exercise capacity, coronary risk factors, behavior, and quality of life in patients with coronary artery disease. South Med J 1997;90:43–49.

63. Fries J, Singh G. The hierarchy of patient outcomes. In: Spilker B, ed. Quality of life and pharmacoeconomics in clinical trails. Philadelphia: Lippincott-Raven, 1996:33–40.

64. Ades PA, Pashkow FJ, Nestor JR. Cost-effectiveness of cardiac rehabilitation after myocardial infarction. J Cardpulm Rehab 1997;17:222–231.

65. Oldridge N, Furlong W, Feeny D, et al. Economic evaluation of cardiac rehabilitation soon after myocardial infarction. Am J Cardiol 1993;72:154–161.

66. Krumholz HM, Cohen BJ, Tsevat J, et al. Cost-effectiveness of a smoking cessation program after myocardial infarction. J Am Coll Cardiol 1993;22:1697–1672.

67. Cummings SR, Rubin SM, Oster G. The cost-effectiveness of counseling smokers to quit. JAMA 1989; 261:75–79.

68. Fiscella K, Franks P. Cost-effectiveness of the transdermal nicotine patch as an adjunct to physicians' smoking cessation counseling. JAMA 1996;275:1247–1251.

69. Kinosian B, Glick H, Schwartz JS. Scandinavian simvastatin survival study (4S): cost-effectiveness (CE) of cholesterol lowering treatment [abstract]. J Am Coll Cardiol 1996;27(Suppl A):165A.

70. Goldman L, Weinstein MC, Goldman PA, et al. Cost effectiveness of HMG-CoA reductase inhibition for primary and secondary prevention of coronary heart disease. JAMA 1991;265:1145–1151.

71. Goldman L, Sia B, Cook EF, et al. Costs and effectiveness of routine therapy with long-term beta-adrenergic antagonists after acute myocardial infarction. N Engl J Med 1988;319:152–157.

72. Kupersmith J, Holmes-Rovner M, Hogan A, et al. Cost effectiveness analysis in heart disease. Prog Cardiovasc Dis 1995;37:243–271 (Pt 2) and 307–346 (Pt 3).

73. Midgette AD, Wong JB, Beshansky JR, et al. Cost-effectiveness of streptokinase for acute myocardial infarction. Med Decis Making 1994;14:108–17.

74. Mark DB, Hlatky MA, Califf RM, et al. Cost effectiveness of thrombolytic therapy with tissue plasminogen activator as compared with streptokinase for acute myocardial infarction. N Engl J Med 1995;332:1418–1424.

75. Weinstein MC, Stason WB. Cost-effectiveness of coronary artery bypass surgery. Circulation 1982;66(Suppl 3):56–66.

76. Wong JB, Sonnenberg FA, Salem DN, et al. Myocardial revascularization for chronic stable angina. Ann Intern Med 1990;113:852–871.

77. Cohen DJ, Breall JA, Kalon KL, et al. Evaluating the potential cost-effectiveness of stenting as a treatment for symptomatic single vessel coronary disease. Circulation 1994;89:1859–1874.

78. Birkmeyer JD, AuBuchon JP, Littenberg B, et al. Cost-effectiveness of preoperative autologous donation in coronary bypass grafting. Ann Thorac Surg 1994;57:161–169.

79. American Heart Association. Heart and stroke facts: 1997 statistical supplement. Dallas, TX.

SECTION II.

Functional Assessment and Prescription of Exercise

Exercise Electrocardiographic Testing

Fredric J. Pashkow, Sharon A. Harvey, and Victor Froelicher
with a section on heart rate by Michael S. Lauer

HISTORICAL OVERVIEW OF EXERCISE ELECTROCARDIOGRAPHIC TESTING

Probably the earliest experience in exercise testing was described by Feil and Siegel (1) in 1928. During electrocardiographic (ECG) monitoring, they had patients perform sit-ups with the goal of reproducing anginal symptoms. Intensity of work was increased by applying resistance to the patient's chest. During this process, they noticed an association between anginal symptoms and changes in the ST segment and T waves. Therefore, they hypothesized that the ECG changes were indicative of reduced blood flow to the heart. Master and Oppenheimer (2) published a paper in 1929 describing the use of exercise hemodynamics (heart rate and blood pressure) in evaluating cardiac capacity. Still, the value of the ECG in identifying ischemia had not yet been recognized. In 1941, Master and Jaffe (3) suggested that an ECG should be taken before and after the Master's step test to detect ECG changes during exercise. Eleven years later, Yu and Soffer (4) delineated criteria still commonly used today to define an ischemic ECG response to exercise: 1) ST-segment depression of more than 1.0 mm; 2) T wave inversion and pseudonormalization of T waves; and 3) increased amplitude of T waves during exercise. However, exercise ECG testing in its current format is probably attributable to Bruce (5). In 1956, he performed exercise tests on a motorized treadmill and established a nomogram for functional capacity. Subsequent research in the area of exercise testing has focused on identification of more accurate diagnostic criteria and development of objective interpretation algorithms for

exercise test data to maximize sensitivity, specificity, and predictive accuracy for coronary artery disease (CAD). Despite the promise of newer technologies, exercise testing continues to hold its own as a diagnostic procedure and actually has grown in its diverse applications (6). Although not the most sensitive noninvasive test for the diagnosis of CAD (7), exercise testing's reliability and cost-effectiveness for monitoring the progression of disease and the determination of therapeutic efficacy are not surpassed by other diagnostic means (8, 9).

The indications for exercise testing have been expanding (10, 11). Although exercise testing cannot reliably predict the location of angiographic findings (12), numerous studies have shown that the response to the exercise test permits prediction of the severity of underlying CAD and the patient's prognosis (11–14).

Exercise testing is extremely useful as a test of functional capacity in those persons with established heart disease. Data now suggest that certain parameters measurable by the exercise test provide reliable expectation for outcome after acute coronary events (12, 15–21). Because survival can be improved only in specific clinical subsets of patients, it is important to select carefully for catheterization and subsequent revascularization only those patients in whom intervention can improve quality and extent of life (22–26).

In asymptomatic persons who have fewer than two risk factors, it appears that the use of exercise tests in screening for CAD is potentially more misleading than previously thought because of the relatively high rate of false-positive results (11, 27–31). However, exercise testing for this population may be useful in evaluating the safety of exercise program participation and formulating an exercise prescription (32).

During the mid to late 1980s, the volume of exercise tests being performed in the United States was on the increase (33). The Health Care Financing Administration reported a 22% increase in the number of exercise tests interpreted and reported between 1986 and 1988. This represented an annual estimated increased cost of about $30 million. Given the popularity of this noninvasive diagnostic test and its role as a "gatekeeper" to more expensive noninvasive and invasive procedures, continued improvement in identification of its appropriate indications for performance can have a huge impact on health care (34).

CARDIOVASCULAR RESPONSE TO EXERCISE

Exercise is the most common human physiologic stress and provides the most practical available means to test cardiac perfusion and function. Dynamic (isotonic) exercise puts a volume load on the heart and is preferred for testing because it can be applied and modulated gradually. Pure isometric exercise is contraction without movement (such as a handgrip), and because of the diversity in size of peripheral muscle groups, isometric stress can impose a disproportionate left ventricular (LV) pressure load. Most physical activities involve both isometric and isotonic exercise in varying degrees.

Oxygen is required for cells to metabolize nutrients. That which is taken up by heart muscle is referred to as myocardial oxygen uptake and by the body (collectively) is referred to as ventilatory or total body oxygen uptake. At the beginning of exercise, there is a temporary lag in oxygen uptake. During this time, anaerobic metabolism fuels immediate energy needs and an oxygen deficit is incurred. Assuming a gradually increasing exercise intensity, oxygen uptake should then plateau, achieving a steady state in 2 to 3 minutes at each given submaximal exercise level. During steady state, heart rate (HR), cardiac output (CO), blood pressure (BP), and pulmonary ventilation maintain constant levels. The point at which increasing work intensity fails to elicit an increase in these variables is called the maximal oxygen uptake ($\dot{V}O_2$max). When strenuous exercise is terminated, recovery to normal resting values is not immediate. This period of recovery oxygen uptake, or oxygen debt, supports the metabolic processes required to return the body and its functions to a resting state and "repay" the oxygen deficit.

Maximal Ventilatory Oxygen Uptake ($\dot{V}O_2$max)

Maximal ventilatory oxygen uptake is the greatest amount of oxygen that a person can extract from inspired air when performing dynamic exercise that involves a large part of the peripheral muscle mass. It is conventional to measure oxygen consumption in multiples of basal resting requirements. The "MET" is a unit of basal oxygen consumption, or approximately 3.5 mL $O_2 \cdot kg^{-1} \cdot min^{-1}$. This value represents the amount of oxygen required to maintain life in the basal resting state.

Maximal ventilatory oxygen uptake is related to age, sex, predisposing genetic factors, health status, and exercise proclivity. Values of $\dot{V}O_2$max peak between 15 and 20 years of age and decline linearly thereafter. In moderately active young men, $\dot{V}O_2$max is about 12 METs, whereas persons who perform aerobic training, such as distance running, can have $\dot{V}O_2$max as high as 18 to 25 METs. By age 60, mean $\dot{V}O_2$max in men is about two-thirds that at the age of 20. With sustained bed rest, there is a 25% decrease in $\dot{V}O_2$max in normal men during a 3-week period.

Maximal $\dot{V}O_2$ is equal to maximal CO times the maximal arteriovenous oxygen (a–v O_2) difference. Because CO is equal to the product of stroke volume and HR, $\dot{V}O_2$ is directly related to HR. The maximal a–v O_2 difference during exercise has a physiologic limit of 15 to 17 vol%; hence, if a maximal effort is given, $\dot{V}O_2$max can be used to estimate maximal CO.

Myocardial Oxygen Consumption

Myocardial oxygen consumption ($M\dot{V}O_2$) is determined by intramyocardial wall tension (LV pressure × end-diastolic volume / LV wall thickness), contractility, and HR. Other less important factors include the external work performed by the heart, as well as the energy necessary for electrical activation, and basal metabolism of the myocardium.

Accurate measurement of $M\dot{V}O_2$ requires cardiac catheterization. Noninvasively, $M\dot{V}O_2$ can be measured by positron emission tomography or roughly estimated by calculating the product of HR and systolic blood pressure (SBP). This has been called the double product, or rate-pressure product (RPP). There is a linear relationship between $M\dot{V}O_2$ and coronary blood flow. During exercise, coronary blood flow increases up to five times the normal resting value. A patient who has obstructive CAD cannot increase coronary blood flow enough to supply the metabolic demands of the myocardium during exercise. As a consequence, myocardial ischemia occurs. Angina and ischemic ST changes usually occur at the same RPP rather than at the same workload.

An important basic principle of exercise physiology is that $\dot{V}O_2$ and $M\dot{V}O_2$ are distinct in their determinants and in the way that they are measured or estimated. Although directly related to each other, this relationship can be altered, for example, by exercise training or β-blockers.

Peripheral Responses to Dynamic Exercise

The response to dynamic exercise consists of a complex series of cardiovascular adjustments that ensure that active muscles receive a blood supply appropriate to their metabolic needs, dissipate the heat generated, and maintain the blood supply to the brain and heart. Because a delivered workload can be calibrated accurately and the physiologic response can be measured easily, dynamic exercise is appropriate for clinical exercise testing.

As CO increases with dynamic exercise, an increase in systemic arterial pressure occurs. Peripheral vascular resistance increases in the tissues that are not functioning in the performance of the ongoing exercise and decreases in active muscles. The net result is a decrease in overall systemic vascular resistance, because although pressure may increase by 25% to 50%, flow can increase by as much as five times during dynamic exercise. Because the denominator (flow) increases much more than the numerator (pressure) in the formula for resistance, the result is a decrease in systemic vascular resistance.

HEART RATE RESPONSE

An increase in HR is the first measurable response of the cardiovascular system to exercise: the sympathetic outflow to the heart and systemic blood vessels is increased, and the vagal outflow to the heart decreases. The increase in HR is the major mechanism to increase CO.

Heart rate accounts for about 60% to 70%, whereas alteration of preload and afterload (stroke volume) accounts for about 30% to 40% of each liter per minute pumped. Heart rate during exercise increases linearly with workload and ventilatory oxygen uptake. During low levels of exercise and at a constant work rate, HR will rise and reach a plateau or steady state within several minutes. At higher workloads, it takes progressively longer to reach a steady state HR.

Mean maximal HR declines as age increases (35). This inverse relationship in age appears to be caused by intrinsic cardiac changes rather than by neural influences. Individuals with good cardiovascular fitness tend to show less rapid declines in maximal HR with age.

Heart rate also is influenced by the type of muscular activity. Dynamic exercise increases HR more so than isometric exercise. Lack of gravitational forces on baroreceptor mechanisms may play a role in the accentuated HR response observed after bed rest. Other factors that influence HR include body position, physical conditions, state of health, blood volume, and environment. Even in normal subjects, a wide array of regression lines have been reported.

The HR response to maximal dynamic exercise depends on numerous factors, but particularly on age and health. Although a regression line of (220 − age) for age-predicted maximal heart rate (APMHR) is fairly reproducible, the scatter around this line is considerable. Such predictions are maximal for some persons and submaximal for others. Therefore, its clinical application is of questionable value.

BLOOD PRESSURE RESPONSE

Systolic blood pressure rises with increasing dynamic work as a result of increasing CO. At each level of work, a more consistent increase in SBP occurs during the first few minutes, and then a steady state is attained. Systolic blood pressure generally correlates with the maximal exercise level achieved. In women, the values are variable and do not relate as well as the level of effort.

An inadequate SBP rise can be caused by aortic outflow obstruction, LV dysfunction, or ischemia. Because it also depends on peripheral resistance, changes of BP reflect more than just the contractile function of the left ventricle. Patients who experience hypotension during exercise frequently have serious heart disease.

After performing maximal exercise, a normal decline occurs in SBP, reaching basal levels usually in 6 minutes, and then often remaining lower than preexercise levels for several hours. In some patients, higher levels of SBP in recovery phase have been observed, exceeding the peak exercise values. Ratios of this rebound phenomenon have been proposed to diagnose CAD. Some normal subjects will have precipitous drops in SBP when exercise is stopped abruptly. This is caused by venous pooling.

During exercise the arteries in active muscles dilate immediately because of the sudden increase in metabolites. Peripheral vascular resistance increases in the tissues that do not participate in the performance of the exercise. The net result is a decrease in overall systemic vascular resistance. Although SBP increases simultaneously, diastolic blood pressure (DBP) usually remains about the same. A rising DBP may be a marker for labile hypertension.

METHODS AND INSTRUMENTATION

Essential or desirable instrumentation features are summarized in Table 5.1.

ECG Monitoring Systems

The revolution that has occurred throughout medicine related to miniaturization of electronics and the use of large-scale, integrated microprocessors has had a significant impact on instrumentation and the technique of exercise electro-

Table 5.1.   Exercise Electrocardiography Instrumentation

Essential
  Display and record more than one channel
  Programmable 12 lead sets
  Full-range frequency response (0.01 Hz to 100 Hz)
Desirable
  ECG display preexercise and current exercise
  Selectable dynamic noise reduction (filter)
  Computer compatibility
  Digital signal conversion
  Digital storage of test data
  Software for data analysis
  Nonproprietary platform using standard database
    package
  Ability to export data to standard software database
    or spreadsheet formats

cardiographic testing. The influence of computerization on the quality of the tracings and the utility of computer-averaged signals currently is being debated. The conversion from analog to digital recording systems has allowed the integration of multiple leads and simultaneous multiple-channel recordings, with an enormous effect on the convenience and simplification of the performance of the technical procedure. As the emphasis on flexibility of data analysis and maintenance of databases continues to increase, ECG stress systems are being developed for use in a personal computer environment.

Electrodes and Cables

Many electrodes are available for performing exercise testing. Silver plate or silver chloride crystal pellets are the best electrode materials with the lowest offset voltage. Electrodes should be constructed with a metal interface that is sunken to create a column to be filled with either an electrolyte solution or a saturated sponge. These fluid column electrodes avoid direct metal-to-skin contact, decreasing motion artifact. Electrodes for exercise testing should be made of a material that easily conforms to the chest and offers greater adhesive quality so that they adhere to the patient despite movement and excessive perspiration.

Connecting cables between the electrodes and recorder should be light, flexible, and properly shielded. Most commercial exercise cables available are constructed to lessen motion artifact. In general, cables have a life span of 1 year or so, depending on use. Eventually, they become a source of noise and electrical discontinuity and must be replaced.

Testing Modalities

Numerous devices have been used to provide the dynamic exercise for exercise testing, including treadmills, cycle ergometers, fixed steps, and ladder mills. Today, the cycle ergometer (36) and treadmill are the most commonly used dynamic exercise devices. The former is more popular in Europe, probably because of its more modest cost, whereas the latter is clearly more popular in the United States.

Mechanical cycles must maintain a constant number of revolutions per minute (rpm), but in electrically braked cycles, this number can range from 40 to 70 rpm without a significant effect on delivered watts. This allows for better workload control as uncooperative or fatigued patients will tend to decrease pedaling speed. The highest values of $\dot{V}O_2$ and HR are obtained when pedaling speeds of 70 rpm are used. Mechanical or electrically braked cycles are calibrated in kiloponds (kp) or watts. One watt is equivalent to 6 $kp \cdot m \cdot min^{-1}$. Because cycle exercise is nonweightbearing, kiloponds or watts equate directly to calories, which correlate directly to liters of oxygen per minute. METs (in milliliters of O_2 per kilogram per minute) are obtained by dividing the oxygen consumption by the body weight (in kilograms) of the patient tested. The cycle ergometer allows the application of uniform power increments graduated on the basis of a patient's body mass. It is easier to obtain BP readings and ECG tracings free of motion artifact with the subject seated and with upper extremities stabilized by the handlebars.

Cycle ergometry is indicated for patients who are unsteady when walking or who are otherwise incapable of exercising on the treadmill. If cycle ergometry is the chosen modality, care must be taken to ensure that isometric exercise is not performed inadvertently by the arms. Patients who are not accustomed to bicycle exercise may be limited by local muscular fatigue before achieving $\dot{V}O_2$max. As maximal aerobic capacity usually is lower when measured by cycle technique, the treadmill is more sensitive for diagnosis (32, 37, 38). Treadmills used for exercise testing should have front and side rails for the patients to steady themselves. Treadmill testing will be discussed in more detail later in the chapter.

Blood Pressure Monitoring Equipment

A standard sphygmomanometer and stethoscope should be used. Although the desire to attempt automated BP monitoring is understandable, this technology requires further validation during exercise before its use can be recommended for exercise testing.

TECHNICAL CONSIDERATIONS FOR OPTIMAL ECG MEASUREMENT

Skin Preparation

The most critical point of the electrode-amplifier recording system is the interface between electrode and skin. Removal of the superficial layer of skin significantly lowers its resistance, decreasing the noise-to-signal ratio. The areas for electrode application are first rubbed with an alcohol-saturated gauze. After the skin dries the electrode sites are rubbed with fine sandpaper or rough material. With these procedures, skin resistance should be reduced to 5000 Ω or less.

Lead Systems

Bipolar lead systems were the first to be used to detect ECG changes during exercise. The relatively short time for placement, freedom from motion artifact, and the ease with which noise problems can be located are the factors that favor their use. The usual positive reference is an electrode placed the same as the positive reference for V_5 (the 5th intercostal space [ICS] at the midclavicular line). The negative reference for V_5 is Wilson's central terminal, which consists of connecting the limb electrodes—right arm (RA), left arm (LA), and left leg (LL). The bipolar lead CM_5 is the most sensitive for ST-segment changes, whereas CC_5 excludes the vertical component included in CM_5 and decreases the influence of the atrial repolarization (Ta), thereby reducing false-positive responses. Electrode placement affects ST-segment slope and amplitude. The various placements do not result in comparable waveforms for analysis.

Because a standard 12-lead ECG with electrodes placed on the limbs cannot be obtained during exercise, other electrode placements have been used. Figure 5.1 illustrates modified limb lead placement for exercise testing. The interpretation of a 12-lead ECG obtained by these recommended exercise electrode sites (39) differs substantially from that of a 12-lead ECG obtained using the standard lead positions (40). Care therefore must be taken to interpret correctly the baseline tracing and not substitute it for the standard diagnostic ECG. The exercise electrode sites cause the QRS vectors to appear to be directed inferiorly, posteriorly, and rightward, producing a marked rightward mean frontal axis shift of $+48°$. Therefore false lateral and apical infarcts can be seen, whereas inferior, posterior, and apical infarcts can disappear falsely on the preexercise tracings (Fig. 5.2). False-positive or false-negative anterior infarctions are not a problem (40).

It is recommended that a lead from each lead group be monitored during the test: a lateral lead such as V_5, an inferior lead such as II, and an

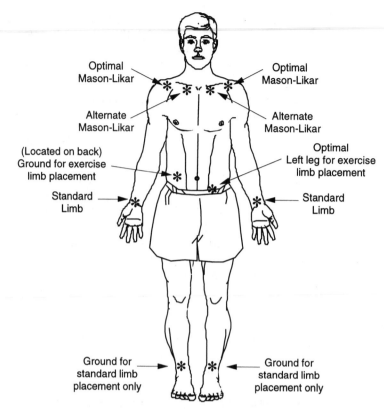

Figure 5.1.   Illustration of exercise electrode placement. Optimal Mason-Likar placement near the acromioclavicular joint may produce motion artifact, so the location marked "Alternate Mason-Likar" is commonly used. The optimal left leg for exercise limb placement is located inferior to the umbilicus (Modified from Froelicher VF, Perdue ST, Atwood JE, et al. Exercise testing of patients recovering from myocardial infarction. Curr Prob Cardiol 1986;11:369–444).

anterior lead such as V_2. This approach allows real-time monitoring for ischemic changes in each of the major lead groups. It is also helpful for the detection and identification of dysrhythmias. A 12-lead ECG should be recorded at the end of each stage of exercise for a more global view of ischemic ST changes. This is particularly important as abnormalities may be absent or considered border-line in V_5 but are clearly present in V_4, V_6, or other precordial leads.

Relative Sensitivity of Leads

The precordial leads are capable of detecting 90% of all ST depression observed in multiple-lead systems. Provided the baseline ECG does not contain Q waves, the most reliable and valid lead for analysis during exercise is V_5, or a similarly configured bipolar lead. Other reports relate that using other leads in addition to V_5 increases the yield of abnormal response by about 10% to 25%; however, the specificity of an abnormal response

in other leads is lower. Isolated inferior ST depression with a normal resting ECG is often a false-positive finding and, therefore, is not predictive of CAD (41).

However, in subsets of patients with a high prevalence of previous myocardial infarction (MI) or symptoms that suggest coronary artery spasm, a more complete lead system is preferable. ST depression in multiple leads (five or more) usually predicts multivessel disease whereas assessment of ischemia caused by spasm can usually be adequately performed using a three-lead system (i.e., V_1, II, and V_5). In asymptomatic persons or those with nonspecific chest pain and a normal resting ECG, recording a single lead such as CC5 is adequate.

Computer Averaging of the ECG Signal

Computer averaging of the ECG signal has been shown to distort information and to increase the incidence of false-positive studies (42).

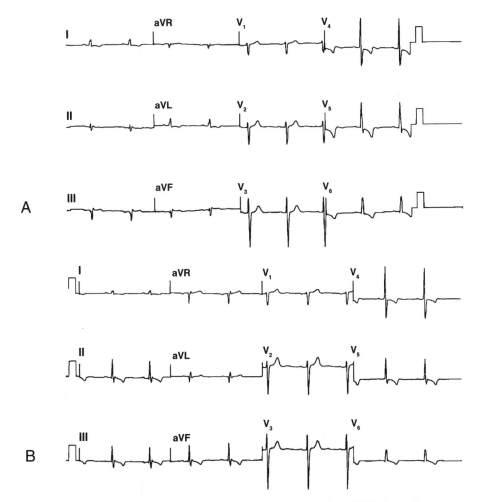

Figure 5.2.   A. An ECG obtained using standard limb lead placement. B. An ECG obtained on the same patient using the Mason-Likar torso-mounted limb lead placement. Note the loss of inferior Q waves in leads III and aVF and appearance of a false Q wave in aVL and false T wave inversion in the inferior leads.

Most clinicians are not aware that the sequential beats displayed are multiple impressions of a single averaged beat, and that these averaged beats may be influenced unduly by signal noise, respiration, and ectopic beats. Often, computer averaging is used to improve the interpretability of poor-quality ECG tracings; however, if significant baseline wander or excessive signal noise is present, the result is a "garbage in, garbage out" phenomenon. The numerical averages also can be misleading. Tall T waves, for instance, can cause doubling of the calculated HR. If computer-averaged data are to be used, they should always be compared with the raw ECG data before interpretation.

INDICATIONS FOR EXERCISE TESTING

In the context of cardiac rehabilitation, exercise testing has three major applications: 1) as a means to assess the extent of myocardial ischemia; 2) as a test of functional capacity in those patients who have established disease; and 3) as a tool for risk stratification. The clinical indications for exercise testing are summarized in Table 5.2.

Evaluation of symptoms, however, remains the most common indication for diagnostic exercise electrocardiography. The history of chest pain alone significantly contributes to pretest

Table 5.2.   Clinical Indications for Exercise Electrocardiography Testing

Evaluation of symptoms
Progression and severity of disease
    Preevent—extent of disease
    Postevent—risk stratification for myocardial infarction, sudden death, or need for revascularization
Selection and evaluation of most effective therapy
Progression of disease
Screening for latent coronary artery disease
Evaluation of dysrhythmias
Evaluation of functional capacity
    Exercise prescription
    Disability evaluation
Evaluation of pacemaker or internal defibrillator function

Table 5.3.   ACC/AHA Guidelines—Indications for Exercise Electrocardiography

Class I—General agreement that the test is justified
Adults with intermediate probability of CAD
Risk/prognostic assessment of patients with symptoms or known CAD
Patients with suspected or known CAD with significant change in clinical status
After AMI for prognostic assessment, activity guidelines, and evaluation of medical therapy as follows: 1) predischarge after AMI (4–7 days); 2) early after discharge after AMI if a predischarge test was not performed (14–21 days); or 3) late after discharge for AMI if the early exercise test was submaximal
Demonstration of ischemia before revascularization
Evaluation of recurrent symptoms after revascularization
Establishing appropriate parameters for rate-responsive pacemakers

Class IIa—Divergence of opinion as to test value; opinion is in favor of test
Patients with vasospastic angina
After discharge for activity recommendation as part of cardiac rehabilitation in patients who have been revascularized
Patients with known or suspected exercise-induced arrhythmias
Evaluation of interventions in patients with exercise-induced arrhythmias

Class IIb—Divergence of opinion as to test's value; efficacy of test is less well supported by opinion
Patients with high and low pretest probability
Diagnosis of CAD with <1.0-mm resting ST depression on digoxin or with LVH
Risk/prognostic assessment in patients with symptoms, known CAD, or after MI who have abnormal resting ECGs, to include preexcitation (WPW), paced rhythms, >1.0-mm resting ST depression, complete left bundle branch block
Patients requiring occasional monitoring to guide treatment
Predischarge localization of ischemia in area of borderline lesions after angiography
Periodic monitoring of patients enrolled in cardiac rehabilitation or exercise programs
Evaluation of patients with multiple risk factors
Evaluation of asymptomatic men >40 y and women >50 y who 1) want to start an exercise program, and 2) are at high risk for CAD because of other diseases
Evaluation of functional capacity in patients with valve disease
Monitoring or detecting restenosis, graft occlusion, or disease progression in high-risk, asymptomatic patients
Evaluation of isolated ventricular ectopic beats in patients without other evidence of CAD

continued

stratification (32). A man older than 40 years with nonspecific chest pain, atypical of ischemia, has a 10% likelihood of showing significant obstructive disease by angiogram. With a classic history of angina, pretest likelihood is an impressive 85% (43). An abnormal exercise test by ECG criteria increases the posttest risk by only 6% to 20%. In a person who has typical angina, an abnormal exercise test adds little to the diagnosis (44). The test is of much greater value in patients with intermediate pretest likelihood. Although controversial, exercise tests also may be justified in asymptomatic persons who have at least one major clinical risk factor (31). In those persons with known CAD, the exercise ECG can add substantially to the estimation of prognosis (45). (This is discussed in more detail in the section on sensitivity and specificity.)

An American College of Cardiology/American Heart Association Task Force on Practice Guidelines (Committee on Exercise Testing) has published guidelines for exercise testing (46). In this schema, class I studies are those in which it is generally agreed that the test is justified. Class II studies are those in which there may be a divergence of opinion about the test's value. Class III studies are those in which there is general agreement that the test is of little or no value, inappropriate, or contraindicated by risk. These classifications are summarized in Table 5.3. The significant implication for these criteria is related mainly to reimbursement for testing.

Some of the criteria are controversial clinically and, in some cases, are misunderstood. For example, we have found the exercise study to be safe and

Table 5.3.   ACC/AHA Guidelines—Indications for Exercise Electrocardiography

Class III—General agreement that the test is not useful and may be harmful

Diagnosis of CAD in patients with abnormal resting ECGs

Presence of comorbidity that may limit life expectancy or alter decision to treat CAD

Routine screening of asymptomatic men and women

Diagnosis of CAD in patients with valve disease

Localization of ischemia for determining site of revascularization

Routine monitoring of patient after revascularization without other indications

ACC/AHA, American College of Cardiology/American Heart Association; AMI, acute myocardial infarction; CAD, coronary artery disease; LVH, left ventricular hypertrophy; MI, myocardial infarction; WPW, Wolff-Parkinson-White syndrome.

of potential value in selected patients with Wolff-Parkinson-White (WPW) syndrome for the "unmasking" of accessory pathways and for follow-up of therapy designed to obliterate these preexcitation pathways. The loss of the delta wave during exercise implies a better prognosis than in those patients whose QRS complexes remain wide.

The class IIb designation of assessments of functional capacity in the setting of a cardiac rehabilitation program refers to the use of formal, serial testing at the program site and is not for initial functional assessment (class I indication). A formal study at the time of "exit" from a cardiac rehabilitation program is worthwhile to assess exercise outcomes.

Reasonable approaches to exercise screening for CAD have been described (27, 28). Refinements in Bayesian methods have led to reports of improved diagnostic ability (30). Although recent reports have suggested that screening exercise tests may be justified in patients who have a total cholesterol:HDL cholesterol ratio of 6.0 or greater (31), others report such a small predictive value for an abnormal test in hypercholesterolemic patients that the effort may not be worthwhile (47).

CONTRAINDICATIONS TO EXERCISE TESTING

Good clinical judgment should be foremost in deciding the contraindications to exercise testing. Whereas absolute contraindications are definitive, in selected cases with relative contraindications, testing can provide valuable information even when performed submaximally.

For instance, persons may undergo testing for evaluation of therapeutic devices or procedures, in which former contraindications may be set aside. An example would be the need to exercise a patient with complex ventricular ectopy at rest and a new implantable cardioverter defibrillator. The need to ensure appropriate device function in a supervised and monitored setting outweighs the risk of provoking a sustained arrhythmia. Table 5.4 lists current absolute and relative contraindications to performing an exercise test.

Safety Issues

In selected patient populations, the American College of Physicians/American College of Cardiology/American Heart Association Task Force on Clinical Privileges in Cardiology stated that exercise testing can be safely supervised by well-trained personnel such as nurses, exercise physiologists, physical therapists, or medical technicians (48) . These individuals must have a good working knowledge of exercise physiology and emergency medical procedures. The testing laboratory must be supervised by a physician who is

Table 5.4.   Contraindication to Exercise Testing

Absolute contraindications

Acute MI (within 2 days)

Acute myocarditis or pericarditis

Pulmonary edema, embolus, or infarction

Severe or symptomatic aortic stenosis

Dissecting aneurysm

Hemodynamically unstable arrhythmias

Uncontrolled or symptomatic heart failure

Unstable angina

Relative contraindications (risks vs. benefits should be considered before proceeding with test)

Recent change in resting ECG suggestive of cardiac event

Left main coronary artery obstruction

Hypertrophic cardiomyopathy with rest gradient

High degree AV block

Moderate stenotic valvular disease

Electrolyte abnormalities

Severe resting hypertension (>200 mm Hg systolic or >110 mm Hg diastolic)

Tachyarrhythmias or bradyarrhythmias

Mental or physical impairment resulting in inability to exercise

Uncontrolled metabolic disease

Advanced or complicated pregnancy

Disorders that are exacerbated by exercise

AV, atrioventricular; MI, myocardial infarction.

in the immediate vicinity and able to respond instantly for emergencies and other medical needs. It is prudent that the resting ECG and a patient case history be discussed with the physician before beginning exercise. Technicians and physicians familiar with both normal and abnormal responses during exercise are best able to recognize or prevent untoward events. Safety precautions indicated by the American Heart Association (AHA) are explicit with regard to exercise testing (49). Everything necessary for cardiopulmonary resuscitation must be readily available.

Although exercise testing is considered a safe procedure, reports exist of acute infarctions and deaths occurring secondary to maximal exercise (50). Multiple surveys have confirmed that up to 10 deaths or MIs can be expected per 10,000 tests. The relative risk of an adverse event during an exercise test compared with usual activity in patients who have CAD is estimated to be 60 to 100 times normal.

EXERCISE TEST PROCEDURE

Explanation of Test and Informed Consent

In any procedure with a risk of complication, it is advisable to make certain that the patient understands the situation and acknowledges the risks. Some physicians believe that informing patients of such risks makes them overly anxious or discourages them from having the test performed. Because of this and the fact that the signed consent form does not protect a physician from legal action, there has been less insistence recently on consent forms. A physician may be held responsible, however, in the event of a major untoward effect if consent is not obtained first. The argument can be made that the patient would not have undergone the procedure had he or she been made aware of the risks associated with the test. A careful explanation of the testing protocol, its risks, and possible complications should be given, and although this often is delegated to the technician or specialist who performs the pretest preparation, legal authorities recommend that informed consent be obtained by the supervising physician (see chapter 25). The patient must be instructed carefully on how to mount and walk on the treadmill and should

be made familiar with the laboratory routine and safety procedures.

Patient Preparation

Preparations for exercise testing include the following: The patient should be instructed not to eat, consume caffeine, or smoke for 3 to 4 hours before the test and should come dressed for exercise. No unusual physical efforts should be performed 12 hours before testing.

A brief history and physical examination should be accomplished to rule out any contraindications to testing or to detect such important clinical signs as cardiac murmur, gallop sounds, pulmonary bronchospasm, or rales. Patients with a history of increasing or unstable angina should not undergo exercise testing until stabilized. A cardiac physical examination should indicate which patients have concurrent valvular or other heart disease (particularly those with severe aortic stenosis, who should not be exercised).

Withdrawal of medications should be considered, depending on the indications of the study, because some drugs interfere with exercise responses and complicate the interpretation of the exercise test. In some exercise laboratories, drugs are withdrawn 24 to 48 hours before performing a test. No formal guidelines exist for tapering medications, and life-threatening rebound phenomena may occur with discontinuance of β-blockers. Most testing is done with patients on their usual medications, although it is important to question which drugs have been taken, to be aware of possible electrolyte abnormalities and other effects. In general, if an exercise prescription is to be performed based on exercise test results, the patient must be on all usual medications, particularly those that may affect ischemic threshold and hemodynamic response.

A standard 12-lead ECG should be obtained. This is essential, particularly for patients who have known heart disease, because an abnormality or a change may prohibit testing. Recording the ECG after hyperventilation before starting the exercise should be avoided because of the association of vigorous hyperventilation with frequent premature ventricular complexes (PVCs) and even angina in CAD patients and because it can cause false-positive results. Additionally, patients with significant functional impairment may not perform as well on the exercise test after hyperventilation. In patients who are believed to have false-positive ST responses, the ECG response to hyperventilation is best observed after exercise or on a day other than the one of the exercise test.

Standing ECG and BP should be recorded to look for vasoregulatory abnormalities, particularly ST depression. The standing ECG should be used as the resting reference for comparison with exercise ECG changes. Orthostatic testing should not be combined with hyperventilation.

Protocols

Exercise ECG is usually performed on a treadmill using a standardized protocol that increases speed and grade in stepwise fashion. Protocol selection is an important consideration. Figure 5.3 illustrates the relationship of workload to stage in the common testing protocols.

The presence of a technician at the side of the treadmill is a prudent safety measure, especially for light support of elderly or unsteady patients. Patients should not grasp the front or side rails or be "held" on the treadmill by a technician as this decreases oxygen uptake and work and increases exercise time and muscle artifact. It is helpful if patients take their hands off the rails and extend one finger, touching the side rails, to maintain balance when walking (after they are accustomed to the treadmill). When a patient is

no longer able to continue exercise without significant handrail or technician support the test should be terminated due to fatigue.

The subject should be started at low speed (1.5 to 2 mph for at least 1 minute), to allow for accommodation to the treadmill. The subject then is exercised on a standardized protocol that should result in 9 or more minutes of work. Exercise tests should be symptom-limited rather than terminated at a mandatory HR limit such as 85% or 100% APMHR. If used appropriately, this would result in a rating of 9 or 10 on the new Borg scale or 17 to 19 on the 6–20 Borg scale.

The many different protocols for clinical use include an initial low load (warm-up), progressive exercise with adequate duration at each level, and a recovery period. The most commonly used protocols are progressive: they are uninterrupted and the workload is increased in stages. For cycle ergometry, the initial workload usually is 10 to 25 W (60 to 150 kp·m·min^{-1}), and is usually followed by increases of 25 W every 2 or 3 minutes until end points are reached.

Numerous treadmill protocols are currently in use, with the most widely used being the Bruce. Although the Bruce protocol has advantages, such as a final stage that cannot be completed by most persons and its wide use by investigators in published studies, it also has several disadvantages. It is often too arduous for elderly or debilitated patients, resulting in peripheral muscle fatigue before the achievement of true cardiopulmonary limitation; it also results in too few data points to be meaningful statistically. Its large increments in work make estimation of $\dot{V}O_2$max less accurate, and the fourth stage can either be run or walked, resulting in divergent oxygen costs. Many patients are forced to terminate exercise prematurely because of orthopedic difficulties or inability to tolerate the high workload increments. Many exercise testing laboratories are now trying to use even MET levels for stage advances and to avoid a situation in which either walking or running can be performed by the patient. An initial "zero" and "half-stages" (1.7 mph at 0% and then 5% grade) can be used for more limited participants. For instance, Okin et al. (51) further modified the Modified Bruce protocol by adding half-stages at 2-minute intervals. This created more gradual, linear work increments yet left intact the familiar landmark stages of the Bruce protocol.

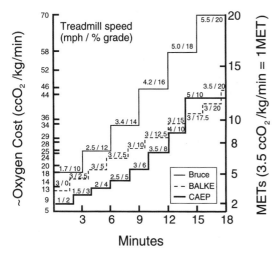

Figure 5.3. Comparison of the Bruce, BALKE, and CAEP protocols. Note the larger number of data points obtained at lower workloads with the CAEP compared with the Bruce protocol.

In an optimally designed protocol, we have observed that a smoother linear relationship should exist between any increase in metabolic reserve (MR) and heart rate reserve (HRR) (52). The observed MET increments of the standard Bruce protocol are large and uneven and limit the number of submaximal responses that may be observed in relation to the exercise stages. For this reason, protocols that provide four or five stages to achieve maximal exercise, such as Balke, Naughton, and the Chronotropic Assessment Exercise Protocol (CAEP), are becoming increasingly prevalent (53). Comparison of the Bruce, Balke, and CAEP protocols is seen in Figure 5.3.

The optimal protocol should be adjusted to the individual patient and should last from 7 to 12 minutes—if the test goes longer, then endurance is tested rather than aerobic capacity. It is more important to report workload achieved in METs rather than in minutes of total exercise. Shorter durations do not give a patient adequate time to warm up, and longer durations result in peripheral fatigue. The protocols should be tailored according to the type of patient tested. Three-minute stages are not necessary to achieve steady state at low workloads or with very small work increments. The oxygen costs of the stages of the major exercise protocols are given in Figure 5.4.

With the availability of computerized, integrated stress testing systems, the use of ramp testing is likely to become more practical in the future. The ramp protocol uses a constant and continuous augmentation in workload by imperceptible changes in speed and grade, allowing for a more steady increase in cardiopulmonary responses to exercise. Ramp testing can also be performed on cycle ergometers interfaced to stress systems with supporting software. Comparison of the ramp with commonly used clinical protocols shows the ramp to result in a more linear relationship between oxygen uptake and a given increase in work (38).

Systolic Blood Pressure Monitoring

Physicians often report that it is difficult to auscultate BP during exercise, but this response is important to the interpretation of results and deserves significant consideration. A mark with a felt-tipped pen over the brachial artery after location by palpation is helpful in locating the point of optimal auscultation during the motion of exercise. The patient's arm should hang relaxed when BP is being taken and during recording; it is important to be certain that the patient neither tenses the muscles of the arm nor rests on the handrail. Care must be taken to minimize bumping and banging of the tubing. The DBP can drop all the way to zero and still be normal, but a drop in SBP below the preexercise value is an important marker for cardiac disease (23).

Test End Points

The patient is instructed to perform without using any specific pretest estimate of maximal predicted heart rate (MPHR), because pretest estimations of MPHR often are misleading related to the use of bradycardia-inducing drugs or common intrinsic dysrhythmias such as atrial fibrillation (54). Perceived exertion responses on the Borg scale are used during the course of the test for this purpose (Table 5.5). The patient is allowed to exercise to a level of maximal effort without adverse signs or symptoms and is encouraged to achieve a 19 or 20 on the 6–20 Borg scale, or 9 or 10 on the 0–10 Borg scale, after which the exercise is discontinued. Indications for termination of an exercise test have been derived from clinical experience and are summarized in Table 5.6.

For the submaximal or predischarge exercise study, one of the following should end the test: signs or symptoms of ischemia; achievement of 6 METs; 85% of APMHR; and a rating of 17 on the 6–20 Borg scale or 7 on the 0–10 Borg scale.

Postexercise Period

Some abnormal responses occur only on recovery after exercise. Subjects are usually allowed a short cool-down walk on the treadmill or low resistance pedaling on the cycle ergometer to minimize postexercise side effects. Having the patient perform too long a cool-down walk after maximal exercise can delay or eliminate the appearance of ST-segment depression. Some testing centers omit the cool-down walk and have the patient assume a supine position immediately after peak exercise. This is based on the law of Laplace, which correlates the increased supine heart volume with increased $M\dot{V}O_2$. When performing diagnostic testing in a population without known CAD, the practice of having the subject stop exercise abruptly and lie supine on an

Figure 5.4. Comparison of oxygen costs, METs, functional class, and clinical status for several of the major exercise protocols.

The figure is a rotated comparison table. Its contents, reconstructed by MET level, are:

Functional Class	Clinical Status	O₂ Cost mL/kg/min	METs	Bicycle Ergometer (1 Watt = 6 kpds; for 70 kg body weight) kpds	Sheffield[1] 3-min stages mph	Sheffield %gr	BALKE 2-min stages mph	BALKE %gr	Naughton 2-min stages mph	Naughton %gr	Cornell 2-min stages mph	Cornell %gr	CAEP[2] 2-min stages mph	CAEP %gr	METs
Normal and I	Healthy, dependent on age, activity	66.5	19										7.0	15	19
		63.0	18		5.5	20									18
		59.5	17										7.0	10	17
		56.0	16		5.0	18	4.0	20.0							16
		52.5	15								5.0	18.0	6.0	10	15
		49.0	14				3.5	20.0			4.6	17.0			14
	Sedentary, healthy	45.5	13	1500	4.2	16	3.0	20.0			4.2	16.0	5.0	10	13
		42.0	12	1350			3.0	17.5			3.8	15.0			12
		38.5	11	1200	3.4	14	3.0	15.0			3.4	14.0	4.0	10	11
		35.0	10	1050			3.0	12.5	2.0	21.0	3.0	13.0			10
		31.5	9	900			3.0	10.0	2.0	17.5	2.5	12.0	3.5	8	9
		28.0	8	750	2.5	12	3.0	7.5	2.0	14.0	2.1	11.0			8
		24.5	7	600			3.0	5.0	2.0	10.5	1.7	10.0	3.0	6	7
		21.0	6	450					2.0	7.0			2.5	5	6
II	Limited	17.5	5		1.7	10	3.0	2.5					2.0	4	5
		14.0	4	300			3.0	0.0	2.0	3.5	1.7	5.0			4
III	Symptomatic	10.5	3	150	1.7	5							1.5	3	3
		7.0	2		1.7	0			2.0	0.0	1.7	0.0	1.0	2	2
IV		3.5	1						1.0	0.0					1

1 This is the Bruce protocol with two additional stages of 1.7/0 and 1.7/5.
2 Cleveland Clinic Chronotropic Assessment Exercise Protocol.

Table 5.5. The Borg Scales of Perceived Exertion During Exercise

10 Point Scale	6–20 Point Scale
0 = Nothing at all	6 = Nothing at all
0.5 = Very, very light	7 = Very, very light
1 = Very light	9 = Very light
2 = Light	11 = Light
3 = Moderate	12
4 = Somewhat hard	13 = Somewhat hard
5 = Hard	15 = Hard
6	16
7 = Very hard	17 = Very hard
8	18
9	19 = Very, very hard
10 = Very, very hard	20

examination table will increase preload and enhance ST-segment abnormality, thereby increasing the diagnostic power of the test (55). This may not be necessary or desirable in patients with known CAD (50), and the cool-down walk may be preferable.

Monitoring should continue for 6 to 8 minutes after exercise or until changes stabilize (32). In the supine position, approximately 85% of patients who show abnormal responses in a large series were abnormal by 4 to 5 minutes into the recovery period. An abnormal response occurring only in the recovery period is not unusual (52). It appears to have nearly the same predictive value (84%) of angiographically significant disease as ST-segment depression during exercise (87%), but in subjects who have no symptoms or risk factors, these responses seem more likely to be false-positives. There are mechanical dysfunctions and electrophysiologic abnormalities in the ischemic ventricle after exercise that can persist from minutes to hours (56–58).

INTERPRETATION OF THE EXERCISE TEST

Clinical Responses

PATIENT APPEARANCE

The patient's appearance is helpful in making a clinical assessment. Patients who have sympathetic dystonia generally are anxious before and after the test, show excessive perspiration, have disproportionate increases in HR, and tend to exaggerate their limitations and symptoms. A drop

in skin temperature, cool and light perspiration, and peripheral cyanosis during exercise can indicate poor tissue perfusion caused by inadequate CO with secondary vasoconstriction. This is an indication for not exhorting a patient to a higher workload. Neurologic manifestations such as lightheadedness or vertigo also can indicate inadequate CO. The use of symptom-rating scales is recommended (59).

PHYSICAL EXAMINATION

Cardiac auscultation made soon after exercise can give some information about ventricular function. Gallop sounds, especially protodiastolic gallop or a precordial bulge, can be caused by LV dysfunction. A mitral regurgitant murmur suggests papillary muscle dysfunction related to transitory ischemia. The physical findings of congestive heart failure (CHF), including rales and neck vein distention, should be encountered rarely in patients referred for exercise testing.

Table 5.6. Indications for Test Termination

Absolute indications

Drop in SBP >10 mm Hg from resting value despite increase in workload with evidence of ischemia
  Moderately severe angina (+3 to +4)
  Central nervous system symptoms (ataxia, dizziness, near syncope)
  Signs of poor perfusion (pallor, cyanosis)
  Serious arrhythmias (sustained VT)
  Technical problems with monitoring ECG or blood pressure
  Patient request to stop
  Marked ECG changes
  ST elevation (>1.0 mm) in leads without diagnostic Q waves (other than V_1 and AVR)

Relative Indications

Drop in SBP >10 mm Hg from resting value despite increasing workload without other evidence of ischemia
>2.0-mm horizontal or downsloping ST-segment depression
Marked axis shift
Less serious arrhythmias
Increasing chest pain
Fatigue, shortness of breath, wheezing, leg cramps, or intermittent claudication
Exaggerated blood pressure response (>250 mm Hg systolic; >115 mm Hg diastolic)
Development of bundle branch block that cannot be distinguished from VT
Second- or third-degree AV block

AV, atrioventricular; SBP, systolic blood pressure; VT, ventricular tachycardia.

Symptoms and Subjective Responses to Exercise

Typical exercise-induced angina is a strong marker for CAD. Ischemic chest pain induced by the exercise test predicts the presence of CAD as well as ST-segment depression. When they occur together, they are even more predictive of CAD than either alone (37). It is important, however, that a careful description of the pain be obtained from the patient to ascertain that it is typical angina rather than nonischemic chest pain.

It is important to remember that the threshold for ischemic symptoms and ECG changes may be increased by administration of many antihypertensive and vasodilating agents. For instance, the use of nitrates before an exercise test will attenuate the anginal and ST-segment response associated with myocardial ischemia. The reason for testing the patient must be carefully considered before advising the patients about use of medication before the test.

Silent ischemia, or ST depression without pain, appears to carry the same prognostic indications as ST depression with pain (12), although it has been suggested that silent ischemia after MI is associated with an adverse prognosis (60).

The use of relative perceived exertion (RPE) scales has helped immeasurably in the clinical monitoring of exercise intensity and duration results (61, 62). The original 6–20 or the newer nonlinear 0–10 scale of Borg represents a subjective scaling system that is reliable and valid and correlates closely to objective measures of physical work. The 0–10 scale uses a logarithmic progression for perceived work, from 0 = "Nothing at all" to 10 = "Very, very heavy" (almost maximal). The original and the newer scales are compared in Table 5.5. In practice, subjects are asked to indicate their perceived value when a chart is held up before them during the last 15 seconds of a given stage of exercise. The scale is useful both in the diagnostic setting (where it provides surprising consistency for the validation of serial results) and in the therapeutic milieu (for use as a self-monitoring parameter for the guidance of the exercise program).

Exercise Capacity or Functional Capacity

It is important to appreciate the relationship between myocardial and ventilatory oxygen consumption and other exercise test variables (40).

Maximal ventilatory oxygen uptake is a measure of the functional limits of the cardiovascular system and provides the best index of exercise capacity. As previously discussed, $\dot{V}O_2max$ depends on many factors and is an indirect estimate of maximal CO. A decline in maximal CO is the major hemodynamic consequence of symptomatic CAD, causing a decrease in exercise capacity. Acute reduction in LV performance, resulting in decreased stroke volume and increasing pulmonary artery pressure, appears to be the mechanism that limits CO. Maximal oxygen uptake is related linearly to maximal CO.

A mean exercise capacity of 10 METs has been observed in nonathletic, normal men. If 10 METs is reached by patients who have CAD, then they have a good prognosis no matter what other exercise test responses occur and appear to do as well in terms of survival when treated medically or surgically. In patients who have an exercise capacity lower than 5 METs, mortality is higher than in those who have higher exercise capacities (12). In a recent study, Snader et al. (63) found impaired functional capacity in patients with known or suspected CAD to be a powerful and independent predictor of cardiac and all-cause mortality, with a three- to fourfold increase in risk within 2 years of the exercise test. When applying these findings, it is important to take age and sex into consideration. Although a functional capacity of 5 METs is clearly abnormal in a 40-year-old man, it shouldn't raise concern in an 82-year-old woman.

A normal exercise capacity does not exclude severe cardiac impairment. Mechanisms proposed to explain normal work performance in patients who have compromised ventricular function include increased peripheral oxygen extraction, preservation of systolic volume and chronotropic reserve, ability to tolerate elevated wedge pressures without dyspnea, ventricular dilatation, and increased levels of plasma norepinephrine at rest and during exercise. Many patients who show decreased ejection fractions at rest are able to perform relatively normal levels of exercise. Some can do this without untoward effects, whereas others report increased fatigue for some time after the test. The expected outcomes associated with various levels of exercise capacity are summarized in Table 5.7.

Exercise capacity should not be reported as

Table 5.7.   Bench Marks of Exercise Capacity

METs	Exercise Capacity
<5	Associated with a poor prognosis in patient <65 years old
5	Equated with limit for ADLs, the usual exercise limit in the immediate post-MI period
10	Considered a normal level of fitness. In patient with angina, there is no improved survival with bypass surgery vs. medical management
13	Indicates good prognosis despite any abnormal exercise response
18	Aerobic master athlete
22	Well-trained competitive athlete

ADLs, activities of daily living; MET, metabolic equivalents; MI, myocardial infarction.

total time exercised but as the $\dot{V}O_2$ or MET equivalent of the workload achieved. This permits the results of diverse exercise testing protocols to be compared with accurate exercise prescription.

In applying results of the exercise test for the purpose of appraising a patient for various occupational or recreational physical activities, caution must be applied when making direct translations between peak MET performance on the test and energy cost estimations in METs available from various published sources or tables. There are many factors that contribute to a wide variability in the MET cost of activities in "real life," including environmental temperature, temporal pace of the activity in question, motor skill level, motivational intensity, and competitiveness. Despite these confounding variables of exercise prescription, as a general rule anyone should be able to maintain a familiar aerobic training activity for 30 to 60 minutes whenever the oxygen requirement does not exceed 50% to 60% of the peak MET level obtained during the exercise test.

Hemodynamic Responses

BLOOD PRESSURE DURING EXERCISE

Blood pressure depends on CO and peripheral resistance. Systolic BP at maximal exertion or at immediate cessation of exertion has been considered a clinically useful first approximation of inotropic capacity of the heart. Because DBP generally remains constant during exercise, the differential BP or systolic pressure gradient should reflect LV function. Cardiac output is the product of HR times stroke volume. An increase in HR alone is not enough to increase the arterial BP significantly. The normal values for

changes in SBP during exercise have been defined: SBP gradient from rest should be 60 ± 25 mm Hg in men 40 to 64 years of age. For women of the same age, it should be 40 ± 20 mm Hg. An inadequate SBP rise or fall during exercise is frequently associated with severe CAD and ischemic dysfunction of the myocardium (64) or LV damage. Exercise-induced hypotension also can identify patients at increased risk for ventricular fibrillation in the exercise laboratory (64). A drop in SBP during exercise below standing resting SBP is associated with increased risk in patients who have had a prior MI or myocardial ischemia (12).

The significance of an exaggerated exercise SBP response remains unclear. In a population with known or strongly suspected CAD, Lauer et al. (65) found an association between exercise hypertension, less severe angiographic disease, and a better prognosis.

HEART RATE DURING EXERCISE

During dynamic exercise, HR increases linearly with workload and oxygen uptake. During low levels of exercise and at a constant workload, HR will rise and gradually reach a plateau or steady state. At higher workloads, it takes progressively longer to reach a steady state.

The issue of chronotropism, or the ability to develop a rate appropriate to a given level of metabolic demand, is receiving a lot of attention. Mathematical models have been developed that define normal and abnormal chronotropic responses (58). Although the presence of absolute chronotropic incompetence generally is considered a primary rhythm anomaly (66), the documentation of relative chronotropic incompetence is increasingly germane (35) and may be a manifestation of ischemia (67). In a study by Brener et al. (68), low peak HR and low percentage of target HR achieved were found to be independent predictors of the presence and severity of CAD, whereas Lauer et al. (69) found failure to achieve target HR and a "blunted" HR response to exercise to predict CAD and total mortality.

Relatively rapid HRs during submaximal exercise or recovery could be caused by vasoregulatory asthenia, any condition decreasing vascular volume or peripheral resistance, prolonged bed rest, anemia, or metabolic disorders. This is a relatively frequent finding soon after MI and coronary artery surgery. Relatively low HR at any point during submaximal exercise could be caused by exercise training, enhanced stroke volume, or drugs. Conditions that affect the sinus node—for instance, inferior wall MI and intrinsic disease of the sinus node—attenuate the normal response of HR during exercise testing.

The common use of β-blockers, which lower HR, has complicated the interpretation of HR responses to exercise. Although the diagnostic value of the test may by reduced by failure to achieve an adequate HR response, it is probably not necessary to discontinue β-blockers before routine testing for evaluation of symptoms or efficacy of medical therapy. However, a normal result when tested on medication is no longer valid if the medical regimen is changed. This may be an indication for retesting. When performing an exercise test for exercise prescription, it is critical that the patient has taken all medications, at their prescribed dosages and times, before the test. In patients who use β-blockers or other bradycardia-inducing medications, or who have chronotropic incompetence, HR is not a good indication of pending fatigue for test termination. In these cases, the Borg scale is a particularly helpful tool in quantifying the patient's level of exertion.

Electrocardiographic Responses

NORMAL RESPONSES

The J point is depressed in lateral leads with maximum depression at peak exercise that gradually returns toward preexercise values in recovery. A dramatic increase in ST-segment slope is observed in all leads and is greatest at 1 minute into recovery. These changes return toward pretest values later in recovery. The normal ST-segment vector response to tachycardia and to exercise is a shift rightward and upward. The degree of this shift appears to have a fair amount of biologic variation. The ST segment, at 60 to 80 ms after the J point, should be less than 0.10 mV above or below the isoelectric line.

A gradual decrease in T wave amplitude is observed in all leads during early exercise. At maximal exercise, the T wave begins to increase, and, at 1-minute recovery, the amplitude is equal to resting values in the lateral leads.

ABNORMAL RESPONSE

The ST-segment abnormalities have been described classically as the major markers of is-chemia. The physiology of cardiac ischemia defines these indicators for measurement. The continuing controversy as to their worth is a consequence of their complexity. All the following physiologic constituents influence the surface ECG configuration: oxygen supply versus demand; pressure relationships; contractility and wall motion; preload and afterload; and HR.

On the surface ECG, exercise-induced myocardial ischemia can result in one of the three ST-segment manifestations: depression, elevation, or normalization. As a general rule, an ST-segment shift of more than 0.10 mV above or below the isoelectric line at 60 to 80 ms after the J point indicates an abnormal response. Confounding factors in interpreting ST-segment depression will be discussed later in the chapter. In patients who have had coronary artery bypass surgery (8) or a recent Q wave MI (70), ST-segment depression does not appear to have prognostic value.

NONDIAGNOSTIC RESPONSE

When resting ECG abnormality worsens during exercise, it is often unclear whether the etiology is ischemia or a nonischemic magnification of the resting changes. Often, tests are called "nondiagnostic" for ischemia when there is resting ECG abnormality. Typically, exacerbation of ST depression during exercise in patients with left bundle branch block (LBBB), even when greater than 1.0 mm, is not ischemic (71). Similarly, in right bundle branch block, ST depression provoked in the anterior leads is not indicative of ischemia (72); however, ST depression noted in the inferior and lateral leads should be considered abnormal.

The presence of left ventricular hypertrophy (LVH) on the resting ECG has long been considered an indication for imaging studies. Meta-analysis has shown that LVH does not affect sensitivity but is associated with a reduction in specificity. Digoxin therapy produces false-positive ST depression in 25% to 40% of apparently healthy individuals (73). Therefore, exercise-induced ST abnormality within 2 weeks of digoxin administration must not be considered diagnostic for ischemia and is an indication for further testing.

The presence of nonspecific resting ST depression of less than 1.0 mm that is not attributable to any of the previously mentioned causes has been associated with adverse cardiac events in patients with and without known CAD. After excluding patients with congenital or valvular heart disease, patients on digitalis, women, and patients with LVH or LBBB on their resting ECGs, Miranda et al. (74) found that those with resting ST depression had nearly twice the prevalence of severe CAD as those without resting changes. Additionally, the presence of an additional 2.0-mm ST depression during exercise or 1.0-mm downsloping ST depression in recovery were good indicators of CAD (likelihood ratio 3.4, sensitivity 67%, specificity 80%).

For diagnostic purposes, it is reasonable to perform an exercise ECG test in the initial work-up. Even when these ECG conditions are present, a negative test result will provide reassurance of decreased likelihood of significant CAD, whereas provocation of additional abnormality would be an indication for further study using other testing modalities.

ST-Segment Analysis

The PR segment is used as the isoelectric line because the TP segment disappears during exercise. ST-segment elevation and depression are defined as the vertical distance in millivolts between the isoelectric line and a predetermined point along the ST segment. The most common definition for abnormal ST depression is more than 1.0-mm depression at 60 to 80 ms after the J point (point at which the QRS complex ends and the ST segment begins). The slope of the ST segment also contributes its strength as a predictor of CAD. Although downsloping ST depression is more significant than horizontal ST depression, both are more predictive of CAD than upsloping ST depression. As an isolated finding, the presence of upsloping ST depression should be considered a "borderline" or perhaps negative result. Upsloping ST depression associated with angina should be considered a positive result. However, the significance of very slowly upsloping ST depression or upsloping ST depression of more than 2.0 mm is less clear. These findings are more likely to be indicative of ischemia than rapidly upsloping ST depression or upsloping ST depression of lesser magnitude. Of course, the increase in sensitivity gained by including upsloping ST depression as an abnormal finding will be at the cost of reducing test specificity.

ST elevation should be measured from the isoelectric line at the J point even in the presence of baseline elevation. Resting ST elevation is usually a result of one of three findings: 1) early repolarization—a normal variant that shifts to isoelectric with exercise; 2) prior MI or ventricular aneurysm—further shift from baseline in the ST segment is not suggestive of ischemia; or 3) injury or infarct—a contraindication to exercise testing. Slope is not measured when there is ST elevation.

ST-segment measurements should be performed using the unprocessed analog data. Use strips of 10 seconds or more with minimal baseline deviation ("wander"). Upward baseline wander may cause depressed ST segments to appear normal, and downward wander may cause normal ST segments to appear depressed. Therefore, ST changes should not be considered significant unless there is a stable baseline and there are three or more beats in a lead. When ST depression is present at rest, it is measured relative to the baseline level of zero. Some of the newer principles of exercise test interpretation are summarized in Table 5.8.

ST-SEGMENT DEPRESSION

ST-segment depression is the most common manifestation of exercise-induced myocardial ischemia. It is a global subendocardial ischemia, with direction determined largely by the placement of the heart in the chest. The standard criterion for this abnormal response is horizontal or downsloping ST-segment depression of more than 0.10 mV at 60 to 80 ms after the J point; however, other criteria have been considered (Fig. 5.5). Downsloping ST-segment depression is more serious than horizontal depression. Upsloping ST depression, without other findings associated with ischemia, should be considered a borderline or negative result. In the presence of baseline abnormalities, exercise-induced ST-segment depression is less specific for ischemia but should not be ignored. Baseline ST abnormalities that worsen with exercise in patients with angina or exertional hypotension probably indicate resting ischemia. Other factors have been related to the probability and severity of CAD, including the amount, time of appearance, duration, and location and number of leads with ST-segment depression.

Table 5.8.   Principles of Exercise Test Interpretation

Ischemic ST depression usually occurs in the lateral leads (I, AVL, V_4–V_6)

Changes in both lateral and inferior leads suggest more severe ischemia

Isolated inferior ST abnormalities are often false-positive changes

ST depression does not localize ischemia to an area of myocardium

ST depression without angina suggests milder CAD and lower risk

ST depression is not interpretable in the face of an abnormal resting ECG (i.e., LVH, LBBB, WPW, Q wave MI, digitalis effect, ventricular paced rhythm)

ST elevation in leads with Q waves is indicative of myocardial damage or aneurysm

ST elevation in leads without Q waves is indicative of transmural ischemia or injury

Markers of poor prognosis or severe CAD

   Exertional hypotension (exercise SBP drops below preexercise value)

   Angina that limits exercise

   Exercise capacity of <6 METs

   Downsloping ST depression, especially in recovery

   ST abnormality or angina starting at a low double product (<15,000)

   ST depression that persists late in recovery

   Chronotropic incompetence in absence of rate-lowering drugs

---

CAD, coronary artery disease; LBBB, left bundle branch block; LVH, left ventricular hypertrophy; MET, metabolic equivalent; MI, myocardial infarction; WPW, Wolff-Parkinson-White syndrome.

The severity of CAD is also related to the time of appearance of ischemic shifts. The lower the workload and double product at which the shift occurs, the worse the prognosis and the more likely the presence of multivessel disease. The persistence of ST depression in the recovery phase, particularly when it becomes downsloping, is also related to the severity of CAD.

ST-SEGMENT ELEVATION

Exercise-induced ST elevation differs in meaning, depending on the status of the myocardium and ECG at baseline (75). ST elevation is classified by whether it occurs over Q waves of an MI or whether it occurs in an ECG area without Q waves. The mechanisms and implications are totally different (70). Early repolarization is a normal variant in healthy persons and usually disappears during exercise.

ST-Segment Elevation Over Q Waves of Prior Myocardial Infarction

Previous MI has been considered the most frequent cause of ST-segment elevation during exercise. The significance of this finding remains controversial and is believed to be related to the presence of dyskinetic areas, ventricular aneurysms, or viable myocardium in the area of the infarct. Approximately 50% of patients who show anterior infarction and 15% of patients who show inferior infarction exhibit this finding during exercise. Those patients with elevation usually have a lower ejection fraction than those without elevation waves over Q waves. The underlying extent of the Q waves for the QRS duration actually determines the amount of ST elevation rather than independently reflecting the amount of dysfunction present. ST-segment elevation has been more frequently observed in anterior leads with Q waves (V_1 through V_2).

ST-Segment Elevation Without Q Waves

In patients who have not had previous MI (absence of Q waves on the resting ECG), ST-segment elevation during exercise is proarrhythmic and frequently localizes the site of severe transient ischemia because of significant proximal disease or spasm (76). ST elevation in V_2 through V_4 indicates left anterior descending coronary artery (LAD) involvement. ST elevation in the lateral leads indicates left circumflex or diagonal artery involvement. ST elevation in the inferior leads indicates right coronary artery involvement. Severe transmural ischemia is the mechanism for such ST-segment elevation during exercise, and the patient should be considered for angiography. An increase in R wave amplitude has been reported in the lateral leads without Q waves when ST-segment elevation occurs.

ST-SEGMENT NORMALIZATION OR ABSENCE OF CHANGE

Another manifestation of ischemia can be no change in or normalization of the ST segment because of cancellation effects. Electrocardiographic abnormalities at rest, including T wave inversion and ST-segment depression, have been reported to return to normal during attacks of angina and during exercise in some patients who have ischemic heart disease. This cancellation effect is a rare occurrence, but it should be kept in mind. Patients who have severe CAD would be most likely to have cancellation occur, yet they have the highest prevalence of abnormal tests. It has been reported that 20% to 25% of patients who have dyskinesia

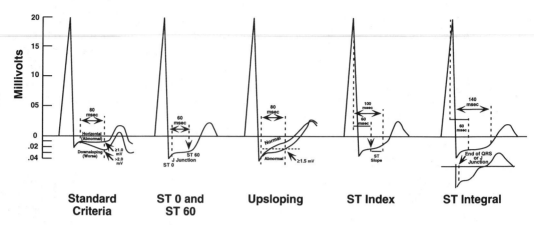

Figure 5.5. Common approaches for the interpretation of ischemia by ST-segment alteration during exercise ECG testing.

and CAD have normal tests or minimal ST-segment elevation during exercise. When exercise testing fails to produce ST-segment depression or elevation in a patient with known CAD, it is hypothesized that two or more equal yet opposing ischemic myocardial segments cause a cancellation of the ST-segment vectors.

DIAGNOSTIC VALUE OF R WAVE CHANGES

A multitude of factors affect the R wave amplitude response to exercise, and the response does not have diagnostic significance (77).

T WAVE AND U WAVE CHANGES

In normal subjects a gradual decrease in the T wave amplitude is observed in all leads during early exercise. At maximal exercise, the T wave begins to increase, and, at 1-minute recovery, the amplitude is equivalent to resting values in lateral leads (78). Inversion of the U wave has been associated with LV hypertrophy, CHD, and aortic and mitral regurgitation. These conditions are associated with abnormal LV distensibility. The U wave inversion induced by exercise in patients who have a normal resting ECG appears to be a marker of myocardial ischemia. Unfortunately, U waves are often difficult to identify as HR reaches higher levels.

COMPUTERIZED ANALYSIS OF THE ST SEGMENT

Computer-generated indices, such as ST/HR slope and ΔST/ΔHR index, have been developed to improve the diagnostic accuracy of the exercise ECG in predicting the presence and severity of CAD (79). However, the results of meta-analysis

(7), as well as other studies (80), have not supported the benefit of their use. Explanations for the discordance in results include population differences, treadmill protocol selection, number of ECG leads analyzed, and accuracy of ST-segment measurement (81). Until further validation has been performed, ST/HR slope and index probably will not be widely used in clinical practice. Therefore, this will be an area of continued focus.

REPORTING EXERCISE TEST RESULTS

Preferably, exercise tests are reported as "normal" or "abnormal." The terminology "negative" or "positive" should be reserved for describing the absence or presence of ischemic changes in the ST-segment portion of the study. Each major element of the test should be described: exercise capacity (in METs), reason for termination, ST-segment response, BP and HRR, arrhythmia and conduction disturbances, and important subjective responses such as RPE, the presence, absence, and quality of pain or discomfort experienced, and other non–fatigue-related signs and symptoms.

The abbreviated criteria currently in use at The Cleveland Clinic Foundation are summarized in Table 5.9.

DIAGNOSTIC USE OF THE EXERCISE TEST

Sensitivity and Specificity

Sensitivity and specificity are the terms used to define how effectively a test separates diseased

Table 5.9. Exercise Electrocardiographic Interpretive Criteria

Normal test
Normal exercise capacity for age
<1.0-mm ST-segment depression from baseline during exercise or recovery
Systolic blood pressure and heart rate increase during exercise
Use "normal except for" to describe potentially important criteria that do not meet criteria for abnormal responses (i.e., ST depression in leads with Q waves, exaggerated BP response, symptoms without ECG changes)

Nondiagnostic test
Abnormal resting ECG (digitalis, LBBB, LVH, WPW, or ventricular pacing)
Failure to achieve adequate heart rate because of suboptimal effort or noncardiac termination points

Abnormal Test
Horizontal or downsloping ST depression >1.0 mm (0.1 mV) from baseline
ST elevation >1.0 mm from baseline in leads without Q waves (except AVR)
Estimated functional capacity of <3 METs
Serious arrhythmias or high-degree AVB provoked by exercise
Decrease in heart rate as exercise increases

AVB, atrioventricular block; BP, blood pressure; LBBB, left bundle branch block; LVH, left ventricular hypertrophy; MET, metabolic equivalent; WPW, Wolff-Parkinson-White syndrome.

from nondiseased persons, that is, how well a test diagnoses disease. For exercise testing, sensitivity is the percentage of those persons with CAD who have an abnormal test. Specificity is the percentage of persons without CAD who will have a normal test result. Table 5.10 summarizes the concepts of sensitivity and specificity.

Sensitivity and specificity are inversely related. When sensitivity is the highest, specificity is the lowest, and vice versa. Any test has a range of inversely related sensitivities and specificities that can be chosen by specifying a certain discriminant or cut-point value.

Complicating the choice of a discriminant value even more is the fact that some of the exercise test responses do not have values established that best separate normals from those who have disease. Once a discriminant value is chosen that determines a test's sensitivity and specificity, then the population tested must be considered. If the population is skewed toward persons who have a greater severity of disease, then the test will have a higher sensitivity. For

instance, the exercise test has a higher sensitivity in persons with three-vessel disease than in those with one-vessel disease. Also a test can have a lower specificity if it is used in persons more likely to give false-positive results. For instance, the exercise test has a lower specificity in persons with mitral valve prolapse and in women.

The sensitivity and specificity of exercise-induced ST-segment depression can be demonstrated by comparing the results of exercise testing and coronary angiography. From these studies, it can be seen that the exercise test cut-point of 0.1 mV horizontal or downsloping ST-segment depression has approximately an 84% specificity for angiographically significant CAD; that is, 84% of those persons who have no significant angiographic disease also had a normal exercise test. These studies demonstrated a mean 66% sensitivity of exercise testing for significant angiographic CAD, with a range of 40% for one-vessel disease to 90% for three-vessel disease.

Bayes' theorem states that the probability of a hypothesis is variably modified as additional data are taken into account (30, 43). For example, if the likelihood of CAD is very low in a given person on the basis of known coronary risk factors, then an abnormal test is likely to be a false-positive. Some statisticians refer to this as "subjective" or "posterior" probability. An understanding of this is especially relevant to the use of exercise testing for the screening of asymptomatic populations in whom the low prevalence (around 4% in asymptomatic men) of disease re-

Table 5.10. Sensitivity and Specificity and Their Relationship to Exercise Electrocardiography

Sensitivity (75% sensitivity means test detects 75% of all people who actually have the disease)[a]
  True-positives: patients with abnormal tests and CAD
  False-positives: patients with abnormal tests and no CAD
Specificity (75% specificity means test is normal in 75% of all people who are actually normal)
  True-negatives: patients with normal tests and no CAD
  False-negatives: patients with normal tests and CAD

CAD, coronary artery disease.
[a]Sensitivity = ratio of patients with positive exercise tests and CAD to all patients with CAD; specificity = ratio of patients with negative tests and no CAD to all patients with no CAD.

sults in a very poor predictive value (about 23%) for a positive result but an excellent predictive value (about 99%) for the negative result (82). For practical purposes, this means that when screening, one must regard positive exercise ECG results with skepticism but may find negative results reassuring.

Factors That Affect Sensitivity and Specificity

Several factors have been shown to affect sensitivity and specificity (7, 37). Sensitivity decreases when equivocal or "nondiagnostic" tests are considered normal or when the testing method is compared with another "superior" method, such as exercise radionuclide imaging using technetium ^{99m}Tc sestamibi. Sensitivity also increases when patients on digitalis are excluded. Specificity is likewise associated with methods of data management and decreases, for example, when upsloping ST depression is reported as abnormal and when preexercise hyperventilation is used. Specificity increases when patients who have had prior MI are included, and when patients who have LBBB are excluded (7). Table 5.11 summarizes some examples of factors that reduce the sensitivity and specificity of exercise testing.

Table 5.11.   Factors That Affect Exercise Test Sensitivity and Specificity

Decreases sensitivity
  Equivocal tests considered normal
  Comparison of exercise ECG to better test
  Defining upsloping ST depression as normal
  Single-vessel disease
  Inclusion of patients on digoxin therapy
  Increased cut-point value for ST depression
  Suboptimal effort
Decreases specificity
  Use of preexercise hyperventilation
  Patients with mitral valve prolapse
  Decreased cut-point value for ST depression
  Abnormal resting ECG (i.e., LVH, LBBB)
  Exclusion of patients with prior MI
  Defining upsloping ST depression as abnormal
  Low prevalence of CAD in population
  Women with ST depression
  High prevalence of vasospasm
  Anemia

CAD, coronary artery disease; LBBB, left bundle branch block; LVH, left ventricular hypertrophy; MI, myocardial infarction.

THE EXERCISE ECG IN WOMEN

The predictive accuracy of ST-segment depression in women has been a major focus of study and controversy. Women, especially those who are premenopausal, have a lower incidence of CAD, resulting in reduced test sensitivity when compared with men (83). The effect of female sex on specificity is also commonly believed to be negative; however, results in this area have been variable. Conflicting conclusions are probably attributable to 1) use of varied criteria to define a positive test result; 2) differences in defining significant CAD; 3) differences in test termination criteria; 4) use of different exercise modalities; 5) varying prevalence of CAD in the study populations; and 6) the presence of referral bias in the study populations. It has been hypothesized that false-positive ST depression in women is caused by a higher prevalence of mitral valve prolapse, microvascular disease and coronary artery spasm, gender difference in coronary and exercise physiology, and hormonal differences (43). Clearly, the interpretation of the exercise ECG presents a clinical challenge to the cardiologist. When other non-ECG indicators of ischemia are present, confidence will increase in the abnormal ST-segment response. An abnormal ECG response without other ischemic indicators at least merits further study with an imaging modality. Although it has been suggested that the initial exercise test in women be performed with imaging (84), further study will be required to confirm that this is a financially advantageous practice. Meanwhile, in the cardiac rehabilitation setting, the value of other information derived from an exercise ECG study, such as functional capacity, hemodynamic response, and symptomatic response, must not be overlooked.

Relative Risk and Predictive Value

Two additional terms that help to define the diagnostic value of a test are its relative risk and predictive value. Relative risk or risk ratio is the chance of having disease if the test is abnormal as compared with the chance of having disease if the test is normal. Predictive value of an abnormal test is the percentage of patients who show an abnormal response who really have disease. It is directly related to the prevalence of disease in the population tested.

PROGNOSTIC USE OF THE EXERCISE TEST

Rationale

There are two principal reasons for estimating prognosis. The first is to provide accurate answers to patients' questions regarding the probable outcome of their illness. Although discussion of prognosis is inherently delicate, and probability statements can be misunderstood, most patients find this information useful in planning their affairs regarding work, recreational activities, personal estate, and finances. The second reason to determine prognosis is to identify those patients in whom interventions might improve outcome and distinguish them from those patients who can be managed without further studies.

Pathophysiology

The basic pathophysiologic features of CAD that determine prognosis are arrhythmic risk, amount of remaining functional myocardium (reflected by LV function), and the amount of myocardium in ischemic jeopardy. These features are summarized in Table 5.12. Arrhythmic risk does not appear to be predicted independently by exercise testing because the prognosis related to arrhythmia is more closely related to LV dysfunction. Exercise test responses caused by myocardial ischemia include angina, ST-segment depression, and ST-segment elevation over ECG areas

Table 5.12. Pathophysiology of Risk Prediction in Coronary Artery Disease

Myocardium in jeopardy
  Amount of viable but underperfused myocardium
    Clinical benchmark—angina pectoris
    Exercise-induced ischemia—ECG, SPECT, PET, echo
Extent of myocardium damaged
  Quantity of myocardium beyond salvage
    Clinical benchmark—heart failure
    Studies—resting ECG (Q waves), radionuclide LVEF, echo, PET
Arrhythmia potential
  Expectation of untoward arrhythmic event
    Clinical benchmark—sudden cardiac death
    Studies—Holter monitoring, signal-averaged ECG, electrophysiologic studies

LVEF, left ventricular ejection fraction; PET, positron emission tomography; SPECT, single-photon emission computed tomography.

without Q waves. Predicting the amount of ischemia (i.e., the amount of myocardium in jeopardy) is difficult (85). The responses related to ischemia or LV dysfunction include chronotropic incompetence or HR impairment, SBP deterioration during exercise, and a poor exercise capacity. Serious exercise-induced dysrhythmias indicate electrical instability.

The only response specifically associated with LV dysfunction is ST elevation over Q waves. This carries an increased risk in patients with Q waves and indicates that they have lower left LV function and, possibly, larger aneurysmal areas compared with those patients with Q waves without ST elevation. Exercise capacity correlates poorly with LV function in patients who show no signs or symptoms of right-sided failure.

Exercise testing is not helpful in identifying patients who have moderate LV dysfunction associated with improved survival after surgical revascularization. This is better recognized by a history and physical findings of CHF, loss of ventricular forces on resting ECG, or estimation of global versus regional LV dysfunction by echocardiogram or radionuclide ventriculography.

POSTMYOCARDIAL INFARCTION EXERCISE TESTING

Purpose

Purposes for performing exercise tests in post-MI patients include assessment of functional capability, determination of an exercise prescription, recognition of the need for modification in the medical regimen, and need for interventions (86). These reasons are detailed in Table 5.13. To submit recovering MI patients to exercise testing may expedite and optimize their discharge from the hospital (87). Ventricular arrhythmias not present at rest can be provoked during exercise (58, 88). The patient's reaction to exercise, the work capacity, and limiting factors at the time of discharge can be assessed (89). An exercise test before discharge is important for giving the patient guidelines for exercise at home, for reassuring the patient about physical status, and for determining the risk of complications (12). This provides a safe basis for advising the patient to resume or increase activity and to return to work.

The test can demonstrate to the patient, the concerned family, and the employer the effect of

Table 5.13. Postmyocardial Infarction
Exercise Testing

Risk stratification, the major indication
Reassurance for the patient and family
Discharge exercise prescription
Baseline functional assessment for future comparison

the MI on the capacity for physical performance (90). Psychologically, it can enhance the patient's self-confidence by lessening any anxiety about performing daily physical activities (91). The test has been helpful in reassuring spouses of post-MI patients of their physical capabilities (92). The psychological impact of performing well on the exercise test is impressive (91). Many patients increase their activity and actually rehabilitate themselves after being encouraged and reassured by their response to this test.

Some investigators use symptom- or sign-limited end points for patients beyond 2 or 3 weeks of infarction; however, a submaximal limited predischarge test appears to be as clinically predictive. Arbitrarily, a HR limit of less than 85% of age-predicted maximal and a MET level of 7 can be used for patients younger than 40 years and less than 85% of APMHR and a MET level of 5 can be used for patients older than 40. Particularly for patients who take β-blockers, a Borg perceived exertion level in the range of 7 to 8 (15 to 16) can be used to end the test before achieving other HR limit criteria. Onset of ischemic ST abnormality or angina are also indications to terminate the test before reaching other termination points. Maximal testing probably is more appropriate at more than 3 weeks after MI, when a patient is ready to return to full activities.

Safety of Exercise Testing After Myocardial Infarction

The trend toward earlier higher level testing is at odds with our understanding of the pathophysiology of the MI process. The duration of the healing phase after MI is about 6 weeks. Traditionally, we have assumed that if the heart is subjected to a major increase in HR or BP during this period, deleterious effects could result. These hypothetical hazards of exertion in MI patients include cardiac rupture, aneurysm formation, extension of infarction, CHF, and serious dysrhythmias. In actual experience, these problems are rarely reported in patients who perform

moderate intensity exercise beyond the first or second week after infarction (17).

Predictors of Poor Outcome After Myocardial Infarction

Twenty-five post-MI exercise test studies that used follow-up for cardiac events to determine which exercise test responses indicate high risk were evaluated by meta-analysis (93). Abnormal ST-segment responses predicted the high-risk patient in only 11 of 25 studies examined. The only test responses associated with high risk more often than by chance were an abnormal SBP and reduced exercise capacity. The ST-segment changes were predictive only for men not taking digoxin who had non-anterolateral Q wave infarctions. Of interest, exclusion from testing seems to identify patients at highest risk, and submaximal predischarge testing appears more predictive than later symptom-limited testing.

Review of these 25 studies of exercise testing in post-MI patients (12) suggests that clinical judgment can be used to identify the high-risk patients, and that ST-segment shifts are not as predictive of high risk as an abnormal SBP response or poor exercise capacity (Table 5.14). Studies that compared angiographic findings and the differential outcome of coronary artery bypass surgery compared with medical therapy have shown the exercise test to have prognostic power in patients with stable CHD (12).

One consistent finding was that patients who met whatever criteria had been set forth for exercise testing were at lower risk than patients not tested. This validates the clinical judgment of a skilled clinician. When the studies were subgrouped by whether testing was done before or after discharge, a high proportion of predischarge test results indicated a poor outcome. Risk predictors from exercise testing best identify the patients who die early after an MI—before later testing can be done. Submaximal testing resulted in the highest proportion of positive associations and the highest risk ratios. Abnormal responses at higher workloads are not as predictive as those at lower workloads.

The failure of exercise-induced ST-segment depression could be a result of population differences and the resting ECG. Exercise-induced ST-segment depression increases risk of subsequent mortality by 11 times when it appears in patients who have relatively normal resting

Table 5.14. Exercise Predictors of Poor Outcome After Myocardial Infarction in 24 Studies

	Abnormal Exercise Test Responses				
	SBP	PVCs	Exercise Capacity	Angina	ST Change
No. studies report results	14	19	13	15	19
No. with positive results[a]	12	13	13	11	12

PVCs, premature ventricular contractions; SBP, systolic blood pressure.
[a]Positive = exercise test response generated a risk ratio for predicting cardiac events.

ECGs (70). Similar findings have been reported by others (19).

Definitive algorithms for intervention after an MI are disappointing, but marked severity of the ST-segment response or a combination of abnormal responses (abnormal SBP response plus 2-mm ST-segment depression) are probably helpful in risk stratification of patients after MI. In post-MI patients, clinical judgment identifies the high-risk patients, and ST shifts are not as predictive as an abnormal SBP response or a poor exercise capability.

PREDICTING IMPROVED SURVIVAL AS A RESULT OF CORONARY ARTERY BYPASS SURGERY USING EXERCISE TESTING

The exercise test variables that indicate which patients would have an improved prognosis if they underwent coronary artery bypass surgery can be presumed only from the studies available because the patients were not randomized to surgery according to their exercise test results, and the analysis is retrospective. From the Seattle Heart Watch, patients who had cardiomegaly, exercise capacity under 5 METs, and maximal SBP less than 130 mm Hg would have a better outcome if treated with revascularization (94). In the European surgery trial, patients who had an exercise test response of 1.5 mm of ST-segment depression had improved survival with surgery. This also extended to those patients with baseline ST-segment depression and those with claudication (95).

From the Coronary Artery Surgery Study (CASS), in more than 5000 nonrandomized patients, the surgical benefit regarding mortality was greatest in the 789 patients who showed 1-mm ST-segment depression at fewer than 5 METs (96). Among the 398 patients who had three-vessel disease with this exercise test response, the 7-year survival rate was 50% in those who were medically managed (versus 81% in those who underwent coronary artery bypass surgery). There was no difference in mortality in patients able to exceed 10 METs exercise capacity.

These studies have indicated that patients who demonstrate marked degrees of ST-segment depression (i.e., more than 2 mm, in multiple leads, prolonged into recovery) accompanied by a poor exercise capacity, exertional hypotension, PVCs, or angina are at increased risk of having three-vessel or left main CAD and a relatively poorer prognosis.

Prognosis in Patients Who Become Symptomatic After Coronary Artery Bypass Surgery

Predicting prognosis of patients who become symptomatic after coronary artery bypass is an important issue because more than 200,000 patients annually undergo this major surgical procedure in the United States. Several studies have documented the functional benefit from coronary artery bypass surgery and have demonstrated more reduced electrocardiographic evidence of ischemia than was demonstrated preoperatively, but no study has addressed prospectively the use of treadmill testing to predict prognosis after coronary artery bypass surgery (97–99). One study has documented the reversal of exercise-induced hypotension, apparently caused by ischemic LV dysfunction after coronary artery revascularization (99).

In a retrospective analysis, MET level and maximal HR were related significantly to prognosis, but the predictive power of these exercise test responses was low and ST-segment depression was not predictive at all (8). The inability of the exercise ECG to predict cardiac events in patients after bypass surgery suggests that other modes of testing are required (i.e., nuclear imaging exercise testing or exercise echocardiographic studies). An exercise capacity of 8 METs or more, however, indicates a good prognosis regardless of other responses (8).

EXERCISE TESTING TO ASSESS PROGNOSIS AFTER THROMBOLYSIS OR PERCUTANEOUS TRANSLUMINAL CORONARY ANGIOPLASTY

Exercise testing in clinically stable patients before percutaneous transluminal coronary angioplasty (PTCA) has been advocated by Weiner and others (100) to confirm the objective presence of myocardial ischemia before performance of the procedure. After PTCA, the presence of an ischemic response similar to that observed before the procedure can be indicative of restenosis. Exercise ECG with radionuclide perfusion imaging provides a useful evaluation of angioplasty results in other more stable patients and can be used to assess ischemia after single-vessel dilation. Multivessel dilation can be associated with restenosis at more than one site, and stress perfusion scanning may be helpful in assessing which region of the myocardium is ischemic (100). Exercise tests should be performed off antianginal medication if possible, and the test should be a sign-limited or symptom-limited one. Weiner and Chaitman (100) advocate elective exercise testing in an asymptomatic patient between 1 and 2 weeks after PTCA to serve as a baseline for future follow-up. In patients who develop restenosis, symptomatic status often suggests a PTCA failure. In asymptomatic patients or patients who have atypical symptoms, the exercise thallium study may be useful (100).

Wijns and colleagues (101) have reported that early detection of restenosis after successful PTCA can be achieved by exercise-redistribution thallium scintigraphy. The presence of a reversible defect on thallium predicts recurrence of ischemia far better than the exercise ECG (ST-segment depression or angina at peak workload). Restenosis was predicted in 74% of patients by thallium scintigraphy but in only 50% of patients by the exercise ECG. Thallium scanning, therefore, was highly predictive but the exercise ECG was not (101, 102).

Deligonul and associates (9) also assessed the prognostic value of early exercise testing after successful coronary angioplasty and found that the exercise ECG did correlate with the presence of multivessel disease. Patients underwent a symptom-limited exercise test within 30 days of the angioplasty procedure. The incidence of exercise-induced ischemic ST-segment depression was significantly greater in patients who had multivessel disease versus single-vessel disease and in patients with multivessel CAD who had incomplete versus complete revascularization. An abnormal exercise ECG result was associated with an increased risk of cardiac events in patients with multivessel disease but not in patients with single-vessel disease. Exercise-induced angina was associated with a higher incidence of follow-up cardiac events in patients with multivessel disease and incomplete revascularization. Exercise duration was significantly lower in patients with multivessel disease who had subsequent cardiac events, compared with patients who did not experience such events.

An abnormal exercise ECG finding within 1 month of successful coronary angioplasty may be predictive of subsequent cardiac events in patients who have multivessel disease (9). In the assessment of long-term benefit of early thrombolytic therapy in patients with acute MI, however, Simoons and associates (103) reported that outcome was more clearly related to LV function at the time of discharge and not to the ischemic activity of underlying CAD.

EXERCISE TESTING FOR EXERCISE PRESCRIPTION

An exercise test is the primary means used to evaluate the safety of participating in an exercise program and to formulate the exercise prescription. Because of the wide scatter of maximal HR when plotted against age, it is much better to determine a person's maximal HR by testing to assign a target for training rather than to give a predicted value. In formal cardiac rehabilitation programs an exercise test can be used to advance a patient safely to a higher level of performance. Also, the improvement in exercise capacity demonstrated by an exercise test can be an effective incentive and can encourage risk factor modification. The methodology for development of exercise prescriptions will be reviewed in chapter 8.

EXERCISE TESTING TO DETERMINE FUNCTIONAL CLASSIFICATION FOR WORK STATUS OR DISABILITY

Exercise testing is used to determine the degree of disability of patients who have various forms of heart disease. Patients who exaggerate their symptoms or who mainly have a psychological impairment often can be identified. Exercise testing can measure more accurately the degree of cardiac impairment than an assessment of exercise capacity by history. Maximal ventilatory oxygen uptake, either directly measured or estimated, is the best noninvasive measurement of the exercise capacity of the cardiovascular system. Being unable to reach 5 METs (less than 18 mL·kg^{-1}·min^{-1}) without signs or symptoms has been used as the criterion for disability by the Social Security Administration. The determination of a patient's exercise capacity affords an objective measurement of the degree of cardiac impairment and can be useful in management.

SUMMARY

The exercise test remains an accessible and cost-effective means of assessing cardiac function. Three features essentially determine the prognosis of CHD: the amount of myocardial ischemia, LV dysfunction, and the arrhythmic potential of the myocardium. For those patients who experience an acute ischemic event, the exercise ECG facilitates identification of the subset for whom intervention is appropriate to improve outcome and to inform the patient fully about this prognosis so that life plans and priorities regarding work or retirement can be adjusted.

Recent advances in exercise testing include an improved understanding of test indications, refinement of methods, and enhancements in the interpretation for diagnosis and physical activity planning. Because of its growing use and the potentially high yield of clinically relevant information, the exercise test will continue to have a significant impact on future cardiovascular health care.

THE HEART RATE RESPONSE TO EXERCISE

Historical Perspective

The term "chronotropic incompetence" refers to an attenuated HR response to exercise. More than 20 years ago, Ellestad (104) performed an exercise test on a 51-year-old athletic man who had a normal exercise tolerance for his age and no symptoms or ST-segment depression during exercise. A short time after the exercise test he experienced sudden cardiac death; an autopsy revealed severe two-vessel CAD with an 80% LAD stenosis. Of note, the patient had only reached a maximum HR of 110 beats per minute during exercise. Later, analyzing follow-up of 2700 patients undergoing exercise testing, Ellestad and Wan (105) noted that patients with a slow HR during exercise were more likely to suffer an acute coronary event than patients with ischemic ST-segment depression and a normal HR response. Other groups also reported on worse prognosis among patients with attenuated exercise heart responses (106), as well as larger burdens of myocardial scar as noted by radionuclide imaging (107).

As imaging modalities, such as thallium scintigraphy and stress echocardiography, became more popular, interest on the HR response to exercise was focused away from prognosis and more toward its impact on test accuracy for the diagnosis of CAD. A number of groups have found that an impaired HR response to exercise is associated with reduced test sensitivity (108–111). Indeed, many exercise laboratories will report out tests in which patients fail to reach 85% of their APMHR as being "nondiagnostic." Although such a term does at least indirectly imply the need for further testing, it does not carry the same ominous connotation as the phrase "evidence of myocardial ischemia."

During the 1980s and 1990s interest in the HR response to exercise has again focused on prognostic implications (112), with particular attention also being directed toward certain patient subsets, such as those with CHF (113, 114) and cigarette smokers (115). Other groups have proposed directly incorporating the HR response to exercise into analysis of ST segments, arguing that doing this improves the usefulness of the exercise ECG for both purposes of diagnosis and prognosis (116, 117).

Definitions of Chronotropic Incompetence

The physiology behind the HR response to exercise is a complex one that relates to perturbations in resting and exercise sympathetic and parasympathetic tone and neurohormonal milieu. A detailed discussion of the mechanisms underlying normal and abnormal HR responses to exercise is beyond the scope of this review, but can be found elsewhere (118).

ABILITY TO REACH AN AGE-PREDICTED MAXIMUM HEART RATE

The most important determinant of HR response to exercise is age, with decreasing maximal HRs achievable as people get older. There is an inverse linear relationship between peak HR and age in healthy individuals; a number of groups have reported on linear equations for estimating peak heart, with 220 minus age in years being one of the more popularly used equations in clinical exercise laboratories. A commonly used definition of chronotropic incompetence is failure to reach 85% of the APMHR. A major limitation of this approach is that the estimated peak HR has a high standard deviation and therefore may be difficult to apply to individuals, as opposed to populations (118).

There are other problems with using ability to reach 85% of the APMHR as a measure of chronotropic incompetence. In addition to age, other important predictors of the HR response to exercise are resting HR and physical fitness, both factors which themselves are predictive of coronary heart disease risk (119–123). Data from the Framingham Heart Study have shown that ability to reach a target HR is influenced by these two variables and even by age itself (112). Therefore, any effort to relate chronotropic incompetence of prognosis or diagnosis suffers an inherent risk of serious confounding.

THE CHRONOTROPIC INDEX—ACCOUNTING FOR AGE, RESTING HEART RATE, AND METABOLIC WORK

Wilkoff and Miller (124) have described a method for describing the exercise HR response, which takes advantage of the linear relation between exercise HR increase and metabolic work. Before exercise, a person has a certain MR, which is the difference between his peak oxygen consumption (or exercise capacity) and his resting oxygen consumption, which is typically 3.5 mL $\cdot$ kg^{-1} $\cdot$ min^{-1}, or 1 MET (metabolic equivalent). As exercise progresses that MR is used up. Analogously, at rest there is a potential HRR, which is the difference between the peak attainable HR (as estimated, for example, by 220 minus age) and the resting HR. As exercise progresses HRR, like the MR, is used up as well.

During any given stage of exercise, the percent MR used can be expressed as:

$$\%MR\ used = [(METs_{stage} - METs_{rest})\ / \\ (METs_{peak} - METs_{rest})] \times 100$$

In an analogous fashion, the percent HRR used at any given stage of exercise can be expressed as:

$$\%HRR\ used = [(HR_{stage} - HR_{rest})\ / \\ (220 - age - HR_{rest})] \times 100$$

Wilkoff and Miller (124) have shown that in a group of healthy, nonhospitalized adults a plot of HRR used to MR used during different stages of exercise reveals a tight linear relationship with a slope of approximately one and a 95% confidence interval (CI) of 0.8 to 1.3 (Fig. 5.6). The calculated value of this slope, which we have termed as the "chronotropic index" (112, 115, 125), is independent of stage of exercise considered. Chronotropic incompetence can thus be defined as a percent HRR used to percent MR used ratio of less than 0.8; this is referred to as a "low chronotropic index." The advantage of using this approach to assess chronotropic response is that it accounts for age, functional capacity, and resting HR; it is not merely a reflection of physical fitness or exercise time.

One possible problem with this method is that except for patients undergoing sophisticated gas-exchange analyses, exercise capacity in METs is estimated and not directly measured. Among patients who undergo symptom-limited testing, one can consider the ratio of HRR used to MR used at peak exercise, when by definition the proportion of MR used has a value of one. Using this approach the chronotropic index is based entirely on directly measured variables, namely resting HR, peak HR, and age (117). Because the value of the chronotropic index is independent of stage of exercise considered, this measure at least indirectly takes into account effects of functional capacity as well (124).

Chronotropic Incompetence and Diagnosis

HEART RATE-ADJUSTED ST-SEGMENT ANALYSES

As previously mentioned, chronotropic incompetence has been shown to adversely affect

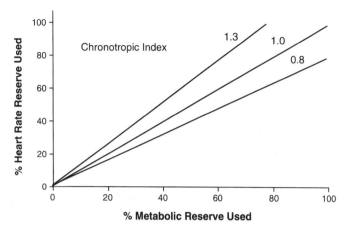

Figure 5.6.   The chronotropic index plotting % heart rate reserve used versus % metabolic reserve used (Adapted from Wilkoff BL, Miller RE. Exercise testing for chronotropic assessment. Cardiol Clin 1992;10:705–717).

the sensitivity of stress imaging tests. Several groups, however, have focused on formally incorporating the HR response into the interpretation of the exercise ECG, thereby improving the accuracy of that test. The rationale for this is based on the well-known relationship between inducible ischemia and workload (126) as well as the impact that varying levels of ischemia have on intramyocardial voltage transients (127).

One approach toward incorporating HR response into ST-segment analysis is to divide the change in ST-segment deviation from the isoelectric line during exercise by the change in HR during exercise; this is known as the ΔST/ΔHR index (116, 128). This approach can be used for stepped protocols with marked increments in workload between stages of exercise, like the traditional Bruce protocol (129). A more precise ST/HR slope can be used in the setting of less-stepped protocols, like the Cornell protocol (116) (Fig. 5.7). Although there is still some controversy, a number of studies have demonstrated that using these HR-adjusted ST-segment analyses improves the diagnostic and prognostic powers of the exercise ECG (130–134).

Chronotropic Response and Angiographic Severity of Coronary Artery Disease

We have reported on the association of chronotropic response to exercise and angiographic severity of CAD (125). Among 475 patients who underwent exercise testing and coronary angiography within 180 days, peak HR, percent target HR achieved, and the chronotropic index were all

closely related to the number of diseased coronary arteries (Fig. 5.8). Also of note, despite the anatomic relationship between the right coronary artery and the sinus node, there was no association between isolated disease of the proximal right coronary artery and chronotropic response. In contrast, after adjusting for age and sex, stenosis in the proximal LAD was strongly associated with peak HR (for each 10 beats per minute decrement, odds ratio [OR] 1.23, 95% CI 1.07 to 1.41, $P = .03$), percent target HR achieved (for each 10% decrement, OR 1.44, 95% CI 1.15 to 1.81, $P = .02$), and chronotropic index (for each 0.2 decrement, OR 1.6, 95% CI 1.03 to 1.54, $P = .02$).

Combined Approach

More recently, we have investigated combining HR-adjusted ST-segment indices with the chronotropic index (117). In a study of 337 patients with angiographically proven CAD and 283 control subjects, the magnitudes of absolute ST-segment depression, the ΔST/ΔHR index, and the ST/HR slope were divided by chronotropic index as measured at peak exercise. At a matched specificity of 96%, this led to improvements in sensitivity of all three measures: for ST-segment depression from 52% to 87%, for ΔST/ΔHR index from 90% to 94%, and for ST/HR slope from 88% to 93%.

Chronotropic Incompetence and Prognosis

The HR response to exercise represents a change in HR in response to a change in physiologic environment. Even at rest, HR is not con-

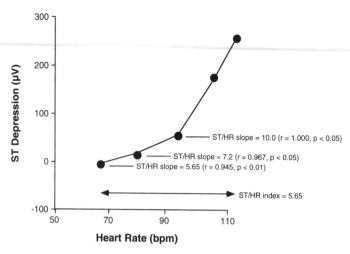

Figure 5.7.   Example of adjusting ST-segment changes for heart rate during exercise (Reprinted with permission from Okin PM, Kligfield P. Heart rate adjustment of ST segment depression and performance of the exercise electrocardiogram: a critical evaluation. J Am Coll Cardiol 1995;25:1726–1735).

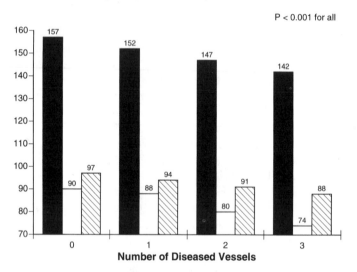

Figure 5.8.   Association between peak heart rate (beats/min) (black bars), chronotropic index (100) (white bars), and percent heart rate achieved (striped bars) and number of diseased coronary arteries (Reprinted with permission from Brener SJ, Pashkow FJ, Harvey SA, et al. Chronotropic response to exercise predicts angiographic severity in patients with suspected or stable coronary artery disease. Am J Cardiol 1995;76:1228–1232).

stant, but varies in a dynamic manner to phases of the respiratory cycle and changes in posture. A number of investigators have shown that HR variability at rest is strongly associated with prognosis among survivors of acute MI (135, 136) and even among healthy adults (137). Combining these observations with the reports of improved estimation of prognosis with HR-adjusted ST-segment analyses (130), we hypothesized that the HR response to exercise can be thought of as a kind of HR variability subject to perturbations

in autonomic function that would also have strong prognostic implications.

We studied 1575 healthy male participants of the Framingham Heart Study who underwent graded exercise testing according to the Bruce protocol (129) and were followed up for nearly 8 years (112). There were 327 who failed to reach 85% of their APMHR; of these 21 (6%) died and 44 (14%) experienced an incident coronary heart disease event. In contrast, of the 1248 subjects who reached their target HR, only 34 (3%) died and only 51 (4%) experienced coronary heart disease events. After adjusting for ST-segment changes and standard cardiovascular risk factors, all-cause mortality was predicted by the change in HR with exercise ($P = .04$) and by the chronotropic index as measured during stage 2 of exercise ($P = .05$); incident coronary artery disease was similarly independently predicted by failure to achieve the target HR ($P = .02$), the change in HR with exercise ($P = .0003$), and the chronotropic index ($P = .001$).

Because nicotine is a sympathomimetic drug that has been shown to cause alterations in autonomic tone and HR variability (138), we also chose to study the relationship between smoking and chronotropic incompetence among healthy subjects in the Framingham Heart Study. In a cohort of 1468 men and 1652 women, smoking was noted to be strongly associated with failure to reach a target HR (in men 25% versus 15%, smokers versus nonsmokers, OR 1.97, 95% CI 1.51 to 2.56; in women 32% versus 18%, OR 2.10, 95% CI 1.63 to 2.61) and with a low chronotropic index (in men 17% versus 12%, OR 1.50, 95% CI 1.12 to 2.03; in women 17% versus 8%, OR 2.28, 95% CI 1.68 to 3.09). A dose–response relationship was also noted in which those who smoked more were more likely to manifest abnormal chronotropic responses (Fig. 5.9). An interesting finding was that smokers who also had an abnormal chronotropic response were at particularly high risk for death and incident coronary events (Tables 5.15 and 5.16).

Mechanisms

It is unclear why chronotropic incompetence is associated with an adverse outcome. Previous investigators had argued that a slower HR during exercise represents a compensatory mechanism for hearts beset by a heavy ischemic burden, but the ability to predict events many years after testing argues that the mechanism must be more complex (104). Nonetheless, there must be some relation to ischemia, given the association of chronotropic incompetence with angiographic severity of CAD (125) and with thallium perfusion defects (107) and the improvement of chronotropic response with myocardial revascularization (139). Another possible mechanism might be that subtle alterations of autonomic tone are themselves markers, if not outright contributors, to the severity and activity of atherosclerosis. Investigations in this area have included consideration of the Bezold-Jarisch reflex (140), decreased vagal activity at rest (141), and the relationship between resting HR and CAD risk (119). Some have argued that the relationship between chronotropic incompetence and outcome may parallel the associations between exercise HR responses and severity of neurohormonal alterations in patients with CHF (113, 114).

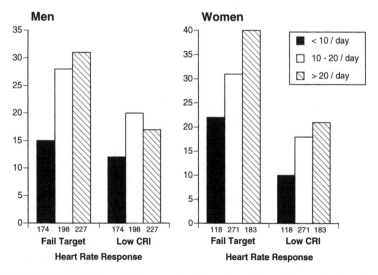

Figure 5.9. Rates of chronotropic incompetence according to number of cigarettes smoked per day on average. The numbers below the bars indicate the number of subjects in each group (Reprinted with permission from Lauer MS, Pashkow FJ, Larson MG, et al. Association of cigarette smoking with chronotropic incompetence and prognosis in the Framingham Heart Study. Circulation 1997;96:897–903).

Table 5.15.   Impact of Failure to Achieve Target Heart Rate on the Association of Smoking with Outcome: Results of Cox Proportional Hazards Analyses

Group	Event No.	8-year Kaplan-Meier Rate	Hazard Ratio (95% CI)[a]
All-cause mortality (48 events)			
Nonsmokers, reached THR	17/740	2%	1.0 (reference group)
Nonsmokers, failed THR	4/128	3%	0.71 (0.23–2.19)
Smokers, reached THR	15/446	3%	1.96 (0.94–4.09)
Smokers, failed THR	12/152	8%	2.45 (1.14–5.24)
Coronary heart disease (90 events)			
Nonsmokers, reached THR	23/740	3%	1.0 (reference group)
Nonsmokers, failed THR	11/128	9%	1.44 (0.68–3.05)
Smokers, reached THR	25/446	6%	2.40 (1.34–4.27)
Smokers, failed THR	31/152	21%	4.92 (2.84–8.53)

THR, target heart rate; FEV_1, forced expiratory volume in 1 second; FVC, forced vital capacity; HDL, high-density lipoprotein.
[a]After adjustment for age, body mass index, blood pressure, antihypertensive medications, physical activity index, diabetes, ratio of total to HDL cholesterol, FEV_1 to FVC ratio, and ST-segment response to exercise.

Table 5.16.   Impact of Low Chronotropic Index on the Association of Smoking with Outcome: Results of Cox Proportional Hazards Analyses

Group	Event No.	8-year Kaplan-Meier Rate	Hazard Ratio (95% CI)[a]
All-cause mortality (48 events)			
Nonsmokers, normal CRI	18/767	2%	1.0 (reference group)
Nonsmokers, low CRI	3/101	3%	1.33 (0.38–4.61)
Smokers, normal CRI	16/499	4%	1.67 (0.82–3.38)
Smokers, low CRI	11/99	10%	5.84 (2.68–12.71)
Coronary heart disease (90 events)			
Nonsmokers, normal CRI	29/767	4%	1.0 (reference group)
Nonsmokers, low CRI	5/101	6%	1.07 (0.41–2.80)
Smokers, normal CRI	40/499	8%	2.76 (1.69–4.50)
Smokers, low CRI	16/99	17%	4.59 (2.47–8.54)

CRI, chronotropic index; FEV_1, forced expiratory volume in 1 second; FVC, forced vital capacity; HDL, high-density lipoprotein.
[a]After adjustment for age, body mass index, blood pressure, antihypertensive medications, physical activity index, diabetes, ratio of total to HDL cholesterol, FEV_1 to FVC ratio, and ST-segment response to exercise.

The Future

Future investigations will need to focus on the applicability of measures of chronotropic response for predicting prognosis and response to therapy in clinical populations. The data that currently exist argue strongly that chronotropic incompetence should be considered as a dire prognostic sign, and not merely a marker of a nondiagnostic or technically inadequate stress test. Methods of routine incorporation of chronotropic response into stress test reporting will need to be developed and tested. Other ripe areas for inquiry include learning more about the pathophysiology underlying chronotropic incompetence and determining whether this impaired HR response to exercise is a potentially modifiable risk factor susceptible to specific therapy.

References

1. Feil H, Siegel M. Electrocardiographic changes during attacks of angina pectoris. Am J Med Sci 1928;175: 225–260.
2. Master AM, Oppenheimer EJ. A simple exercise tolerance test for circulatory efficiency with standard tables for normal individuals. Am J Med Sci 1929; 177: 223–243.
3. Master AM, Jaffe HL. The electrocardiographic changes after exercise in angina pectoris. J Mt Sinai Hosp 1941; 7:629–632.
4. Yu PNG, Soffer A. Studies of electrocardiographic changes during exercise (modified double two step test). Circulation 1952; 6:183–192.

5. Bruce RA. Evaluation of functional capacity and exercise tolerance of cardiac patients. Mod Concepts Cardiovasc Dis 1956;25:321–326.

6. DeBelder M, Pumphrey CW, Skehan JD, et al. Relative power of clinical, exercise test, and angiographic variables in predicting clinical outcome after myocardial infarction: the Newham and Tower Hamlets study. Br Heart J 1988;60:377–389.

7. Gianrossi R, Detrano R, Mulvihill D, et al. Exercise-induced ST depression in the diagnosis of coronary artery disease. A meta-analysis. Circulation 1989;80: 87–98.

8. Dubach P, Froelicher V, Klein J, et al. Use of the exercise test to predict prognosis after coronary artery bypass grafting. Am J Cardiol 1989;63:530–533.

9. Deligonul U, Vandormael MG, Shah Y, et al. Prognostic value of early exercise stress testing after successful coronary angioplasty: importance of the degree of revascularization. Am Heart J 1989;117:509–514.

10. Fuller T, Movahed A. Current review of exercise testing: application and interpretation. Clin Cardiol 1987;10:189–200.

11. Detrano R, Froelicher VF. Exercise testing: uses and limitations considering recent studies. Prog Cardiovasc Dis 1988;31:173–204.

12. Froelicher VF, Duarte GM, Oakes DF, et al. The prognostic value of the exercise test. Dis Mon 1988;34: 677–735.

13. Gibson RS. Comparative analysis of the diagnostic and prognostic value of exercise ECG and thallium-201 scintigraphic markers of myocardial ischemia in asymptomatic and symptomatic patients. Cardiol Clin 1989;7:565–575.

14. Do D, West JA, Morise A, et al. A consensus approach to diagnosing coronary artery disease base on clinical and exercise test data. Chest 1997;111:1742–1749.

15. Weld FM, Chu KL, Bigger JJ, et al. Risk stratification with low-level exercise testing 2 weeks after acute myocardial infarction. Circulation 1981;64:306–314.

16. DeBusk RF. Specialized testing after recent acute myocardial infarction. Ann Intern Med 1989;110:470–481.

17. Saunamaki KI. Early post-myocardial infarction exercise testing. Exercise response and clinical value. Dan Med Bull 1988;35:549–564.

18. Hamm LF, Stull GA, Crow RS. Exercise testing early after myocardial infarction: historic perspective and current uses. Prog Cardiovasc Dis 1986;28:463–476.

19. Krone RJ, Dwyer EJ, Greenberg H, et al. Risk stratification in patients with first non-Q wave infarction: limited value of the early low level exercise test after uncomplicated infarcts. The Multicenter Post-Infarction Research Group. J Am Coll Cardiol 1989;14:31–37.

20. Schechtman KB, Capone RJ, Kleiger RE, et al. Risk stratification of patients with non-Q wave myocardial infarction. The critical role of ST segment depression. The Diltiazem Reinfarction Study Research Group. Circulation 1989;80:1148–1158.

21. Kuchar DL, Thorburn CW, Freund J, et al. Noninvasive predictors of cardiac events after myocardial infarction. Complementary value of exercise testing and signal-averaged electrocardiography. Cardiology 1989;76: 18–31.

22. Bogaty P, Dagenais GR, Cantin B, et al. Prognosis in patients with a strongly positive exercise electrocardiogram. Am J Cardiol 1989;64:1284–1288.

23. Dubach P, Froelicher VF, Klein J, et al. Exercise-induced hypotension in a male population. Criteria, causes, and prognosis. Circulation 1988;78:1380–1387.

24. Nielsen JR, Mickley H, Damsgaard EM, et al. Predischarge maximal exercise test identifies risk for cardiac death in patients with acute myocardial infarction. Am J Cardiol 1990;65:149–153.

25. Do D, West JA, Morise A, et al. An agreement approach to predict severe angiographic coronary artery disease with clinical and exercise test data. Am Heart J 1997;134:672–679.

26. Marcus R, Lowe R III, Froelicher VF, et al. The exercise test as a gatekeeper: limiting access or appropriately directing resources? Chest 1995;107:1442–1446.

27. Bruce RA, Hossack KF, DeRouen TA, et al. Enhanced risk assessment for primary coronary heart disease events by maximal exercise testing: 10 years' experience of Seattle Heart Watch. J Am Coll Cardiol 1983;2:565–573.

28. Detrano R, Froelicher V. A logical approach to screening for coronary artery disease. Ann Intern Med 1987; 106:846–852.

29. Hindman MC. Is exercise tolerance testing indicated for diagnoses and/or screening in family practice? An opposing view. J Fam Pract 1989;28:476–480.

30. Morise AP, Duval RD. Comparison of three Bayesian methods to estimate post-test probability in patients undergoing exercise stress testing. Am J Cardiol 1989;64:1117–1122.

31. Sox HJ, Littenberg B, Garber AM. The role of exercise testing in screening for coronary artery disease. Ann Intern Med 1989;110:456–469.

32. Froelicher V, Marcondes G. A manual of exercise testing. Chicago, IL: Year Book Medical Publishers, 1989.

33. Schlant RC, Blomqvist CG, Brandenburg RO, et al. Guidelines for exercise testing. A report of the Joint American College of Cardiology/American Heart Association Task Force on Assessment of Cardiovascular Procedures. Circulation 1986;74:653A–667A.

34. Wigton RS, Nicolas JA, Blank LL. Procedural skills of the general internist. Ann Intern Med 1990;111:1023–1034.

35. Wilkoff BL, Beck G, Pashkow FJ, et al. Confidence interval calculation of chronotropic incompetence. Pacing Clin Electrophysiol 1990;13:1215.

36. Deckers JW, Rensing BJ, Tijssen JG, et al. A comparison of methods of analyzing exercise tests for diagnosis of coronary artery disease. Br Heart J 1989;62:438–444.

37. Detrano R, Janosi A, Lyons KP, et al. Factors affecting sensitivity and specificity of a diagnostic test: the exercise thallium scintigram. Am J Med 1988;84:699–710.

38. Myers J, Buchanan N, Walsh D, et al. Comparison of the ramp versus standard exercise protocols. J Am Coll Cardiol 1991;17:1334–1342.

39. Mason RE, Likar I. A new system of multiple-lead exercise electrocardiography. Am Heart J 1966;71:196–205.

40. Sevilla DC, Dohrmann ML, Somelofski CA, et al. Invalidation of the resting electrocardiogram obtained via exercise electrode sites as a standard 12-lead recording. Am J Cardiol 1989;63:35–39.

41. Miranda CP, Liu J, Kadar A, et al. Usefulness of exercise-induced ST segment depression in the inferior leads during exercise testing as a marker for coronary artery disease. Am J Cardiol 1992;69:303–307.

42. Milliken JA, Abdollah H, Burggraf GW. False-positive treadmill exercise tests due to computer signal averaging. Am J Cardiol 1990;65:946–948.

43. Chaitman BR. The changing role of the exercise electrocardiogram as a diagnostic and prognostic test for chronic ischemic heart disease. J Am Coll Cardiol 1986;8:1195–1210.

44. Weiner DA, Ryan TJ, McCabe CH, et al. Exercise stress testing. Correlations among history of angina, ST segment response and prevalence of coronary artery disease in the Coronary Artery Surgery Study. N Engl J Med 1979;301:230–235.

45. Ellestad MH. Stress testing: principles and practice. 3rd ed. Philadelphia: FA Davis, 1996.

46. Gibbons RJ, Balady GJ, Beasley JW, et al. ACC/AHA guidelines for exercise testing. A report of the American College of Cardiology/American Heart Association Task Force on Practice Guidelines (Committee on Exercise Testing). J Am Coll Cardiol 1997;30:260–315.

47. Ekelund LG, Suchindran CM, McMahon RP, et al. Coronary heart disease morbidity and mortality in hypercholesterolemic men predicted from an exercise test: the Lipid Research Clinics Coronary Primary Prevention Trial. J Am Coll Cardiol 1989;14:556–563.

48. Schlant RC, Friesinger GC II, Leonard JJ. Clinical competencies in exercise testing: a statement for physicians from the ACP/ACC/AHA Task Force on Clinical Privileges in Cardiology. J Am Coll Cardiol 1990;16:1061–1065.

49. Piña IL, Balady GJ, Hanson P, et al. Guidelines for clinical exercise testing laboratories: a statement for health care professionals from the Committee on Exercise and Cardiac Rehabilitation. Circulation 1995;91:912–921.

50. Gibbons L, Blair SN, Kohl HW, et al. The safety of maximal exercise testing. Circulation 1989;80:846–852.

51. Okin PM, Ameisen O, Kligfield P. A modified treadmill exercise protocol for computer-assisted analysis of the ST segment/heart rate slope: methods and reproducibility. J Electrocardiol 1986;19:311–318.

52. Wilkoff BL, Corey J, Blackburn G. A mathematical model of the chronotropic response to exercise. J Electrophysiol 1989;3:176–180.

53. Froelicher VF. Exercise and the heart: clinical concepts. Chicago, IL: Year Book Medical Publishers, 1993;16–17.

54. Corbelli R, Masterson M, Wilkoff BL. Chronotropic response to exercise in patients with atrial fibrillation. Pacing Clin Electrophysiol 1990;13:179–187.

55. Lachterman B, Lehmann KG, Abrahamson D, et al. "Recovery only" ST-segment depression and the predictive accuracy of the exercise test. Ann Intern Med 1990;112:11–16.

56. Weiner DA, Levine SR, Klein MD, et al. Ventricular arrhythmias during exercise testing: mechanism, response to coronary bypass surgery and prognostic significance. Am J Cardiol 1984;53:1553–1557.

57. Detry JM, De Jonge D. Exercise testing in the evaluation of ventricular arrhythmias in coronary artery disease [review]. Eur Heart J 1987;8:55D–59D.

58. Podrid PJ, Venditti FJ, Levine PA, et al. The role of exercise testing in evaluation of arrhythmias. Am J Cardiol 1988;62:24H–33H.

59. Borg G, Holmgren A, Lindblad I. Quantitative evaluation of chest pain. Acta Med Scand 1981;644(Suppl): 43–45.

60. Erikssen J. Prognostic importance of silent ischemia during long-term follow-up of patients with coronary artery disease. A short review based on own experience and current literature. Herz 1987;12:359–368.

61. Borg G, Ottoson D. The perception of exertion in physical work. Dobbs Ferry, NY: Sheridan House Publishers, 1986.

62. Borg GAV, Hassmen P, Lagerstrom M. Perceived exertion related to heart rate and blood lactate during arm and leg exercise. Eur J Appl Physiol Occup Physiol 1987;56:679–685.

63. Snader CE, Marwick TH, Pashkow FJ, et al. Importance of estimated functional capacity as a predictor of all-cause mortality among patients referred for exercise thallium single-photon emission computed tomography: report of 3,400 patients from a single center. J Am Coll Cardiol 1997;30:641–648.

64. Weiner DA, McCabe CH, Cutler SS, et al. Decrease in systolic blood pressure during exercise testing: reproducibility, response to coronary bypass surgery and prognostic significance. Am J Cardiol 1982;49: 1627–1631.

65. Lauer MS, Pashkow FJ, Harvey SA, et al. Angiographic and prognostic implications of an exaggerated exercise systolic blood pressure response and rest systolic blood pressure in adults undergoing evaluation for suspected coronary artery disease. J Am Coll Cardiol 1995;26:1630–1636.

66. Wilkoff BL, Blackburn G, Pashkow FJ, et al. Exercise testing in identification of sinus node dysfunction. Proc Eur Pacing Clin Electrophysiol Soc 1993;6:105–111.

67. Wiens RD, Lafia P, Marder CM, et al. Chronotropic incompetence in clinical exercise testing. Am J Cardiol 1984;54:74–78.

68. Brener SJ, Pashkow FJ, Harvey SA, et al. Chronotropic response to exercise predicts angiographic severity in patients with suspected or stable coronary artery disease. Am J Cardiol 1995;76:1228–1232.

69. Lauer MS, Okin PM, Larson MG, et al. Impaired heart rate response to graded exercise: prognostic implications of chronotropic incompetence in the Framingham Heart Study. Circulation 1996;93:1520–1526.

70. Klein J, Froelicher VF, Detrano R, et al. Does the rest electrocardiogram after myocardial infarction determine the predictive value of exercise-induced ST depression? A 2 year follow-up study in a veteran population. J Am Coll Cardiol 1989;14:305–311.

71. Whinnery JE, Froelicher VF, Stuart AJ. The electrocardiographic response to maximal treadmill exercise in asymptomatic men with left bundle branch block. Am Heart J 1977;94:316–324.

72. Whinnery JE, Froelicher VF, Longo MR, et al. The electrocardiographic response to maximal treadmill

exercise in asymptomatic men with right bundle branch block. Chest 1977;71:335–340.

73. Sketch MH, Mooss AN, Butler ML, et al. Digoxin-induced positive exercise tests: their clinical and prognostic significance. Am J Cardiol 1981;48:655–659.

74. Miranda CP, Lehmann KG, Froelicher VF. Correlation between resting ST segment depression, exercise testing, coronary angiography, and long-term prognosis. Am Heart J 1991;122:1617–1628.

75. Nosratian FJ, Froelicher VF. ST elevation during exercise testing. Chest 1989;96:653–654.

76. Mark DB, Hlatdy MA, Lee KL, et al. Localizing coronary artery obstructions with the exercise treadmill test. Ann Intern Med 1987;106:53–55.

77. Voyles WF, Smith ND, Abrams J. Directional variability in the R wave response during serial exercise testing in patients with coronary artery disease. Am Heart J 1984;108:983–988.

78. Surawicz B. ST-segment, T-wave, and U-wave changes during myocardial ischemia and after myocardial infarction. Can J Cardiol 1986;2:71A–84A.

79. Okin PM, Kligfield P. Computer-based implementation of the ST-segment/heart rate slope. Am J Cardiol 1989;64:926–930.

80. Lachterman B, Lehmann KG, Detrano R, et al. Comparison of ST segment/heart rate index to standard criteria for analysis of exercise electrocardiogram. Circulation 1990;82:44–50.

81. Okin PM, Kligfield P. Heart rate adjustment of ST segment depression and performance of the exercise electrocardiogram: a critical evaluation. J Am Coll Cardiol 1995;25:1726–1735.

82. Sheffield LT. Exercise stress testing for coronary artery disease. In: Braunwald E, ed. Heart disease. A textbook of cardiovascular medicine. 3rd ed. Philadelphia: WB Saunders, 1988:223–241.

83. Hlatdy MA, Pryor DB, Harrell FE, et al. Factors affecting sensitivity and specificity of exercise electrocardiography: multivariable analysis. Am J Med 1984;77:64–71.

84. Marwick TH, Anderson T, Williams MJ, et al. Exercise echocardiography is an accurate and cost-efficient technique for detection of coronary artery disease in women. J Am Coll Cardiol 1995;26:335–341.

85. Hamby RI, Davison ET, Hilsenrath J, et al. Functional and anatomic correlates of markedly abnormal stress tests. J Am Coll Cardiol 1984;3:1375–1381.

86. DeBusk RF, Dennis CA. "Submaximal" predischarge exercise testing after acute myocardial infarction: who needs it? Am J Cardiol 1985;55:499–500.

87. Topol EJ, Juni JE, O'Neill WW, et al. Exercise testing three days after onset of acute myocardial infarction. Am J Cardiol 1987;60:958–962.

88. Sainiv, Graboys TB, Towne V, et al. Reproducibility of exercise-induced ventricular arrhythmia in patients undergoing evaluation for malignant ventricular arrhythmia. Am J Cardiol 1989;63:697–710.

89. Hammond HK, Kelly TL, Froelicher VF, et al. Use of clinical data in predicting improvement in exercise capacity after cardiac rehabilitation. J Am Coll Cardiol 1985;6:19–26.

90. Oren A, Sue DY, Hansen JE, et al. The role of exercise testing in impairment evaluation. Am Rev Respir Dis 1987;135:230–235.

91. Fein SA, Klein NA, Frishman WH. Exercise testing soon after uncomplicated myocardial infarction. Prognostic value and safety. JAMA 1981;245:1863–1868.

92. Taylor CB, Bandura A, Ewart CK, et al. Exercise testing to enhance wives' confidence in their husbands' cardiac capability soon after clinically uncomplicated acute myocardial infarction. Am J Cardiol 1985;55:635–638.

93. Froelicher VF, Perdue S, Pewen W, et al. Application of meta-analysis using an electronic spread sheet to exercise testing in patients after myocardial infarction. Am J Med 1987;83:1045–1054.

94. De Rouen TA, Hammermeister KE, Dodge HT. Comparison of the effects on survival after coronary artery surgery in subgroups of patients from the Seattle Heart Watch. Circulation 1981;63:537–545.

95. Akhras F, Upward J, Keates J, et al. Early exercise testing and elective coronary artery bypass surgery after uncomplicated myocardial infarction. Effect on morbidity and mortality. Br Heart J 1984;52:413–417.

96. Weiner DA, Ryan TJ, McCabe CH, et al. Value of exercise testing in determining the risk classification and the response to coronary artery bypass grafting in three-vessel coronary artery disease: a report from the Coronary Artery Surgery Study (CASS) registry. Am J Cardiol 1987;60:262–266.

97. Gohlke H, Gohlke BC, Samek L, et al. Serial exercise testing up to 6 years after coronary bypass surgery: behavior of exercise parameters in groups with different degrees of revascularization determined by postoperative angiography. Am J Cardiol 1983;51:1301–1306.

98. Weiner DA, McCabe CH, Roth RL, et al. Serial exercise testing after coronary artery bypass surgery. Am Heart J 1981;101:149–154.

99. Sarma RJ, Sanmarco ME. Reversal of exercise-induced hemodynamic and electrocardiographic abnormalities after coronary artery bypass surgery. Circulation 1982;65:684–689.

100. Weiner DA, Chaitman BR. Role of exercise testing in relationship to coronary artery bypass surgery and percutaneous transluminal coronary angioplasty. Cardiology 1986;73:242–258.

101. Wijns W, Serruys PW, Reiber JH, et al. Early detection of restenosis after successful percutaneous transluminal coronary angioplasty by exercise-redistribution thallium scintigraphy. Am J Cardiol 1985;55:357–361.

102. Wijns W, Serruys PW, Simoons ML, et al. Predictive value of early maximal exercise test and thallium scintigraphy after successful percutaneous transluminal coronary angioplasty. Br Heart J 1985;53:194–200.

103. Simoons ML, Vos J, Tijssen JG, et al. Long-term benefit of early thrombolytic therapy in patients with acute myocardial infarction: 5 year follow-up of a trial conducted by the Interuniversity Cardiology Institute of The Netherlands. J Am Coll Cardiol 1989;14:1609–1615.

104. Ellestad MH. Chronotropic incompetence. The implications of heart rate response to exercise (compensatory parasympathetic hyperactivity?). Circulation 1996;93:1485–1487.

105. Ellestad MH, Wan MK. Predictive implications of stress

testing. Follow-up of 2700 subjects after maximum treadmill stress testing. Circulation 1975;51:363–369.

106. Hinkle LE Jr, Carver ST, Plakun A. Slow heart rates and increased risk of cardiac death in middle-aged men. Arch Intern Med 1972;129:732–748.

107. Hammond HK, Kelly TL, Froelicher V. Radionuclide imaging correlatives of heart rate impairment during maximal exercise testing. J Am Coll Cardiol 1983;2: 826–833.

108. Beleslin BD, Ostojic M, Stepanovic J, et al. Stress echocardiography in the detection of myocardial ischemia. Head-to-head comparison of exercise, dobutamine, and dipyridamole tests. Circulation 1994;90: 1168–1176.

109. Marwick TH, Nemec JJ, Pashkow FJ, et al. Accuracy and limitations of exercise echocardiography in a routine clinical setting. J Am Coll Cardiol 1992;19:74–81.

110. Heller GV, Ahmed I, Tilkemeier PL, et al. Influence of exercise intensity on the presence, distribution, and size of thallium-201 defects. Am Heart J 1992;123:909–916.

111. Huang PJ, Chieng PU, Lee YT, et al. Exercise thallium-201 tomographic scintigraphy in the diagnosis of coronary artery disease: emphasis on the effect of exercise level. J Formosan Med Assoc 1992;91:1096–1101.

112. Lauer MS, Okin PM, Larson MG, et al. Impaired heart rate response to graded exercise. Prognostic implications of chronotropic incompetence in the Framingham Heart Study. Circulation 1996;93:1520–1526.

113. Colucci WS, Ribeiro JP, Rocco MB, et al. Impaired chronotropic response to exercise in patients with congestive heart failure. Role of postsynaptic beta-adrenergic desensitization. Circulation 1989;80: 314–323.

114. Francis GS, Goldsmith SR, Ziesche S, et al. Relative attenuation of sympathetic drive during exercise in patients with congestive heart failure. J Am Coll Cardiol 1985;5:832–839.

115. Lauer MS, Pashkow FJ, Larson MG, et al. Association of cigarette smoking with chronotropic incompetence and prognosis in the Framingham Heart Study. Circulation 1997;96:897–903.

116. Okin PM, Kligfield P. Heart rate adjustment of ST segment depression and performance of the exercise electrocardiogram: a critical evaluation. J Am Coll Cardiol 1995;25:1726–1735.

117. Okin PM, Lauer MS, Kligfield P. Chronotropic response to exercise. Improved performance of ST-segment depression criteria after adjustment for heart rate reserve. Circulation 1996;94:3226–3231.

118. Hammond HK, Froelicher VF. Normal and abnormal heart rate responses to exercise. Prog Cardiovasc Dis 1985;27:271–296.

119. Dyer AR, Persky V, Stamler J, et al. Heart rate as a prognostic factor for coronary heart disease and mortality: findings in three Chicago epidemiologic studies. Am J Epidemiol 1980;112:736–749.

120. Paffenbarger RS, Hale WE. Work activity and coronary heart mortality. N Engl J Med 1975;292:545–550.

121. Lakka TA, Venalainen JM, Rauramaa R, et al. Relation of leisure-time physical activity and cardiorespiratory fitness to the risk of acute myocardial infarction. N Engl J Med 1994;330:1549–1554.

122. Willich SN, Lewis M, Lowel H, et al. Physical exertion as a trigger of acute myocardial infarction. Triggers and mechanisms of Myocardial Infarction Study Group. N Engl J Med 1993;329:1684–1690.

123. Mittleman MA, Maclure M, Tofler GH, et al. Triggering of acute myocardial infarction by heavy physical exertion. Protection against triggering by regular exertion. Determinants of Myocardial Infarction Onset Study Investigators. N Engl J Med 1993;329:1677–1683.

124. Wilkoff BL, Miller RE. Exercise testing for chronotropic assessment. Cardiol Clin 1992;10:705–717.

125. Brener SJ, Pashkow FJ, Harvey SA, et al. Chronotropic response to exercise predicts angiographic severity in patients with suspected or stable coronary artery disease. Am J Cardiol 1995;76:1228–1232.

126. Holland RP, Arnsdorf MF. Solid angle theory and the electrocardiogram: physiologic and quantitative interpretations. Prog Cardiovasc Dis 1977;19:431–457.

127. Mirvis DM, Ramanathan KB. Alterations in transmural blood flow and body surface ST segment abnormalities produced by ischemia in the circumflex and left anterior descending coronary arterial beds of the dog. Circulation 1987;76:697–704.

128. Okin PM, Kligfield P. Solid-angle theory and heart rate adjustment of ST-segment depression for the identification and quantification of coronary artery disease. Am Heart J 1994;127:658–667.

129. Doan AE, Peterson DR, Blackmon JR, et al. Myocardial ischemia after maximal exercise in healthy men. One year follow-up of physically active and inactive men. Am J Cardiol 1966;17:9–19.

130. Okin PM, Anderson KM, Levy D, et al. Heart rate adjustment of exercise-induced ST segment depression. Improved risk stratification in the Framingham Offspring Study. Circulation 1991;83:866–874.

131. Okin PM, Kligfield P. Identifying coronary artery disease in women by heart rate adjustment of ST-segment depression and improved performance of linear regression over simple averaging method with comparison to standard criteria. Am J Cardiol 1992;69:297–302.

132. Okin PM, Kligfield P. Gender-specific criteria and performance of the exercise electrocardiogram. Circulation 1995;92:1209–1216.

133. Okin PM, Grandits G, Rautaharju PM, et al. Prognostic value of heart rate adjustment of exercise-induced ST segment depression in the multiple risk factor intervention trial. J Am Coll Cardiol 1996;27: 1437–1443.

134. Okin PM, Prineas RJ, Grandits G, et al. Heart rate adjustment of exercise-induced ST-segment depression identifies men who benefit from a risk factor reduction program. Circulation 1997;96:2899–2904.

135. Bigger JT Jr, Fleiss JL, Rolnitzky LM, et al. Frequency domain measures of heart period variability to assess risk late after myocardial infarction [published correction appears in J Am Coll Cardiol 1993;21:1537]. J Am Coll Cardiol 1993;21:729–736.

136. Kleiger RE, Miller JP, Krone RJ, et al. The independence of cycle length variability and exercise testing on predicting mortality of patients surviving acute myocardial infarction. The Multicenter Postinfarction Research Group. Am J Cardiol 1990;65:408–411.

137. Tsuji H, Venditti FJ Jr, Manders ES, et al. Reduced heart rate variability and mortality risk in an elderly cohort. The Framingham Heart Study. Circulation 1994;90:878–883.

138. Stein PK, Rottman JN, Kleiger RE. Effect of 21 mg transdermal nicotine patches and smoking cessation on heart rate variability. Am J Cardiol 1996;77: 701–705.

139. Chin CF, Messenger JC, Greenberg PS, et al. Chronotropic incompetence in exercise testing. Clin Cardiol 1979;2:12–18.

140. Mark AL. The Bezold-Jarisch reflex revisited: clinical implications of inhibitory reflexes originating in the heart. J Am Coll Cardiol 1983;1:90–102.

141. Hayano J, Yamada A, Mukai S, et al. Severity of coronary atherosclerosis correlates with the respiratory component of heart rate variability. Am Heart J 1991;121:1070–1079.

Cardiopulmonary Exercise Testing

Ileana L. Piña

Cardiopulmonary (metabolic) exercise testing is defined as an exercise testing procedure during which gas exchange is measured. The advent of up-to-date computerized systems coupled with rapid-response gas analyzers have taken this procedure from a cumbersome test performed in research laboratories to an acceptable and simple form of testing for the clinical arena. Much information can be processed in a short interval allowing a "view" into the physiology of the exercise response. The test can be reliable and reproducible if basic procedures are followed with consistency. Oxygen uptake ($\dot{V}O_2$) measured directly is much more accurate than assessing functional capacity simply by exercise time (1, 2). The information derived from cardiopulmonary testing (CPX) can be useful clinically as shown on Table 6.1.

DEFINITIONS

To better understand the process of cardiopulmonary testing and to interpret test results accurately, some basic definitions are necessary. The following are the most commonly used terms and variables measured during cardiopulmonary exercise testing (3).

Oxygen Uptake ($\dot{V}O_2$)

This is the amount of oxygen used while breathing room air whether at rest or during activity. Oxygen uptake is the product of the cardiac output (CO) and the arteriovenous oxygen (a–v O_2) difference. Hence, $\dot{V}O_2 = CO \times (a–v\ O_2)$. Oxygen uptake is expressed as volume in time, or flow, as mL/min or, when normalized to body weight, as $mL \cdot kg^{-1} \cdot min^{-1}$

Maximal Oxygen Uptake ($\dot{V}O_2 max$)

Also known as maximal aerobic capacity, this is a plateauing in the increase of $\dot{V}O_2$ with exercise in spite of increasing workload. It is closely related to maximal cardiac output with exercise, and influenced by age, sex, physical conditioning, obesity, and genetics. The average $\dot{V}O_2 max$ for untrained middle-aged adults ranges between 30 and 40 $mL \cdot kg^{-1} \cdot min^{-1}$.

Peak Oxygen Uptake (Peak $\dot{V}O_2$)

This is the highest $\dot{V}O_2$ achieved during an exercise test. It may not be the same as the $\dot{V}O_2 max$.

Anaerobic or Ventilatory Threshold

The anaerobic (AT) or ventilatory threshold (VT) is the $\dot{V}O_2$ at which anaerobic metabolism supersedes aerobic metabolism during exercise. It is also the point at which lactate increases in plasma during exercise indicating a limitation in oxygen transport. The AT or VT occurs at 50% to 60% of $\dot{V}O_2 max$ in sedentary individuals. There are multiple methodologies used to assess the AT. Some of these will be discussed below.

$\dot{V}CO_2$

Carbon dioxide production is measured in the expired gas. It is expressed as a flow measurement in mL/min and closely parallels $\dot{V}O_2$ before the anaerobic threshold. The $\dot{V}CO_2$ increases more steeply beyond the anaerobic threshold.

O_2 Pulse

The O_2 pulse equals the $\dot{V}O_2$ divided by heart rate which equals stroke volume times (a–v O_2) difference. The O_2 pulse reflects the capacity of the heart to deliver O_2 per beat. A value of less than 80% predicted based on height, weight, age, and sex at peak effort is considered abnormal.

Respiratory Exchange Ratio

The respiratory exchange ratio (RER) is the ratio of $\dot{V}CO_2$ to $\dot{V}O_2$. The RER can be used as an

Table 6.1. Clinical Applications of Cardiopulmonary Exercise Testing

Complement a standard exercise test for diagnostic purposes
Complement nuclear studies, e.g., thallium imaging
Evaluate the source of dyspnea
Assess true functional capacity of patients with heart failure
Assess prognosis in patients with heart failure
Evaluate patients for listing for cardiac transplantation
Review patients listed for cardiac transplantation
Assess effects of therapeutic interventions
Assign an accurate exercise prescription
Assess sports fitness
Determine disability
Evaluate before surgery, e.g., valvular replacement

assessment of effort. An RER of greater than 1.1 nearly always assures that the AT has been achieved. Values approaching or exceeding 1.3 are highly unusual in patients with cardiac disease and may signal gas-analyzing system problems that need to be addressed.

Minute Ventilation ($\dot{V}E$)

Minute ventilation is a measure of the ventilatory response to exercise expressed as liters per minute. The maximum $\dot{V}E$ achieved must be related to the amount of work performed. The maximum voluntary ventilation (MVV) can be approximated by age, height, weight, and sex or measured during pulmonary function tests. The MVV is often also referred to as the maximal ventilatory capacity.

Ventilatory Equivalent for $\dot{V}CO_2$ ($\dot{V}E/\dot{V}CO_2$)

$\dot{V}E/\dot{V}CO_2$ can serve as a measure of abnormal ventilation–perfusion relation and as an estimator of dead space ventilation. It is a noninvasive assessment of the appropriateness of minute ventilation.

Breathing or Ventilatory Reserve

The relationship of $\dot{V}E$max to MVV is the ventilatory reserve. It can be expressed as either MVV $-$ $\dot{V}E$max or 1 $-$ $\dot{V}E$max/MVV. The latter expression in normal subjects is usually 20% to 50%. Extremely well-conditioned athletes may have a breathing reserve of close to 100%. The breathing reserve is a very important parameter to measure in cardiopulmonary testing particularly if a ventilatory reason for symptoms is sought.

PRINCIPLES OF GAS EXCHANGE

To better understand the derivation of gas exchange parameters, it is worthwhile reviewing basic cardiopulmonary physiology. The concept of the cardiopulmonary unit aptly defines the contributions of the respiratory (cellular and pulmonary) and the cardiovascular systems to support the increasing metabolic rate and gas exchange of contracting muscles while performing exercise. This concept was described by Wasserman and colleagues (3) and is depicted in Figure 6.1. The gas transport system couples cellular or internal respiration to pulmonary or external respiration using the cardiovascular system in a direct and integrated fashion. The energy necessary for muscle contraction is derived primarily from the mitochondria in the form of ATP. Phosphocreatine is a shuttle for high-energy phosphate but the stores of phosphocreatine are limited. To sustain muscle activity, therefore, ATP must be regenerated primarily aerobically. Aerobic production of ATP requires oxygen in increasing quantities during exercise and is reflected by an increasing $\dot{V}O_2$. The increased utilization of O_2 during exercise requires an increased delivery of O_2 and is achieved by increased O_2 extraction at the muscle site, dilation of the selected vascular beds, an increase in cardiac output, an increase in pulmonary blood flow, and an increase in ventilation.

The increased delivery of O_2 to the mitochondria also includes an increase in the removal of CO_2 as shown in the first gear of Figure 6.1. The excess CO_2 is eliminated during ventilation. Therefore, $\dot{V}O_2$ and $\dot{V}CO_2$ rise in parallel during exercise until the point at which O_2 delivery lessens and anaerobic metabolism ensues, thereby increasing the rate of CO_2 production to exceed $\dot{V}O_2$.

At the point when the circulation can no longer deliver more O_2 to sustain exercise, the production of ATP will also slow down and will be reflected by a slowing of the $\dot{V}O_2$ rate of increase with the appearance of ATP generated anaerobically. At this point, lactic acid will be-

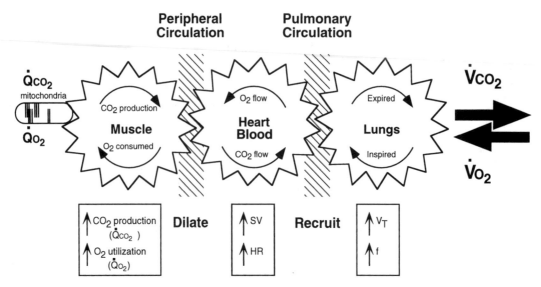

Figure 6.1. The gas transport mechanism that joins cellular or internal respiration to pulmonary or external respiration. There is interdependence of muscle, heart and blood, and lungs. To do work, O_2 is extracted from blood, which perfuses working muscle. The increase in O_2 is also facilitated by peripheral vasodilation, an increase in cardiac output, an increase in pulmonary blood flow, and an increase in ventilation. Ideally $\dot{V}o_2$ is equal to $\dot{Q}o_2$ so that the amount of oxygen uptake matches the amount of oxygen required by the mitochondria. Ventilation (tidal volume and breathing frequency) will increase in response to the CO_2 produced. $\dot{Q}o_2$, utilization of O_2 by muscles; $\dot{Q}co_2$, CO_2 produced at the muscle site; SV, stroke volume; HR, heart rate; Vt, tidal volume; f, breathing frequency.

gin to accumulate, buffered by HCO_3^- and increased CO_2 production measured in the expired gases. Therefore, the appearance of excess lactic acid in the periphery has been identified at the point of rapid increase of $\dot{V}co_2$ in relation to $\dot{V}o_2$.

Ventilatory Parameters

A description of ventilation-related responses to exercise forms an essential core of cardiopulmonary testing. The appropriateness of ventilation depends on its effectiveness in producing the appropriate gas exchange and how it regulates acid–base balance. Therefore, ventilation needs to increase in proportion to the metabolic rate to accommodate CO_2 exchange. The amount of ventilation necessary to clear a certain amount of CO_2 depends on the CO_2 concentration in the alveolar gas. Not all respired air, however, ventilates the lung completely because some air goes to the large airways not involved in gas exchange and to the nonperfused alveoli. The ratio of ventilatory dead space and the tidal volume (VD/VT) determines the difference between the volume of air respired and the theoretical ideal alveolar ventilation. The $\dot{V}E$ is thus closely coupled to the

$\dot{V}co_2$. If the $\dot{V}E$ does not rise in concordance with the appearance of CO_2, respiratory acidosis would ensue. Conversely, if $\dot{V}E$ rises out of proportion to the production of CO_2, respiratory alkalosis would occur. However, exercise at moderate work intensities keeps a steady Pao_2, $Paco_2$, and pH (see Fig. 6.2). The slope of the relationship between $\dot{V}E$ and $\dot{V}co_2$ has been described in normal subjects and is higher in patients with heart failure (see Fig. 6.3) (3–5). More recently, a steeper $\dot{V}E/\dot{V}co_2$ slope has been described in older healthy adults between the ages of 55 and 86 years (6).

The behavior of $\dot{V}E$ with exercise will indicate a component of dyspnea from ventilatory causes. In ordinary exercise, the maximum $\dot{V}E$ remains below 60% of the maximum ventilation. The breathing reserve is expressed as the MVV − $\dot{V}E$max but can also be defined as 1 − $\dot{V}E$max/MVV. Patients with a pulmonary disease entity, e.g., pulmonary fibrosis, will encroach on the ventilatory reserve early in exercise (3).

Anaerobic or Ventilatory Threshold

The amount of oxygen required for any given amount of work is approximately 10 mL/W regardless of fitness, age, or sex (2). Once the car-

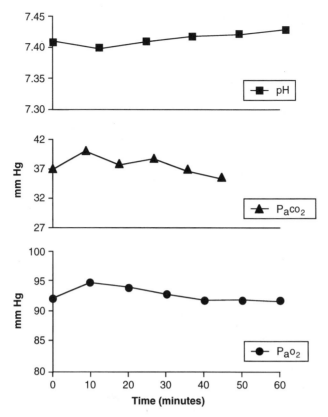

Figure 6.2. Exercise at moderate intensities maintains PaO_2, $PaCO_2$, and pH relatively steady. Should exercise increase beyond this point, $\dot{V}E$ increases in proportion to the CO_2 produced. PaO_2 and $PaCO_2$ are in mm Hg, and the x axis is time in minutes.

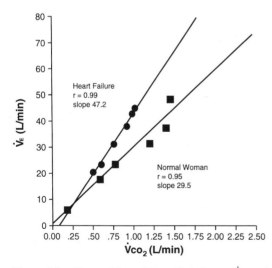

Figure 6.3. Slope of the relationship between $\dot{V}E$ and $\dot{V}CO_2$. The slope of a normal healthy 46-year-old woman and that of a 62-year-old man with moderate heart failure are illustrated. The slope of $\dot{V}E$ versus $\dot{V}CO_2$ has been consistently shown to be higher in patients with heart failure.

diopulmonary unit can no longer deliver adequate O_2 to sustain work, lactic acid accumulates. The work rate at which lactic acid increases is usually unique for an individual and is a measure of the degree of fitness. The $\dot{V}O_2$ point, or threshold above which anaerobic metabolism exceeds aerobic metabolism, is termed the AT. More recently, the term "ventilatory threshold" has been preferred, because the measurement of this point is performed by gas exchange in expired air.

$\dot{V}O_2$ kinetics below the VT reach a steady state at approximately 3 minutes in normal subjects exercising at a moderate work intensity. Before the VT, the $\dot{V}CO_2$ is slightly lower than the $\dot{V}O_2$. Once the VT is achieved at higher work intensity, the rate of rise of $\dot{V}O_2$ slows down and may not reach a steady state, whereas the rate of $\dot{V}CO_2$ accelerates. It is reasonable, thus, to use the rate of $\dot{V}CO_2$ versus $\dot{V}O_2$ to assess the VT. This explanation forms the basis of the V-slope method of VT measurement (7).

The VT usually occurs at 50% to 60% of $\dot{V}O_2$max but will be higher in fit individuals. In patients with cardiac disease, e.g., heart failure, the VT may occur earlier. The VT is reproducible in any given individual regardless of testing protocol (8), and should improve with a conditioning program. In any test given for derivation of an exercise prescription before training, the VT should be recorded and assessed once again during the posttraining test.

The V-slope method of VT determination is widely used today although there are still controversies surrounding its general applicability in all disease states (see Fig. 6.4) (7). Another method includes determination of the nadir of $\dot{V}E/\dot{V}O_2$ (ventilatory equivalent of O_2) in relation to the $\dot{V}E/\dot{V}CO_2$ (ventilatory equivalent of CO_2) curve (see Fig. 6.5) (2). Generally, $\dot{V}E$ and $\dot{V}CO_2$ accelerate in a proportional manner above the VT, but there is a short period when $\dot{V}E/\dot{V}CO_2$ does not change while $\dot{V}E/\dot{V}O_2$ increases. As the VT is exceeded, $\dot{V}E$ increases in relation to O_2 but not to CO_2. The increase in $\dot{V}E/\dot{V}O_2$ with no increase in $\dot{V}E/\dot{V}CO_2$ is an indication that VT has been attained.

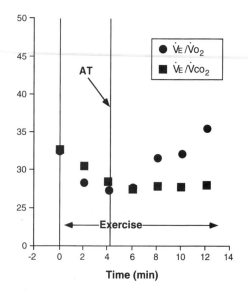

Figure 6.5. Determination of the anaerobic (AT) or ventilatory (VT) threshold by the ventilatory equivalents for $\dot{V}O_2$ and $\dot{V}CO_2$. The AT or VT is defined as the initial point of systematic increase in $\dot{V}E/\dot{V}O_2$ without a concomitant increase in $\dot{V}E/\dot{V}CO_2$.

CARDIOPULMONARY EXERCISE TESTING EQUIPMENT: BASIC PRINCIPLES, CALIBRATION, AND SETUP

A diagram of the process of measuring expired gases is depicted in Figure 6.6. Figure 6.7A is a photograph of a metabolic computer system. Metabolic systems are capable of measuring three variables (9):

1. The fraction of O_2 and CO_2 in the inspired air.
2. The fraction of O_2 and CO_2 in the expired air.
3. The volume of inspired or expired air and breathing rate.

More commonly, only the fraction of CO_2 and O_2 in expired air is measured in the systems that are widely available today. With these variables, minute ventilation $\dot{V}E$, oxygen uptake $\dot{V}O_2$, and CO_2 production $\dot{V}CO_2$ are derived. Thus, $\dot{V}O_2$ (mL/min) $= \dot{V}E \times (FIO_2 - FEO_2)$ where FIO_2 is the fraction of O_2 in inspired air and FEO_2 is the fraction of O_2 in expired air. Although mixing chambers for collection of expired gases were the rule in the past, current technology makes breath-by-breath measurements feasible and reliable.

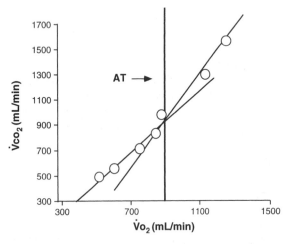

Figure 6.4. The V-slope method of determining the anaerobic or ventilatory threshold (AT or VT). The production of CO_2 is less influenced by oscillatory changes in ventilation and directly influenced by lactate production and accumulation. The regression of $\dot{V}CO_2$ versus $\dot{V}O_2$ is shown for a healthy man. The point of inflection at which $\dot{V}CO_2$ increases relative to $\dot{V}O_2$ is labeled as AT.

Metabolic System Basics

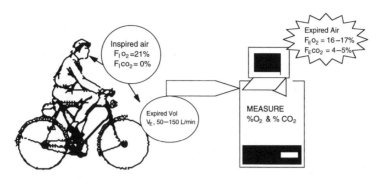

Figure 6.6. Diagram demonstrating the basic concept of a metabolic system. The fractions of inspired oxygen and carbon dioxide (F_{IO_2} and F_{ICO_2}) are known. The expired volume is measured as well as the concentration of both O_2 and CO_2 in the expired air (F_{EO_2} and F_{ECO_2}). In a simplified manner, $\dot{V}_{O_2}$ (mL/min) = $\dot{V}_E \times (F_{IO_2} - F_{EO_2})$.

Calibration

It is essential to calibrate the system daily, at the beginning of the testing period, and to check systems before each test. A copy of the initial calibration report should be filed in a separate binder for quality assurance purposes. The calibration report for each test should be added to the testing report to attest to the validity of the measurements. Gas analyzers are also calibrated according to the specifications of the manufacturer. Most metabolic systems will also calibrate for airflow with a syringe of known volume. Because each system carries its own calibration peculiarities, the reader is advised to follow the instructions of the gas exchange system's manufacturer for the best testing results.

EXPIRED VENTILATION

Expired air is collected through a mouthpiece with a tight seal and a nose clip. If the patient cannot tolerate the mouthpiece, an air-tight mask is recommended. The usual dead space found in most mouthpieces is 100 mL. The smaller the dead space, although permitting a greater accuracy of ventilation, the higher the resistance through the mouthpiece.

PNEUMOTACHOMETERS

The pneumotachometer measures flow, which is proportional to changes of airflow pressure, through a tube or a series of wire screens. A picture of a modern pneumotachometer is seen in Figure 6.7B. This mouthpiece is light and comfortable.

GAS ANALYZERS

Today's gas analyzers are rapid responding with a zirconium cell for oxygen and an infrared analyzer for carbon dioxide. The rapidity of response (less than or equal to 100 ms) allows the systems to read $\dot{V}_{O_2}$ and $\dot{V}_{CO_2}$ on line with breath-by-breath measurements. The response of both gas analyzers is linear and allows calibration with only one certified gas mixture. The usual calibrations gases have a concentration of 5% to 7% for CO_2 and 12% to 16% for O_2.

Because O_2 concentration varies with ambient temperature, barometric pressure, and humidity, most metabolic systems allow for correction of ambient O_2 concentration. At an ideal temperature of 22°C the relationship between O_2 and humidity is shown on Figure 6.8 (9).

PHASE DELAY

The difference in time from the moment that the pneumotachometer measures air volume (almost instantaneously) to the moment the gas analyzers measure the gas concentrations is the phase delay. Once measured, the phase delay is used to adjust the time course of each volume received to match the time course of gas concentration changes.

SYSTEM VALIDATION

Validation includes not only the daily calibration report but also a periodic series of tests to verify reproducibility. Reproducibility can be demonstrated either by repeated maximal testing on normal subjects or by exercising normal

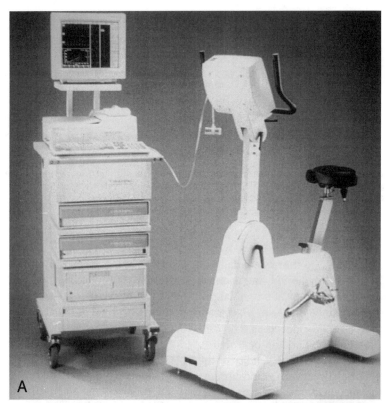

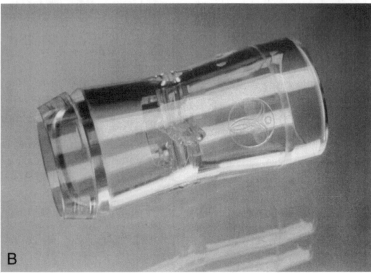

Figure 6.7.   A. A modern metabolic gas exchange system is compact and includes the desktop computer system. An electronically braked bicycle ergometer is shown. **B.** Disposable pneumotachometer is pictured. Ventilation volume is measured as the difference in pressure between the two sides of a small strut placed in the middle of the clear cylinder. (Compliments of Medical Graphics Corporation, St. Paul, MN.)

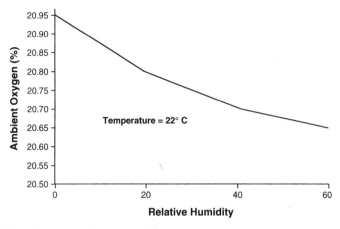

Figure 6.8. The relationship between O_2 and humidity. O_2 is expressed as a percent and the relative humidity at a temperature of 22°C. The importance of adjusting O_2 concentration to ambient temperature and humidity is evident. The slope of this line changes with temperature as well. (Reprinted with permission from Piña IL, Balady GJ, Hanson P, et al: Guidelines for clinical exercise testing laboratories. Circulation 1995;91:912–919.)

subjects at a steady workload state and comparing the $\dot{V}O_2$ with the O_2 costs of predicted submaximal workloads. Suggested limits of variability among tests are shown in Table 6.2 (9).

CONDUCTING THE CARDIOPULMONARY TEST

Equipment and Techniques

LABORATORY PHYSICAL FACILITY

The CPX testing laboratory should be set up according to American Heart Association standards (10). The room should be well-ventilated with sufficient space to hold all equipment. Patient privacy during testing is essential. A barometer, thermometer, and hygrometer should be available in the testing area to adjust gases during calibration of the metabolic testing system (see below). Ideally, room temperature should be kept at 22°C with a humidity of 50%.

Treadmill testing is the most common form of ergometry used clinically for CPX, but a bicycle should be available for patients who cannot use the treadmill or for stabilization of catheters when performing CPX in conjunction with hemodynamic monitoring. A suitable electrocardiographic system is necessary for evaluation of arrhythmias and ECG changes during exercise. Some modern metabolic testing systems are available with electrocardiographic monitoring built-in. If not, most standard ECG recording exercise systems can be connected to the metabolic

cart so that speed, grade, workload, and heart rate are read directly into the gas exchange system. In addition, blood pressure cuffs of various sizes should be available to accommodate different arm sizes. A large-print scale of the Borg or Modified Borg scale (11) will allow communication with the patient to determine perceived effort. An additional scale of symptom severity can also be useful. Emergency equipment should include a "crash cart" with all appropriate medications and a defibrillator.

All equipment should be placed under a routine maintenance schedule including inspection and calibration. Ergometer calibration is outside of the scope of this chapter. However, the reader is referred to the Guidelines for Clinical Exercise Testing Laboratories of the American Heart Association for a more thorough discussion (10).

PERSONNEL

Administering and interpreting the CPX test requires skill and competency. Although require-

Table 6.2. Variability: Repeated Testing— Steady State

Variable	Limit ($\pm$)
Oxygen uptake	5.1%
Carbon dioxide output	6.2%
Ventilation	5.0%
Heart rate	4.7%
Mixed venous P_{CO_2}	2.7%
Cardiac output	8.9%

(Adapted from Jones NL. Clinical Exercise Testing 1988.)

ments for physician competency in exercise testing have been clearly defined, strict requirements for interpretation of CPX testing by physicians have not been so clearly specified. Staff members administering the test must receive basic life support training. It is highly recommended that physicians have advanced cardiac life support training.

It is the responsibility of the physician to interpret the test in a timely fashion. Preliminary reports should be provided immediately after testing. Suggestions for test interpretation will be presented later in this chapter.

PATIENT PREPARATION

A written consultation for CPX testing is strongly encouraged. The request should include the patient's diagnosis and list of medications as well as the reason for testing. As in any other diagnostic procedure, taking at least a brief history is essential. The history should include the type of activities that the patient is accustomed to, including job-related activities and any recreational sports. The time when medications were last taken should be noted. Timing of drug therapy is especially important for β-blockers, which can alter rest and exercise heart rate and may also decrease peak $\dot{V}O_2$max (12). Patient instructions should include abstinence from food for at least 3 hours before testing. Clothing should be loose and comfortable, and include secure footwear.

INFORMED CONSENT

The informed consent should be made part of the testing record. Taking informed consent includes an explanation of testing procedures and any discomfort that the patient may experience. The mouthpiece for gas exchange may cause dryness of the oral mucosa and give the sensation of resistance. The patient should be advised of these usual occurrences as normal and to be expected. If patients cannot tolerate a mouthpiece, a mask should be available. The written and verbal informed consent needs to include all risks involved in testing. The patient should clearly understand that the test will be stopped at the patient's request but that an adequate exercise response is crucial for adequate interpretation of the data. A sample informed consent is included in appendix 6.A.

ELECTRODES AND SKIN PREPARATION

The electrodes used should be identical to those used for standard exercise testing. Skin prepara-

tion should be optimal to obtain the best tracing. The reader is once again referred to the Guidelines for Clinical Exercise Testing Laboratories published by the American Heart Association (10).

RESTING DATA

Usual resting parameters such as blood pressure, sitting and standing, and resting heart rate should be recorded. To ensure accurate data during exercise testing, it is essential that an adequate collection of gases be performed at rest. A minimum of 2 minutes of a stable baseline $\dot{V}O_2$ is optimal. Any potential problems with the metabolic system are likely to be observed during this resting collection, allowing time for correcting the problem before initiating the exercise portion of testing. This resting period also allows the patient to become accustomed to the mouthpiece or mask.

EXERCISE DATA

Testing of patients with gas exchange measurements can be performed either on a treadmill or bicycle ergometer. The bicycle ergometer offers the convenience of a stable sitting position, which allows more accurate measurements of blood pressure and particularly of concomitant hemodynamic measurements. Walking, however, is more familiar to the average U.S. population and patients may be capable of performing at a higher level. The exercise testing results, however, will vary with the testing mode. More specifically, peak $\dot{V}O_2$, the anaerobic threshold, and minute ventilation will be higher with treadmill testing than with bicycle ergometry. On the other hand, heart rate, systolic blood pressure, RER, and rate of perceived exertion (RPE) can be identical with both testing modalities (13).

The choice of protocol will often depend on the functional status of the patient including any other conditions that could limit exercise. Protocols with stages of 2 or 3 minutes' duration will show an increment in $\dot{V}O_2$ until a steady state is achieved at each stage and therefore may have the appearance of a stepwise increase in $\dot{V}O_2$ (see Fig. 6.9). Ramp protocols change workload at each minute or at 30-second intervals and give a much smoother $\dot{V}O_2$ curve. Ramp protocols can also be tailored to the ability of the patient being tested. It may be more important to select protocols by patient and not rely solely on one or two protocols that may not allow enough time at a

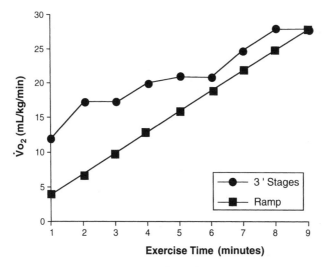

Figure 6.9. Oxygen uptake expressed as $mL \cdot kg^{-1} \cdot min^{-1}$ for two protocols. The protocol with 3-minute stages shows a plateau effect at each stage whereas the progressively increasing ramp protocol shows a smooth increase in $\dot{V}O_2$. The plateau effect lessens as the AT is approached or exceeded.

relatively low workload to observe all the necessary measurements. The Bruce protocol has been commonly used in exercise testing laboratories that use radionuclide imaging. The Bruce protocol may be too challenging from Stage 1 for more deconditioned patients or for those patients with impaired left ventricular function.

In most patients, exercise duration alone is not nearly as reproducible as measurements of gas exchange. Oxygen uptake and anaerobic threshold are highly reproducible (14). In patients with heart failure, the Modified Naughton protocol has been used extensively in published works of exercise response in this specific patient population (15). Thus, the Modified Naughton became the rule rather than the exception when choosing exercise protocols. Exercise testing, however, can be performed using a variety of published protocols. The protocol chosen often depends on the experience of the testing physician and on the norms of any specific testing facility.

However, the selection of protocols for cardiopulmonary testing should follow the same criteria as when choosing protocols for other testing purposes, e.g., ischemia. An exercise protocol should yield the maximum amount of information and truly assess a patient's maximal or near-maximal function with a high degree of confidence and reproducibility. Breathlessness may be the salient symptom when exercise is of sudden onset, whereas fatigue predominates at slow but longer-lasting activity. A fast protocol

(high workload presented rapidly) will generally yield a higher $\dot{V}O_2$max, cardiac output, and a greater degree of breathlessness. In contrast, a slow protocol will most likely provoke fatigue at a lower $\dot{V}O_2$max and cardiac output (16). Protocols lasting longer than 10 to 12 minutes may also be associated with boredom and lack of motivation on the part of the patient.

It is more crucial that the patient be able to perform a certain workload comfortably to determine a true level of functional capacity for that individual. Subsequently, the Balke, Ellestad, and modified Astrand protocols apply speeds that may be too difficult for a patient with known cardiac disease and deconditioning (17). Similarly, the Bruce protocol may be too challenging and difficult because of its large increments in workload per stage, and although patients with heart failure can perform this protocol, the duration of exercise may be short-lived (18).

Ramp protocols provide an interesting alternative to the standard 2 and 3 minutes per stage protocols. In addition, ramp protocols can be created across various levels of difficulty, thus ensuring the patient's ability to perform in accordance with individual capabilities. Most ramp protocols are in 1-minute stages with constant speed and increasing elevations allowing a desirable time of completion of less than 10 minutes. An additional benefit to ramp protocols lies in the linear increase in $\dot{V}O_2$ versus time allowing a better visualization of a maximum $\dot{V}O_2$ or "plateau," if attained.

When using gas exchange in addition to ECG monitoring, it is more important to achieve, at the very least, an anaerobic threshold and, preferably, as close to a true maximum $\dot{V}O_2$ as possible than to use the same protocol routinely. Exercise that is sufficient to reach an anaerobic threshold demonstrates a significant level of effort on the part of the patient. Furthermore, the anaerobic threshold is effort- and protocol-independent and should be a minimal target in testing (18). If properly measured, the anaerobic threshold is also reproducible in repeated testing and can be used as a clinical and prognostic tool as well (14). By using the V-slope method among others (7), the anaerobic threshold can be adequately measured in most patients with heart failure. The V-slope methodology will be discussed subsequently. The Weber classification (A through D) has been applied to the level of functional capacity as defined by $\dot{V}O_2$max and by anaerobic threshold in patients with impaired left ventricular function with a range of cardiac indices (see Table 6.3).

REASONS FOR STOPPING THE TEST

It is advantageous in most instances to allow the patient to exercise to a maximum point of fatigue. Although this point may be difficult to assess in ordinary exercise testing, the addition of gas exchange measurements simplifies it. Minimum exercise should include the achievement of a ventilatory (anaerobic) threshold. Only then can repeated testing serve for comparison. The ventilatory threshold should be reproducible in stable clinical conditions. This important level of $\dot{V}O_2$ should also increase in parallel with $\dot{V}O_2$ maximum on completion of a cardiac rehabilitation program. Therefore, every effort should be made to encourage the patient to continue beyond an RER of 1.0 to assure that the VT has been reached. Although the appearance of a plateau indicates the approximation of maximum exercise, patients who are deconditioned or have significant ventricular impairment may find the sensation of maximum exercise difficult to tolerate and may not be able to achieve it.

Patients with ischemia induced by exercise may also not be able to attain a maximum test by RER criteria. Nonetheless, the information acquired as to the onset of ischemia by ECG or by symptoms will have clinical relevance and allow an exercise prescription to be written within the asymptomatic period. In addition, there are other clinical entities that limit exercise, such as peripheral vascular disease with claudication, neuromuscular impediments, and pulmonary disease, among others.

As in standard exercise testing, clinical observation of the patient is essential as well as careful monitoring of the blood pressure during exercise along with the heart rate and the exercise ECG. Testing should always be stopped if the patient wishes to do so or if the physician responsible for the testing process feels that it is necessary for the patient's well-being.

Because verbal communication with the gas exchange system in place is not feasible, a printed scale of perceived exertion, e.g., the Borg Scale or a scale indicating symptoms, should be available and placed before the patient. It is crucial that the patient understand that communication of symptoms and effort level will be possible in spite of the lack of verbalization. A small amount of time spent during pretesting to adequately explain the Borg scale will be rewarded by a better patient assessment of personal effort. Perceived exertion scales can be important for patients whose heart rate may be blunted by β-adrenergic blocking agents or in cardiac transplant recipients whose lack of vagal input results in a flat chronotropic response.

REPORTING THE TEST RESULTS

A preliminary report should be immediately available. Most cardiopulmonary exercise systems have the ability to print a basic report eas-

Table 6.3.   Functional Impairment During Incremental Treadmill Testing: The Weber Classification

Class	Severity	Peak $\dot{V}O_2$ (mL·kg^{-1}·min^{-1})	AT	CL max (L·min^{-1}·m^{-2})
A	Mild to none	>20	>14	>8
B	Mild to moderate	16–20	11–14	6–8
C	Moderate to severe	10–16	8–11	4–6
D	Severe	6–10	5–8	2–4
E	Very severe	<6	<4	<2

$\dot{V}O_2$, oxygen uptake; AT, anaerobic threshold; CI, cardiac index.

ily. Some systems will also completely analyze the test. Because the input of a patient's history or an interpretation based on the clinical question is difficult to extract from a computerized system, we recommend a separate written report that synthesizes the entire test, including blood pressure, heart rate, exercise ECG, and the gas exchange interpretation. An example of a test report is included as appendix 6.B.

INTERPRETATION OF THE CARDIOPULMONARY TEST

When a cardiopulmonary test is ordered, the physician should have a clinical question concerning exercise limitations or symptoms that the test may help to elucidate. Seeking to answer a specific question will help to focus the interpretation of the test.

Wasserman and colleagues (3) have presented a logical algorithm for test interpretation. Analysis should begin with a decision on whether the $\dot{V}O_2$ achieved is normal or abnormal. The testing center must decide on a range of normal values using either a standardized predictive equation or by derivation from a center-specific set of normal subjects. Table 6.4 represents three methodolo-

gies for age- and sex-adjusted predicted maximal $\dot{V}O_2$ (3, 19, 20). Not all available predicted equations have been equally tested in both extremes of age, i.e., the very young and the elderly, particularly older women. If the $\dot{V}O_2$ is normal and the patient complains of exercise intolerance, possible causes may be early cardiovascular disease, obesity, or anxiety. If the $\dot{V}O_2$ is low, an analysis of anaerobic or ventilatory threshold should follow. A normal AT should prompt an assessment of the ventilatory reserve. If the ventilatory reserve is normal, the patient may have provided a poor effort, could be deconditioned or in the presence of an abnormal ECG, or have ischemia. If the breathing reserve is abnormal, pulmonary disease is probably present. If the AT is low and the breathing reserve is normal, cardiovascular disease or peripheral vascular disease is probably present. On the other hand, if the breathing reserve is also abnormal, the patient may have a mixed condition of cardiovascular and pulmonary limitations. Figure 6.10 will be helpful to keep as an analysis algorithm tree. As in any other diagnostic test, the analysis must be made in light of the patient's clinical picture and known disease entities.

INDICATIONS FOR CARDIOPULMONARY TESTING

The indications for the assessment of cardiopulmonary parameters with exercise testing are multiple and are shown in Table 6.1. The following sections will discuss briefly some of those applications.

Assessment of Ischemia

Although not commonly used in clinical practice, the use of gas exchange indices in patients with coronary artery disease will add another dimension to regular exercise testing. Myocardial ischemia can lead to a reduced maximum $\dot{V}O_2$ and anaerobic threshold. In these cases, the breathing reserve is normal unless there is concomitant pulmonary disease. Exertional breathlessness can accompany ischemia but could be caused by deconditioning or respiratory impairment. Predicting $\dot{V}O_2$max can be influenced by a variety of factors including the treadmill experience of the patient, inherent inaccuracies of predictive equations, and the design of the testing protocol. Therefore, when the evaluation of true functional capacity or response to therapy is needed, the objective assessment of $\dot{V}O_2$ will provide accurate results. In addi-

---

Table 6.4. Predicted Maximum Oxygen Uptake

Equations from Wasserman et al.

The following equations normalize weight to height:

Men:　W = 0.79H − 60.7

Women: W = 0.79H − 68.2

Overweight is defined as weight in excess of weight calculated from the above equations.

Men

Overweight:　$\dot{V}O_2$max = (0.79H − 60.7) × (56.36 − 0.413A)

Not overweight: $\dot{V}O_2$max = W × (56.36 − 0.413A)

Women

Overweight:　$\dot{V}O_2$max = (0.79H − 68.2) × (44.37 − 0.413A)

Not overweight: $\dot{V}O_2$max = W × (44.37 − 0.413A)

Equations from Jones et al.

Men:　4.2 − 0.032A

Women: 2.6 − 0.14A

Equations from Bruce et al.

Sedentary men:　57.8 − 0.445A

Sedentary women: 41.2 − 0.343A

W, weight in kg; H, height in cm; A, age in years.

(Wasserman K, Hansen JE, Sue Dy, et al. Principles of exercise testing and interpretation. Philadelphia: Lea & Febiger, 1987. Jones NL, Campbell EJM, Edwards RHT, et al. Clinical exercise testing, Philadelphia: WB Saunders, 1975:202.)

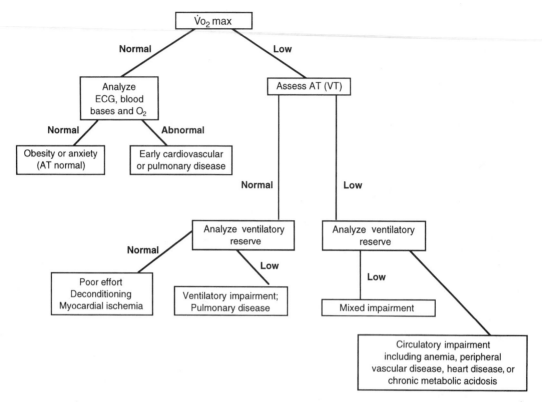

Figure 6.10.   Algorithm for analysis of cardiopulmonary testing. See text for full details. First, an assessment of $\dot{V}_{O_2}$ is necessary to determine whether the value is normal or low for age, sex, height, and weight. If the $\dot{V}_{O_2}$ is low, an evaluation of AT is next. After AT assessment, the behavior of ventilation in light of the work performed and the effort expended is reviewed. (Reprinted with permission from Wasserman K, Hansen JE, Sue DY, et al. Principles of exercise testing and interpretation. Philadelphia: Lea & Febiger, 1987.)

tion, as noted above, patients with coronary artery disease may also experience respiratory symptoms. Objective assessment of gas exchange will help to clarify the clinical situation and rule out the presence of pulmonary disease.

After myocardial infarction, many studies have shown that exercise testing is predictive of mortality (21, 22). Most studies however, have set a level of submaximal exercise such as MET, workload, or heart rate. More recently, peak oxygen uptake has been shown to provide independent prognostic information in patients with coronary artery disease (23). In addition, maximal exercise testing is a more potent predictor of mortality than testing to a set value of METs or a predetermined heart rate (24, 25). Using cardiopulmonary parameters, the level of effort can be better assessed to approach a maximal test.

Determination of peak $\dot{V}_{O_2}$ and anaerobic threshold has also been used to evaluate the development of heart failure in patients treated with an angiotensin-converting enzyme inhibitor after myocardial infarction (26). The peak $\dot{V}_{O_2}$ and anaerobic threshold of a captopril-treated group showed a small difference in favor of the angiotensin-converting enzyme inhibitor–treated group when compared with placebo, as well as fewer heart failure events.

In patients with silent ischemia, the use of gas exchange testing has identified that this group of patients has a significantly higher peak $\dot{V}_{O_2}$, anaerobic threshold, and oxygen pulse than patients with symptomatic ischemia regardless of the severity of coronary artery disease (27). In fact, the peak $\dot{V}_{O_2}$ of patients with silent ischemia approaches that of normals.

Valvular Heart Disease

Cardiopulmonary exercise testing can provide valuable information in patients with known valvular disease especially after surgical or percutaneous interventions.

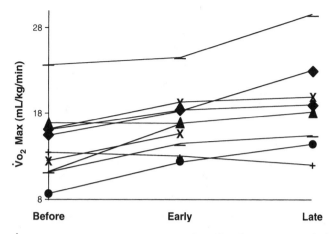

Figure 6.11. Exercise $\dot{V}O_2$max before and early (12 ± 4.2 days) and late (15 ± 2.3 weeks) after balloon mitral valvu-loplasty in a group of 10 patients. Note that the majority of patients exhibit an increase early after the intervention. The subtle changes would not be found by exercise testing alone without gas exchange.

In patients with severe mitral stenosis, $\dot{V}O_2$max can increase acutely by approximately 10% with an improvement in ventilation after balloon valvuloplasty (28, 29). The exercise data of a group of 10 patients before and early and late after balloon mitral valvuloplasty are shown in Figure 6.11 (28). These relatively small changes would not be evident by standard exercise testing without gas exchange. More significant changes could be expected with time in these patients. A baseline test before and after the procedure will serve well as a comparison point.

Pacemaker Programming

The use of cardiopulmonary testing to determine the optimal settings of rate-adaptive pacemakers has been extensively described. Because chronotropic incompetence can limit exercise performance and aerobic capacity, appropriate settings to simulate the normal heart rate/workload to $\dot{V}O_2$ relationship are recommended. Using a ramp protocol, an ideal heart rate/work rate (HR/WR) slope of 0.37 ± 13 beats per minute per watt is recommended so that the pacemaker should generate an average of 5 beats per minute for each 10 W of external treadmill work (30). Others have described a rate increase of 2 to 5 beats per minute to effect an increase of 1 mL·kg^{-1}·min^{-1} of oxygen uptake (31). Patients with the lowest intrinsic maximum sinus rate are those that will benefit the most from rate-adaptive pacing as shown in Figure 6.12. By dividing patients into groups according to their intrinsic sinus rate

(group I, less than or equal to 90 beats per minute; group II, 90 to 110 beats per minute; group III, more than 110 beats per minute), Alt and colleagues (32) have demonstrated the improvement in both $\dot{V}O_2$max and anaerobic threshold.

Heart Failure

Exercise testing provides a unique tool to assess the functional capacity of patients with heart failure. Cardiopulmonary testing for direct measurement of $\dot{V}O_2$ with exercise adds a valuable dimension to the evaluation of patients with heart failure in determining the source of symptoms induced by activity and currently plays a major role in prognostic assessment (33–35). Furthermore, the use of gas exchange allows derivation of an objective exercise prescription for rehabilitation in a group of patients that may be significantly debilitated.

Markedly impaired exercise tolerance places the patient with heart failure in a high-risk category for a poor outcome. The New York Heart Association classification system is imprecise owing to its inherently subjective nature. Consequently, direct measurement of oxygen uptake by cardiopulmonary testing appears to be the preferred assessment of exercise capacity to predict survival. A peak $\dot{V}O_2$ of less than 14 mL·kg^{-1}·min^{-1} generally identifies a group of patients with a poor 1-year prognosis, and this group should be considered for transplantation evaluation if otherwise deemed possible candidates (34). Currently, most cardiac transplantation programs use $\dot{V}O_2$ deter-

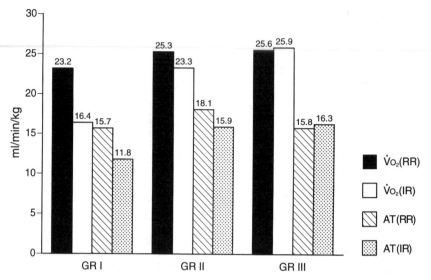

Figure 6.12. Maximum oxygen uptake ($\dot{V}o_2$) and anaerobic threshold (AT) during treadmill testing with rate-adaptive pacing (RR) and the patients' intrinsic rate (IR). Values shown are means. Group I, less than or equal to 90 beats per minute; group II, 90 to 110 beats per minute; group III, more than 110 beats per minute. See text for details.

mination in the selection of transplant recipients. Some heart failure/transplant centers use percent predicted $\dot{V}o_2$ in consideration of candidacy for cardiac transplantation. Patients with more than 50% predicted $\dot{V}o_2$max have a good short-term prognosis and may be able to be managed with medical treatment, thus deferring transplantation (36).

Recently, a subgroup of patients with $\dot{V}o_2$ less than 14 mL·kg^{-1}·min^{-1} has been identified who may have preserved cardiac function with exercise but who are extremely deconditioned (37). In this patient cohort, a program of directed cardiac rehabilitation can successfully improve peak $\dot{V}o_2$.

Evaluating the Source of Dyspnea

In cases in which the source of dyspnea on exertion is unclear, cardiopulmonary testing, with a proper interpretation, will often clarify the clinical picture. Deconditioning alone can cause symptoms of breathlessness on exertion and produce a decreased $\dot{V}o_2$max. In this setting, however, the cardiorespiratory responses should be normal. Patients become limited with a reduced $\dot{V}o_2$ as a result of one of three major reasons: 1) a cardiovascular limitation that includes the heart, pulmonary and systemic circulations, and blood; 2) a respiratory limitation that includes mechanical ventilation and

gas exchange; and 3) peripheral factors including musculoskeletal limitations that could impact on O_2 utilization at the tissue level (see Fig. 6.1) (3).

When cardiovascular disease limits exercise, the $\dot{V}o_2$ is abnormal because of decreased O_2 delivery to the periphery. In that case, the ventilatory reserve or "breathing" reserve should be normal, i.e., 1 − VEmax/MVV should range from 20% to 50% in normal subjects. In the presence of cardiac disease, oxygen uptake is depressed, anaerobic metabolism ensues earlier, and the patient is limited at low workloads yet with a high respiratory reserve. Conversely, those patients who are limited by pulmonary causes will approach or exceed their respiratory reserve although their cardiac system remains understressed. Minute ventilation in these situations will be excessive for the workload achieved. In addition, MVV is often reduced by obstruction or restriction to airflow. It is advisable in these instances to obtain pulmonary function tests to complement the cardiopulmonary test and to assess a true MVV rather than accept the predicted values as fact. Should desaturation be a consideration, the test can be performed with simultaneous pulse oximetry. Table 6.5 reviews some of the differences in the differential diagnosis of pulmonary versus cardiac exercise limitation.

Table 6.5. Exertional Dyspnea

	Cardiac	Pulmonary (Ventilatory)
$\dot{V}O_2$max	Yes, but low	Not achieved
Peak $\dot{V}O_2$	Reduced	Reduced
AT	Yes, but low	Rarely achieved
$\dot{V}E$max	>50% true MVV	>50% true MVV
SaO_2	Normal	May drop <90%
CO	Normal or low	Normal

$\dot{V}O_2$max, maximum oxygen uptake; AT, anaerobic threshold; $\dot{V}E$max, maximum minute ventilation; MVV, maximum voluntary ventilation; SaO_2, arterial oxygen saturation; CO, cardiac output.

How To Develop an Exercise Prescription

The cardiopulmonary test provides the best assessment of functional capacity and therefore serves as an excellent basis from which to derive an exercise treatment plan. The exercise prescription should be individualized according to the results of the cardiopulmonary exercise test. In our laboratory we have used the heart rate at AT as the heart rate for intensity recommendation. Generally, however, one must be sure that the heart rate at AT is safe and that the patient does not exhibit symptoms of angina or moderate dyspnea at that level. Alternatively, a heart rate 10 beats per minute less than that at AT may be a reasonable starting point for patients with severe symptoms or marked debilitation. Exercise is recommended three times per week for 20 to 30 minutes at the assigned intensity. Initially, aerobic training modalities are advised.

For patients after cardiac transplantation, the Borg scale rating at the AT is used to assign intensity because the heart rate will be flat early in exercise (38). The remainder of the exercise prescription remains the same.

The Agency for Health Care Policy and Research has provided an in-depth review of the published data on exercise prescription in cardiac disease and its derivation (39).

EXAMPLES

Normal Woman

A 46-year-old woman was tested for atypical chest pain using the Modified Naughton protocol (weight, 77.1 kg; height, 165.1 cm; predicted $\dot{V}O_2$max, 1610 mL/min or 20.88 mL·kg^{-1}·min^{-1}; MVV, 111 L/min) (Table 6.6).

Analysis: The patient has a normal $\dot{V}O_2$ for age, sex, height, and weight. The anaerobic threshold is also normal, occurring at 64% of the $\dot{V}O_2$max. The minute ventilation is normal with a ventilatory reserve of 60% using $1 - \dot{V}E$max/MVV. The blood pressure at rest is not normal and repeat blood pressure measurements were recommended. The maximum predicted heart rate is $220 - $ age, or 174. The patient reached 94% of predicted maximum heart rate.

Patient with Severe Triple-vessel Coronary Artery Disease

A 63-year-old man with a history of severe coronary artery disease and a coronary bypass surgical procedure 3 years previously was tested. The patient complained of chest discomfort and shortness of breath with exertion. The ejection fraction was 35%. The Modified Naughton protocol was used (weight, 71.2 kg; height, 172.7 cm; predicted $\dot{V}O_2$max, 1943 mL/min or 27.28 mL·kg^{-1}·min^{-1}; MVV, 125 L/min). The test was stopped owing to chest pain and moderate dyspnea. The RER was 1.07 (Table 6.7).

Analysis: The patient has a low $\dot{V}O_2$ for age, sex, height, and weight. The anaerobic threshold is also low but occurs at 71% of the $\dot{V}O_2$max. The minute ventilation is normal with a ventilatory reserve of 30% using $1 - \dot{V}E$max/MVV. The blood pressure at rest is low and remains relatively flat during exercise. The maximum predicted heart rate is $220 - $ age, or 157. The patient reached 82% of predicted maximum heart rate. The level of effort was submaximal (RER 1.07) owing to the onset of symptoms. In addition, the $\dot{V}O_2$ of 13.1 mL·kg^{-1}·min^{-1} places the patient in a Weber class C, indicative of a poor prognosis, which is also confirmed by a percent predicted $\dot{V}O_2$ of less than 50%. From Figure 6.10, the analysis leads to circulatory impairment, which includes myocardial ischemia and left ventricular dysfunction, among others. In patients such as the one illustrated above, myocardial perfusion imaging can be used simultaneously to supplement the cardiopulmonary test.

Patient with Heart Failure—Evaluation for Cardiac Transplantation

A 61-year-old physician was referred for transplant evaluation with a severe ischemic cardiomyopathy and an ejection fraction of 15%. A bypass

Table 6.6.   Normal Woman

	Systolic BP (mm Hg)	Heart Rate (bpm)	$\dot{V}O_2$ (mL·kg^{-1}·min^{-1})	Time (min)	$\dot{V}E$ (L/min)
Rest	150	77	3.4	0	6
Maximal exercise	195	164	22.4 (107% predicted)	15.45	66
Ventilatory threshold	180	118	14.3 (64% $\dot{V}O_2$max)	6.1	18

BP, blood pressure; $\dot{V}O_2$, oxygen uptake; $\dot{V}E$, minute ventilation; $\dot{V}O_2$max, maximum oxygen uptake.

Table 6.7.   Patient with Severe Triple-vessel Coronary Artery Disease

	Systolic BP (mm Hg)	Heart Rate (bpm)	$\dot{V}O_2$ (mL·kg^{-1}·min^{-1})	Time (min)	$\dot{V}E$ (L/min)
Rest	92	68	3.3	0	8
Maximal exercise	118	130	13.1 (47% predicted)	7.8	37
Ventilatory threshold	110	97	9.3 (71% $\dot{V}O_2$max)	4.5	21

BP, blood pressure; $\dot{V}O_2$, oxygen uptake; $\dot{V}E$, minute ventilation; $\dot{V}O_2$max, maximum oxygen uptake.

surgical procedure had been performed 10 years before presentation. There was no active ischemia by radionuclide perfusion imaging, which had been obtained before referral. The test was performed after maximization of medical therapy, especially angiotensin-converting enzyme inhibitors, using Modified Naughton protocol (weight, 76.8 kg; height, 175.3 cm; predicted $\dot{V}O_2$max, 2153 mL/min or 28.03 mL·kg^{-1}·min^{-1}; MVV, 134 L/min). The test was stopped owing to moderate dyspnea. The RER was 1.11 (Table 6.8).

Analysis: The patient has a low $\dot{V}O_2$ for age, sex, height, and weight. The anaerobic threshold is also low but occurs at 75% of the $\dot{V}O_2$max. The minute ventilation is normal with a ventilatory reserve of 42% using 1 − $\dot{V}E$max/MVV. The blood pressure at rest is low and remains relatively flat during exercise. The maximum predicted heart rate is 220 − age, or 151. The patient reached 82% of predicted maximum heart rate. The level of effort was submaximal (RER 1.11) owing to the onset of symptoms but adequate to assess the AT. In addition, the $\dot{V}O_2$ of 13.5 mL·kg^{-1}·min^{-1} places the patient in a Weber class C, indicative of a poor prognosis, which is also confirmed by a percent predicted $\dot{V}O_2$ of less than 50%. From Figure 6.10, the analysis leads to circulatory impairment, which includes myocardial ischemia and left ventricular dysfunction, among others. In this case there was no evidence of ischemia either by symptoms or by ECG.

Patient After Cardiac Transplantation

A 64-year-old man who had cardiac transplantation 2 weeks previously was tested. The patient had undergone inpatient cardiac rehabilitation. The Modified Naughton protocol was used (weight, 94.8 kg; height, 172.7 cm; predicted $\dot{V}O_2$max, 2039 mL/min or 21.51 mL·kg^{-1}·min^{-1}; MVV, 124 L/min). The test was stopped owing to moderate dyspnea. The RER was 1.17 (Table 6.9).

Analysis: The patient has a low $\dot{V}O_2$ for age, sex, height, and weight. The anaerobic threshold is also low and occurs at 66% of the $\dot{V}O_2$max. The minute ventilation is normal with a ventilatory reserve of 47% using 1 − $\dot{V}E$max/MVV. Chronotropic incompetence is a common finding in transplanted patients with absence of vagal innervation. The patient's heart rate increase of 15 beats per minute is abnormal for the workload used. The level of effort was submaximal (RER 1.17) owing to the onset of leg fatigue but adequate to assess the AT. Using the Weber class to describe the functional capacity of this patient is not appropriate because the A through D classification was not developed for the transplant population. This test was used to derive an exercise prescription because the AT occurred at a low level of work. The RPE at the AT was 12. An exercise prescription was given for an intensity commensurate with an RPE of 12, because heart rate is not useful in this patient. Exercise was recommended three times per week for at least 20 to 30 minutes with progression as tolerated.

Table 6.8.   Patient with Heart Failure—Evaluation for Cardiac Transplantation

	Systolic BP (mm Hg)	Heart Rate (bpm)	$\dot{V}O_2$ (mL·kg^{-1}·min^{-1})	Time (min)	$\dot{V}E$ (L/min)
Rest	90	82	3.8	0	8
Maximal exercise	110	131	13.5 (48% predicted)	10	57
Ventilatory threshold	102	120	10.2 (75% $\dot{V}O_2$max)	7.5	30

BP; blood pressure; $\dot{V}O_2$, oxygen uptake; $\dot{V}E$, minute ventilation; $\dot{V}O_2$max, maximum oxygen uptake.

Table 6.9.   Patient After Cardiac Transplantation

	Systolic BP (mm Hg)	Heart Rate (bpm)	$\dot{V}O_2$ (mL·kg^{-1}·min^{-1})	Time (min)	$\dot{V}E$ (L/min)
Rest	128	85	3.6	0	7.2
Maximal exercise	148	100	11.2 (52% predicted)	9.8	58
Ventilatory threshold	132	86	7.4 (66% $\dot{V}O_2$max)	8	36.3

BP, blood pressure; $\dot{V}O_2$, oxygen uptake; $\dot{V}E$, minute ventilation; $\dot{V}O_2$max, maximum oxygen uptake.

References

1. Mahler D, Franco M. Clinical applications of cardiopulmonary exercise testing. J Cardpulm Rehabil 1996;16:357–365.
2. Neuberg GW, Friedman SH, Weiss MB, et al. Cardiopulmonary exercise testing: the clinical value of gas exchange data. Arch Intern Med 1988;148:2221–2226.
3. Wasserman K, Hansen JE, Sue DY, et al. Principles of exercise testing and interpretation. Philadelphia: Lea & Febiger, 1987.
4. Al-Rawas OA, Carter R, Richens D, et al. Ventilatory and gas exchange abnormalities on exercise in chronic heart failure. Eur Respir J 1995;8:2022–2028.
5. Weisman IM, Zeballos RJ. An integrated approach to the interpretation of cardiopulmonary exercise testing. Clin Chest Med 1994;15:421–445.
6. Poulin MJ, Cunningham DA, Paterson DH, et al. Ventilatory response to exercise in men and women 55 to 86 years of age. Am J Respir Crit Care Med 1994;149:408–415.
7. Beaver WL, Wasserman K, Whipp BJ. A new method for detecting anaerobic threshold by gas exchange. J Appl Physiol 1986;60:2020–2027.
8. Smith TD, Thomas TR, Londeree BR, et al. Peak oxygen consumption and ventilatory thresholds on six modes of exercise. Can J Appl Physiol 1996;21:79–89.
9. Myers J. Ventilatory gas exchange in heart failure: techniques, problems and pitfalls. In: Balady GJ, Piña IL, eds. Exercise and heart failure. Armonk, NY: Futura, 1997:213–241.
10. Piña IL, Balady GJ, Hanson P, et al. Guidelines for clinical exercise testing laboratories. Circulation 1995;91:912–919.
11. Borg G. Psychophysical basis of perceived exertion. Med Sci Sports Exer 1982;14:377–381.
12. Wolfel EE, Bristow MR. Effects of long-term beta adrenergic blockade on exercise capacity in patients with chronic heart failure. In: Balady GJ, Piña IL, eds. Exercise and heart failure. Armonk, NY: Futura, 1997:141–170.
13. Page E, Cohen-Solal A, Jondeau G, et al. Comparison of treadmill and bicycle exercise in patients with chronic heart failure. Chest 1994;106:1002–1006.
14. Weber KT, Janicki JS. Lactate production during maximal and submaximal exercise in patients with chronic heart failure. J Am Coll Cardiol 1985;6:717–724.
15. Weber KT, Kinasewitz GT, Janicki JS, et al. Oxygen utilization during exercise in patients with chronic cardiac failure. Circulation 1982;65:1213–1223.
16. Lipkin DP, Canepa-Anson R, Stephens MR, et al. Factors determining symptoms in heart failure: comparison of fast and slow exercise tests. Br Heart J 1986;55:439–445.
17. Pollock ML, Bohannon RL, Cooper KH, et al. A comparative analysis of four protocols for maximal treadmill stress testing. Am Heart J 1976;92:39–46.
18. Piña IL, Karalis DG. Comparison of four exercise protocols using anaerobic threshold measurement of functional capacity in congestive heart failure. Am J Cardiol 1990;65:1269–1271.
19. Jones NL, Campbell EJM, Edwards RHT, et al. Clinical exercise testing, Philadelphia: WB Saunders, 1975:202.
20. Bruce RA, Kusumi F, Hosmer D. Maximal oxygen uptake and nomographic assessment of functional aerobic impairment in cardiovascular disease. Am Heart J 1973;85:546–562.
21. Waters DD, Bosch X, Bouchard A, et al. Comparison of clinical variables and variables derived from a limited predischarge exercise test as predictors of early and late mortality after myocardial infarction. J Am Coll Cardiol 1985;5:1–8.
22. Hossack KF, Bruce RA. Prognostic value of exercise testing: the Seattle Heart Watch experience. J Cardpulm Rehabil 1985;5:9–19.
23. Vanhees L, Fagard R, Thijs L, et al. Prognostic significance of peak exercise capacity in patients with coronary artery disease. J Am Coll Cardiol 1994;23:358–363.

24. Vanhees L, Schepers D, Fagard R. Comparison of maximum versus submaximum exercise testing in providing prognostic information after acute myocardial infarction and/or coronary artery bypass grafting. Am J Cardiol 1997;80:257–262.

25. Vanhees L, Fagard R, Thijs L, et al. Prognostic value of training-induced change in peak exercise capacity in patients with myocardial infarcts and patients with coronary bypass surgery. Am J Cardiol 1995;76:1014–1019.

26. Kleber F, Sabin G, Winter U, et al. Angiotensin-converting enzyme inhibitors in preventing remodeling and development of heart failure after acute myocardial infarction: results of the German multicenter study of the effects of captopril on cardiopulmonary exercise parameters (ECCE). Am J Cardiol 1997;80(3A):162A–167A.

27. Klainman E, Kusniec J, Stern J, et al. Contribution of cardiopulmonary indices in the assessment of patients with silent and symptomatic ischemia during exercise testing. Int J Cardiol 1996;53:257–263.

28. Kolling K, Lehmann G, Dennig K, et al. Acute alterations of oxygen uptake and symptom-limited exercise time in patients with mitral stenosis after balloon valvuloplasty. Chest 1995;108:1206–1213.

29. Barlow C, Long J, Brown G, et al. Exercise capacity and skeletal muscle structure and function before and after balloon mitral valvuloplasty. Am J Cardiol 1995; 76:684–688.

30. Lewalter T, MacCarter D, Jung W, et al. Heart rate to work rate relation throughout peak exercise in normal subjects as a guideline for rate-adaptive pacemaker programming. Am J Cardiol 1995;76:812–816.

31. Wilkoff BL, Corey J, Blackburn G. A mathematical model of the cardiac chronotropic response to exercise. J Electrophysiol 1989;3:176–180.

32. Alt EU, Schlegl MJ, Matula MM. Intrinsic heart rate response as a predictor of rate-adaptive pacing benefit. Chest 1995;107:925–930.

33. Szlachcic J, Massie B, Kramer B, et al. Correlates and prognostic implications of exercise capacity in chronic congestive heart failure. Am J Cardiol 1985;55: 1037–1042.

34. Mancini DM, Eisen H, Kussmaul W, et al. Value of peak exercise oxygen consumption for optimal timing of cardiac transplantation in ambulatory patients with heart failure. Circulation 1991;83:778–786.

35. Cohn JN, Johnson GR, Shabetal R, et al. Ejection fraction, peak exercise oxygen consumption, cardiothoracic ratio, ventricular arrhythmias, and plasma norepinephrine as determinants of prognosis in heart failure. Circulation 1993;87(Suppl 6):VI24–VI31.

36. Stelken AM, Younis LT, Jennison SH, et al. Prognostic value of cardiopulmonary exercise testing using percent achieved of predicted peak oxygen uptake for patients with ischemic and dilated cardiomyopathy. J Am Coll Cardiol 1996;27:345–352.

37. Wilson JR, Rayos G, Keoh TK, et al. Dissociation between peak exercise oxygen consumption and hemodynamic dysfunction in potential heart transplant candidates. J Am Coll Cardiol 1995;26:429–435.

38. Scott CD, Dark JH, McComb JM. Evolution of the chronotropic response to exercise after cardiac transplantation. Am J Cardiol 1995;76:1292–1296.

39. Wenger NK, Froelicher ES, Smith LK, et al. Cardiac rehabilitation. Clinical practice guideline No. 17. Rockville, MD: US Department of Health and Human Services, Public Health Service, Agency for Health Care Policy and Research and the National Heart, Lung and Blood Institute. AHCPR Publication No. 96–0672, October 1995.

40. Imbriaco M, Cuocolo A, Pace L, et al. Ambulatory monitoring of left ventricular functions during cardiopulmonary exercise tests in normal sedentary subjects. J Nucl Med 1995;36:564–568.

41. Bhadha K, Walter JD, DiMarzio D, et al. Comparison of the Bruce and ramp protocols in the assessment of left ventricular performance during exercise in healthy women. Am J Cardiol 1995;75:963–966.

42. Panton LB, Graves JE, Pollock ML, et al. Relative heart rate, heart rate reserve, and VO_2 during submaximal exercise in the elderly. J Gerontol A Biol Sci Med Sci 1996;51:M165–M171.

43. Meyer K, Stengele E, Westbrook S, et al. Influence of different exercise protocols on functional capacity and symptoms in patients with chronic heart failure. Med Sci Sports Exerc 1996;28:1081–1086.

44. Serra R. A new metabolic simulator system for routine cardiopulmonary exercise test equipment: technical specifications and validation. Monaldi Arch Chest Dis 1997;2:189–194.

45. Meyers K, Samek L, Pinchas A, et al. Relationship between ventilatory threshold and onset of ischaemia in ECG during stress testing. Eur Heart J 1995;16: 623–630.

46. Sullivan M, Froelicher V. Maximal oxygen uptake and gas exchange in coronary heart disease. J Cardiac Rehabil 1983;3:549–560.

47. Weber KT, Kinasewitz GT, Janicki JS, et al. Oxygen utilization and ventilation during exercise in patients with chronic cardiac failure. Circulation 1982;6:1213–1223.

48. Bogaard HJ, Woltjer HH, van Keimpema AR, et al. Comparison of the respiratory and hemodynamic responses of health subjects to exercise in three different protocols. Occup Med (Oxf) 1996;46:293–298.

Sample Informed Consent

To determine the response of my heart, circulation, and lungs to exercise, I voluntarily agree to perform a cardiopulmonary exercise test. The information obtained about my heart and circulation will be used to help my doctor understand more about any problems related to my heart and advise me about activities in which I may engage.

I have been told that before I undergo the test, I will be interviewed and examined by a physician in an attempt to determine if I have a condition indicating that I should not engage in this test.

I am told that the test I will undergo will be performed on a (treadmill or bicycle) with gradually increasing effort until symptoms such as fatigue, shortness of breath, or chest discomfort may appear, indicating to me that I should stop. My heart rhythm will be monitored at all times.

I will also have a small mouthpiece through which I will breathe room air and all the air I exhale will be collected and analyzed to determine the amount of oxygen that my body uses with exercise. I will also have a plastic clip placed on my nose.

I have been told certain changes may occur during the test, including abnormal blood pressure, fainting, abnormal cardiogram showing heart "strain," disorders of the heart rhythm (too fast, too slow, or not effective), and possible heart attack and death.

I have read the above and understand it and my questions have been answered to my satisfaction.

Patient _____

Date _____

Physician supervising the test_____

_____

Witness_____

PATIENT NAME _____
DATE _____
RESTING: HEART RATE_____
HEIGHT _____ WEIGHT _____
 BLOOD PRESSURE _____
 OXYGEN UPTAKE _____

The patient exercised for _____minutes on a _____protocol to a peak heart rate of _____beats per minute and a peak blood pressure of _____mm Hg. The rate of perceived exertion was ____using the Borg scale. The test was stopped owing to _____.
The peak $\dot{V}O_2$ was ____$mL \cdot kg^{-1} \cdot min^{-1}$. The peak $\dot{V}CO_2$ was _____ $mL \cdot kg^{-1} \cdot min^{-1}$. The RER was _____. The anaerobic threshold was _____ $mL \cdot kg^{-1} \cdot min^{-1}$ (*could also state "not attained"*). The minute ventilation was _____L/min.

ECG RESULTS:
The resting ECG had _____.
During exercise there was _____.
_____arrhythmias were (*noted or not noted*). The ECG returned to baseline at _____minutes into recovery.

IMPRESSION: Functional capacity is ____normal or abnormal for patient's age and sex (____% predicted). (*Use the Weber Class if indicated.*)
The blood pressure response was _____.
The heart rate response was _____.

RECOMMENDATIONS:
(*Cardiac rehabilitation exercise prescription can be provided*)

_____

DIRECTOR EXERCISE LABORATORY

Other Noninvasive Diagnostic Tools: Test of Left Ventricular Function, Perfusion, and Metabolism

Thomas H. Marwick

The noninvasive assessment of cardiac function after myocardial infarction (MI) is based on several considerations. First, the patient's functional state and prognosis need to be established—this is very important with respect to plans for rehabilitation. Second, patients with residual jeopardized tissue should be detected early and referred for intervention—thus, patients selected for rehabilitation should be able to undergo the process safely. Third, as rehabilitation extends into the arena of risk factor modification, studies identifying the extent of atherosclerotic plaque may be of value.

The use of thrombolytic therapy has accelerated the reduction of acute MI mortality witnessed during the last three decades (1). The mechanisms that underlie postinfarction mortality, however, have remained the same. Factors determining prognosis after MI may be classified as extrinsic and intrinsic to the cardiovascular system. Extrinsic factors, such as age and the presence of diabetes, cannot be influenced. The main intrinsic factors are infarct size and the extent of residual jeopardized tissue supplied by stenosed coronary vessels. This ischemic tissue is characterized by normal perfusion at rest, but failure of its blood supply to be augmented in response to the increased oxygen requirement of the myocardium with stress. Such tissue includes that which is at a distance from the infarcted site (in the territory of another stenosed coronary artery), that which is subject to peri-infarct ischemia (a border zone that surrounds truly infarcted tissue), and that which is subject to homozonal ischemia (within the infarct serum itself). The prognostic role of the residual is-

chemic burden has been evidenced by studies that demonstrate a correlation between prognosis and the number of diseased coronary vessels (2), or with the extent of ischemia at myocardial perfusion imaging (3). These problems are readily treated by revascularization. The extent of infarction (evidenced by ejection fraction [EF] or size of perfusion defects) has long been appreciated to be of prognostic importance (4, 5). Some of this damaged tissue is potentially salvageable, despite the presence of "nonreversible" perfusion defects, or resting wall-motion abnormalities (6). This viable tissue has been categorized as stunned and/or hibernating myocardium. Myocardial stunning describes a state of contractile dysfunction after ischemic episode, in the presence of normal coronary flow: this recovers spontaneously (7). Hibernating myocardium describes a heterogeneous state of severe resting hypoperfusion, with impaired myocardial contractility, which may be partially or completely restored to normal function by improvement of oxygen supply or by reduction of demand (8).

Although coronary angiography remains a vital component in the decision-making process regarding coronary intervention, noninvasive cardiac imaging modalities have more to offer from the standpoint of risk stratification (9). Early submaximal exercise testing (5) has some value for the identification of ischemia, but it cannot be used to identify viable myocardium and does not give information regarding the site of jeopardized tissue, which may be important in management decisions. Consequently, this discussion will focus on imaging tests used in the postinfarction patient, including dobutamine echocardiography, myocardial perfusion scintigraphy, and metabolic imaging using positron emission tomography (PET).

EVALUATION OF RESTING LEFT VENTRICULAR FUNCTION

The importance of left ventricular (LV) function as a prognostic determinant after MI is well-established; right ventricular function is more difficult to measure, but also appears to be important. Although EF is the most widely used index of global LV function, LV volumes are probably more predictive of outcome (Fig. 7.1) (10). Because more severely damaged hearts are less able to sustain the insult of another ischemic event, the degree of dysfunction modulates the prognostic importance of further ischemia (4, 5). Numerous techniques are available for the assessment of LV function, including contrast and nuclear ventriculography, two-dimensional and M-mode echocardiography, magnetic resonance imaging (MRI), and computed tomography (CT). The latter two techniques offer excellent three-dimensional definition of regional myocardial function, but they are expensive, have limited availability, and are largely restricted to research settings. In centers in which all postinfarction patients undergo cardiac catheterization, contrast ventriculography offers a moderately accurate assessment of LV function, although it is somewhat nonphysiologic (because of the injection of the contrast bolus), and the nature of its silhouette image may be suboptimal for visualizing all myocardial segments.

Nuclear Ventriculography

At institutions in which the selection of postinfarction patients for angiography is based on risk stratification, practical alternatives for the noninvasive assessment of ventricular function are nuclear ventriculography and echocardiography. Nuclear ventriculography has traditionally been performed using a gated approach after injection of labeled red blood cells (11). After the subtraction of background activity, the EF is determined by dividing the stroke volume (the difference between the end-systolic and end-diastolic counts) by the end-diastolic volume (end-diastolic counts within the LV region of interest). This calculation of EF is independent of LV geometry, although some inaccuracy is inherent because of soft tissue attenuation. Moreover, the acquisition of these data during a number of cardiac cycles blurs the definition of the LV wall, compromising the assessment of regional LV function. Important technical influences include the need for good red blood cell labeling, careful background subtraction, and choice of an appropriate region of interest for the ventricle. Reporting LV function as an apparently objective measure (EF) may thus be inappropriately reassuring. Nonetheless, measurements of LV function correlate closely with those achieved at angiography (12). Increasingly, these data are gathered in the course of technetium-99m sestamibi injection for perfusion imaging (13).

Echocardiography

Two-dimensional echocardiography also has become widely used for the assessment of ven-

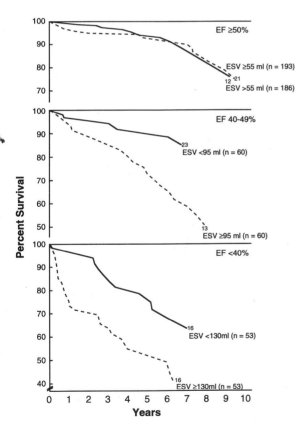

Figure 7.1. Influence of left ventricular (*LV*) end-systolic volume (*ESV*) and ejection fraction (*EF*) on estimated survival (expressed in a life-table analysis). (Reproduced with permission from Hamer et al. Circulation 1994; 90:2899–2904.)

tricular function after MI. The particular benefits in relation to nuclear ventriculography relate to its versatility (allowing ready use in the coronary care and emergency room settings), lower cost, and good discrimination of regional ventricular function. It also is effective for the detection of nonischemic cardiac disease, including valvular and pericardial disease, although these benefits are more pertinent to the early evaluation of patients with MI than in the rehabilitation phase. The major disadvantage of echocardiography is that the calculation of LV volumes and EF depends on assumptions of ventricular geometry, which may be inappropriate after infarction (14). The fewest assumptions regarding geometry are made by application of Simpson's rule, but this requires assessment from the apical views, introducing technical problems caused by "foreshortening" of the ventricular cavity and inadequate detection of the endocardial border. These limitations may be reduced by new technologies, such as lateral gain control and acoustic quantification (15), or avoided by new Doppler techniques, such as automated cardiac output measurement (ACOM) (16). Nonetheless, in most instances, good correlation exists between echocardiographic and nuclear EF (17). In contrast to nuclear ventriculography, echocardiography is a very reliable technique for analysis of regional LV function. Thus, an alternative approach to the assessment of global function is to evaluate the left ventricle by the sum of its parts, as a regional wall-motion score or score index (representing the mean score). This index correlates with Killip class and carries prognostic value analogous to the EF (18, 19).

Paradoxically, although the technical aspects of echocardiography are almost the opposite of the considerations used for nuclear ventriculography, little separates the accuracy of the techniques for assessing LV function at rest. Such choices may therefore reflect considerations of cost, local availability, and expertise.

ASSESSMENT OF VENTRICULAR FUNCTION AFTER STRESS

The assessment of resting LV function stratifies risk, but does not identify risk that can be modified by intervention. Detection of ischemic or viable myocardium requires evaluation during or after stress. Numerous alternatives are available for this purpose, but the practical choice in the routine clinical setting is between nuclear ventriculography and echocardiography.

Stress Nuclear Ventriculography

Evaluation of global ventricular responses to stress using nuclear ventriculography has made this a powerful prognostic tool (20–22). However, the optimal predictors of subsequent events have varied among studies, and include the change of EF with exercise, and absolute levels of exercise EF. From a diagnostic standpoint, however, nuclear ventriculography is less attractive for two reasons: first, because hyperkinesis in nonischemic regions may compensate for areas of ischemia unless these are extensive, and second, because an exercise-induced deterioration of global LV function is not specific for ischemia (23). These limitations may be avoided by the examination of regional wall motion, but this is a strength of two-dimensional echocardiography rather than gated nuclear ventriculography. Moreover, exercise echocardiography has the ability to examine myocardial thickening in addition to endocardial excursion. In light of these differences, it is not surprising that exercise echocardiography has been found to be more accurate for the diagnosis of coronary disease than its nuclear counterpart (24).

Stress Echocardiography

PRACTICAL CONSIDERATIONS

The performance of stress echocardiography involves acquisition and comparison of images obtained at rest and during or after stress. Good quality images are essential, requiring the best available echocardiographic equipment. Image digitization enhances definition of the endocardium, improves the quality of stop-frame images, and permits display of wall motion in a cine-loop format, with rest and stress images side-by-side (25).

Stress echocardiography may be performed using the exercise or pharmacologic stress techniques. Because of the prognostic importance of exercise capacity, and the relevance of these data to rehabilitation decisions, the exercise approach is desirable in active patients. Treadmill testing is the most common modality used for exercise echocardiography in the United States, but this protocol necessarily involves postexercise imaging, as images cannot be obtained during peak treadmill exercise. Bicycle ergometry permits the acquisition of peak exercise images. These may be more sensitive than postexercise images for the detection of mild ischemia, but less specific because of the presence of more movement artifact at peak stress imaging (26). The benefits and disadvantages of bicycle exercise are summarized in Table 7.1. The main disadvantages are unfamiliarity to many patients and limitations of exercise by fatigue before ischemia is induced.

Although most cardiac rehabilitation patients are able to exercise, many cannot exercise adequately enough to provoke ischemia. For this group, pharmacologic and pacing stimuli have been used for echocardiographic stress testing. Dipyridamole has been used extensively for myocardial perfusion imaging, and the development of ischemia caused by coronary steal at higher doses has made this procedure useful for stress echocardiography (27). Dobutamine has been used as an alternative approach to induce ischemia by raising myocardial oxygen requirements (28). This approach is also desirable if stress testing is planned very early after myocardial infarction, or if questions arise in relation to myocardial viability.

INTERPRETATION

The interpretation of stress echocardiography is based on comparison of regional function at rest and during and after stress in each segment of the left ventricle (Fig. 7.2). The normal response of wall motion to exercise is the development of hyperkinesis: failure to increase function or deterioration of function is consistent with the presence of ischemia. Resting wall-motion abnormalities, particularly if associated with echodensity and mural thinning, are relatively specific for the presence of previous MI. Myocardial viability is recognized in this setting as improvement of regional function in response to low-dose dobutamine, particularly if the function subsequently deteriorates because of the development of ischemia. In addition to the diagnosis of ischemia, the degrees of wall-motion disturbance may be quantified by use of a wall-motion score or score index. Although such scores better define the extent and severity of wall-motion disturbance, the current use of this qualitative or subjective interpretation is a significant limitation. This approach has important influences on the need for special training, as well as limiting reproducibility (29, 30).

A quantitative, centerline approach has been pioneered by Ginzton et al. (31) with favorable results. This requires high-quality images for endocardial definition, is time-consuming, and may be influenced by translational moment. In the experience of most centers, this is currently impractical for routine use. However, recent advances in tissue Doppler imaging have given some promise that this modality could be used as a quantitative index of regional LV function (32).

DIAGNOSTIC ACCURACY

A number of studies (Table 7.2) have shown that exercise and dobutamine echocardiography, using digital acquisition techniques and qualitative wall-motion scoring, are accurate tests for the diagnosis of coronary disease (33–45). These tests exceed the accuracy of routine exercise testing.

The calculation of sensitivity and specificity depends on comparison with the coronary angiogram. Clearly, not all moderate stenoses are flow-limiting (especially if they are bypassed by adequate collaterals), and this may cause some apparently false-negative results if the stress echocardiogram identifies absence of ischemia correctly, despite the presence of significant coronary disease. False-negative findings may occur owing to failure to provoke ischemia because of submaximal exercise (37), continuing antianginal

Table 7.1.   Advantages and Disadvantages of Treadmill and Bicycle Exercise Echocardiography

	Treadmill	Bicycle
Acceptance	High—familiar to most patients	Less—unfamiliar to many
Adequacy of stress	Maximal stress in most patients	Leg fatigue may provoke premature termination
		Patient compliance required to obtain maximal stress
Imaging	Postexercise only	Peak exercise and postexercise

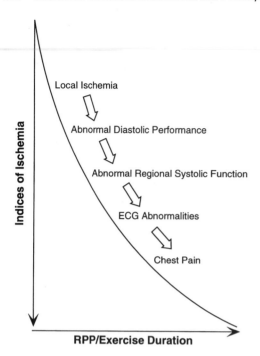

Figure 7.2.   Ischemic cascade: relationship between onset of angina and ischemic changes with increasing levels of stress. *RPP,* rate-pressure product. (Reproduced with permission from Topol EJ, Textbook of Cardiovascular Medicine Philadelphia: Lippincott-Raven Publishers, 1998:1271.)

medications, poor image quality, or a delay before postexercise imaging. The specificity of exercise echocardiography may be impaired by inclusion in the study group of patients who have small-vessel coronary disease or noncoronary heart disease, especially if changes in end-systolic volume or global EF are used as diagnostic features.

Viable myocardium is defined as tissue that shows improvement of regional function after revascularization or spontaneous recovery of stunned myocardium. Using this as an end point, the accuracy of dobutamine echocardiology for the prediction of viable myocardium has generally been in the range of 80% to 85% (46).

However, sensitivity and specificity are of limited application to the postinfarction patient, in whom coronary disease has already been diagnosed. Indeed, previous MI is known to inflate the sensitivity of stress echocardiography, because resting wall-motion abnormalities are readily identified. However, the identification of ischemia is more of a problem in the setting of resting wall-motion abnormalities, because the recognition of minor differences in degrees of hypokinesia is dif-

ficult. Nonetheless, exercise echocardiography accurately identifies multivessel disease (ischemia at a distance) in post-MI patients. In our experience of patients undergoing maximal exercise (37), the sensitivity of exercise echocardiography for distant ischemia was 82%. The ability to recognize augmentation of function within hypokinetic, viable segments has enhanced the ability of dobutamine echocardiography to identify ischemia in the setting of MI (47). Nonetheless, a better approach is probably to examine the ability of the technique to identify patients at risk of events.

PROGNOSTIC ASSESSMENT

A number of studies have addressed the ability of stress echocardiography to predict patients at high risk of cardiac events after MI. Interestingly, only two, involving small populations, have evaluated exercise stress for this purpose. In contrast, pharmacologic stress has been extensively studied, the attraction of this approach being the ability to study the patient relatively early after the event. The variation in the reported findings reflects differences in the duration of follow-up and the nature of the events studied. Generally, the studies have shown that patients without ischemia have a favorable prognosis, and those with ischemia can be further stratified by assessment of the extent of ischemia and the ischemic threshold.

FUTURE DEVELOPMENTS

Adequate images for the purpose of qualitative reporting are obtained in about 95% of stress echocardiograms. Nonetheless, technical problems are a major limitation of this technique, and developments aimed at improving image quality will alleviate this issue. Those under active development include the use of edge-detection algorithms to enhance the definition of the endocardial border, myocardial Doppler, and echocardiographic contrast agents to opacify the LV cavity. Myocardial contrast echocardiography is likely to offer the acquisition of simultaneous perfusion data as a routine clinical tool in the near future.

MYOCARDIAL PERFUSION IMAGING

Hemodynamically significant coronary stenoses have the consequence of reducing coronary blood flow reserve. Myocardial perfusion imaging at rest and after stress identifies regional varia-

Table 7.2.   Accuracy of Exercise and Dobutamine Echocardiography for Identification of Coronary Artery Disease[a]

Author	Ref	Stress	n	Multivessel (% all CAD)	MI (% all CAD)	Sensitivity—overall	Sensitivity—SVD pts	Specificity
Quinones	33	Tml	112	45 (52%)	—	74% (n=86)	58% (n=41)	81% (n=26)
Armstrong	34	Tml	123	59 (58%)	50 (50%)	88% (n=101)	81% (n=42)	86% (n=22)
Roger	35	Tml	127			88% (n=107)		72% (n=20)
Beleslin	36	Tml	136	11 (9%)	41 (34%)	88% (n=119)	88% (n=108)	82% (n=17)
Marwick	37	Tml	150	54 (47%)	55 (48%)	84% (n=114)	77% (n=60)	86% (n=36)
Hecht	38	S/Bike	180	82 (60%)	38 (28%)	93% (n=137)	84% (n=55)	86% (n=43)
Crouse	39	Tml	228	106 (61%)	—	97% (n=175)	92% (n=66)	64% (n=53)
Ryan	40	U/Bike	309	126 (60%)	132 (63%)	91% (n=211)	86% (n=85)	78% (n=98)
Pingitore	41	$40 \mu g \cdot kg^{-1} \cdot min^{-1}$ + atro	110	42 (46%)	25 (27%)	84% (n=92)		89% (n=18)
Takeuchi	42	$30 \mu g \cdot kg^{-1} \cdot min^{-1}$	120	37 (50%)	62 (84%)	85% (n=74)	73% (n=37)	93% (n=46)
Beleslin	36	$40 \mu g \cdot kg^{-1} \cdot min^{-1}$	136	11 (9%)	41 (34%)	82% (n=119)	82% (n=108)	77% (n=27)
Marcovitz	43	$30 \mu g \cdot kg^{-1} \cdot min^{-1}$	141	47 (43%)	—	96% (n=109)	95% (n=62)	66% (n=32)
Ostojic	43	$40 \mu g \cdot kg^{-1} \cdot min^{-1}$	150	16 (12%)	38 (29%)	75% (n=131)	—	79% (n=19)
Ling	45	$40 \mu g \cdot kg^{-1} \cdot min^{-1}$	183			93% (n=162)	84% (n=66)	62% (n=21)
Marwick	44	$40 \mu g \cdot kg^{-1} \cdot min^{-1}$	217	74 (52%)	0 (0%)	72% (n=142)	66% (n=68)	83% (n=75)

CAD, coronary artery disease; SVD, single vessel disease; Tml, treadmill; S/Bike, stationary bicycle; U/Bike, unstationary bike; atropine.
[a]Confined to studies of > 100 patients.

tions of myocardial perfusion in patients with ischemic heart disease. Perfusion and wall-motion imaging address different physiologic consequences of coronary stenoses; regional reduction of hyperemia at peak stress may not be sufficient to induce abnormal wall motion, and abnormal function is not necessarily specific for ischemia. According to the "ischemia cascade" paradigm (Fig. 7.3), alterations in myocardial perfusion precede changes in function. Perfusion imaging may therefore identify mildly abnormal flow reserve, even when flow is sufficient to avoid myocardial ischemia in a functional or metabolic sense.

Despite the differences in the underlying principles of these investigations, perfusion imaging provides analogous information to functional imaging in the postinfarction setting with respect to defining infarct size and the presence, extent, and localization of residual ischemia. The extent and severity of resting perfusion defects after MI are prognostically important: a moderate or greater reduction of perfusion in more than 40% of the left ventricle has been found to be a better predictor of cardiac events than clinical parameters or even left ventricular ejection fraction (LVEF) (48). Similarly, in a comparison of submaximal exercise testing, coronary angiography, and planar thallium imaging, the prediction of "high risk" by perfusion imaging correlated best with the occurrence of nonfatal cardiac events during a 15-month follow-up (9).

PRACTICAL ASPECTS OF MYOCARDIAL PERFUSION IMAGING WITH SINGLE PHOTON EMISSION COMPUTED TOMOGRAPHY (SPECT)

Although much of the prognostic data with myocardial perfusion imaging has been described using the planar approach, most centers in the United States are currently using the tomographic approach SPECT. The superior spatial resolution of SPECT has improved the ability of perfusion imaging to address aspects important to postinfarction patients, including assessing the localization of ischemia, and its extent (49, 50).

Single photon emission computed tomography is performed using either thallous chloride Tl 201 or technetium Tc 99m sestamibi. Unfortunately, ^{201}Tl has a number of properties unfavorable to its use as an imaging agent, including its long half-life, dose limitations based on radiation dosimetry, and the low intensity of its emissions, which are prone to "scatter" and attenuation by overlying tissue. The clinical sequelae of these considerations are absence of a true resting scan, reduction of available counts because of low doses, production of false-positive defects because of attenuation by soft tissue, and

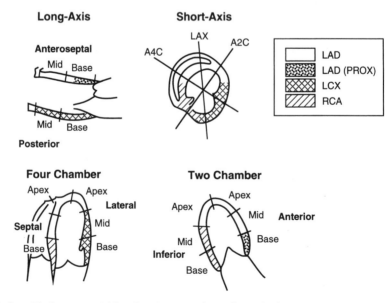

Figure 7.3.   Left ventricular segmental function at stress echocardiography (16-segment model of the American Society of Echocardiography). *A4C,* apical four-chamber; *LAX,* long axis; *A2C,* apical two-chamber; *LAD,* left anterior descending coronary artery; *LCX,* left circumflex artery; *RCA,* right coronary artery; *PROX,* proximal. (Reproduced with permission from Topol EJ, Textbook of Cardiovascular Medicine. Philadelphia: Lippincott-Raven Publishers, 1998:1279.)

difficulty with imaging the inferoposterior part of the heart (where low counts and scatter may lead to false-negative results). The longer half-life and photon energy of technetium Tc 99m are more favorable for imaging, and the isonitriles have alleviated but not resolved many of these limitations of [201]Tl.

As in the case of stress echocardiography, the performance of maximum stress is an important determinant of the reliability of myocardial perfusion imaging (51). Again, exercise stress is preferable if the patient is able to exercise maximally. In patients unable to exercise, dipyridamole or adenosine SPECT has been shown to have a sensitivity similar to that with exercise stress (52–54) with a high level of safety (55, 56).

PRACTICAL ASPECTS OF POSITRON EMISSION TOMOGRAPHY

This technique uses the same tracer kinetic principles as SPECT. However, the principles of imaging are different, because photons released during the annihilation of positrons simultaneously activate opposing detectors (57). In contrast with SPECT, PET offers greater spatial resolution and better contrast resolution owing to higher available counts and attenuation correction. However, the technique is expensive and not widely available.

Positron emission tomography myocardial perfusion imaging protocols may involve exercise or pharmacologic stress, depending on the choice of radionuclide. The usual imaging sequence involves the acquisition of attenuation correction data, followed by a resting scan, stress, and stress imaging. Examination of rubidium (Rb) washout may address the issue of myocardial viability (58), although this is usually addressed with metabolic imaging (see below).

INTERPRETATION

The detection of myocardial ischemia depends on comparison of relative activity in stress and rest images. Infarction produces a persistent ("fixed") perfusion defect, because the tissue is malperfused at all times. Ischemic myocardium demonstrates a perfusion defect on the stress images, which dissipates as thallium is taken up from the blood pool (to which it returns from extracardiac sites after stress). An experienced observer is necessary, as a number of potential artifacts may influence the results, especially with SPECT

imaging (59). Sequential short-axis images may be combined into a "bull's-eye" format (polar map), so that perfusion may be compared with a population standard (60). The feasibility of this quantitative evaluation is in contrast to echocardiography. High-risk patients with multivessel disease may be detected by multiple perfusion defects, transient dilatation of the left ventricle, and increased lung thallium uptake (61, 62).

The long half-life of ^{201}Tl precludes the performance of a true resting scan, unless a significant interval is possible between this and the stress image. If a stress-induced perfusion defect is present, this will dissipate with time, as long as the myocardium is viable and blood flow continues to deliver thallium to the tissue (63). Conventional thallium protocols require redistribution imaging after a delay of 4 to 6 hours; this process may be delayed in the presence of severe ischemia (64, 65). Reversibility therefore may be demonstrated by rescanning some fixed defects at 24 hours (66), or by reinjection of thallium (67). Delayed redistribution is unique to thallium protocols and is important in the distinction of scar from ischemia in postinfarction patients. Assessment of viability with other agents (^{99m}Tc sestamibi, PET perfusion tracers) is dependent on assessment of relative or absolute flow or kinetic measurements that describe wash-in or wash-out of the tracers.

DIAGNOSTIC ACCURACY

Thallium SPECT has a sensitivity of 90% and a specificity of 70% in comparison with coronary angiography (68). The accuracy of MIBI-SPECT and dual-isotope techniques has been comparable, but new techniques, such as gated SPECT, may avoid some artifacts and further enhance specificity. Positron emission tomography is highly accurate for the detection of coronary artery disease (69). Attenuation correction restricts false-positive scans caused by interposed soft tissue. The high-energy emissions and recording of only coincident photons reduce scatter, producing high-quality images of the inferoposterior area. Good contrast resolution (from high counts) enable the detection of mild ischemia, as well as the detection of relatively small foci of ischemia.

As in the case of stress echocardiography, the population studied influences the accuracy of data, and sensitivities are inflated in postinfarction patients. Nonetheless, these parameters may be used to compare different techniques against a separate "gold standard," coronary angiography. Such studies have shown stress echocardiography and perfusion scintigraphy to have similar sensitivity and specificity for the identification of coronary artery disease (70). Nonetheless, in the rehabilitation population, analysis of the sensitivity and specificity of tests is limited because this binary approach ("positive" or "negative" test results) does not discriminate between the diagnoses of scar and ischemia (both "positive"). A more appropriate means of comparison involves assessment of the degree of concordance between the tests in the categorization of coronary disease (into normal ischemic and scar tissue) on a regional basis. Most published series report approximately 80% agreement between the techniques (33, 44, 71). Compared with exercise echocardiography, SPECT thallium imaging may be superior for the identification of ischemia in regions of previous infarction (33). On the other hand, dobutamine echocardiography may avoid the problems of exercise stress in this context (47) and may avoid the problems posed by delayed thallium redistribution. Both the rest-reinjection and stress-redistribution-reinjection techniques are sensitive for the detection of viable tissue, but their specificity has been variable.

PROGNOSTIC VALUE

A number of studies have addressed the prognostic implications of myocardial perfusion imaging with planar and SPECT techniques. These data indicate that the total stress defect extent (reflecting scar, viable, and ischemic myocardium), reversible defect extent, and the presence of factors suggesting severe disease (transient dilatation and increased lung uptake) are predictive of subsequent events (72). Similarly, total defect extent has been a powerful prognostic determinant with PET imaging (73).

Apart from patients with completely normal electrocardiograms (74)—which are uncommon in the rehabilitation population—myocardial perfusion imaging has been shown to supply prognostic data incremental to that provided by exercise testing (75). There are scant published data comparing the prognostic aspects of stress echocardiography and myocardial perfusion imaging. A small study in patients after MI has

suggested that ischemia documented by stress echocardiography is a more potent predictor of subsequent events than abnormal perfusion imaging (76). The benefits of providing simultaneous flow and function data, using gated SPECT, remain unclear from a prognostic standpoint.

MYOCARDIAL METABOLIC IMAGING

Historically, PET has been the technique most associated with assessment of myocardial metabolism. The initial methodology used [^{18}F]-fluorodeoxyglucose (FDG) to trace the myocardial uptake of glucose (77). Subsequent studies have examined aerobic metabolism (78). Recent advances promise to offer comparable data using SPECT to assess either FDG uptake (79) or fatty acid metabolism using free fatty acids (FFAs) labeled with iodine 123 (80). As these modalities have yet to move into widespread clinical use, this discussion will focus on PET as the method of choice for the performance of myocardial metabolic imaging.

Methodology

The most widely used FDG protocol involves glucose loading before FDG injection. The aim of this is to increase cellular glucose (and thereby FDG) uptake. However, the uptake of FDG depends on the glucose and insulin response, and some centers have opted for a euglycemic glucose-clamp approach to standardize the hormonal milieu (81). The alternative approach, fasting or post-exercise imaging, may identify both viable and ischemic myocardium (82) at the same scan. This is technically difficult and is now rarely performed.

Although most centers perform myocardial perfusion imaging to define a "metabolism-perfusion mismatch" (83), a consensus is lacking on how this should be defined. This is an important issue, because the *presence* of viable tissue may be less important in terms of management than its *extent*.

Accuracy of FDG-PET for Assessment of Viability

The sensitivity of FDG-PET for the detection of viable segments is usually reported as more than 90%. The specificity is more variable, with some reports in the range of 50% (78). To confer significant improvements in symptom status, EF, and exercise capacity, extensive viable myocardium (probably more than 20% to 25% of LV mass) is required (84). From a prognostic standpoint, failure to revascularize viable tissue may be associated with adverse events (85–87).

CONCLUSIONS

The safe selection of patients for rehabilitation is based on the premise that those who show residual ischemic tissue will be identified so that they can be rehabilitated in their most effective functional state. The investigation of these patients also is directed toward tailoring rehabilitation techniques to the patient's functional state and, therefore, to their degree of infarct burden. In both these respects, determination of residual ischemia and the degree of myocardial viability are important considerations. Functional assessment using myocardial perfusion imaging or wall-motion imaging with stress should be considered mandatory for patients who are suitable for revascularization after infarction.

References

1. Groupo Italiano per lo studio della streptokinasi nell'infarcto miocardio (GISSI). Effectiveness of intravenous thrombolytic treatment in acute myocardial infarction. Lancet 1986;1:397–402.
2. Sanz G, Castaner A, Betriu A, et al. Determinants of prognosis in survivors of myocardial infarction: a prospective clinical angiographic study. N Engl J Med 1982;306:1065–1070.
3. Machecourt J, Longere P, Fagret D, et al. Prognostic value of thallium-201 single photon emission computed tomographic myocardial perfusion imaging according to extent of myocardial defect. J Am Soc Cardiol 1994;23:1096–1106.
4. Vlietstra RE, Assad-Morrell JL, Frye RL, et al. Survival predictors in coronary artery disease: medical and surgical comparisons. Mayo Clin Proc 1977;52:85–90.
5. Multicenter Postinfarction Research Group. Risk stratification and survival after myocardial infarction. N Engl J Med 1983;309:331–336.
6. Fudo T, Kambara H, Hashimoto T, et al. F-18 Deoxyglucose and stress N-13 ammonia positron emission tomography in anterior wall healed myocardial infarction. Am J Cardiol 1988;61:1191–1197.
7. Braunwald E, Kloner RA. The stunned myocardium: prolonged postischemic ventricular dysfunction. Circulation 1982;66:1146–1149.
8. Rahimtoola SH. The hibernating myocardium. Am Heart J 1989;117:2113–2115.
9. Gibson RS, Watson DD, Craddock GB, et al. Prediction of cardiac events after uncomplicated myocardial infarction: a prospective study comparing predischarge exercise thallium-201 scintigraphy and coronary angiography. Circulation 1983;68:321–336.

10. Hamer AW, Takayama M, Abraham KA, et al. End-systolic volume and long-term survival after coronary artery bypass graft surgery in patients with impaired left ventricular function. Circulation 1994;90:2899–2904.
11. Parker DA, Thrall JH, Froelich JW. Radionuclide ventriculography: methods. In: Gerson MC, ed. Cardiac nuclear medicine. New York: McGraw-Hill, 1987:67–84.
12. Burow RD, Strauss HW, Singleton R, et al. Analysis of left ventricular function from multiple gated acquisition cardiac blood pool imaging: comparison to contrast angiography. Circulation 1977;56:1024–1030.
13. Palmas W, Friedman JD, Diamond GA, et al. Incremental value of simultaneous assessment of myocardial function and perfusion with technetium-99m sestamibi for prediction of extent of coronary artery disease. J Am Soc Cardiol 1995;25:1024–1031.
14. Stamm RB, Carabello BA, Mayers DL, et al. Two-dimensional echocardiographic measurement of left ventricular ejection fraction: prospective analysis of what constitutes an adequate determination. Am Heart J 1982;104:136–144.
15. Gorcsan J, Lazar JM, Schulman DS, et al. Comparison of left ventricular function by echocardiographic automated border detection and by radionuclide ejection fraction. Am J Cardiol 1993;72:810–815.
16. Sun JP, Pu M, Fouad FM, et al. Automated cardiac output measurement by spatiotemporal integration of color Doppler data: in vitro and clinical validation. Circulation 1997;95:932–939.
17. Starling MR, Crawford MH, Sorensen SG, et al. Comparative accuracy of apical biplane cross-sectional echocardiography and gated equilibrium radionuclide ventriculography for the estimation of left ventricular size and performance. Circulation 1981;63:1075–1084.
18. Kan G, Visser CA, Koolen JJ, et al. Short and long term predictive value of admission wall motion score in acute myocardial infarction. A cross-sectional echocardiographic study of 345 patients. Br Heart J 1986;56:422–427.
19. Nishimura RA, Reeder GS, Miller FA, et al. Prognostic value of predischarge 2-dimensional echocardiogram after acute myocardial infarction. Am J Cardiol 1984;53:429–432.
20. Morris KG, Palmeri ST, Califf RM, et al. Value of radionuclide angiography for predicting specific cardiac events after acute myocardial infarction. Am J Cardiol 1985;55:318–325.
21. Kuchar D, Freund J, Yeates M, et al. Enhanced prediction of major cardiac events after myocardial infarction using exercise radionuclide ventriculography. Aust NZ J Med 1987;17:228–233.
22. Abraham RD, Harris PJ, Roubin GS, et al. Usefulness of ejection fraction response to exercise one month after acute myocardial infarction in predicting coronary anatomy and prognosis. Am J Cardiol 1987;60:225–230.
23. Rozanski A, Diamond GA, Berman D, et al. The declining specificity of exercise radionuclide ventriculography. N Engl J Med 1983;309:518–522.
24. Limacher MC, Quinones MA, Poliner LR, et al. Detection of coronary artery disease with exercise two-dimensional echocardiography. Description of a clinically

applicable method and comparison with radionuclide ventriculography. Circulation 1983;67:1211–1218.

25. Feigenbaum H. Exercise echocardiography. J Am Soc Echocardiogr 1988;1:161–166.

26. Presti CF, Armstrong WF, Feigenbaum H. Comparison of echocardiography at peak exercise and after bicycle exercise in evaluation of patients with known or suspected coronary artery disease. J Am Soc Echocardiogr 1988;1:119–126.

27. Picano E. Dipyridamole-echocardiography test: historical background and physiologic basis. Eur Heart J 1989;10:365–376.

28. Sawada SG, Segar DS, Ryan T, et al. Echocardiographic detection of coronary artery disease during dobutamine infusion. Circulation 1991;83:1605–1614.

29. Orlandini A, Picano E, Lattanzi F, et al. Stress echocardiography and the human factor: the importance of being an expert. J Am Coll Cardiol 1990;15:52–58.

30. Hoffmann R, Lethen H, Marwick T, et al. Analysis of interinstitutional observer agreement in interpretation of dobutamine stress echocardiograms. J Am Soc Cardiol 1996;27:330–336.

31. Ginzton LE, Conant R, Brizendine M, et al. Quantitative analysis of segmental wall motion during maximal upright dynamic exercise: variability in normal adults. Circulation 1986;73:268–275.

32. Katz WE, Gulati VK, Mahler CM, et al. Quantitative evaluation of the segmental left ventricular response to dobutamine stress by tissue Doppler echocardiography. Am J Cardiol 1997;79:1036–1042.

33. Quinones MA, Verani MS, Haichin RM, et al. Exercise echocardiography versus 201Tl single-photon emission computed tomography in evaluation of coronary artery disease. Analysis of 292 patients. Circulation 1992;85:1026–1031.

34. Armstrong W, O'Donnell W, Ryan T, et al. Effect of prior myocardial infarction and extent and location of coronary disease on accuracy of exercise echocardiography. J Am Soc Cardiol 1987;10:531–538.

35. Roger VL, Pellikka PA, Oh JK, et al. Identification of multivessel coronary artery disease by exercise echocardiography. J Am Soc Cardiol 1994;24:109–114.

36. Beleslin BD, Ostojic M, Stepanovic J, et al. Stress echocardiography in the detection of myocardial ischemia. Head-to-head comparison of exercise, dobutamine, and dipyridamole tests. Circulation 1994; 90:1168–1176.

37. Marwick TH, Nemec JJ, Pashkow FJ, et al. Accuracy and limitations of exercise echocardiography in a routine clinical setting. J Am Soc Cardiol 1992;19:74–81.

38. Hecht HS, DeBord L, Sotomayor N, et al. Supine bicycle stress echocardiography: peak exercises imaging is superior to postexercises imaging. J Am Soc Echocardiogr 1993;6:265–271.

39. Crouse LJ, Harbrecht JJ, Vacek JL, et al. Exercise echocardiography as a screening test for coronary artery disease and correlation with coronary arteriography. Am J Cardiol 1991;67:1213–1218.

40. Ryan T, Segar DS, Sawada SG, et al. Detection of coronary artery disease with upright bicycle exercise echocardiography. J Am Soc Echocardiogr 1993;6:186–197.

41. Pingitore A, Picano E, Colosso MQ, et al. The atropine factor in pharmacologic stress echocardiography. Echo Persantine (EPIC) and Echo Dobutamine International Cooperative (EDIC) Study Groups. J Am Soc Cardiol 1996;27:1164–1170.

42. Takeuchi M, Araki M, Nakashima Y, et al. Comparison of dobutamine stress echocardiography and stress thallium-201 single-photon emission computed tomography for detecting coronary artery disease. J Am Soc Echocardiogr 1993;6:593–602.

43. Ostojic M, Picano E, Beleslin B, et al. Dipyridamole-dobutamine echocardiography: a novel test for the detection of milder forms of coronary artery disease. J Am Soc Cardiol 1994;23:1115–1122.

44. Marwick T, D'Hondt AM, Baudhuin T, et al. Optimal use of dobutamine stress for the detection and evaluation of coronary artery disease: combination with echocardiography or scintigraphy, or both? J Am Soc Cardiol 1993:22:159–167.

45. Ling LH, Pellikka, PA, Mahoney DW, et al. Atropine augmentation in dobutamine stress echocardiography: role and incremental value in a clinical practice setting. J Am Soc Cardiol 1996;28:551–557.

46. Vanoverschelde JL, Pasquet A, Melin JA. Echocardiographic techniques for assessment of myocardial viability. In: Marwick TH, ed. Cardiac stress testing and imaging. New York: Churchill Livingstone, 1996: 475–490.

47. Senior R, Lahiri A. Enhanced detection of myocardial ischemia by stress dobutamine echocardiography utilizing the "biphasic" response of wall thickening during low and high dose dobutamine infusion. J Am Soc Cardiol 1995:26:26–32.

48. Silverman K, Becker L, Bulkley B, et al. Value of early thallium-201 scintigraphy for predicting mortality in patients with acute myocardial infarction. Circulation 1980;61:996–1003.

49. Fintel DJ, Links JM, Brinker JA, et al. Improved diagnostic performance of exercise thallium-201 single photon emission computed tomography over planar imaging in the diagnosis of coronary artery disease: a receiver operating characteristic analysis. J Am Coll Cardiol 1989;13:600–612.

50. De Pasquale EE, Nody AC, De Puey EG, et al. Quantitative rotational thallium-201 tomography for identifying and localizing coronary artery disease. Circulation 1988;77:316–327.

51. Iskandrian AS, Heo J, Kong B, et al. Effect of exercise level on the ability of thallium-201 tomographic imaging in detecting coronary artery disease: analysis of 461 patients. J Am Coll Cardiol 1989;14: 1477–1486.

52. Timmis AD, Lutkin JE, Fenney LJ, et al. Comparison of dipyridamole and treadmill exercise for enhancing thallium-201 perfusion defects in patients with coronary artery disease. Eur Heart J 1980;1:275–280.

53. Josephson MA, Brown BG, Hecht HS, et al. Noninvasive detection and localization of coronary stenoses in patients: comparison of resting dipyridamole and exercise thallium-201 myocardial perfusion imaging. Am Heart J 1982;103:1008–1018.

54. Coyne EP, Belvedere DA, Vande Streek PR, et al. Thallium-201 scintigraphy after intravenous infusion of

adenosine compared with exercise thallium testing in the diagnosis of coronary artery disease. J Am Soc Cardiol 1991;17:1289–1294.

55. Ranhosky A, Kempthorne-Rawson J. The safety of intravenous dipyridamole thallium myocardial perfusion imaging. Circulation 1990;81:1205–1209.

56. Cerqueira MD, Verani MS, Schwaiger M, et al. Safety profile of adenosine stress perfusion imaging: results from the Adenoscan Multicenter Trial Registry. J Am Soc Cardiol 1994;23:384–389.

57. Phelps, ME, Hoffman EJ, Mullani NA, et al. Application of annihilation coincidence detection into transaxial reconstruction tomography. J Nucl Med 1975;16:210–218.

58. Gould L, Yoshida K, Hess M, et al. Myocardial metabolism of fluorodeoxyglucose compared to cell membrane integrity for the potassium analog rubidium-82 for assessing infarct size in man by PET. J Nucl Med 1991;32:1–9.

59. DePuey EG, Garcia EV. Optimal specificity of thallium-201 SPECT through recognition of imaging artifacts. J Nucl Med 1989;30:441–449.

60. Maddahi J, Garcia EV, Berman DS, et al. Improved non-invasive assessment of coronary artery disease by quantitative analysis of regional stress myocardial distribution and washout of Tl-201. Circulation 1981; 64:924–935.

61. Boucher CA, Zir LM, Beller GA, et al. Increased lung uptake of Tl-201 during exercise myocardial imaging: clinical, hemodynamic and angiographic implications in patients with coronary artery disease. Am J Cardiol 1980;46:189–196.

62. Weiss AT, Berman DS, Lew AS, et al. Transient ischemic dilation of the left ventricle on stress thallium-201 scintigraphy: a marker of severe and extensive coronary artery disease. J Am Coll Cardiol 1987;9:752–759.

63. Beller GA, Pohost GM. Mechanisms for Tl-201 redistribution after transient myocardial ischemia. Circulation 1977;56:141–148.

64. Gutman J, Berman DS, Freeman M, et al. Time to completed redistribution of thallium-201 in exercise myocardial scintigraphy: relationship to the degree of coronary artery stenosis. Am Heart J 1983;106:989–995.

65. Cloninger K, DePuey EG, Garcia EV, et al. Incomplete redistribution in delayed thallium-201 single photon emission computed tomographic (SPECT) images: an overestimation of myocardial scarring. J Am Coll Cardiol 1988;12:955–962.

66. Kiat H, Berman DS, Maddahi J, et al. Late reversibility of tomographic myocardial Tl-201 defects: an accurate marker of myocardial viability. J Am Coll Cardiol 1988;12:1456–1463.

67. Dilsizian V, Rocco TP, Freedman NM, et al. Enhanced detection of ischemic but viable myocardium by the reinjection of thallium after stress-redistribution imaging. N Engl J Med 1990;323:141–146.

68. Maddahi J, Rodrigues E, Berman DS, et al. State of the art myocardial perfusion imaging. In: Verani MS, ed. Nuclear cardiology: state of the art. Philadelphia: WB Saunders, 1994; 199–222.

69. Schwaiger M. Myocardial perfusion imaging with PET. J Nucl Med 1994;35:693–698.

70. O'Keefe JH Jr, Barnhart CS, Bateman TM. Comparison of stress echocardiography and stress myocardial perfusion scintigraphy for diagnosing coronary artery disease and assessing its severity. Am J Cardiol 1995;75: 25D–34D.

71. Pozzoli MM, Fioretti PM, Salustri A, et al. Exercise echocardiography and technetium 99m MIBI single photon emission computed tomography in the detection of coronary artery disease. Am J Cardiol 1991;67: 350–355.

72. Heller GV, Brown KA. Prognosis of acute and chronic coronary artery disease by myocardial perfusion imaging. Cardiol Clin 1994;12:271–287.

73. Marwick TH, Shan K, Patel S, et al. Incremental value of rubidium-82 positron emission tomography for prognostic assessment of known or suspected coronary artery disease. Am J Cardiol 1997;80:865–870.

74. Christian TF, Miller TD, Bailey KR, et al. Exercise thallium-201 imaging in patients with severe coronary artery disease and normal electrocardiograms. Ann Intern Med 1994;121:825–832.

75. Hachamovitch R, Berman DS, Kiat H, et al. Exercise myocardial perfusion SPECT in patients without known coronary artery disease: incremental prognostic value and use in risk stratification. Circulation 1996;93:905–914.

76. van Daele ME, McNeill AJ, Fioretti PM, et al. Prognostic value of dipyridamole sestamibi single photon emission computed tomography and dipyridamole stress echocardiography for new cardiac events after an uncomplicated myocardial infarction. J Am Soc Echocardiogr 1994;7:370–380.

77. Phelps ME, Hoffman EJ, Selin C, et al. Investigation of [F-18] 2-fluoro-2-deoxyglucose for the measure of myocardial glucose metabolism. J Nucl Med 1978;19: 1311–1319.

78. Gropler RJ, Geltman EM, Sampathkumaran K, et al. Comparison of carbon-11-acetate with fluorine-18-fluorodeoxyglucose for delineating viable myocardium by positron emission tomography. J Am Soc Cardiol 1993;22:1587–1597.

79. Bax JJ, Cornel JH, Visser FC, et al. Prediction of improvement of contractile function in patients with ischemic ventricular dysfunction after revascularization by fluorine-18 fluorodeoxyglucose single-photon emission computed tomography. J Am Soc Cardiol 1997;30:377–383.

80. Franken PR, De Geeter F, Dendale P, et al. Abnormal free fatty acid uptake in subacute myocardial infarction after coronary thrombolysis: correlation with wall motion and inotropic reserve. J Nucl Med 1994;35: 1758–1765.

81. Knuuti MJ, Nuutila P, Ruotsalainen U, et al. Euglycemic hyperinsulinemic clamp and oral glucose load in stimulating myocardial glucose utilization during positron emission tomography. J Nucl Med 1992;33: 1255–1262.

82. Marwick TH, MacIntyre WJ, Salcedo EE, et al. Identification of ischemic and hibernating myocardium: feasibility of post-exercise F-18 deoxyglucose positron emission tomography. Cath Cardiovasc Diagn 1991; 22:100–106.

83. Schelbert HR. Blood flow and metabolism by PET. Cardiol Clin 1994;12:303–315.

84. Marwick TH, Nemec JJ, Lafont A, et al. Prediction by postexercise fluoro-18 deoxyglucose positron emission tomography of improvement in exercise capacity after revascularization. Am J Cardiol 1992;69:854–859.

85. Di Carli MF, Davidson M, Little R, et al. Value of metabolic imaging with positron emission tomography for evaluating prognosis in patients with coronary artery disease and left ventricular dysfunction. Am J Cardiol 1994;73:527–533.

86. Lee KS, Marwick TH, Cook SA, et al. Prognosis of patients with left ventricular dysfunction, with and without viable myocardium after myocardial infarction: relative efficacy of medial therapy and revascularization. Circulation 1994;90:2687–2694.

87. Eitzman D, Al Aouar Z, Kanter HL, et al. Clinical outcome of patients with advanced coronary disease after viability studies with positron emission tomography. J Am Coll Cardiol 1992;20:559–564.

Exercise Prescription Development and Supervision

Gordon G. Blackburn, Sharon A. Harvey, William A. Dafoe, and Ray W. Squires

Part A. Perspectives on the Formulation of Exercise Prescriptions
Gordon G. Blackburn and
Sharon A. Harvey

Historically, activity guidelines, or restrictions, were the cornerstone of cardiac rehabilitation. Today, cardiac rehabilitation has evolved beyond such a simplistic approach and recognizes that rehabilitation, just like the disease process itself, is multifactorial. Exercise is just one component of a program designed to reduce a patient's risk factors for future cardiac events, while maximizing the patient's potential to carry on a satisfying and active lifestyle. Exercise does remain a key component of the rehabilitation program, however, and the application of appropriate guidelines for activity has become more complex and challenging as the benefits of regular activity have been demonstrated in high-acuity patients, as new procedures and technologies are introduced, and as the medication armamentarium continues to expand drastically.

The development of an exercise prescription must be based not only on a comprehensive understanding of the patient's medical history, current status, and medication regimen but also on a solid understanding of exercise physiology as it relates to recreational and vocational activities. In addition, insight into the patient's interests and expectations regarding activity is essential. Application of the basic scientific principles of exercise prescription allows the clinician to create an appropriate exercise prescription, but there also is an art to developing an effective ex-

ercise prescription. This chapter addresses the basic scientific principles of exercise prescription, but the sterile application of these principles across all patients is likely to result in less than satisfactory outcomes for the patient and the clinician alike. Experience and individualization of the exercise prescription are essential for optimal success in activity programming. This, like any other clinical skill, cannot be learned solely from a textbook.

EXERCISE PROGRAM DESIGN

Despite the increased complexity of patients referred to cardiac rehabilitation programs, the basics of exercise prescription remain unchanged. Before the subtleties of exercise prescription can be applied to individual patients, the basics must be mastered. Every activity program should consist of a warm-up, conditioning, and cool-down period (1).

Warm-up Period

The warm-up period is literally that, a period of between 5 and 15 minutes, during which time the musculature and joint structures are stimulated gently with a series of static stretches and dynamic range-of-motion (ROM) activities. Lack of flexibility has been associated with increased risk for orthopedic complications. A goal of the warm-up stretches is to promote a normal ROM. Persons with above-average ROMs should not be assumed to have less orthopedic risk. They actually may be at increased risk for injury if the musculature to stabilize the joint is inadequate.

The type of specific stretching activity varies, depending on orthopedic limitations or special needs. Typically, the large muscle groups of the lower and upper extremities, as well as the lower back, are included in the warm-up stretches. Emphasis should be given to the muscle groups to be used in the conditioning activity. Range-of-motion activities should be conducted slowly with gradually increasing ROM about the joint. Static stretches should be conducted only to the point at which a gentle pull sensation is felt in the musculature being stretched. The stretch should be held for approximately 15 to 30 seconds and should not elicit discomfort or pain. During static stretches, it is important to encourage the patient to continue to breathe to avoid a Valsalva maneuver that can cause exaggerated blood pressure (BP) responses. The patient should also be counseled to avoid "bouncing" or "jerking" during the stretch. This prevents activation of the muscle spindle reflex that would cause muscle contraction, thus limiting the impact of the stretching activity and increasing the chance for muscle tears.

Low-level, dynamic aerobic activity at approximately 25% to 40% of the patient's functional capacity (FC) also should be included as part of the warm-up. This may not be necessary if the patient's FC is very low because the ROM activities may provide adequate stimulus. For most patients, however, a 3- to 5-minute period of casual to moderate walking is recommended before more vigorous activity. This activity allows muscle temperature to rise, aiding in stretching and contraction; offsets the initial oxygen debt that would occur if more vigorous activity were engaged in without warm-up; and has been shown to extend the anginal/ischemic threshold during activity (2). All this combines to make the activity more enjoyable while minimizing the risk of orthopedic and cardiovascular complications.

There is very limited research on the optimal structure of the warm-up period. It generally is recommended that if stretching activities are done before the low-level aerobic activity, they be performed with care. However, warm-up activities are recommended before engaging in more vigorous aerobic activity.

Conditioning Period

The conditioning period is the part of the exercise session in which the activity stimulus increases or is maintained to bring about the desired changes. The conditioning period may be designed to focus on the following activities:

1. To increase caloric expenditure to aid with weight management
2. To improve overall functional capacity
3. To delay the onset of symptoms
4. To maintain current functional ability
5. To improve muscle tone or strength
6. To optimize job or avocational abilities
7. To optimize recreational activity performance
8. To optimize ability to perform activities of daily living (ADL)

Regardless of the goal for the conditioning period, it must address five key factors:

1. Frequency
2. Intensity
3. Mode
4. Duration
5. Rate of progression

The focus of the program should determine the emphasis placed on each of these factors.

FREQUENCY

The frequency with which the conditioning stimulus is applied can vary from several times per day to just a few times per week. It is affected by the overall goal of the program but must be modified by the functional ability of the patient, the type and intensity of activity, and the patient's interests and level of personal commitment and recent activity history. Typically, the exercise stimulus must be applied at least three times per week to cause any improvement. If the patient's functional ability is extremely low, however, short bouts of activity offered two to three times daily may be more beneficial. The latter is true for most patients engaged in cardiac rehabilitation immediately after their surgery or infarction or for persons who have functional capacities less than 5 metabolic equivalents (METs.)

The standard recommendation for frequency of formal activity is three to five times per week. If the activity is engaged in only three times per week, it is recommended that the sessions be spaced equally throughout the week. If the intensity of the activity is relatively low, and especially if caloric expenditure is a major goal of the activity program, more frequent activity sessions, up to six to seven times per week, will prove beneficial providing the orthopedic stress can be tolerated. From an FC improvement standpoint, there is minimal gain by extending the program beyond five days per week.

The majority of cardiac rehabilitation patients are mature adults who have family, community, and business commitments in addition to their rehabilitation programs. Couple this with the fact that many patients have been inactive for several years, are obese, and have concomitant osteoarthritic/osteoporotic conditions or low back pain, and it is likely that an overly aggressive exercise prescription with respect to frequency will result in poor compliance and increased risk. It is recommended that the average rehabilitation program begin with an exercise frequency of three times per week for at least the first 3 to 6 months. If after this time the patient has remained free of orthopedic complications and expresses an interest in increasing the frequency, the program can be extended to four to five times per week (3).

INTENSITY

Intensity describes the absolute and relative vigor with which an activity is performed. Ideally, the intensity of the exercise should be set at a level that allows the desired improvements to occur but is not high enough to cause clinical symptoms, patient discomfort, or disenchantment with the activity program. According to the American College of Sports Medicine (ACSM) guidelines (4), the intensity threshold for healthy adults is between 60% and 90% of maximum heart rate (HRmax) or between 50% and 85% of maximal oxygen uptake ($\dot{V}O_2$max) or heart rate (HR) reserve. Those with lower initial levels of fitness, such as many cardiac patients, however, may initiate their conditioning at 40% to 50% of $\dot{V}O_2$max. The typical range of exercise intensity for patients involved in cardiac rehabilitation is between 40% and 85% (4). Generally, the lower the patient's functional capacity and the higher the risk of future cardiac events, the lower the exercise intensity. Some studies suggested that for patients with large anterior wall infarctions and poor left ventricular (LV) function, formal aerobic conditioning at approximately 70% of functional capacity can lead to worsening of LV function (5). However, this should not exclude all cardiac patients from exercising at higher intensities. In low-risk cardiac popula-

tions, exercise intensities of up to 90% have been shown to be effective at increasing LV performance as well as overall FC (6, 7).

One approach to selecting the most appropriate exercise intensity for the patient is to use the "sliding scale" of intensity, as described in the ACSM guidelines (8) and referred to by Franklin et al. (9). The baseline exercise intensity was set at 60% of functional capacity. The patient-specific exercise intensity was determined by adding functional capacity, expressed in METs, to the base 60%. For example, if a patient had a peak FC of 7 METs, the exercise intensity would be as follows:

$$\text{Training Intensity} = (60 + \text{Max METs})\%$$
$$= (60 + 7)\%$$
$$= 67\%$$

This rendition of the sliding scale is appropriate for persons at low risk and with average to above-average FCs, but it is inappropriate to apply to the patient at high risk who has a low FC.

We have developed and used a more versatile version of the sliding scale for calculating exercise intensity. Instead of a base of 60%, we use a base of 40% and add twice the FC to the base. Thus the person who has an FC of only 5 METs would exercise at an intensity of 50% instead of 65%, whereas the patient at low risk, with a peak FC of 12 METs, would exercise at an intensity of 64% instead of 72%.

Exercise intensity is not static. The cost of the activity varies slightly from day to day, depending on the time of day, environmental factors, and time since medications were last taken. It is recommended that a window of exercise intensities be set that ranges 10% above and below the calculated or desired exercise intensity.

It should be noted that although emphasis has been on the selection of an exercise intensity based on the patient's peak FC, the ability to determine peak FC accurately is not as straightforward as one might have been led to believe. Peak FC can be measured directly by using gas exchange systems. The equipment for this is expensive, requires a degree of technical expertise to use, and adds a time factor to the study. Therefore, in most testing laboratories FC is estimated based on prediction formulas that consider treadmill speed and grade or workload on a cycle ergometer or from nomograms based on exercise duration time for given exercise protocols (10, 11). These methods have been shown to be accurate in healthy, young to middle-aged populations who do not have orthopedic limitations and do not take any cardiac medication (12). A significant volume of research has shown, however, that for persons who have coronary artery disease (CAD), poor LV function, or pacemakers, or those who are post-transplantation or on β-blockers, the prediction methods can drastically overestimate the peak FC (13–15). This appears to be related to altered oxygen kinetics in these populations.

Test technique also has been shown to have a significant impact on the ability to estimate FC from nomograms or prediction formulas (16, 17). If patients are allowed to use the front handrail in any way, including light contact, oxygen uptake can be overestimated by up to 31%. These overestimations impact significantly on the intensity selection for the exercise program.

For many patients it is unrealistic to expect that they can walk safely on the treadmill without some support. With a brief orientation and practice period, however, the majority of patients are able to walk with confidence by resting one hand on a side handrail for support. This method allows for a more accurate prediction of peak FC.

Medications, especially β-blockers, can alter the patient's FC significantly. Patients are often weaned off β-blockers before an exercise test, β-blockers might be prescribed after the exercise test, or patients on once-a-day β-blockers are tested at a time of day different from the time that they will be exercising. In each scenario, the FC determined from the exercise test can differ significantly from the FC of the patient during the rehabilitation program. If possible, to avoid errors in prescribing exercise intensity, it is desirable to conduct the exercise test for the exercise prescription on all usual medications and at the same approximate time of day as the patient exercises.

Methods of Applying Exercise Intensity

Once the appropriate exercise intensity has been determined for the patient, the next task is to translate that into specific activities. This can be accomplished in various ways.

WORKLOAD AND METS

Perhaps the most straightforward method is to calculate an exercise level based on METs. If the patient has a peak FC of 10 METs and the selected exercise intensity is 70%, then the appropriate MET level of exercise would be 7 METs. Assuming a 10% window on either side of the target intensity, a range of 6.3 to 7.7 METs would be appropriate. Speeds and grades, or workloads, to elicit these MET levels can be calculated using the ACSM formulas for walking or jogging on the treadmill or outside and for cycle or arm-crank ergometry (4).

For example, in the scenario already described, the desired range of 6.3 to 7.7 METs could be achieved by setting the treadmill at 3.5 mph and using a grade setting between 5.5% and 8.5%. These workloads can be determined using the treadmill walking formula as follows:

$$\text{METs} = [(\text{speed in m/min} \times 0.1) + (\text{grade as a decimal} \times \text{speed in m/min} \times 1.8) + 3.5]/3.5$$

When calculating workloads for the cycle ergometer, it is essential that the patient's weight be factored into the equation. Treadmill walking is weight-dependent; however, cycle and arm-crank activities are weight-independent. At a given workload on the cycle or arm ergometer, the absolute cost of performing the work is the same, but the cost of doing the work expressed per kilogram of body weight, or in METs, varies with total body weight. Therefore, when prescribing absolute workloads for the cycle or arm ergometer the patient's body weight must be factored into the equation. Cycle ergometer workloads are calculated using the leg ergometer formula as follows:

$$\text{Cycle Workload (kpm/min)} = [(\text{MET})(3.5)(\text{body weight}) - (3.5)(\text{body weight})]/2$$

Therefore, the leg ergometer setting to achieve 7 METs for a patient weighing 50 kg would be

$$\text{Cycle Workload (kpm/min)} = [(7)(3.5)(50) - (3.5)(50)]/2 = 525 \text{ kpm/min}$$

If, however, the patient weighed 100 kg, the cycle workload to achieve 7 METs would be

$$\text{Cycle Workload (kpm/min)} = [(7)(3.5)(100) - (3.5)(100)]/2 = 1050 \text{ kpm/min}$$

The advantage of using the ergometer settings to control exercise intensity is that specific workloads can be set that place the patient in the desired exercise range. However, such settings do not allow for fluctuations in environmental conditions or individual differences in exercise efficiency. The greatest drawback to using ergometer settings is the inability to account for improvement with time.

Not all activities lend themselves to specific workload settings. A list of common household and leisure activities are listed in the tables in appendix A. The average range of metabolic costs for these activities is graphically displayed. Although these are less specific than the cycle workload calculation, they can also be used in prescribing activities of the appropriate intensity. A major limitation of the MET tables is the inability to account for the skill level and competitive nature of a person for a given activity. Although the average cost of the activity may be appropriate, there may be extreme fluctuations in the cost of sporting activities.

HEART RATE AND EXERCISE INTENSITY

For most persons, a linear relationship exists between $\dot{V}O_2$ (or METs) and HR; therefore, HR can be used to prescribe exercise intensity. Three methods of determining appropriate exercise HRs to set exercise intensities have been described by the ACSM (1, 4). The first method involves plotting individual HRs during each stage of the exercise test against the predicted or measured MET cost of the activity. The target exercise intensity in METs is calculated using the treadmill or cycle ergometer formulas. The HRs achieved at the desired MET levels are used to guide the exercise intensity.

A second method relies on the established and relatively stable relationship between the percent of $\dot{V}O_2$ and the percent of peak HR. Although linear, the relationship does not follow the line of identity. The accepted relationship is 70% to 85% of peak HR corresponds to 60% to 80% of peak $\dot{V}O_2$. This relationship is stable for most patients and under a variety of conditions. The straight percentage of peak HR is easy to apply and accounts for improvements in FC. As the absolute $\dot{V}O_2$ increases, the relative relationship remains unaltered. Therefore, if clinical conditions remain stable and no medications that impact the chronotropic response to activity (such as β-blockers or amiodarone) are changed, the patient can use the same HR range to guide exercise intensity and rate of progression for an extended time.

The drawback of the straight HR percentage method is that it inherently accounts for HR response that ranges from zero beats per minute to the patient's actual peak HR. This causes the HR versus $\dot{V}O_2$ relationship to deviate from the line of identity, and the person who prescribes the activity must always be aware of the relationship that requires a different correction factor at $\dot{V}O_2$ of approximately 40%, compared with $\dot{V}O_2$ of 80%. The shortcomings of this method are especially apparent in the congestive heart failure (CHF) patient who has an elevated resting HR and a blunted peak HR. These patients continue to have a linear response in HR against $\dot{V}O_2$, but because the range is so small, the relationship between percent peak HR and percent peak $\dot{V}O_2$ is drastically altered.

For example, consider the patient with CHF who has a resting HR of 104 beats per minute and a peak HR of 134 beats per minute. Although the linear relationship between $\dot{V}O_2$ and HR exists, if a direct 80% of peak HR was taken, the calculated exercise HR would be 107 beats per minute, essentially the resting HR. If a more conservative intensity of 65% was selected, the recommended HR would be 87 beats per minute, a value lower than the patient's resting HR.

Calculations of the target HR that use the true dynamic range of HR response, or heart rate reserve, represent a third method of determining exercise intensity based on HR. This is known as the Karvonen method and is based on the linear and near one-to-one relationship between the percentage of HR reserve and percentage of $\dot{V}O_2$ (18). Using the Karvonen method, the exercise intensity HR, or target HR, is calculated by subtracting the resting HR from the peak HR, multiplying the difference by the desired exercise intensity (expressed as a percentage) and then adding the calculated value to the resting HR. For a patient with a resting HR of 70 beats per minute, a peak HR of 160 beats per minute, and a target exercise intensity of 60%, the calculations are as follows:

Peak HR:	160 beats per minute
Resting HR:	− 70 beats per minute
HR reserve:	90 beats per minute
Training intensity:	× 0.6 (or 60%)
	54
Resting HR:	+ 70 beats per minute
Target HR:	124 beats per minute

The clinician who develops exercise prescriptions needs to be aware that, consistent with metabolic load which needs to be adjusted for varying functional capacities on different modes of activity, the exercise HR also requires adjustment. As a general rule, the exercise HR response for the cycle is 6 beats per minute lower than for treadmill activity, and arm work is approximately 12 beats per minute lower.

For patients who show normal chronotropic responses to activity and who can palpate their own pulse rate accurately, the Karvonen method of directing the exercise intensity is accurate and reliable. For patients who have atrial fibrillation, sick sinus syndrome, or fixed or rate-responsive pacemakers, or who have received a heart transplant, the linear and consistent relationship between $\dot{V}O_2$ and HR does not exist, and HR cannot be used to guide exercise intensity. Patients who are unable to determine their own HR reliably, whether or not it is secondary to frequent arrhythmias, weak peripheral pulses, or decreased peripheral tactile sensation, or patients who cannot coordinate pulse counting with counting time, should not have exercise intensity prescribed using target HRs unless they are also monitored.

RATINGS OF PERCEIVED EXERTION AND EXERCISE INTENSITY

Another popular method to help guide exercise intensity is the use of the rating of perceived exertion (RPE) scales. There are two scales, both of which were developed by Borg (19, 20). Both scales are displayed in chapter 5 of this text (see Table 5.5). The first scale developed by Borg ranges from 6 to 20 and is linear, with word anchors that describe the exercise intensity equally spaced along the length of the scale. When the scale was first released, Borg identified a close relationship between HR and the RPE. Further investigation revealed that the relationship of perceived exertion was also affected by respiratory variables and lactate levels. The second scale has an exponential design to the spacing of the word anchors and runs from 0 to 10.

The relationship between a patient's perception of exertion and the exercise intensity has been shown to be valid. On average, a perceived exertion of 12 to 16, on the 6 to 20 scale, corresponds with a HR response of between 60% and 85%, respectively. Therefore, it is usually recommended that exercise be maintained at an intensity between these values. For ratings on the 10-point scale, values between 3 and 6 correspond to a similar HR response.

The RPE scales are convenient and easy to administer, but there are individual variations with respect to their use. Also, there is no method of validating the patient's rating with true feelings. Therefore, it is important to recognize these outliers and ensure that if RPE is used to guide exercise intensity, the RPE range is appropriate for that patient.

ONSET OF SYMPTOMS AND EXERCISE INTENSITY

Any or all of the previously described methods can be used to help control exercise intensity, but the onset of symptoms during activity should be an absolute determinant of the upper limit of the exercise intensity. If significant yet stable ischemic changes or symptoms occur with activity, the exercise intensity must be established at a level adequately below the threshold for these findings. Usually a 10- to 12-beats per minute buffer, below the onset of the ischemic changes, is selected as the upper intensity level of activity. Heart rate alone cannot predict the ischemic threshold. The rate-pressure-product (RPP) threshold, however, can be used to set upper limits of exercise intensity because it predicts myocardial $\dot{V}O_2$ more accurately. However, not even the RPP ischemic threshold is a fixed number because the ischemic threshold varies not only between activities but also within the same mode of activity, depending on whether an adequate warm-up was used. Without an adequate warm-up angina can occur at a lower double product (21).

DURATION

The duration of the conditioning period typically lasts between 15 and 60 minutes. The specific duration is determined by the goal of the program and the patient's ability and interests. A minimum of 15 minutes of aerobic activity is necessary to achieve an improvement in FC. The optimal duration of the conditioning period for most cardiac patients is between 20 and 40 minutes. This can be extended if the intensity is reduced and a goal of the program is increased caloric expenditure.

For most patients, the goal is to achieve continuous activity during the conditioning period at the prescribed intensity; however, patients with significant claudication, low FC, or marked weakness may not be able to maintain the prescribed intensity for the desired duration. These patients may require an interval program. With an interval program patients exercise until they are limited by symptoms (e.g., claudication, fatigue, or dyspnea). The program then is interrupted until the symptoms subside, after which time it is resumed until the symptoms return. This pattern is repeated until the total exercise time of all intervals equals the prescribed duration.

Interval programs also may be used by persons who are training at intensities too high for a comfortable walk but too low for continuous jogging. Patients without orthopedic complications and an FC of between 10 and 12 METs most often fall into this category. The highest MET level they can achieve walking outside is 4 to 5 METs, which would be below their recommended conditioning intensity. A slow jog on the level at a 12-minute-mile pace is too high to be sustained at 8.6 METs. Therefore, these patients can continue to benefit from an alternating conditioning stimulus of walk and jog periods. Although the body does not respond in a square wave fashion to the onset and offset of activity, a simplistic mathematical averaging of the MET cost of the two exercise intensities, weighted for the duration at each intensity, approximates the average MET cost of the session. For example, for a patient with a 10-MET FC and a training intensity range of 65% to 75%, continuous walking would be too low and continuous jogging would be too high. However, if the patient jogs at a 5-mph pace on the level (8.6 METs) for 4 minutes and walks at a 3-mph pace on the level for 1 minute, the average MET cost for the activity would be

$$\text{Average MET} = [(\text{Cost of activity A} \times \text{Duration of A}) + (\text{Cost of activity B} \times \text{Duration of B})]/\text{Total activity time}$$

$$= [(8.6 \text{ METs} \times 4 \text{ min}) + (3.3 \text{ METs} \times 1 \text{ min})]/5 \text{ min}$$

$$= 7.5 \text{ METs}$$

This equates to 75% of FC. If the pattern is repeated six times, the patient would achieve 30 minutes of activity at approximately the desired intensity.

MODE

Any activity that uses a large muscle group in a rhythmical and repetitive fashion at the appropriate intensity and duration results in an improved FC. Selection of the most appropriate activity depends on the specific goals, needs, and abilities of the patient. Arguably, the most common forms of activity used in cardiac rehabilitation are walking and, if appropriate, jogging. These activities are familiar to all patients and represent the primary mode of self-ambulation in North America. Advantages of walking programs are that the exercise level can be maintained easily and accurately and the exercise intensity range is extremely wide.

Cycling is another popular type of conditioning activity used in cardiac rehabilitation programs. For persons who have low back pain, marked obesity, or joint instability, the stationary cycle can be an excellent mode of exercise. The cycle offers many of the same advantages as walking. The range of exercise intensities is almost unlimited and the activity is easily performed. Cycling is likely to lead to greater local muscle fatigue because of the increased resistance the legs must work against. In addition, caloric expenditure for cycle activity is lower than that for walking. This is owing to increased mechanical efficiency coupled with lower peak FC, resulting in lower absolute exercise intensities.

To optimize the benefits of exercise, it is critical, especially in cardiac rehabilitation in which central improvements are small or nonexistent, that the musculature used during vocational and recreational activities be used during the conditioning period. This follows the law of specificity of conditioning, which states simply that improvements occur in the muscles used during the conditioning activity and there is no crossover benefit to unused muscle groups. Therefore, if a patient's job or recreational hobbies depend heavily on the repetitive use of the upper extremities, then a significant portion of the conditioning activity should focus on these muscle groups. Seated-arm cycling, the Schwinn Air-Dyne® or a similar upper-extremity cycle, rowing, or, perhaps, stationary cross-country skiing devices could be included in the conditioning program.

Limitations of upper-extremity activity include significant local muscle fatigue, low caloric expenditure, and an unfamiliarity with most of the apparatus. In addition, the activity intensity guidelines must be modified significantly if a treadmill exercise test was conducted to develop the exercise prescription.

Variations in Functional Capacity Based on Test Mode

In North America, the primary mode of exercise testing is the treadmill. For most persons, the treadmill yields the highest FC, measured or estimated, as well as the highest peak HR. Cycle ergometry yields an FC that is only about 85% of that obtained on the treadmill, and peak HR observed is usually about 95% of that measured at peak exercise for treadmill activity. For arm ergometry, the observed peak FC falls off even more, reaching only 50% to 70% of treadmill values whereas peak HRs for arm cranking achieve only 85% to 90% of values achieved for treadmill exercise (22). These differences are important to consider when prescribing activity for various exercise modes based on the results of one exercise test. For example, consider the patient who has a peak FC on the treadmill of 10 METs and a desired exercise intensity of 70% of that value, or 7 METs. The patient decides to exercise using the cycle ergometer. If the difference in peak FC between the treadmill and cycle is not accounted for when the exercise intensity is transferred, the 7-MET absolute exercise intensity on the cycle would represent 82% of the FC on the cycle.

Treadmill FC	= 10 METs
Training Intensity	= 70%
	= (0.7 × 10 METs)
Desired Work load	= 7 METs
Estimated Cycle FC	= (Treadmill FC × 0.85) METs
	= (10 × 0.85) METs
Estimated Cycle FC	= 8.5 METs
Actual training intensity for cycle	= (7/8.5) × 100 = 82%

For persons unaccustomed to cycle or arm activity, for those who have small muscle masses, or for many geriatric patients, the reductions in FC between the treadmill and the cycle or arm ergometer are even greater than those already reported. If appropriate corrections are not applied, the patient may be asked to exercise at intensities beyond those recommended as appropriate.

Because of the differences in peak FC and peak HR between modes of exercise, it is recommended that the primary mode of exercise used in the rehabilitation program be used for the exercise test. In reality, a patient may use various exercise modes during the rehabilitation program, and it is impractical to think that an exercise test would be conducted for each activity. Therefore, conversion factors can be applied to develop appropriate exercise intensities for cycle and arm ergometry exercise.

For cycle exercise at a 70% intensity, based on a 10-MET maximal treadmill exercise study, take 85% of the treadmill FC to determine cycle peak FC and to calculate the cycle exercise level using the appropriate training intensity for the patient.

$$Cycle\ exercise\ level = (0.85 \times treadmill\ FC)$$
$$(training\ intensity)$$
$$= (0.85 \times 10\ METs)\ (0.7)$$
$$= 5.95\ METs$$

For arm exercise prescribed from cycle exercise study, take 60% of the cycle training exercise level.

$$Arm\ exercise\ level = (0.6 \times cycle\ exercise\ level)$$
$$METs$$
$$= (0.6 \times 5.95)$$
$$= 3.57\ METs$$

or take 50% of the cycle workload. If the appropriate cycle workload was 630 kpm/min, then

$$Arm\ workload = (0.5 \times cycle\ workload)$$
$$= (0.5 \times 630\ kpm/min)$$
$$= 315\ kpm/min$$

If a cycle-graded exercise test was conducted but the patient was supposed to exercise on the treadmill in the rehabilitation program, the treadmill exercise level can be calculated from the cycle exercise level using the following formula (23):

$$Treadmill\ METs = (0.98 \times cycle\ METs) + 1.85$$
$$= (0.98 \times 5.95) + 1.85$$
$$= 7.7\ METs$$

Absolute exercise intensities must be modified as the patient moves between exercise modes to ensure optimal safety and effectiveness.

Resistive Weight Activities

Historically, weight-training activities were felt to be contraindicated in a cardiac rehabilitation program secondary to the high increase in blood pressure and rapid rise in myocardial oxygen demand. Recent studies, however, have demonstrated the safety and benefit of isotonic and circuit weight-training programs (24–27). It is currently thought that dynamic isotonic exercise for the upper and lower extremities can be incorporated safely into the cardiac rehabilitation program for many patients. The activity should closely match the tasks that patients perform in their daily jobs and recreational activities. After open heart surgery and a passive recuperative period after a cardiac event, patients often lack the strength and confidence to perform what had been regular activities. If a patient plans to return to a lifestyle that includes moderate manual labor, including frequent lifting of weights, the cardiac rehabilitation program should document the safety of these activities and prepare the patient to return to them through a program of resistive exercise training (28, 29).

To begin with, light weights that can be lifted at 15 to 20 times without fatigue should be used. The weight can be increased after 1 to 2 weeks if the patient is asymptomatic and tolerates the activity. Depending on the goal of the resistive weight program, weight can be increased and the repetitions decreased to 12 to 15 per set. Slightly higher weights and fewer repetitions per set add more muscle strength, whereas lower weights and higher repetitions result in muscle toning and smaller strength gains. Large muscle groups should be used, simulating activities that the patient typically would be expected to perform. Two sets per activity and 2 to 3 sessions of resistive weight lifting per week are recommended (30).

Although the literature shows that resistive weight training is safe and is beneficial to the patient who lacks the strength to conduct normal ADL or vocational tasks, the benefits (with respect to reduced cardiovascular risk) have not proven to be as beneficial as regular aerobic activity. Therefore, resistive weight training should function as a supplement to the standard activity program for selected patients who could benefit from this form of conditioning.

RATE OF PROGRESSION

Perhaps the most difficult aspect of the exercise prescription to master is the rate and amount at which to advance a patient. The rate of progression of the activity in the conditioning period is determined by factors such as current level of fitness, prior activity history, health status, age, personal preferences of the patient, and goals of the rehabilitation program (1).

Patients who have not been active before their entry into the rehabilitation program are at high risk for orthopedic complications. Those who have low FCs should begin the activity portion of the rehabilitation program at the low end of the ranges prescribed (e.g., 10% below the target exercise intensity calculated and at the low end of the activity duration and frequency ranges). The use of HR response to modify the exercise workload downward if target HRs are being exceeded is valuable during the first few sessions of activity.

Patients should be advised regarding the symptoms of delayed muscle soreness that are all too common in persons who are just starting an activity program. They should know that this is common during the 24- to 48-hour period after the exercise session, that it is a transient condition as the musculature adjusts to a more active lifestyle, and that the soreness can be relieved by gentle static stretching to the sore muscle groups.

A major goal of rehabilitation activity is to have an appropriate level of regular activity incorporated into the patient's lifestyle. Overly aggressive activity early in the program is likely to be less enjoyable for the patient, thus leading to poor long-term compliance as well as increased likelihood of complications. If the exercise specialist who develops and implements the exercise program accepts the fact that the goal of rehabilitation is long-term impact, then there is little to no advantage in beginning the program aggressively. The patient must also be made aware that adaptation is a gradual process, and improvements cannot be expected or achieved quickly. If patients are counseled at the start of the program not to expect significant changes for approximately 3 months, then they are more likely to be realistic in their expectations.

Initially, the duration of exercise should be the component of the activity program to be increased (rather than intensity or frequency). If the initial duration of the conditioning period is less than 15 minutes, the focus should be on increased duration toward 20 to 30 minutes of activity. For asymptomatic patients, duration increases of 10% to 30% weekly or biweekly during the initial part of the rehabilitation program are realistic until the goal of 30 to 40 minutes of activity is achieved. Higher percentage increases usually apply to the shorter duration programs, and smaller percentage increases are used as the duration approaches 30 minutes of activity or greater.

Patients with activity-limiting angina, claudication, or pulmonary disease may not be able to achieve 15 minutes of continuous activity. These persons may require interval activity throughout the entire program, and the increases in duration of the entire conditioning session may be much slower than what already has been described. For these persons, the onset of symptoms is the best guide regarding the rate of progression.

After the duration of the conditioning period has reached 20 to 40 minutes, the intensity can be increased gradually from the lower end of the intensity range prescribed into the mid to upper range. Again, the patient's HR response, RPE ratings, and symptoms are excellent guides to the rate and amount of progression appropriate for each patient. As a general rule, only one aspect of the conditioning period should be increased at a time, and the rate of change should be made no more frequently than weekly. Changes every 2 to 3 weeks are more likely (1).

The greatest and most rapid improvements in functional ability are observed in the first 4 to 6 months of the program. After this period the rate of progression and the amount of change slow significantly as the patient enters a plateau or "maintenance" stage. It is important that the patient be made aware that the rate of progression normally declines or plateaus at this time and that the emphasis of the activity program is on maintaining the gains achieved to date.

Cool-down Period

The cool-down period should immediately follow the conditioning period in an activity session. This period lasts approximately 3 to 10 minutes, depending on the patient's interests and needs and on the intensity of the conditioning activity. The patient should perform low-level, rhythmic, aerobic activities during this period, such as casual walking or low-resistance cycling, allowing BP and HR return to preexercise warm-up levels. These activities enhance venous return and minimize

the likelihood of postexercise hypotension and arrhythmias (31). In addition, an active recovery is beneficial in removing lactate, which reduces the likelihood of delayed muscle soreness (32).

After the active aerobic cool-down, static stretching and gentle ROM activities may be included again, especially if a specific muscle group is stiff or has a limited ROM.

Caloric Expenditure Estimates

Weight loss is a rehabilitation goal for many patients. For the majority of patients, this translates to a simple, yet difficult to implement, matter of caloric balancing. If weight loss is to occur, the calories coming into the body must be less than the calories expended. The role of exercise to enhance caloric expenditure is an integral component of the overall weight-loss strategy. The exercise program and the dietary restructuring program should be coordinated to optimize the benefits and likelihood of success.

Guidelines for weight loss for most patients should include behavior-modification suggestions acceptable to the patient for the long term that are medically and nutritionally sound. Weight-loss goals of no more than 1 to 2 pounds per week are recommended. The behavioral changes required to achieve these goals can be realistic for most patients and will not result in loss of lean body mass and the dehydration observed in excessively restrictive diets (1). These goals translate into a caloric deficit of 3500 to 7000 kcal per week, or an average of 500 to 1000 kcal per day. The person who develops the activity guidelines should also review the nutritional plans, and both programs should be coordinated to ensure that the caloric deficit is adequate but not excessive.

The American College of Sports Medicine recommends that weight-loss programs observe the following guidelines (1):

1. Caloric intake should be balanced and not lower than 1200 kcal/day.
2. A negative caloric balance should not exceed 500 to 1000 kcal/day.
3. The use of behavior modification should be included to identify and eliminate diet habits that contribute to improper nutrition.
4. Exercise programs that provide daily caloric expenditures of more than or equal to 300 kcal/day should be included.

5. The weight-loss program should be structured to show how new eating habits, exercise habits, and associated weight loss can be maintained.

To calculate the caloric expenditure associated with activity prescriptions, use the following formula (1):

$$1 \text{ MET} = 1 \text{ kcal/kg (body weight) per hour of activity}$$

For example, for a 120-kg patient with a peak FC of 10 METs, exercising at 5 METs (50% intensity) for 30 minutes, the caloric expenditure per session would be

$$\text{kcal/session} = (5 \text{ METs}) \times (120 \text{ kg}) \times (0.5 \text{ hr}) = 300$$

SUMMARY

Exercise is one key component in a comprehensive cardiac rehabilitation program. The structure and implementation of the exercise prescription should be tailored to the patient's medical status, interests, and goals. The exercise prescription should address the following essential components of exercise:

Frequency
Intensity
Mode
Duration
Rate of progression

Every activity session should include warm-up, conditioning, and cool-down periods that adhere to established guidelines. The specifics of each component should be developed with the specific patient in mind and should not be applied in a sterile or rigid "cookbook" fashion.

Part B. Application of Exercise Principles to Routine Work and Recreational Activities
William A. Dafoe

GENERAL PRINCIPLES

A common concern among all cardiac patients is the feasibility of resuming various domestic, recreational, and vocational tasks. The cardiac rehabilitation phase is an opportune time to provide such information because appropriate prognostic information is available, including knowledge of the patient. Unfortunately, patients often are given vague advice, such as "take it easy," or "listen to your body," which does little to allay anxieties or to provide guidelines. When a cardiac patient is given approval for a particular activity, the following is assumed:

1. There is minimal risk of a subsequent cardiac event, such as a myocardial infarction (MI).
2. There will be minimal, if any, ischemia (silent or perceived). Although Foster et al. (1) have shown that mild ischemia may be tolerated during steady-state exercise, ischemia and exercise training are associated with an increase in adverse events in cardiac rehabilitation programs, as well as a lowering of the fibrillatory threshold (2). Animal data suggest that intermittent ischemia may cause myocardial necrosis (3). Thus, prudence still dictates activities with minimal if any ischemia.
3. The activity will be within the tolerance level of the patient.
4. Resumption of the activity will pose no threat to others.

It should be acknowledged that assurance of safety is at best an estimate because the disease process can change abruptly (plaque rupture), further atherosclerosis may ensue with time, or the ischemic threshold may vary during the day as seen with silent ischemia during daily tasks.

FACTORS TO CONSIDER

The decision about whether to approve a certain activity is complex and should be considered on an individual basis. Factors that involve the environment, the task, and the medical characteristics of the patient should be part of the decision-making process. These factors are summarized on a Cardiac Activity Work Sheet (Fig. 8.1).

Environmental Factors

Various environmental factors can influence the physical demands of an activity. Extremes of temperature are relatively common for outdoor pursuits. Heat stress induces vasodilation of the

Cardiac   Activity   Work   Sheet

Name - _____   **Task -**_____

R i s k

Environment	**L o w**	**M o d e r a t e**	**H i g h**
Heat/cold	ambient temp	30-50 deg F 75-85 deg F	< 30 deg F > 85 deg F
Safety of others	no risk	possible risk	high risk
Remoteness	help available	> 2 hours for medical care	no help available
Task			
Isometric (% max force)	low	< 20 %	> 20%
Competitive	low	some competition	highly
Rest/work periods	yes	some	not at all
Energy req (% maximal capacity)	< 50%	50 - 80%	> 80%
Duration ˙of task	< 30 sec	< 2 min	> 2 min
Individual			
Myocardial function	normal	moderate impairment	marked impairment
Myocardial jeopardy	none	moderate	severe
Myocardial ischemia	none	moderate	severe
Risk factor control (smoking, lipids, BP)	optimal control	1 factor elevated	> 2 factors elevated
Ability to pace	able	variable	unable
Obesity	normal weight	BMI 27- 30	BMI > 30
Physical condition	exercising regularly	moderate	sedentary
Skill level (for task)	high	medium	low
Functional capacity (from stress test)	> 7 METs	4 - 7 METs	< 4 METs

Recommended -___   **Not Recommended -** ___   **Reviewed by:** _____

Figure 8.1.   The Cardiac Activity Work Sheet allows the physician to summarize the relevant factors that pertain to the decision regarding approval for a certain task.

skin vasculature to maintain core temperature. This redistribution of blood flow leads to a relative decrease in venous return and a compensatory tachycardia to maintain cardiac output (4). Activities in a warm environment therefore require an increase in myocardial oxygen requirements to maintain thermal regulation. In a similar manner, a humid environment increases the metabolic requirements for a task because the normal thermal regulation is less effective. At the other end of the continuum, cold weather also can affect the physiologic demands for various tasks. Cold exposure can increase the myocardial oxygen requirements for any task. Other physiologic changes include an increase in total peripheral resistance, elevated arterial pressure, and greater left ventricular (LV) work (5). Exercise-induced ischemia in the cold may be provoked at levels 30% less than that seen at ambient temperatures (6). Surfaces that are covered with snow or ice increase the energy requirements for walking. The usual winter garments increase total weight and impede the efficiency for the task at hand. Angina may be provoked by vasoconstriction from stimulation of tracheal nerve endings by cold air. It is important to note that cardiac rehabilitation patients have been able to exercise successfully in the cold with appropriate training, education, and clothing (7). For the Cardiac Activity Work Sheet, a higher risk for temperature has been defined as less than 30°F or greater than 85°F.

It is important to consider the safety of the patient and others in the event of an anginal episode or arrhythmias. For example, if a scuba diver with cardiac problems suddenly becomes incapacitated, the safety of the diver and a "diving buddy" is threatened. If cardiac problems recur, how accessible is medical care? If a cardiac patient requires more than 2 hours' transportation to hospital, thrombolytics are of less benefit in the event of a recurrent MI. Activities such as fishing or hunting in remote areas may require days to reach appropriate medical care. The availability of medical care assumes importance for patients who are at moderate to high risk for subsequent cardiac events. Equally important, however, is not to create medical dependency for low-risk cardiac patients.

Task-specific Factors

The actual task needs to be analyzed to determine the factors that will influence energy capac-

ity or safety. Isometric tasks (see discussion on myocardial demands in chapter 17) can elicit the pressor response with a concomitant increase in afterload. The magnitude of the response is proportional to the percent of the maximum voluntary contraction and the total muscle mass used. In general, loads of less than 20% of maximal force elicit minimal response. A normal ventricle usually can tolerate static or static/dynamic tasks with no deleterious effects. An impaired ventricle may decompensate with time when challenged with an isometric challenge.

Competition or time-urgent tasks make it difficult to incorporate adequate rest periods. The superimposed adrenaline from competition increases myocardial demands above those required for the physiologic task at hand (8). It is difficult to maintain the heart rate (HR) intensity within a predefined range under such circumstances. Tasks that can be regulated with an activity/rest cycle have lower net work requirements. A patient with a low FC of 4 METs may still be able to perform a 4-MET task if the work is accomplished intermittently (9). Thus, strict adherence to the MET concept may underestimate tasks that are safe and within the tolerance provided that an appropriate work/rest cycle can be followed.

The energy requirements for various activities are listed in appendix A. It should be appreciated that the energy costs for various tasks are, at best, only estimates. These values taken from the literature need to be viewed with the following points in mind:

1. Most of the data was acquired in the 1960s, using young healthy normal volunteers, mostly men of a 70-kg weight. It has been shown that a number of recreational tasks listed on the traditional charts may be accomplished with less energy (8). New data are increasingly available by the study of cardiac patients, using modern gas analysis equipment.
2. The values are expressed in terms of METs or metabolic equivalents. The same absolute MET value may represent different relative requirements for different patients. For example, a 3-MET task is only 30% of the maximal force for a person with a 10-MET capacity; however, for the patient with a significantly compromised left ventricle (4 METs), this same task now represents 75% of capacity (10).
3. Most activities vary in terms of the energy re-

quirements during the actual task. For example, during the game of tennis, the HR may vary as much as 40 beats per minute during the playing period. Thus, a patient may exceed the proscribed limit during a small percentage of the actual event (8).

4. There is, in general, a linear relationship between total oxygen body requirements and myocardial oxygen demands. The traditional energy-cost charts are in METs and indirectly indicate the myocardial energy requirements. The myocardial oxygen demands increase disproportionately when tasks use small muscle groups, such as in the arms, and when there is an isometric component.

5. If a task is performed in an uncomfortable position, the energy requirements may be increased by as much as 30% (10).

Although the risk of various activities depends on many factors, the Cardiac Activity Work Sheet uses the percentage of maximal capacity as an indicator of risk. The maximum METs for the task is taken from the published values for various tasks (see appendix A). The maximal capacity is determined by the stress test. The percent of maximal capacity is determined by

$$\text{Maximum METs for task/Maximum METs on stress test} \times 100\%$$

In terms of the Cardiac Activity Work Sheet, a task that requires less than 50% of the maximal capacity can be considered at low risk; from 50% to 80% maximal capacity can be considered moderate risk; and more than 80% can be considered high risk.

Tasks that are short in duration are tolerated more readily than prolonged tasks. The pressor response rises in a linear fashion with time and depends on many factors, including the percent of the maximal force, the total muscle mass used, and the muscle fiber types. For ease of use, the Cardiac Activity Work Sheet uses an isometric activity greater than 30 seconds as low risk, from 30 seconds to 2 minutes as moderate risk, and more than 2 minutes as high risk.

Individual Characteristics

It is important to know all the relevant clinical information about the patient. An impaired my-ocardial function can be ascertained by the presence of one or more of the following characteristics: congestive heart failure, poor functional class (New York Heart Association classification), diuretic or digitalis use, cardiomegaly, S3 gallop, prior MI, flattened or falling systolic blood pressure response to exercise, poor exercise capacity (less than 4 METs), ventricular arrhythmias, ejection fraction less than 30%, impaired wall-motion score, or increased LV end-diastolic pressure (11). Myocardial jeopardy refers to the probability that further myocardium may be damaged. Characteristics of increased myocardial jeopardy include angina frequency, duration of angina, a low level of exercise-induced angina, greater than 2 mm of ST-segment depression during exercise, a flattened or falling systolic pressure on exercise, reversible thallium perfusion defects, and a significant number and distribution of obstructed coronary vessels. Characteristics of marked myocardial ischemia include angina that is present at rest, nocturnal, unstable, or progressive; failure to respond to nitroglycerin; and ST-segment depression at rest or with minimal exercise.

The angiographic regression trials have shown not only a retardation of disease progression, but also a reduction in cardiac events (12). The presumed mechanism is stabilization of the vulnerable atherosclerotic plaque by appropriate lipid lowering. Burke et al. (13) showed that elevated cholesterol concentrations predisposed patients to rupture of vulnerable plaques, and cigarette smoking predisposed patients to an acute thrombosis. A postmortem of men with hypercholesterolemia who had sudden death during physical exertion suggested that the cause was rupture of vulnerable plaques (14). Similarly, for hypertensives, Burke et al. (15) have found that LV hypertrophy is associated with plaque rupture for sudden cardiac death. Most of the literature to date implicates optimal control of lipids for plaque stabilization. For the purpose of the Cardiac Activity Work Sheet, low risk will be considered for a nonsmoker who is normotensive and has an optimal control of lipids. Moderate risk will be considered when one or more of these risk factors is elevated. High risk will be considered when two or more of these risk factors are elevated.

The person who has the capacity to control the pace of an activity is able to accomplish the task with less energy cost. The inability to pace is more commonly seen in persons with marked type A characteristics, or in those who are unable to assess adequately their own perceived level of exertion.

The obese person has a greater body mass to move, and any activity that requires stooping, bending, or climbing will require more energy than for a lean person. Obese people may be less efficient at performing various tasks with a resultant higher energy requirement.

If a person has been exercising regularly for at least 3 months, the training effect will be reflected in an increased anaerobic threshold and capacity for endurance activities. A regular exerciser therefore is considered to be at a lower risk and a sedentary person at a higher risk (16).

The skill that a person has for activities such as swimming or cross-country skiing affects the energy requirements. Novices may expend large amounts of energy when learning such activities. It is important, therefore, to determine the previous experience of a cardiac patient who wishes to pursue a skill-related activity.

The functional capacity can be obtained from a stress test (see chapter 17). It should be noted that the HR for the onset of signs or symptoms from the stress test may not represent the HR for similar end points during the actual task. The characteristics of the stress test that may include lack of warm-up, performance anxiety, and a hypertensive response to exercise may lead to earlier symptoms than would normally be observed. In general, an FC of less than 4 METs can be considered a high risk; 4 to 7 METs, a moderate risk; and more than 7 METs, a low risk.

CARDIAC ACTIVITY WORK SHEET

The Cardiac Activity Work Sheet (Fig. 8.1) allows the physician to summarize the relevant factors that pertain to the decision regarding approval for a certain task. It should be noted that this form is descriptive only and provides no quantitative score. It should be appreciated that there is overlap between the various categories, and certain categories carry more weight regarding overall risk. For example, the myocardial function is more important than the presence of humidity. The risk criteria established for low-, medium-, and high-risk categories are arbitrary and, in most cases, form a continuum.

As an example, consider Mr. Jones, who is a 50-year-old man with a recent inferior wall MI. He wants to chop wood at his cottage during summer vacation. His course in the hospital was uncomplicated, and he is proceeding well in his cardiac rehabilitation program. A recent stress test shows that he accomplished 8 METs, but he had ischemic changes at 7 METs. The various factors that are considered are indicated by a check mark for the appropriate category of low-, moderate-, or high-risk (Fig. 8.2). First, the various environmental factors are considered. The temperature may exceed 85°F at that time of the year. There is little risk to anyone else if angina or syncope occurs. The cottage is about 150 miles from the nearest hospital; thus, Mr. Jones has a moderate risk in the event of another MI. There is some isometric component when gripping the ax handle, but this is considered less than 20% of maximal force. There is no competition or time urgency for the task and rest/work periods are certainly possible. Chopping wood requires from 7 to 8 METs (i.e., up to 100% of capacity). This places the activity in the higher risk category and the task most likely will be longer than 2 minutes. This particular patient's characteristics show that he has moderate impairment of his ventricle. There is no indication of myocardial jeopardy, but the database is incomplete because an angiogram was not performed. Ischemia was present at 7 METs, indicating a moderate risk. Mr. Jones has been observed in the rehabilitation program and he is able to pace himself. His body mass index is 28, placing him in the moderate-risk zone. In terms of other risk factors, he has not been doing very well. Unfortunately, he is still smoking half a pack of cigarettes a day, and his lipid profile shows that his LDL cholesterol is still elevated at 160 mg/dL (4.14 mmol/L). Thus, he is at a high risk in terms of "risk factor control." He is exercising regularly in rehabilitation, placing him in the low-risk zone. He has not chopped wood for a few years; thus, his skill level will be considered medium risk. Finally, his FC is at 7 METs (onset of ischemia); thus, his FC puts him in the moderate-risk zone.

It was felt that woodchopping was not appropriate because the workloads are high (7 to 8 METs) and exceed the patient's exercise capacity. Environmental factors such as high tempera-

Cardiac   Activity   Work   Sheet

Name - *Ed Jones*   Task - *Chopping Wood*

R i s k

	L o w	**M o d e r a t e**	**H i g h**
<u>Environment</u>			
Heat/cold	ambient temp	30-50 deg F 75-85 deg F	✓ < 30 deg F > 85 deg F
Safety of others	✓ no risk	possible risk	high risk
Remoteness	help available	✓ > 2 hours for medical care	no help available
<u>Task</u>			
Isometric (% max force)	low	✓ < 20 %	> 20%
Competitive	✓ low	some competition	highly
Rest/work periods	yes	✓ some	not at all
Energy req (% maximal capacity)	< 50%	50 - 80%	✓ > 80%
Duration of task	< 30 sec	< 2 min	✓ > 2 min
<u>Individual</u>			
Myocardial function	normal	✓ moderate impairment	marked impairment
Myocardial jeopardy	✓ none	moderate	severe
Myocardial ischemia	none	✓ moderate	severe
Risk factor control (smoking, lipids, BP)	optimal control	1 factor elevated	✓ > 2 factors elevated
Ability to pace	✓ able	variable	unable
Obesity	normal weight	✓ BMI 27- 30	BMI > 30
Physical condition	✓ exercising regularly	moderate	sedentary
Skill level (for task)	high	✓ medium	low
Functional capacity (from stress test)	> 7 METs	✓ 4 - 7 METs	< 4 METs

Recommended -___   Not Recommended - ✓   Reviewed by: *W. Dafoe , MD*

Figure 8.2.   Example of the use of the Cardiac Activity Work Sheet. This activity was deemed inadvisable because of extremes of temperature, ischemia at 7 METs, the remote location of the activity, and poor control of risk factors. Knowledge of the myocardial jeopardy was incomplete (no angiogram).

tures and humidity increase the workloads. The myocardial jeopardy is not known because the information is not available, and, in the event of a recurrent MI during the activity, a significant delay in obtaining appropriate medical care is anticipated.

SPECIFIC ACTIVITIES

Snow Shoveling

Snow shoveling is a common task in northern climates. Cardiac patients often wish to resume this activity because it is a common household task and signals to some a return to all "normal activities." There are a number of characteristics of snow shoveling that cause it to be an activity with considerable exertion. The moisture content of snow can vary considerably with heavy, wet snow requiring high energy requirements for its removal. Franklin et al. (17) showed that for healthy, untrained males, shoveling heavy, wet snow required 86% to 97% of maximal HR. Systolic blood pressure was elevated with a mean of 200 mm Hg. They concluded that heavy snow shoveling was similar to workloads achieved by maximal treadmill and arm-ergometer testing.

Sheldahl et al. (18) evaluated 16 men with asymptomatic coronary artery disease and good functional work capacity. They were assessed for hemodynamic and metabolic responses during snow shoveling at a self-paced rate. The average work load was 5.3 METs and corresponded to 60% of peak METs and 75% of peak HR achieved on a stress test. Arrhythmias were similar to those seen during dynamic exercise. In a later study (19), a similar asymptomatic cohort with coronary artery disease was assessed for workload requirements for snow blowing and shoveling. Both snow shoveling and snow blowing required approximately 5.3 METs of exertion. Younger men with no disease used 7.4 METs of exertion at a self-paced rate.

Most patients who commence snow shoveling continue until the job is completed. Thus, the task may require a considerably longer time than the usual accustomed exercise period. Upper extremities are used, which may elicit a higher rate-pressure product than lower-extremity exercise. Cold temperatures and wind may initiate vasospasm. The person performing the task often may have just finished a meal and may be time pressured to complete the task to go to work.

Despite these limitations, snow shoveling at a self-paced rate has only moderate exertional demands (i.e., 5.3 METs) (19) and can be safe for selected (see Cardiac Activity Work Sheet, Fig. 8.1) low-risk patients. Advice for such low-risk patients would include the following:

1. Consider snow shoveling as an activity for exercise. Arrange for another person to be responsible for the complete job of clearing the driveway. Then, if circumstances permit, the cardiac patient can help with the task.
2. Do not shovel after a large meal.
3. Perform the usual warm-up activities as with any exercise.
4. Use a smaller shovel or push the snow to the side of the driveway.
5. Intersperse frequent rest periods with shoveling.

Scuba Diving

Scuba diving places unique physiologic demands on the cardiovascular system (20). In 1989, there were 114 fatalities during scuba diving (21). Myocardial infarction was suspected in 13 cases, representing 11.4% of the total fatalities. It should be noted, however, that only 3 cases had a previous history of heart disease. It is suggested that cardiac patients should be able to obtain 13 METs with no signs or symptoms of ischemia if scuba diving is to be considered. Contraindications to diving include symptomatic coronary heart disease or significant dysrhythmias. Relative contraindications include a patent foramen ovale (increased risk of brain lesions owing to paradoxical gas emboli), asthma, diabetes (20), and panic disorders (22).

Consideration of risk should be not only for the cardiac patient but also for the other diver who may be a "buddy" during a dive. Cold water may invoke a vagal response with bradycardia. Emergency situations may arise quickly (caught in a current), requiring peak energy expenditures. The medical clearance for diving is complex and the interested reader is referred to comprehensive texts on the subject (23, 24).

Hot Tubs and Saunas

Hot tubs and saunas represent intense forms of heat stress. As discussed previously, thermal stress results in compensatory mechanisms in an attempt to cool the body; thus, there is vasodilation with shunting of the blood to the periphery. Blood pressure tends to fall because of the vasodilation and water loss. Compensatory mechanisms include an increased HR and preferential shunting of blood away from visceral organs. The added stress to the heart is equivalent to vigorous walking. Exposure to repeat saunas results in habituation with less sympathetic stimulation. Traditional wisdom has indicated that thermal stress should be avoided in circumstances in which vasodilation and decreased cardiac output would be deleterious, e.g., congestive heart failure. However, Tei and colleagues (25) studied 34 patients with chronic heart failure with exposure to a warm water bath for 10 minutes at 41°C, or a sauna bath for 15 minutes at 60°C. They found that cardiac and stroke indices increased and systemic vascular resistance decreased significantly during and after the thermic exposure. It was thought that the improvement in hemodynamics was caused by the reduction in cardiac preload and afterload.

Hyperthermia has been found to increase the absorption and concentration of transdermally delivered nicotine (26). The pharmacokinetics of propranolol were studied after a sauna, and it was found that hyperthermia increased the plasma propranolol concentration (27).

From 1970 to 1986, there were 230 deaths in Finland attributable to hyperthermia (usually during a sauna). Alcohol consumption was detected in most of the victims (28). In 1990 there were 158 deaths in the United States that occurred in spas, Jacuzzis, or hot tubs. Heart disease was implicated in 31% of these deaths alone or in combination with alcohol (29). Allison et al. (30) evaluated 15 men with stable coronary artery disease who had hot tub immersion at 40°C for 15 minutes and reported no ischemic electrocardiographic changes. On the other hand, for patients with ischemia provoked by exercise testing, Giannetti et al. (31) found ischemic changes as assessed by technetium Tc 99m sestamibi in 55% of subjects exposed to a sauna bath for 15 minutes.

The practice of rapid cooling by a cold bath or rolling in snow results in marked cutaneous vasoconstriction with an increased blood pressure and central venous blood flow. This sudden increased volume and pressure load can be deleterious to a compromised myocardium (32).

Thus, the following recommendations may be made about hot tubs and saunas. Saunas may be appropriate

1. For low-risk patients with minimal ischemia.
2. By limiting the time exposure and the heat.
3. For patients with habituation.
4. For heart failure patients with due attention to the time exposed and the amount of thermal stress (25).

Saunas are *not* recommended

1. Immediately after exercise or with alcohol.
2. In combination with rapid cooling, such as a cold shower.
3. For moderate- to high-risk patients.

In those for whom saunas may be appropriate, transdermal patches should be removed during the thermal exposure.

High-altitude Activities

It is not unusual for people to visit locations that are at altitudes in excess of 8,000 ft. Skiing holidays in Colorado or camping trips to the Rockies can expose the cardiac patient to these altitudes. The inspired oxygen tension at sea level is 150 mm Hg; 125 mm Hg at 5,000 ft; and 100 mm Hg at 10,000 ft. Fortunately, the fall in saturation of O_2 is less than 10% because of the characteristics of the sigmoid curve for saturation. Even with a partial pressure of 50 mm Hg, the O_2 saturation is greater than 85%. There is a short-term decrease in the arterial concentration of O_2 until a compensatory increase in hematocrit restores the arterial content to normal. This change in hematocrit takes 1 full week, but after 2 days is partially restored. Heart rate is increased because of relative hypoxia and stimulation of the sympathetic nervous system (4). The rate-pressure product for ischemic changes (signs of symptoms) are similar for high versus low altitudes; however, the ischemic changes occur at a lower absolute work load (33). It appears that the same level of exercise is accomplished by an increase in HR. Grover et al. (4) found that skiing altitudes of 10,000 to 12,000 ft elicited an HR response of more than 80% of age-predicted maximums in the majority of subjects. They concluded that there was no increased cardiac risk with activities at higher altitudes for low-risk patients.

Exercise at higher altitudes has not been reported as posing an added risk; however, any activity that requires a higher HR may not be tolerated by a compromised myocardium or by those patients with severe anemia. In addition, coronary artery spasm can theoretically be provoked by alkalosis and sympathetic stimulation with exercise at higher altitudes. In general, it is recommended that at least 2 days be devoted to acclimatization before vigorous exercise is undertaken. Patients should monitor their exercise by the HR prescription established at normal altitudes (34).

Part C. Exercise Prescription for Cardiac Transplant Patients
Ray W. Squires

After cardiac transplantation, regular exercise training provides important benefits for patients as outlined in chapter 9. Most patients adapt to exercise with an improvement in peak oxygen uptake and submaximal exercise endurance as well as experience improvements in psychological function.

PRETRANSPLANT EXERCISE TESTING AND PRESCRIPTION

Before transplantation, in many centers, ambulatory transplant candidates undergo cardiopulmonary exercise testing as part of the pretransplant evaluation to determine peak exercise oxygen uptake, which is a powerful prognostic indicator (1). Patients with exercise capacities below 4 METs (14 mL·kg^{-1}·min^{-1}) experience a markedly reduced 1-year survival, independent of left ventricular ejection fraction, compared with patients with better preserved peak oxygen uptakes.

From the results of the exercise test, an exercise prescription may be developed for the patient to improve or maintain cardiovascular fitness while waiting for a donor organ. Some patients have responded so well to pretransplant exercise training that peak oxygen uptake has improved to levels that are associated with a reasonable probability of survival, and the patient has been removed from immediate consideration of transplantation (2). The exercise program ideally should be carried out under medical guidance, at least initially, although many patients

have performed home-based exercise training successfully (3). The exercise prescription given for patients with severe chronic heart failure is generally conservative in nature. Modes of activity include walking (free walking indoors or outdoors, motorized treadmill ambulation) or cycle ergometry at perceived exertion levels of 11 to 13 (approximately 40% to 60% of exercise capacity or the heart rate reserve). Duration of exercise is generally 5 to 30 minutes per session, with a frequency of three or more sessions per week. For patients with limited endurance who cannot exercise more than 5 to 10 minutes per session, multiple short sessions each day are recommended (4).

For patients who require continuous hospitalization preoperatively, range-of-motion (ROM) exercises and limited ambulation or cycle ergometry may be performed with direct supervision, as the clinical condition of the patient permits.

INPATIENT POSTOPERATIVE PHYSICAL ACTIVITY

The postoperative inpatient physical activity program may begin at the time of extubation, usually within 24 hours, with passive and active ROM exercises for the upper and lower extremities, performed while sitting in a chair or standing, and slow ambulation (5). Activity may be progressed by levels as given in Table 8.1. Ambulation and cycle ergometry may be gradually increased to 20 to 30 minutes per session. Exercise intensity may be guided using Borg perceived exertion scale ratings of 11 to 13 ("fairly light" to "somewhat hard") with a frequency of two or three sessions per day supervised by a physical therapist or exercise specialist. Typically, patients remain hospitalized for 1 to 2 weeks after transplantation.

During this stage of rehabilitation, as well as at any later stage of the postoperative period, episodes of acute rejection of moderate or greater severity require alteration of the exercise training program. If the rejection is rated as moderate, physical activity may be continued at the present level, but not progressed in intensity or duration until after the rejection has been successfully treated. Severe acute rejection necessitates suspension of physical activity with the exception of passive ROM exercises (5).

Table 8.1.   Inpatient Physical Activity Levels for Heart Transplant Patients

Level 1
   Reeducation of neuromuscular relaxation to counteract muscle tension
   Reeducation of thoracic and diaphragmatic breathing
   Review of posture principles, body mechanics, and transfer techniques
   Exercises (up to 10 repetitions, supine):
      Shoulder flexion[a]
      Shoulder abduction[a]
      Shoulder horizontal abduction[a]
      Hip/knee flexion and extension
      Hip abduction
      Ankle pumps
   Up in chair 20–30 minutes
Level 2
   Breathing and relaxation techniques
   Exercises (up to 10 repetitions, seated):
      Wand exercises as per level 1
      Shoulder circles
      Trunk rotation
      Hip/knee flexion (seated marching)
      Knee extensions
      Ankle pumps
      Gait: standing pregait activities (dips, weight shifting)
   Up in chair 30–60 minutes
Level 3
   Exercises (up to 10 repetitions, standing):
      Head circles
      Arm circles
      Trunk rotation
      Trunk lateral flexion
      Dips
      Toe raises
      Wand exercises, as above
  Gait: short walks in the room, as tolerated
  Up in chair ad libitum
Level 4
   Exercises (up to 10 repetitions, standing)
      Head circles
      Arm circles
      Trunk rotation
      Trunk lateral flexion
      Toe raises
      Wand exercises, as above
   Elbow flexion/extension with 1-lb wrist weights
   Gait: walk in room ad libitum
   Stationary cycle: 5 minutes, minimal resistance
Level 5
   Exercises and walking as per level 4
   Stationary cycle: 10 minutes, minimal resistance
   Cool-down stretches for quadriceps, heel cords
Level 6
   Exercises and walking as per level 4
   Stationary cycle: 15 minutes, minimal resistance
   Cool-down stretches as per level 5 plus hamstring stretch
Level 7
   Exercises and walking as per level 4
   Stationary cycle: 20 minutes, moderate resistance (keep RPE between 11 and 13, include 2–3 minutes of slower
      cadence warm-up and cool-down)
   Cool-down stretches as per level 6

RPE = rating of perceived exertion.
[a]Performed with a wand.

OUTPATIENT POSTOPERATIVE EXERCISE TRAINING

Cardiac transplant patients may enter an outpatient cardiac rehabilitation program within the first few days after hospital dismissal (6). Patients are generally required to remain near the transplant center for 2 to 3 months after hospital dismissal for close follow-up by the transplant team, and ideally should exercise in both a supervised program (up to three sessions per week for a minimum of 6 weeks) and independently (at least three sessions per week).

Continuous monitoring of the ECG during the first several supervised exercise sessions is standard practice. It is not necessary to perform graded exercise testing before beginning the outpatient exercise program. Exercise testing is much more useful for exercise prescription purposes and general physical activity counseling when the patient has sufficiently recovered from surgery, usually 1 to 2 months after the operation.

Patients who have received transplants are immunosuppressed and are at risk for acquiring an infection. Cardiac rehabilitation staff, patient family members, and other cardiac rehabilitation patients who have active infectious diseases must avoid direct contact with transplant patients.

Exercise prescription for patients with heart transplants follows similar methods to those used with other patients who have undergone cardiothoracic surgery, with the exception of not using a target heart rate. As discussed in chapter 9, the transplanted heart rate response to exercise is unique. The rise in heart rate usually observed at the onset and during the first 1 to 3 minutes of exercise is delayed in heart transplant patients. During constant-load submaximal exercise, the heart rate may drift upwards with time or may reach a plateau after several minutes. Heart rates measured during exercise training sessions lasting 30 or more minutes usually exceed 85% of the peak heart rates achieved during symptom-limited graded exercise testing. Occasionally, exercise session heart rates exceed the maximum heart rate observed during graded exercise testing (7). These characteristics make prescribing a precise target heart rate difficult, at best, for these patients. As discussed in chapter 9, cardiac reinnervation may occur in some patients weeks to months after surgery, and this results in a more normal heart rate response to dynamic exercise. In some of these patients, a target heart rate may be prescribed in the manner used for other cardiac patients.

Early experience with exercise prescription for cardiac transplant patients determined that ratings of perceived exertion, using the Borg scale, were very useful in prescribing exercise intensity (8). Ratings of between 12 and 14 ("somewhat hard") are appropriate for outpatient exercise sessions for transplant patients. The exercise prescription includes a period of 5 to 10 minutes of warm-up and cool-down activities, and a gradual increase in aerobic exercise duration to 30 to 60 minutes, with a frequency of three to six sessions per week.

Modes of aerobic exercise commonly used during the early outpatient rehabilitation phase include walking (either outdoors or shopping center or school during inclement weather), motor-driven treadmill walking, cycle ergometry, and limited stair climbing. Because of the sternal incision, special emphasis on upper-extremity ROM exercises is needed, which may be started while the patient is hospitalized and continued in the outpatient program. After approximately 6 to 8 weeks from the surgery date, when sternal healing is nearly complete, rowing, arm cranking, combination arm and leg ergometry, outdoor cycling, hiking, and swimming are additional exercise options for selected patients. More aggressive activities such as racquet sports, jogging, and basketball may be performed if patient fitness is adequate (directly measured peak exercise oxygen uptake of at least 5 METs for racquet sports, minimum of 8 to 9 METs for jogging or basketball) and sternal healing is nearly complete.

Patients with accelerated graft coronary artery disease may develop exercise-related myocardial ischemia. The vast majority of transplant patients will not experience typical angina pectoris with ischemia because of cardiac denervation. Some patients may report exertional dyspnea (anginal equivalent). Case reports of cardiac reinnervation with subsequent development of typical angina in the setting of graft atherosclerosis are rare.

Although life-threatening exercise-related ventricular arrhythmias are rare in transplant patients, acute rejection episodes may present with complex ventricular arrhythmia. Periodic ECG monitoring during cardiac rehabilitation exercise sessions is recommended.

Most transplant patients are very deconditioned before surgery and are required to take corticosteroids postoperatively. In addition, chronic heart failure may result in skeletal muscle dysfunction independent of the effects of inactivity. Skeletal muscle weakness is usually present. Skeletal muscle strengthening exercises are helpful and should be incorporated into the exercise rehabilitation program. For the first 6 weeks after surgery, bilateral lifting using the arms is restricted to less than 10 pounds to avoid sternal nonunion. However, mild strengthening exercises using elastic bands or hand-held weights may be performed within the first 2 weeks after surgery. After 6 weeks of recovery and if the sternum is well-healed, patients may be started on weight-training machines, emphasizing moderate resistance, 10 to 20 repetitions per set, one to three sets of exercises for the major muscle groups on a two- to three-session-per-week basis (6, 9). Because of the high prevalence of hypertension in transplant patients resulting from treatment with cyclosporine, periodic blood pressure measurement during strengthening exercises is prudent.

GRADED EXERCISE TESTING

Exercise testing is extremely useful in measuring the exercise capacity, prescribing exercise training intensity, and providing objective data regarding the timing of return to work and resumption of avocational activities after cardiac transplantation. Because of the stress of surgery and the associated convalescence, as well as the deconditioned state of most patients before transplantation, it is prudent to wait 4 to 8 weeks after surgery before performing graded exercise testing to an end point of maximal effort. In patients with complicated postoperative courses, a longer period of recovery may be necessary before testing is performed.

Treadmill or cycle ergometer protocols with either 2- to 3-minute stages or ramp tests may be used. Arm-cranking protocols may also be used, after sternal healing, for a specific upper-extremity fitness assessment or arm exercise prescription (9). The initial exercise intensity should be set at approximately 2 METs with 1- to 2-MET increments per stage (9, 10). Continuous ECG monitoring with periodic blood pressure measurement and Borg perceived exertion scale ratings for each stage of exercise is recommended.

For precise determination of aerobic capacity and the ventilatory anaerobic threshold, direct measurement of oxygen uptake and associated variables throughout the test is highly desirable. Estimates of exercise capacity for transplant patients using treadmill speed and grade or cycle power may be quite inaccurate.

The end points of the test should be maximal effort (symptom-limited maximum) or signs of exertional intolerance. After the performance of a graded exercise test, exercise prescription for intensity of effort may be based on a given percentage of the measured peak oxygen uptake (exercise intensity corresponding to 60% to 70% of the aerobic capacity, for example) or just below the ventilatory anaerobic threshold.

References

Part A.

1. American College of Sports Medicine. Guidelines for exercise testing and prescription. 4th ed. Philadelphia: Lea & Febiger, 1991.
2. Carleton R, Siconolfi S, Shafique M, et al. Delayed appearance of angina pectoris during low level exercise. J Card Rehabil 1983;3:141–148.
3. Pollock M, Gettman L, Milesis C, et al. Effects of frequency and duration of training on attrition and incidence of injury. Med Sci Sports 1977;9:31–36.
4. American College of Sports Medicine. Guidelines for exercise testing and prescription. 5th ed. Baltimore: Williams & Wilkins, 1995.
5. Jugdutt BI, Michorowski BL, Kappagoda CT. Exercise training after anterior Q wave myocardial infarction: importance of regional left ventricular function and topography. J Am Coll Cardiol 1988;12:362–372.
6. Hagberg J, Ehsani A, Holloszy J. Effect of 12 months of intense exercise training on stroke volume in patients with coronary artery disease. Circulation 1983;67:1194–1199.
7. Ehsani A, Biello D, Schultz J, et al. Improvement of left ventricular contractile function by exercise training in patients with coronary artery disease. Circulation 1986;74:350–358.
8. American College of Sports Medicine. Guidelines for graded exercise testing and prescription. 3rd ed. Philadelphia: Lea & Febiger, 1986.
9. Franklin BA, Hellerstein HK, Gordon S, et al. Cardiac patients. In: Franklin BA, Gordon S, Timmis GC, eds. Exercise in modern medicine. Baltimore: Williams & Wilkins, 1989:44–80.
10. Bruce RA, Kusumi F, Hosmer D. Maximal oxygen intake and nomographic assessment of functional aerobic impairment on cardiovascular disease. Am Heart J 1973;85:546–562.
11. Balke B, Ware RW. An experimental study of physical fitness of Air Force personnel. US Armed Forces Med J 1959;10:675–688.
12. Blackburn G, Harvey S, Wilkoff B. A chronotropic as-

sessment exercise protocol to assess the need and efficacy of rate responsive pacing [abstract]. Med Sci Sports Exerc 1988;20(Suppl):S21.

13. Sullivan M, McKirnan MD. Errors in predicting functional capacity for postmyocardial infarction patients using a modified Bruce protocol. Am Heart J 1984; 107:486–492.

14. Adams GE, Marlon AM, Quinn EJ. O$_2$ uptake in cardiac patients during treadmill testing. CVP 1980;8:14–24.

15. Hughson RL, Smyth GA. Slower adaptation of V̇o$_2$ to steady state of submaximal exercise with beta adrenergic blockade. Eur J Appl Physiol 1983;52:107–110.

16. McConnell TR, Clark BA. Prediction of maximal oxygen consumption during handrail-supported treadmill exercise. J Cardpulm Rehabil 1987;7:324–331.

17. Zeimetz G, McNeill J, Hall J, et al. Quantifiable changes in oxygen uptake, heart rate, and time to target heart rate when handrail support is allowed during treadmill exercise. J Cardpulm Rehabil 1985;5:525–539.

18. Karvonen M, Kentala K, Mustal O. The effects of training on heart rate: a longitudinal study. Ann Med Exp Biol Fenn 1957;35:307–315.

19. Borg G, Linderholm H. Perceived exertion and pulse rate during graded exercise in various age groups. Acta Med Scand Suppl 1967;472:194–206.

20. Borg GA. Physiological bases of perceived exertion. Med Sci Sports Exerc 1982;14:377–381.

21. Garber CE, Carleton RA, Camione DN, et al. The threshold for myocardial ischemia varies in patients with coronary artery disease depending on the exercise protocol. J Am Coll Cardiol 1991;17:1256–1262.

22. Blackburn GG. Cardiorespiratory responses to six-week limb-specific exercise conditioning programs [doctoral thesis]. College Park, PA: The Pennsylvania State University, 1984.

23. Foster C, Pollock ML, Rod JL, et al. Evaluation of functional capacity during exercise radionuclide angiography. Cardiology 1983;70:85–93.

24. Butler RM, Beierwaltes WH, Rogers FJ. The cardiovascular response to circuit weight training in patients with cardiac disease. J Cardpulm Rehabil 1987;7:402–409.

25. Haennel RG, Quinney HA, Kappagoda CT. Effects of hydraulic circuit training following coronary artery bypass surgery. Med Sci Sports Exerc 1991;23:158–165.

26. Stewart KJ, Mason M, Kelemen MH. Three-year participation in circuit weight training improves muscular strength and self-efficacy in cardiac patients. J Cardpulm Rehabil 1988;8:292–296.

27. Vander LB, Franklin BA, Wrisley D, et al. Acute cardiovascular responses to Nautilus® exercise in cardiac patients: implications for exercise training. Ann Sports Med 1986;2:165–169.

28. Wilke NA, Sheldahl LM, Levandoski SG, et al. Transfer effect of upper extremity training to weight carrying in men with ischemic heart disease. J Cardpulm Rehabil 1991;11:365–372.

29. Squires RW, Muri AJ, Anderson LJ, et al. Weight-training during phase II (early outpatient) cardiac rehabilitation. J Cardpulm Rehabil 1991;11:360–364.

30. Verill D, Shoup E, McElveen G, et al. Resistive exercise training in cardiac patients. Sports Med 1992;13:171–193.

31. Dimsdale JE, Hartley H, Guiney T, et al. Plasma catecholamines and exercise. JAMA 1984;251:630–632.

32. Belcastro AN, Bonen A. Lactic acid removal rates during controlled and uncontrolled recovery exercise. J Appl Physiol 1975;39:932–936.

Suggested Readings

American Association of Cardiovascular and Pulmonary Rehabilitation. Guidelines for cardiac rehabilitation programs. 2nd ed. Champaign, IL: Human Kinetics, 1995.

American College of Sports Medicine. Resource manual for guidelines for exercise testing and prescription. 2nd ed. Philadelphia: Lea & Febiger, 1993.

Fletcher GF, Balady G, Froelicher VF, et al. Exercise standards: a statement for healthcare professionals from the American Heart Association. Circulation 1995;91:580–615.

Fletcher GF, Balady G, Blair SN, et al. Statement on exercise. Benefits and recommendations for physical activity programs for all Americans. A statement for health professionals by the Committee on Exercise and Cardiac Rehabilitation of the Council on Clinical Cardiology, American Heart Association. Circulation 1996;94:857–862.

Fletcher GF. How to implement physical activity in primary and secondary prevention. A statement for healthcare professionals from the Task Force on Risk Reduction, American Heart Association. Circulation 1997;96:355–357.

Part B.

1. Foster C, Gal R, Murphy P, et al. Left ventricular function during exercise testing and training. Med Sci Sports Exerc 1996;29:297–305.

2. Hohnloser S, Kasper W, Zehender M, et al. Silent myocardial ischemia as a predisposing factor for ventricular fibrillation. Am J Cardiol 1988;61:461–464.

3. Geft I, Fishbein M, Ninomiya K, et al. Intermittent brief periods of ischemia have a cumulative effect and may cause myocardial necrosis. Circulation 1982;66:1150–1153.

4. Grover R, Reeves J, Rowell L, et al. The influence of environmental factors on the cardiovascular system. In: Schlant R, Alexander R, O'Rourke R, et al., eds. The heart. 8th ed. New York: McGraw-Hill, 1994:2117–2132.

5. Epstein S, Stampfer M, Beiser G, et al. Effects of a reduction in environmental temperature on the circulatory response to exercise in man. N Engl J Med 1969;180:7–11.

6. Lassvik C, Areskog N. Angina pectoris during inhalation of cold air reactions to exercise. Br Heart J 1980;43:661–667.

7. Kavanagh T. Physiologic reactions to cold. J Card Rehabil 1983;43:661–667.

8. Foster C, Thompson N. Functional translation of exercise test responses to recreational activities. J Cardpulm Rehabil 1992;11:373–377.

9. Franklin B, Hellerstein H, Gordon S, et al. Exercise prescription for the myocardial infarction patient. J Cardpulm Rehabil 1986;6:62–79.

10. Aronov DM, Rosykhodzhajeva GA. Energy expenditure and cardiovascular response to daily activities in pa-

tients with coronary heart disease of different functional classes. J Cardpulm Rehabil 1992;12:56–62.

11. Pryor DB, Bruce RA, Chaitman BR, et al. Task Force I. Determination of prognosis in patients with ischemic heart disease. J Am Coll Cardiol 1989;14:1016–1025.

12. Maher V. Coronary atherosclerosis stabilization: an achievable goal. Atherosclerosis 1995;118 (Suppl): S91–S101.

13. Burke A, Farb A, Malcom G, et al. Coronary risk factors and plaque morphology in men with coronary disease who died suddenly. N Engl J Med 1997;336:1276–1282.

14. Burke A, Farb A. Strenuous exercise provokes rupture of vulnerable plaques in dyslipidemic men with severe coronary disease [abstract]. Circulation 1997; 96:8.

15. Burke A, Farb A, Liang Y, et al. Effect of hypertension and cardiac hypertrophy on coronary artery morphology in sudden cardiac death. Circulation 1996;94: 3138–3145.

16. Siscovick D, Weiss N, Fletcher R, et al. The incidence of primary cardiac arrest during vigorous exercise. N Engl J Med 1984;311:874–877.

17. Franklin B, Hogan P, Bonzheim K, et al. Cardiac demands of heavy snow shoveling. JAMA 1995;273: 880–882.

18. Sheldahl L, Wilke N, Dougherty S, et al. Effect of age and coronary artery disease on response to snow shoveling. J Am Coll Cardiol 1992;20:1111–1117.

19. Sheldahl L, Wilke N, Dougherty S, et al. Snow blowing and shoveling in normal and asymptomatic coronary artery diseased men. Int J Cardiol 1994;43:233–238.

20. Bove AA. Medical aspects of sport diving. Med Sci Sports Exerc 1996;28:591–595.

21. Dovenbarger J, Mebane GY, Corson K, et al. Divers Alert Network 1989 report on diving accidents and fatalities. Durham, NC: Divers Alert Network—Duke University Medical Center, 1991.

22. Morgan W. Anxiety and panic in recreational scuba divers. Sports Med 1995;20:398–421.

23. Bennett P, Elliott D. The physiology and medicine of diving. Philadelphia: WB Saunders, 1993.

24. Bove A, Davis J. Diving medicine. Philadelphia: WB Saunders, 1990.

25. Tei C, Horikiri Y, Park J, et al. Acute hemodynamic improvement by thermal vasodilation in congestive heart failure. Circulation 1995;91:2582–2590.

26. Vanakoski J, Seppala T, Sievi E, et al. Exposure to high ambient temperature increases absorption and plasma concentrations of transdermal nicotine. Clin Pharmacol Ther 1996;60:308–315.

27. Vanakoski J, Seppala T. Effects of a Finnish sauna on the pharmacokinetics and haemodynamic actions of propranolol and captopril in healthy volunteers. Eur J Clin Pharmacol 1995;48:133–137.

28. Kortelainen M. Hyperthermia deaths in Finland in 1970–1986. Am J Forensic Med Pathol 1991;12: 115–118.

29. Press E. The health hazards of saunas and spas and how to minimize them. Am J Public Health 1991;81: 1034–1037.

30. Allison T, Miller T, Squires R, et al. Cardiovascular responses to immersion in a hot tub in comparison with exercise in male subjects with coronary artery disease. Mayo Clin Proc 1993;68:19–25.

31. Giannetti N, Juneau M, Arsenault A, et al. Sauna induced myocardial ischemia in coronary patients: assessment with Tc sestamibi [abstract]. Can J Cardiol 1997;13(Suppl C):95C.

32. Vuori I. Sauna bather's circulation. Ann Clin Res 1988;20:249–256.

33. Pandolf K, Young A. Altitude and cold. In: Pollock M, Schmidt D, eds. Heart disease and rehabilitation. 3rd ed. Champaign, IL: Human Kinetics, 1995:309–326.

34. Squires R. Moderate altitude exposure and the cardiac patient. J Cardpulm Rehabil 1985;5:421–426.

Part C.

1. Mancini DM, Eisen H, Kussmaul W, et al. Value of peak oxygen consumption for optimal timing of cardiac transplantation in ambulatory patients with heart failure. Circulation 1991;83:778–786.

2. Meyer K, Gornandt L, Schwaibold M, et al. Predictors of response to exercise training in severe chronic congestive heart failure. Am J Cardiol 1997;80: 56–60.

3. Squires RW, Lavie CJ, Brandt TR, et al. Cardiac rehabilitation in patients with severe ischemic left ventricular dysfunction. Mayo Clin Proc 1987;62:997–1002.

4. Hanson P. Exercise testing and training in patients with chronic heart failure. Med Sci Sports Exerc 1994;26:527–537.

5. McGregor CGA. Cardiac transplantation: surgical considerations and early postoperative management. Mayo Clin Proc 1992;67:577–585.

6. Squires RW. Cardiac rehabilitation issues for heart transplantation patients. J Cardpulm Rehabil 1990;10: 159–168.

7. Keteyian S, Ehrman J, Fedel F, et al. Heart rate-perceived exertion relationship during exercise in orthotopic heart transplant patients. J Cardpulm Rehabil 1990;10:287–293.

8. Squires RW, Arthur PR, Gau GT, et al. Exercise after cardiac transplantation; a report of two cases. J Cardpulm Rehabil 1983;3:570–574.

9. Keteyian S, Brawner C. Cardiac transplant. In: American College of Sports Medicine. ACSM's exercise management for persons with chronic diseases and disabilities. Champaign, IL: Human Kinetics, 1997:54–58.

10. Kavanagh T. Physical training in heart transplant recipients. J Cardiovasc Risk 1996;3:154–159.

Medical Considerations in Cardiovascular Rehabilitation

Rehabilitation of Patients with Heart Failure

Suzanne M. Rodkey and James B. Young
with a special section on transplant by Ray W. Squires

INTRODUCTION

Heart failure resulting from ventricular dysfunction is a serious problem throughout the world. In the United States, congestive heart failure (CHF) alone accounts for more than 43,000 deaths every year. There are about 400,000 new cases diagnosed annually, and it is estimated that 4.9 million Americans currently have CHF (1). Of greater concern is that symptomatic, chronic CHF only accounts for approximately one-half of the patients with severe left ventricular dysfunction (2). With improved management of other cardiovascular disorders, such as myocardial infarction, hypertension, and valvular heart disease, the prevalence of heart failure is anticipated to increase even further. Health-care professionals caring for this growing patient population need a better understanding of the pathophysiology of heart failure and how various treatment modalities, including cardiac rehabilitation and exercise, can decrease morbidity and possibly mortality.

The treatment of heart failure has changed dramatically during the years. The original focus of medical management was aimed at improving hemodynamics and volume overload. It was believed that if the "numbers" obtained from right heart catheterization were optimized with vasodilators, diuretics, and inotropic agents, the patient would symptomatically improve and have longer survival. This philosophy has proved to be at times inaccurate and short-sighted. The experiences gained from oral inotropic agents and vasodilators such as vesnarinone, flosequinan, and prazosin have proven that short-term improvements do not necessarily translate into decreased mortality (3–5). The radical change in the use of β-blockers is another example of how the treatment of heart failure has evolved in an unanticipated fashion (6). It was only a few years ago that one would be bitterly criticized for using a β-blocking drug in a patient with systolic ventricular dysfunction; however, several trials have now demonstrated a substantive benefit with their use (7–11). Exercise and physical activity in the setting of heart failure is another treatment area being completely readdressed and revised.

Fothergill (12), in 1872, offered one of the first accounts of bed rest for the treatment of heart failure, noting improvement in symptoms, particularly in milder cases. Burch (13), in 1969, stressed strict and complete bed rest, sometimes for periods lasting more than a year. Patients were not even allowed to get up to use the bathroom or make a telephone call. "This regimen of bed rest is enforced until patients notice an improvement in their symptoms or are symptom free. They are then allowed to ambulate judiciously and only after careful deliberation." Failure to improve on absolute bed rest was interpreted as either noncompliance with the prescribed treatment or as an ominous sign of the irreversibility of the disease (14). There were many physiologic advantages to bed rest. The supine position promoted diuresis by increasing renal blood flow and decreasing systemic vascular resistance, an especially beneficial therapy in an era when potent loop diuretics did not exist. This led to an eventual reduction in ventricular volume and pulmonary congestion. The workload of the heart was decreased by reducing blood pressure, cardiac output, and heart rate. Total oxygen consumption was also decreased. The diminished metabolic demands of the myocardium lowered the chances of precipitating ischemia. In addition, there were concerns about the potential detrimental effects of physical activity, further promoting the utility of bed rest. For example, worsening left ventricular dilatation that might occur would result in a progressive decline in systolic function. Dysrhythmias could be induced. Decreased renal blood flow could activate the renin-angiotensin system, thus resulting in an exacerbation of fluid retention and symptoms. Sympathetic nervous system activation was also known to be detrimental. Finally, preexisting symptoms such as shortness of breath and fatigue frequently made physical activity difficult to perform, and a sedentary lifestyle was often the easiest therapy.

In 1990, a bold challenge was offered to reconsider bed rest as a treatment for heart failure and even to consider promoting exercise therapy (15). Clearly, there were many known risks of inactivity, including further reductions in exercise tolerance (16, 17), decubiti, venous thrombosis, pulmonary embolism, and muscular atrophy. Many of the benefits previously obtained from bed rest, such as decreased systemic vascular resistance, diuresis, and diminished adrenergic activity, could now be accomplished with drug therapy. Preliminary observations and studies from the 1970s and early 1980s suggested that exercise was feasible, improved peak exercise performance, and probably diminished sympathetic activation, even in patients with heart failure (18–20). This led to the current understanding that inactivity is generally more harmful than beneficial and that exercise should be considered part of the routine treatment of chronic heart failure, particularly in the earlier stages of the syndrome. Indeed, the American Heart Association and the United States Department of Health and Human Services now recommend routine exercise in patients with chronic, stable heart failure (21–23).

PATHOPHYSIOLOGY OF LEFT VENTRICULAR DYSFUNCTION

The intolerance to physical activity well-demonstrated in heart failure patients was previously thought to be secondary to the hostile hemodynamic milieu resulting from left ventricular systolic and diastolic dysfunction. The shortness of breath with exertion was believed to be caused by increased pulmonary capillary wedge pressure (so-called backward failure), and the fatigue patients experienced was from low cardiac output (so-called forward failure). It is mysterious, though, that symptoms vary markedly among patients and even within the same patient at different times, despite the fact that quantifiable hemodynamics remained unchanged (24–26). Certainly, the type and intensity of activity may contribute specific patterns of limiting symptoms, as can the degree of volume overload and medication treatment protocol (27). We now realize, though, that there are more complex physiologic changes than strictly the cardiac hemodynamics that contribute to exercise limitations in heart failure, including pulmonary, peripheral vascular, and skeletal muscle alterations (Fig. 9.1) (28, 29). A better understanding of each of these individual factors may allow for a more scientific approach to guiding and counseling patients regarding physical activity and exercise and will help direct future investigations of exercise physiology (Table 9.1).

Cardiac and Hemodynamic Derangements

Heart failure or cardiomyopathy caused by systolic left ventricular impairment is traditionally defined as an ejection fraction less than 50% (30). There are other forms of heart failure, for example those involving high-output or restrictive states, that can actually have normal or supranormal ejection fractions; however, this chapter is focused on the more common types of cardiomyopathy involving systolic dysfunction. Impairment of function can involve the left, right, or both ventricles. Classically, patients will have myocyte hypertrophy, progressive dilatation of the ventricular cavity, and impaired ventricular contraction (31). The gross anatomic changes that occur are caused by alterations of the myocardium at the molecular and cellular

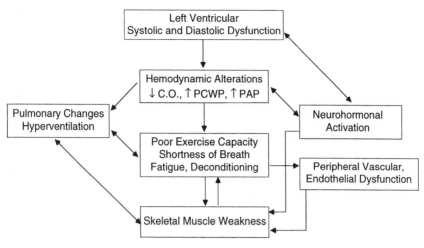

Figure 9.1.   Some of the physiologic changes that occur in heart failure patients, with suggestions of ways that these alterations interact to produce exercise limitations, shortness of breath, and fatigue.

levels and are best characterized as a return to fetal phenotypic states (32–35). Despite increasing knowledge of the mechanisms of myocyte failure, and hope of using this knowledge to devise methods to improve myocardial performance, it has been observed that there is a poor correlation between the resting ejection fraction and exercise capacity (36–39). Similarly, pulmonary capillary wedge pressure and other resting and exercise hemodynamic measurements also correlate poorly with exercise ability and peak oxygen uptake ($\dot{V}O_2$) (40–43). Even asymptomatic patients with left ventricular systolic dysfunction, but with relatively preserved hemodynamics, have their exercise capacity diminished by 30% to 40% (44). Additionally, acute improvements in hemodynamics occasionally, but not uniformly, increase exercise performance (45–47). It may be that cardiac output is the primary determinant of peak performance, but other factors contribute to submaximal exercise tolerance (48).

Pulmonary Changes

Because dyspnea is frequently the limiting symptom of exercise performance with heart failure, the pulmonary system is a natural place to explore for possible explanations of the many dyspnea syndromes seen in patients with heart failure. There have been many pulmonary alterations noted with heart failure. Increased respiratory muscle work mediated by hyperventilation and decreased lung compliance may be a significant contributing factor in the development of exertional dyspnea (49). It has been shown that ventilation and the ratio of minute ventilation to carbon dioxide production ($\dot{V}E/\dot{V}CO_2$) is increased in patients with heart failure when compared with control subjects at rest and at any given workload and oxygen consumption (50, 51), and is an independent prognostic marker of survival (52). These alterations may influence the tolerance to perform even the routine activities of daily living (53). The mechanism for this hyperventilation is unclear, but may be related to several factors (54). In heart failure, physiologic dead space and the dead space:tidal volume ratio are increased (55). Anaerobic metabolism has an earlier onset. The pulmonary ventilation/perfusion mismatches that occur in heart failure may also contribute to the hyperventilation (56). Indeed, the magnitude of the mismatch is directly related to the severity of chronic heart failure (57). Cardiomegaly itself produces atelectasis and shunting, resulting in further mismatches. Enhanced hypoxic and central hypercapnic chemoreceptor sensitivity may also play a role in the hyperventilatory state (58). Other pulmonary changes present in heart failure patients include restrictive patterns that develop from chronic pulmonary hypertension, respiratory muscle weakness and fatigue (59–61), histochemical respiratory muscle alterations (62, 63), and a decrease in lung compliance, which can lead to shallow breathing and

Table 9.1.   Possible Limitations to Exercise in Chronic Heart Failure

Hemodynamics
  Low ejection fraction and cardiac output
  Increased systemic vascular resistance
  Increased pulmonary capillary wedge pressure
  Increased right atrial and pulmonary artery pressures
Pulmonary
  Hyperventilation and increased respiratory muscle work
  Ventilation/perfusion mismatches and increased dead space
  Decreased lung compliance
  Respiratory muscle weakness
  Enhanced central chemoreceptor sensitivity
Neurohormonal
  Sympathetic activation
  Increased renin-angiotensin-aldosterone and arginine vasopressin systems
  Elevated atrial and brain natriuretic peptides
  Increased prostaglandins, tumor necrosis factor-alpha, and growth hormone
  Presence of other cytokines
Peripheral vascular/endothelial
  Increased vasoconstriction/venous tone
  Diminished endothelium-dependent vasodilation
  Increased endothelin
  Impaired nitric oxide release
Skeletal muscle
  Decreased blood flow and nutrient delivery
  Decreased skeletal muscle mass
  Diminished oxidative capacity
  Smaller mitochondrial size and density
  Deconditioning
Psychosocial
  Fear and anxiety
  Instructions not to exercise
  Perception that exercise is harmful or not possible in current state

consequently further increase the physiologic dead space. Still, all of these changes do not completely explain the reduction in exercise performance that is encountered in patients with heart failure. For example, the ventilatory reserve is generally normal in heart failure patients, even in those limited by dyspnea (64). The pulmonary capillary wedge pressure is elevated in heart failure patients at rest and often more markedly during exercise; however, this does not always correlate with exercise performance, indices of dyspnea, fatigue, hypoxemia, or altered carbon dioxide tension (65). It may be that dyspnea and fatigue are central interpretations of the same peripheral signal (66, 67) and that the pul-

monary changes are less likely to be the major factors limiting maximal exercise performance.

Neurohormonal Disturbances

The decreased cardiac output of chronic left ventricular dysfunction leads to hypoperfusion of vital organs, with the body inappropriately perceiving a hypovolemic state. This results in activation of the sympathetic nervous, renin-angiotensin-aldosterone, and arginine vasopressin systems. Consequently, there are many neurohormones increased in chronic heart failure, including aldosterone, angiotensin II, atrial natriuretic factor, endothelin, epinephrine, growth hormone, norepinephrine, prostaglandins, renin, tumor necrosis factor-alpha (TNF-α), and vasopressin. Many of these neurohormones are beneficial in acute settings; however, they are also known or suspected to have detrimental effects on the myocardium chronically and can play a significant role in the progressive decline of ventricular function (68, 69). The current pharmacologic aims in the treatment of heart failure involve suppressing these substances in an attempt to improve the long-term outcomes. One unanswered question that remains is whether excessive neuroendocrine activation results in impairment of exercise tolerance or whether it is strictly a manifestation of the severity of heart failure. Further, the response of neurohormones to exercise in heart failure patients is unclear.

Although the renin-angiotensin-aldosterone system is activated at rest with heart failure, little is known about its function with exercise. In one study, moderate exercise did not immediately change plasma renin activity in normal subjects or in heart failure patients; however, strenuous exertion substantially increased the renin activity in the heart failure group acutely (70). Plasma vasopressin levels were elevated at rest, but did not change with exercise. Normal control subjects had an increase in vasopressin levels with exercise that was comparable to resting levels of the CHF patients. In another study, plasma aldosterone levels increased during exercise in heart failure patients (71).

Increased plasma norepinephrine levels have been demonstrated at rest and with exercise in patients with heart failure. Many believe that this sympathetic response has a supportive role during exercise to maintain arterial blood pressure

(72). This increase has been shown to occur abruptly even with minimal exercise (73); however, the peak levels in heart failure patients do not reach the much higher levels observed in normal subjects. This may be partially explained by the fact that heart failure patients achieve a much lower peak $\dot{V}O_2$. Brain and atrial natriuretic peptides increase with exercise (74, 75) and, recently, peak exercise atrial natriuretic peptide levels have been shown to be a significant independent marker of cardiovascular death (76). However, very few studies that look at the effect of medical treatment on catecholamine release in exercise have been performed. It is perplexing to note that drugs such as angiotensin-converting enzyme inhibitors and carvedilol have a rather dramatic effect on the heart failure neurohumoral milieu, improve systolic ventricular function, decrease mortality, and improve quality of life, but only minimally increase exercise tolerance (77–83).

Peripheral Circulation Abnormalities

Changes in the peripheral circulation are thought to contribute to the decrease in exercise tolerance and symptoms experienced by heart failure patients. The blood vessels are more vasoconstricted in the resting state, which is related to increases in norepinephrine, angiotensin II, and vasopressin and to impaired endothelium-dependent vasodilation (84). There also may be increased endothelin, a potent vasoconstrictor (85). This vasoconstriction is a protective, but inappropriate, response to maintain blood pressure in the face of lowered cardiac output. Increased nitric oxide production may partially compensate for this excessive vasoconstriction in heart failure at rest. There is, however, the suggestion that nitric oxide release is impaired in the setting of heart failure, which may account for the inadequate vasodilator response witnessed during exercise (86). Numerous studies have demonstrated impaired arterial vasodilatory capacity and augmented venous tone in heart failure. Maximum vasodilation is also reduced in this setting. This presumably occurs because of increased vessel wall stiffness, endothelial dysfunction, and other chronic, structural vascular changes. Sodium and fluid retention can further impair vasodilation perhaps by tissue compression of the capillaries or intrinsic vascular

changes (87, 88). Dysfunction of the endothelium may worsen as heart failure progresses, leading to further reductions in exercise ability.

Skeletal Muscle Alterations

Peripheral skeletal muscle alterations accompanying heart failure are primary impediments to physical activity, particularly with submaximal exercise, and have been underappreciated (89, 90). Originally, this restriction in exercise was attributed to inadequate blood flow and nutrients to the skeletal muscles during exercise, because heart failure patients have increases in blood lactate levels earlier than exercising control subjects, reduced cardiac outputs, and augmented limb oxygen extraction (25, 48, 91). However, many pharmacologic therapies aimed at increasing limb blood flow and cardiac output did not improve maximal exercise capacity, fatigue, or lactate levels (92–96). This led to further investigations, which subsequently demonstrated the presence of many ultrastructural muscle changes in heart failure patients, indicative of decreased oxidative capacity and excessive dependence on glycolytic metabolism leading to the earlier onset of anaerobic metabolism. First, a decrease in the total skeletal muscle mass has been noted (97). This decrease in muscle mass may actually be a cause of diminished limb blood flow, rather than vice versa (98). Muscle wasting may explain why strength is reduced in heart failure, but maximal force per unit muscle remains relatively normal. Insulin resistance is present in CHF and may also contribute to muscle catabolism (99). Second, there is a shift in muscle fiber type distribution from type I slow twitch fibers to more type IIb fast twitch fibers. Unfortunately, muscle fiber atrophy, again particularly of type II fibers, has been seen. There is a reduction in the number of capillaries per fiber for type I and IIa fibers. Some of these observations help explain why muscle strength in heart failure is generally more preserved than muscle endurance (100). Third, total mitochondrial size and density are decreased. These decreases have been correlated with reductions in the peak $\dot{V}O_2$ and $\dot{V}O_2$ at anaerobic threshold (101). Further, there are decreases in mitochondrial-based enzyme oxidative activity, such as with 3-hydroxyacyl-CoA-dehydrogenase, succinate dehydrogenase, and cytochrome oxidase (102, 103). Finally, a link via a neural signal may exist between skeletal muscle metabolic dysfunction and the abnormally increased ventilatory response witnessed in heart failure patients (104). Researchers are currently evaluating why biochemical and histologic changes in muscle occur with CHF. Numerous mechanisms have been postulated, including the effects of tissue underperfusion, corticosteroids, growth hormone, TNF-α, and other neurohormones. For instance, it is known that TNF-α (also referred to as cachectin) is increased in heart failure. This same substance can also cause muscle atrophy in other conditions (105–108) and may play a similar role in heart failure patients. However, in the end, it may be that deconditioning and inactivity are the primary reasons for most of these muscle alterations, and an exercise program could potentially reverse or prevent these changes.

Other Obstructions to Exercise

When examining why heart failure patients are limited in their activities, it is important to consider obstructions to exercise other than the obvious hemodynamic, peripheral, and skeletal muscle changes. There are many psychosocial impediments to exercise as well. Patients are frequently instructed by their physician and warned by well-meaning family and friends that they should limit activities. There is the perception that anyone with a "heart condition" should remain inactive. There are also fears of becoming short of breath, precipitating chest discomfort or a heart attack, and increasing the risk of sudden cardiac death. In reality, patients are more likely to die of sudden cardiac death in their sleep rather than while exercising. Deconditioning can easily occur, especially during a hospitalization or decompensation, and patients are often reluctant to resume previous activities, frequently misinterpreting deconditioning for worsening of their heart problem and again assuming that they cannot or should not be active.

EXERCISE IN THE TREATMENT OF HEART FAILURE

There are several benefits of a regular exercise training program in patients with heart failure (Table 9.2). This group can attain all the more commonly recognized benefits of a regular exercise program similar to healthy individuals or other cardiac disease patients with normal left

Table 9.2. Possible Benefits to Exercise in Chronic Heart Failure

Hemodynamics
  Increased maximal and submaximal exercise capacity
  Delay in onset of anaerobic metabolism
  Increased cardiac output and stroke volume
  Decreased systemic vascular resistance
  No worsening of pulmonary and right atrial pressures
Pulmonary
  Decreased minute ventilation
  Decreased minute ventilation to carbon dioxide production ratio
  Improvement in sensation of shortness of breath
Neurohormonal
  Diminished sympathetic tone
  Improved chronotropic competence and heart rate variability
  Decreased resting heart rate
  Decreased cytokines and neurohormones
Peripheral vascular/endothelial
  Improved endothelial function
  Increased nitric oxide synthase
  Decreased platelet aggregation
Skeletal muscle
  Increased muscle strength, mass, and peak power output
  Improved muscle perfusion and capillary density
  Increased oxidative capacity and mitochondrial density
Psychosocial
  Improved quality of life
  Sense of well-being
Other
  Decreased comorbidities such as hypertension and coronary artery disease
  Weight loss
  Improved lipid profile
  Increased insulin sensitivity

ventricular function, including decreased hypertension, improvement of lipid profile with increases in high-density lipoproteins and lowering of triglycerides, increased insulin sensitivity, and decreased death from coronary artery disease. Regular exercise promotes weight loss and reduces the risk from other comorbidities. There are additional benefits that can be realized involving each of the activity-limiting parameters previously described. By understanding and focusing on the various physiologic changes brought about by heart failure, a regular exercise program can be designed to minimize and possibly reverse many of these alterations. A reduction in heart failure symptoms and improvement in well-being and quality of life have repeatedly been shown. Further, the number of hospitalizations is reduced with routine exercise (109).

Cardiac and Hemodynamic Parameters

It has been demonstrated that exercise capacity closely correlates with survival in CHF (110, 111). Patients can have significant increases in maximal and submaximal exercise capacity as seen by increases in peak $\dot{V}O_2$ and exercise tolerance and a delay in the change to anaerobic metabolism with exercise training (112, 113). Consequently, it is believed that an increase in exercise capacity from a training program will lead to improvements in survival. An improvement in exercise endurance is also important because it impacts on tolerance to perform the submaximal workloads encountered during activities of daily life. It is believed that some of the improvement in exercise capacity, particularly with peak exercise, is caused by increased cardiac output (114). Of the factors contributing to the improvement of cardiac output, an increase in stroke volume is the predominant mechanism at submaximal exercise levels, but an elevation of heart rate may also contribute to enhancements in maximal exercise. It is unknown whether the increase in stroke volume results from increases in left ventricular mass, contractile performance, or augmented diastolic recoil. There can also be an increase in ejection fraction with training (115). Training can reduce the rate-pressure product at submaximal workloads (116).

Much debate has occurred about the effects of exercise training on ventricular remodeling. Preliminary animal and human studies suggested that exercise adversely affected the myocardium (117–119). Recent studies, though, employing newer methods of measurement, report no deleterious effects on ventricular volume, wall thickness, or function (115, 120). There was no worsening of hemodynamic pressures, including right atrial, pulmonary arterial, pulmonary capillary wedge, or systemic arterial pressures, with chronic exercise (114, 121). One animal study has demonstrated that chronic dynamic exercise improves the functional abnormality of the G stimulatory protein, which may translate into augmented left ventricular contractility (122). These observations must be placed into the context of what is known about the bradycardic, hypertrophic heart of a world-class athlete, whose hemodynamic performance can support astounding

levels of physical endurance. Exercise-induced cardiac remodeling, then, may be distinct from pathologic cardiac remodeling. Intuitively, aerobic exercise training in heart failure must have benefits at the molecular biodynamic level.

Pulmonary Status

Exercise training reduces excessive minute ventilation and the minute ventilation to carbon dioxide production ratio (113, 123–125). Physical training leads to an improvement in ventilatory performance in patients with chronic heart failure, although this is not present in healthy exercising individuals (126). This improvement may explain why patients report less shortness of breath at rest and with activity after exercise. Other interventions directed at lessening the work of breathing may be of additional benefit (127).

Neurohormonal Disturbances

During acute exercise, sympathetic nervous activity is increased, yet chronic changes in neurohormonal levels occurring with a regular exercise program have not been fully elucidated. Precisely how to measure parameters such as sympathetic activation is still being debated; however, there are trends showing that regular exercise chronically decreases sympathetic tone and neurohormonal activation (128). Regular exercise also increases parasympathetic tone and improves chronotropic incompetence (129). A reduction in resting heart rate is seen. Studies have also demonstrated decreases in norepinephrine levels and increases in heart rate variability (112, 130), both previously documented as being independent predictors of survival (131, 132). A decreased susceptibility to ventricular dysrhythmias also occurs with exercise (133). Additionally, another study showed a significant decrease in angiotensin II, aldosterone, atrial natriuretic peptide, and vasopressin after a training program (134). Finally, there may be decreases in some cytokines (135), but trials are needed to explore this further.

Peripheral Circulation Abnormalities

With training, blood flow to active muscles increases, in part because of a decrease in systemic vascular resistance. Some of the enhanced blood flow in exercising limbs has also been suggested to be related to a reduction of circulating norepinephrine (136). Some evidence exists that endothelial function is also improved (137). For example, there is increased expression of nitric oxide synthase (138) and decreased platelet aggregation. Furthermore, endothelial nitric oxide may play a role in the regulation of mitochondrial oxidation in skeletal muscles (139), causing additional improvements in exercise performance.

Skeletal Muscle Improvement

Exercise promotes an increase in muscle strength and peak power output. Improvements in muscle perfusion, mass, and metabolism contribute to these increases. Capillary density in skeletal muscle increases. Additional improvements occur on the cellular level. One study showed that a training program resulted in an increase in the total volume density of mitochondria and volume density of cytochrome c oxidase–positive mitochondria (140). These increases in oxidative capacity correlated with an increase in maximal exercise tolerance and delayed anaerobic metabolism during submaximal exercise. The remarkable improvement in oxidative capacity with exercise training has also been demonstrated by others (141–145). A reduction in the afferent neural link between skeletal muscles and the central nervous system has been postulated to be involved in a decrease in sympathetic activity with exercise training (146).

THE EXERCISE PRESCRIPTION

Preexercise Cardiac Evaluation

Similar to other cardiac patients, CHF patients should be referred for formal stress testing before starting exercise to identify high-risk individuals and to help guide and tailor the exercise prescription (Table 9.3). The best time to appraise exercise limitations in heart failure patients is when they are maximally treated with an appropriate pharmacologic regimen, so they may be assessed at their best. Information obtained during or immediately after recovering from an episode of congestive failure underestimates the patient's capabilities and may overestimate risk. The stress test may be either symptom-limited or submaximal in design. For patients with severe heart failure, metabolic stress testing, in which maximal $\dot{V}O_2$ and $\dot{V}O_2$ at anaerobic threshold are determined, provides additional useful information. The testing protocol should be modified in degree of workload with

Table 9.3.   Benefits to Stress Testing for Exercise Prescription

Detection of high-risk individuals
   Inducible ischemia
   Dysrhythmias and electrocardiographic changes
   Drop in systolic blood pressure
   Development of gallops, bronchospasm, and
      pulmonary edema
Determine exercise capabilities
   Determine $\dot{V}O_2$ at anaerobic threshold and peak
      $\dot{V}O_2$
   Identify other limitations to exercise such as
      claudication or back pain
Assess heart rate response to exercise
   Detect chronotropic incompetence
   Determine maximum heart rate
   Determine heart rate at anaerobic threshold or at
      various stages of test
Patient education
   Learn rating of perceived exertion scale
   Reassurance of safety of exercise

slower speeds and smaller increments between stages, yet reach the targeted goals between 8 and 10 minutes (147, 148). Standard protocols such as the Balke, Ellestad, Bruce, and modified Astrand may be too difficult for heart failure patients (149). Instead, protocols such as the modified Naughton and Branching allow for better assessment of the true functional capacity of the patient. It is important to watch for hypotensive systolic blood pressure responses, changes in rhythm, and ST-segment changes during exercise testing. It is also useful to examine the patient immediately after the stress test to assess for the presence of a new S3 or S4 gallop, pulmonary rales, or bronchospasm. The rating of perceived exertion (RPE) and heart rate response at the various levels during the exercise protocol will aid in formulating an adequate and safe program for the patient. Most heart failure patients benefit from starting exercise in a supervised cardiac rehabilitation setting. Certainly, moderate- and high-risk individuals should be followed up closely in a monitored program, especially those with a functional capacity of less than 8 metabolic equivalents (METs) or an ejection fraction of less than 30% (150, 151). Home-based programs have been shown to be feasible for stable chronic heart failure patients, even those with severe left ventricular dysfunction (116). Long-term effects of training on morbidity and mortality do not yet exist (152), and it would be prudent to first establish a solid exercise prescription in a supervised setting in all but the most stable and functionally preserved patients.

The Exercise Regimen

The formal exercise prescription consists of four components: type of activity, intensity, duration, and frequency. This has been described in other chapters, but deserves mention regarding how CHF patients differ from other cardiac patients (Table 9.4). The ideal guidelines and programs for heart failure have not yet been determined because it is unknown how to best optimize cardiovascular and skeletal performance in heart failure while avoiding possible adverse effects. From an understanding of the alterations of the periphery in heart failure and how they impact functional capacity, exercise protocols should be aimed primarily at reversing these limiting derangements. This is in contrast with healthy individuals, in whom the focus is also placed on enhancing the cardiac output response to activity.

The most commonly recommended type of activity is isotonic aerobic exercise such as walking or cycling. Walking is very popular because it requires no special training or equipment and can be done almost anywhere. Walking at 2 miles per hour (mph) on a flat surface is about equal to 2.5 METs, 3 mph is about 3.3 METs, and 4 mph is about 4.5 METs. Cycling at a slow speed is about 3.5 METs. Although swimming and rowing are excellent, non–weight-bearing exercises, they may initially be too strenuous for most heart failure patients. For example, swimming slowly using the breast stroke requires about 5 METs. This would require a patient to have an anaerobic threshold greater than approximately $16 \text{ mL} \cdot \text{kg}^{-1} \cdot \text{min}^{-1}$. Typically, exercise is performed in a continuous manner; however, there are some studies demonstrating that an interval method of training can result in a greater increase in aerobic capacity, with minimal cardiac stress and strain (153–155). This method involves cycles of short (10 to 30 seconds) bursts of activity followed by 60 seconds of recovery and may be particularly useful in patients who have more peripheral muscle weakness.

Isometric (static) body-building types of exercise place a greater pressure load on the left ventricle, in contrast to isotonic activities that cause a greater volume load. This results in immediate increases in ventricular wall stress and peripheral vascular resistance and may worsen hemodynamics, precipitate serious dysrhythmias, and increase endothelin levels (156). This type of activity should be avoided. Resistance training (isometric and isotonic) can increase muscle strength, tone, and endurance (157). If the exercise capacity is greater than 5 METs, this form of activity may be done carefully with light weights. Some groups advocate "segmental" rehabilitation in heart failure patients, which is aimed at isolating specific muscle groups, such as respiratory muscles or arms, rather than a "global" total body workout to improve the activities in daily living most impacted by heart failure (158–161). This may be particularly beneficial in more functionally impaired patients and does not put the same type of stress on the heart as more traditional isometric exercises.

The most favorable intensity level has not been agreed on. Lower intensity workloads for longer durations and high intensity for shorter durations have increased the exercise tolerance of patients and have been shown to be acceptable and improve compliance (162). Ideally, when heart failure patients exercise, they should stay below their anaerobic threshold. Trained normal individuals reach anaerobic threshold at 80% to 90% of their peak $\dot{V}O_2$ and untrained normal individuals reach this at 60% to 70% of their peak; however, this may occur at 50% or less in people with heart failure. Having the data from the metabolic stress test can be extremely useful in

Table 9.4.   Exercise Prescription in Chronic Heart Failure

Type
  Aerobic, isotonic exercise
  Light resistance training
  Avoid isometric, body-building type activities
Intensity
  Stay below anaerobic threshold
  Aim for 50% to 70% of peak $\dot{V}O_2$
  Rating of perceived exertion Borg scale
    approximately 13 to 15
  Heart rate 60% to 80% maximum HR or heart rate at
    Borg scale 13 to 15
Duration
  May need to start at only 10 to 20 min/session
  Work up to 30- to 40-minute sessions
Frequency
  3 to 5 times/wk

designating a reasonable intensity level for the patient. Conventionally, patients have been instructed to exercise at approximately 70% of their peak $\dot{V}O_2$. It has been shown that peak aerobic capacity, however, can be enhanced at workloads of less than 50% of peak. This may actually be a safer and equally beneficial approach to exercise, as this does diminish left ventricular diastolic wall stresses when compared with more conventional programs (163, 164).

Once the desired level of intensity is determined, the patient can then adjust the exercise routine based on RPE. The Borg Scale, which ranges from 6 (very, very light exertion) to 20 (very, very hard exertion), is a useful guide. It has been shown that anaerobic threshold usually occurs at a Borg RPE of 13 to 15 (somewhat hard to hard). Instructing patients to aim for a level of intensity just less than 13 to 15 is very practical, especially if exercising in an unsupervised, unmonitored setting. Heart rate can also be used to help guide exercise intensity. Patients should aim for 60% to 80% of their maximum heart rate as determined at stress testing or at the heart rate corresponding to an RPE of 13 to 15. Alternatively, a target heart rate of 50% to 75% of the heart rate reserve (HRR) plus resting heart rate can be used. (The HRR is defined as maximal heart rate minus resting heart rate multiplied by 50% to 75%.) Heart rate guides are somewhat less practical, but still possible for heart failure patients who may be taking medications such as β-blockers, digoxin, or amiodarone which control or limit heart rate. Similarly, many chronic heart failure patients have blunted and reduced chronotropic responses to exercise and this should also be taken into account when giving recommendations. Heart failure patients with atrial fibrillation, whose rate may not be well controlled with exertion, may also have difficulty following heart rate guidelines. In these cases, the Borg scale may be the best alternative. Guiding intensity of the workout by RPE or heart rate also allows patients to adjust the work rate up as they become more conditioned or down on occasions when they might not be feeling as good. Flexibility in the program is essential. Finally, heart failure patients should be instructed and reminded to watch for symptoms of overexertion, such as chest discomfort, exhaustion (rather than mild fatigue), extreme shortness of breath, and dizziness.

The recommended duration and frequency of activity has varied widely in the literature. Ideally, 30- to 40-minute sessions three to five times per week is the target range. Lower intensity or shorter duration activities should have a greater frequency (165). The schedule should remain flexible, especially when first starting out. Realistically, many heart failure patients can only complete 10 to 20 minutes at a time and it is better for long-term compliance to have a regimen that the patient can tolerate and complete successfully. This is particularly true immediately after a decompensation or hospitalization. Portions of the exercise program that are frequently understressed are the warm-up and cool-down periods. The warm-up period is used to stretch the muscles and ligaments to decrease the risk of injury. An adequate cool-down period is critical for heart failure patients, especially if vasodilators or diuretics are being used, because this will help avoid serious, symptomatic hypotension. It is also unknown for how many weeks a patient should minimally exercise. Most rehabilitation programs and trials reported in the literature describe programs ranging between 3 and 24 weeks. No long-term studies have yet been conducted to determine whether there is further incremental benefit or possible harm for exercise beyond 6 months. The best recommendation is that the patient continue a regular exercise routine for as long as tolerated, preferably for life.

SPECIAL CONCERNS AND LIMITATIONS OF EXERCISE

Complications of Exercise

Many concerns have been raised about possible deleterious effects of exercise. It is known that with time the ventricle undergoes progressive remodeling leading to dilatation and alteration of cardiac geometry, further impairing functioning. Until recently, it was feared that physical exercise could accelerate this response, especially after a myocardial infarction (117, 166). Three randomized, controlled trials indicate that long-term training may actually attenuate the unfavorable remodeling process and perhaps even improve ventricular function (115, 167). Others have raised concerns about increasing the incidence of dysrhythmias and sudden cardiac death or precipitating myocardial ischemia or infarction in patients with ischemic cardiomyopathy. There is no evidence to support an increase in any of these adverse effects and with proper preexercise evaluation and supervision these potential problems can be minimized. Because exercise training improves heart rate variability and neurohumoral activation, it is possible that exercise may actually decrease the incidence of sudden cardiac death. Finally, musculoskeletal injuries are theoretically more likely to occur in heart failure patients, presumably because of deconditioning and preexisting skeletal muscle alterations. Again, proper evaluation, supervision, and warm-up and cool-down periods will decrease the risk of an adverse event.

Contraindications to Exercise in Heart Failure

There are some contraindications to exercise in certain patients with ventricular dysfunction (Table 9.5). Patients who have ischemic cardiomyopathy with ejection fractions less than 40% and documented ischemia on a pretraining treadmill stress test have been shown to have poor exercise performance in terms of exercise time, peak oxygen consumption, and submaximal heart rate (168). This group is unlikely to benefit from training and is also at higher risk for complications. Individuals with unstable angina should undergo revascularization if at all possible or have symptoms controlled with aggressive medical management before exercising. Uncorrected or unstable valvular disease, particularly aortic stenosis, severe left ventricular outflow tract obstruction, and severe hypertension, are also contraindications to exercise. Moderate left ventricular outflow tract obstruction is a relative contraindication. Heart failure patients with uncontrolled dysrhythmias should avoid exercise. Those with exercise-induced minor dysrhythmias should, at a minimum, keep the heart rate 10 beats per minute less than the heart rate at which rhythm problems first begin. Those with more serious, untreated rhythm disturbances should refrain from exercise altogether. Patients with active myocarditis and intercurrent febrile illnesses should also abstain from exertion. Patients with true New York Heart Association (NYHA) class IV symptoms are most likely unable to perform any meaningful exercise. In contrast, patients who are dependent on inotropic agents, but compensated

Table 9.5.   Contraindications to Exercise in Chronic Heart Failure

Absolute contraindications
    Unstable angina and significant ischemia detected during stress testing
    Uncorrected/unstable valvular disease, particularly aortic stenosis
    Severe left ventricular outflow tract obstruction
    Uncontrolled/untreated dysrhythmias
    Active myocarditis
    Intercurrent febrile illness
Relative contraindications
    New York Heart Association class IV congestive heart failure
    Moderate left ventricular outflow tract obstruction
Requires additional consideration
    New York Heart Association class III congestive heart failure
    Minor, exercise-induced dysrhythmias
Not a contraindication
    Age
    Absolute ejection fraction
    Presence of pacemaker or implanted cardioverter/defibrillator

on therapy, are capable of exercise and should be encouraged to do so. Likewise, patients with left ventricular assist devices can train under close supervision and demonstrate a consistent training response. Patients with NYHA class III symptoms should have their exercise routine individualized and also carefully supervised.

There are certain criteria that are frequently considered to be contraindications to exercise, but are not justified. First, increased age is not a reason to avoid exercise. It is important, however, to tailor a program that takes into account physiologic changes in an older individual. Balance and sight may be impaired, making certain forms of exercise less safe. Arthritis may be problematic, with weight-bearing activities being less comfortable. Second, the absolute ejection fraction is not a contraindication to exercise. There is no set "number" below which one is no longer able to exercise. What is more important is that the patient is compensated and fluid status is controlled. Occasionally, patients may notice fluid accumulation in the first few weeks after starting an exercise program. This usually responds to an adjustment of the diuretic regimen and is not serious enough to warrant stopping exercise. Finally, the presence of a pacemaker or implanted cardioverter/defibrillator (ICD) is not a contraindication. Optimizing the programming capabilities of the pacemaker, such as upper rate limit and rate responsiveness, may maximize patients' abilities to successfully perform activities. Many patients fear receiving an inappropriate shock from their ICD during exercise. It is essential to check the patient's response to exercise against the programming parameters of the device. There are very sophisticated programming capabilities to help ensure that shocks are delivered appropriately. It will be necessary to keep the exercise heart rate below a certain threshold level to avoid activation of the device.

SUMMARY AND FUTURE PERSPECTIVE

In the past, heart failure was treated with strict bed rest, and any exertion was strongly discouraged. It is now appreciated that regular exercise can improve functional capacity and that the benefits once derived from bed rest can now be attained with medical therapy. Heart failure patients are limited by both shortness of breath and fatigue when performing activities of daily living, as well as with more strenuous activities. These limiting symptoms result from more than just abnormal cardiac hemodynamics, such as elevated pulmonary capillary wedge pressure and low cardiac output. Cardiac output is one of the primary determinants of peak performance in normal individuals and may also be so for heart failure patients; however, other factors determine submaximal exercise tolerance. It is the submaximal exercise tolerance that more closely reflects the ability of the patient to carry out the routine activities of daily life.

Several peripheral changes occur in patients with heart failure. It is likely that many of these abnormalities contribute to diminished exercise tolerance, rather than one factor accounting for all the disability. There are numerous pulmonary alterations with heart failure that can contribute to the symptoms of shortness of breath and fatigue. Heart failure is characterized by a state of excessive ventilation, ventilation/perfusion mismatches, and decreased lung compliance, leading to increased respiratory muscle work. The sympathetic nervous, renin-angiotensin-aldosterone, and arginine vasopressin systems are all activated with heart failure and chronically have

detrimental effects on the myocardium and ventricular performance. The peripheral circulation has an impaired ability to adequately increase flow to skeletal muscle, with increased vasoconstriction and impaired vasodilatory capacity. There are numerous intrinsic abnormalities of skeletal muscles, ranging from genetic and intracellular alterations to gross muscular atrophy. There is clearly diminished oxidative metabolic functioning of the cells. There are also psychosocial impediments to exercise, including previous medical instructions and fear of a potential adverse event. Finally, and importantly, patients can easily become deconditioned.

Exercise therapy is prescribed to improve submaximal and, to a lesser extent, maximal performance. Heart failure patients can also have improvements in sense of well-being, control of other comorbidities, decreased heart failure symptoms, and presumably increased survival. Physical training should be targeted at improving the peripheral changes that occur with heart failure, such as reducing the hyperventilation and increasing skeletal muscle strength and endurance, while minimizing the stress to the heart. Before writing an exercise prescription for a patient with reduced ventricular function, the patient should undergo formal stress testing, preferably metabolic stress testing. This testing should be done only when the patient is well compensated and medical therapy maximized. The results of this testing will help guide and instruct the patient and identify high-risk individuals.

There have been no strictly determined sets of parameters to follow for exercise, but some general guidelines have been suggested. Aerobic exercise, usually walking or cycling, is one of the best forms of activity. Strenuous isotonic exertion should be avoided because of the increased strain placed on the heart. Light resistance training is beneficial in higher functioning individuals. The intensity should remain below anaerobic threshold and may be less than 50% of peak $\dot{V}O_2$ in this group of patients. Intensity can be guided by an RPE scale, heart rate, or predetermined settings based on the preexercise stress test results. Patients should aim for a duration of activity of 30 to 40 minutes 3 to 5 days a week. Initially, many heart failure patients can only complete 10 to 20 minutes but can gradually increase the time and intensity. It is of paramount importance that an exercise prescription for the heart failure patient be flexible and guided by symptoms.

There are many unanswered questions regarding regular exercise in chronic heart failure patients. Little is still known regarding the effects of exercise on neurohormones, the pulmonary system, and the vascular endothelium. The type, intensity, duration, and frequency of exercise that will best optimize functioning and minimize adverse outcomes is also unknown. And most important, does routine activity decrease mortality, as it is hoped? Recently one small study demonstrated improved survival in patients with systolic ventricular impairment who participated in a routine exercise training program.(169) We await the results of large-scale exercise studies.

TRANSPLANT

The era of human cardiac transplantation began in 1967 with Christiaan Barnard's successful operation in Cape Town, South Africa (170). However, because of poor long-term survival, the operation did not enjoy widespread application during the 1960s and 1970s. Pioneering work, primarily by investigators at Stanford University, resulted in acceptance of the procedure in the 1980s. In particular, the development of the transvenous endomyocardial biopsy technique for early detection of acute rejection, the introduction of the powerful immunosuppressant cyclosporine, both of which resulted in a marked improvement in survival, and funding of the operation and aftercare by the insurance industry were important milestones.

For eligible patients with end-stage heart failure, cardiac transplantation is now the accepted form of surgical therapy, with 1-year and 5-year survival of approximately 85% and 75%, respectively (171). Orthotopic transplantation, depicted in Figure 9.2, is by far the most commonly used technique, with excision of the recipient's diseased heart and anastomosis of the donor heart to the great vessels and atria of the recipient (172). Both the recipient and donor heart sinoatrial nodes may be intact and functioning, and the electrocardiogram may include two distinct P waves. For patients with severe pulmonary hypertension or for unusually large recipients who are difficult to match in terms of donor body size, a heterotopic or "piggyback"

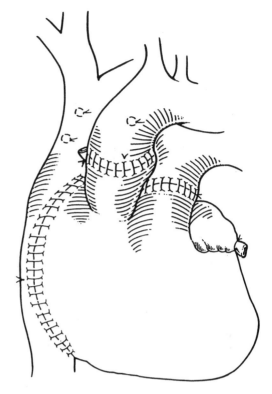

Figure 9.2. Orthotopic cardiac transplantation. (Reprinted with permission from Squires RW: Exercise training after cardiac transplantation. Med Sci Sports Exerc 1991; 23:686–694.)

transplant, as shown in Figure 9.3, may rarely be performed with the donor heart anastomosed to the great vessels without removal of the recipient's heart. This procedure results in the unusual electrocardiographic appearance of two separate QRS complexes on the electrocardiogram (Fig. 9.4). Survival after heterotopic transplantation is inferior to that with the orthotopic technique. Approximately 3000 cardiac transplant operations are performed annually in the United States. Unfortunately, the number of potential candidates for transplantation far exceeds the available supply of donor organs.

The goals of cardiac transplantation are improved survival, reduced symptoms, and an increased exercise capacity. The majority of patients who require transplantation suffer from chronic heart failure resulting from coronary artery disease (ischemic cardiomyopathy) and idiopathic dilated cardiomyopathy (173). Additional diseases that may result in severe heart failure warranting transplantation include hypertension, valvular

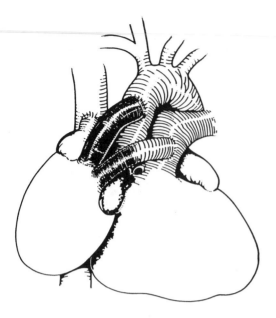

Figure 9.3. Heterotopic cardiac transplantation. (Reprinted with permission from Squires RW: Exercise training after cardiac transplantation. Med Sci Sports Exerc 1991; 23:686–694.)

heart disease, myocarditis, alcohol abuse, chemotherapy-induced myocardial dysfunction, acquired immunodeficiency syndrome, complex congenital heart diseases, infiltrative diseases of the myocardium, pericardial disease, and peripartum. The age range of transplant recipients is from newborn to the eighth decade of life. After transplantation, most patients report a favorable quality of life. Many patients return to work, school, and most avocational activities.

IMMUNOSUPPRESSANTS, ACUTE REJECTION, AND RISK OF INFECTION

Immunosuppressant medications, usually cyclosporine, azathioprine, and prednisone, are given to prevent acute rejection of the donor heart. Acute rejection is characterized by T-lymphocyte infiltration of the myocardium, which potentially results in myocyte injury and necrosis if not detected early in its course and treated aggressively with additional immunosuppressants. Routine, periodic endomyocardial biopsies are performed as a surveillance measure against acute rejection. Rejection is graded from mild to severe,

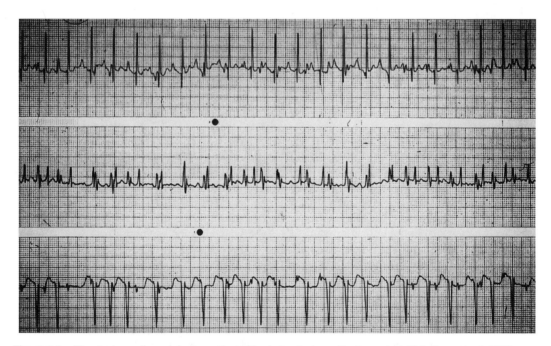

Figure 9.4. The electrocardiogram from a patient with a heterotopic cardiac transplant. Note the separate QRS complexes from the donor and recipient hearts. (Reprinted with permission from Squires RW: Exercise training after cardiac transplantation. Med Sci Sports Exerc 1991; 23:686–694.)

as shown in Table 9.6, based on biopsy-derived tissue sample analysis. Acute rejection occurs in most patients during the first several months after transplantation, with a decreasing incidence thereafter. Severe acute rejection, resulting in substantial myocyte necrosis and fibrosis, may produce left ventricular dysfunction (174).

Immunosuppressants enable the patient to tolerate the donor heart, but they are associated with several common side effects. Skeletal muscle cramping is a common complaint of patients. Cyclosporine may result in renal dysfunction, and the drug possesses general vasopressor activity, resulting in hypertension requiring drug treatment for the majority of transplant patients (175). Additional side effects include tremor, hirsutism, sexual dysfunction, acne, gum hyperplasia, hepatocellular injury, and malignancy. Side effects associated with azathioprine include leukopenia, anemia, and thrombocytopenia. Prednisone alters body fat distribution with resultant truncal obesity and a "moon" faced appearance for many patients. It may also cause mood swings, skeletal muscle atrophy and weakness, osteoporosis, and aseptic necrosis of bone. If possible, prednisone is tapered and stopped during the first 1 to 2 years after surgery to minimize these potential devastating side effects.

Table 9.6.   Standardized Cardiac Biopsy Acute Rejection Grading Scale

Grade	Findings
0	No rejection
1	Mild rejection
1A	Focal infiltrate without necrosis
1B	Diffuse, sparse infiltrate, no necrosis
2	Moderate rejection, one focus with aggressive infiltration and/or myocyte damage
3	Moderate rejection
3A	Multifocal aggressive infiltrates and/or myocyte damage
3B	Diffuse inflammatory process with necrosis
4	Severe rejection, diffuse aggressive polymorphous infiltrates with necrosis

Modified from Perlroth MG, Reitz BA: Heart and heart-lung transplantation. In: Braunwald E, ed. Heart disease: a textbook of cardiovascular medicine. 5th ed. Philadelphia: WB Saunders, 1997;515–533.

Immunosuppressed transplant recipients are at higher risk for opportunistic infections and malignancy than the general population of patients with cardiovascular diseases. During the first several weeks after surgery, pulmonary bacterial infection is common. Late after transplantation, viral, bacterial, and fungal infections pose a threat. Special precautions must be taken to minimize the chances of exposure to infectious agents and to individuals with active infections. Transplant patients are encouraged to wear a surgical mask and gloves in public places, particularly during the first 3 months after surgery, as a barrier to infectious organisms. Recurrent hospitalizations for treatment of acute rejection or infection are common during the first year after transplantation. Acute rejection and infection are the most common causes of early mortality in these patients.

ACCELERATED GRAFT CORONARY ARTERY DISEASE

Accelerated graft coronary artery disease, also called graft vasculopathy or chronic rejection, is characterized by diffuse intimal thickening that often leads to obstructive lesions. It may occur as early as 3 months after transplantation and is commonly seen in patients within 1 to 5 years after surgery. This disease process may result in acute myocardial infarction, congestive heart failure, and sudden cardiac death. It constitutes the major limiting factor in long-term survival after transplantation. The origin of the disease is controversial and is probably multifactorial (175). The classic coronary risk factors of dyslipidemia, cigarette smoking, and hypertension do not appear to play a major role in the disease process. Cytomegalovirus infection is associated with an earlier onset of the disease (176). A complex immune process is likely involved. After transplantation a reduced coronary flow reserve during exercise caused by progressive endothelial dysfunction has been reported and may be involved in the etiology of this disease (177). In addition, plasma homocysteine concentration, an established risk factor for vascular disease, increases dramatically after cardiac transplantation and may play a causative role (178). The process occurs in both pediatric and adult transplant recipients with equal regularity.

Annual coronary angiography is performed for

detection of accelerated graft disease. If severe disease is present, most patients will not experience typical angina pectoris because of the cardiac denervation that occurs at the time of surgery. Revascularization with catheter-based techniques or coronary artery bypass graft (CABG) surgery may be effective treatment for some affected patients with discrete obstructive lesions (179). However, owing to the usual diffuse nature of most lesions, retransplantation is the usual treatment of choice.

The use of hydroxymethylglutaryl-CoA reductase inhibitor medications (statins) in cardiac transplant patients has been demonstrated to reduce the incidence of episodes of acute rejection, improve 1-year survival, decrease the incidence of accelerated graft coronary artery disease, and improve left ventricular systolic function (176, 180). These beneficial effects appear to be independent of the effect of the statin drugs on improving the blood lipid profile.

PSYCHOSOCIAL FACTORS

The psychological reaction to the transplant process is understandably intense for most patients and their significant others (181). During the period of waiting for the operation after being listed as a transplant candidate, emotions range from relief and happiness to anxiety and thoughts of death. During the past several years the average waiting time for a transplant has increased, and as many as 25% of eligible candidates die before a donor becomes available (171, 182).

Immediately after transplantation, patients are usually joyous at the prospect of a longer, better-quality life. As the convalescence continues, patients must adjust to the tedium of taking medications, waiting for appointments, and undergoing procedures. The first episode of acute rejection may result in anxiety and possibly depression.

Denial, directed either toward the graft or the donor, appears to be a defense mechanism for some patients (183). A few cardiac transplant patients develop severe anxiety and behavioral problems that require psychiatric treatment (184).

After hospital discharge, patients should gradually become more independent. As the recovery process continues and the degree of medical supervision decreases, patients generally shift their attention from transplant-related activities to becoming more independent and resuming family activities and avocational and vocational pursuits. Cardiac rehabilitation programs may greatly assist patients and families in this transition. This readjustment to life after transplantation generally requires months, and the first anniversary after surgery is an important milestone in this process.

After recovery from surgery, most patients report an improvement in psychological status compared with pretransplant and early posttransplant conditions (185). However, significant psychosocial problems not uncommonly may persist for 3 or more months after surgery, including mood alteration; marital distress; altered body image; altered family roles; compliance with medications, procedures, and appointments; recommended lifestyle changes; and decreased libido (186). Continued appreciation of psychosocial issues during long-term rehabilitation is needed.

ABNORMAL EXERCISE PHYSIOLOGY AFTER TRANSPLANTATION

The responses of cardiac transplant patients to acute exercise are unique and related to the following factors:

The transplanted heart is denervated at the time of organ harvesting and, at least during the first several weeks to months after surgery, receives no direct efferent activity from the autonomic nervous system and provides no afferent input to the central nervous system.

The donor heart has undergone ischemic time and reperfusion.

There is no intact pericardium.

The donor heart may have suffered a degree of myocyte necrosis resulting from episodes of acute rejection (172).

With cardiac denervation at the time of transplantation and the subsequent loss of parasympathetic innervation, the heart rate at rest is elevated to approximately 95 to 115 beats per minute and represents the inherent rate of depolarization of the sinoatrial node (187). There is no direct sympathetic innervation of the heart, but humoral regulation of heart rate occurs via circulating catecholamines (188). With graded exercise testing, the rate of increase in heart rate is slower and the peak exercise heart rate is slightly lower than normal (approximately 150 beats per minute) (188, 189). Some patients do not increase their heart rate during the first 1 to 3 minutes of exercise. Many transplant patients achieve their peak exercise heart rates during the first few minutes of recovery from exercise, rather than at the highest exercise intensity. Figure 9.5 shows the heart rate response of the same patient to graded exercise before and after orthotopic transplantation. Note the delayed increase in heart rate at the onset of exercise. During recovery from exercise, the heart rate of the transplanted heart remains elevated and slowly returns to preexercise levels as the concentrations of circulating catecholamines return to baseline. The chronotropic or heart rate reserve (difference between rest and peak exercise heart rate) is less than normal. With exercise, transplant patients exhibit normal elevations of plasma catecholamines and, from studies of isoproterenol infusion, possess normal sensitivity to β-adrenergic stimulation (190).

Figure 9.6 shows the unusual heart rate response of a heterotopic transplant patient during exercise. At rest, the heart rate of the innervated recipient heart is lower than that of the denervated donor heart. During exercise, both hearts increase their rates in unison, attaining comparable peak exercise heart rates. During recovery from exercise, the heart rates of the two organs become dissimilar, with the transplanted heart displaying the typical delayed return to preexercise values (191).

Blood pressure at rest may be normal or moderately elevated, and most patients receive antihypertensive medications, as mentioned previously. During exercise, systolic blood pressure

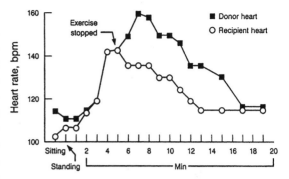

Figure 9.6. Heart rates at rest, during, and after exercise in the donor and recipient heart in a patient with a heterotopic cardiac transplant. (Reprinted with permission from Yusuf S, Mitchell A, Yacoub MH: Interrelation between donor and recipient heart rates during exercise after heterotopic cardiac transplantation. Br Heart J 1985;54:173–178.)

usually increases appropriately, although peak exercise blood pressure may be slightly lower than expected for normal individuals (192).

Afferent denervation apparently results in impaired renin-angiotensin-aldosterone regulation of vasomotion and fluid balance, as well as reducing the vasoregulatory response to changes in cardiac filling pressures (193). Vascular resistance is elevated and intracardiac and pulmonary vascular pressures (particularly right-sided pressures) are generally elevated in transplant patients (194).

Left ventricular systolic function, as measured by ejection fraction, is in the normal range at rest and during exercise (194). Episodes of acute rejection or of myocardial ischemia or necrosis resulting from accelerated graft coronary artery disease may result in left ventricular systolic dysfunction. Most transplant patients have diastolic dysfunction as evidenced by elevated filling pressures for a given end-diastolic volume. This results in a subnormal stroke volume increase during exercise. This, coupled with the below-normal heart rate reserve discussed above, results in an impaired exercise cardiac output.

With the onset of exercise, cardiac output in transplant recipients is increased initially by augmentation of the stroke volume by an enhanced Frank-Starling mechanism and subsequently by an acceleration in heart rate (195). Figure 9.7 shows the greater increase in left ventricular end-diastolic volume index (enhanced Frank-Starling effect) during exercise observed in transplant patients relative to normal con-

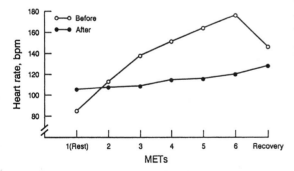

Figure 9.5. Heart rates of the same patient measured during graded exercise 1 year before and 3 months after orthotopic cardiac transplantation. Note the elevated resting heart rate and the delayed increase in heart rate after transplantation. (Reprinted with permission from Squires RW: Cardiac rehabilitation issues for heart transplantation patients. J Cardpulm Rehabil 1990;10:159–168.)

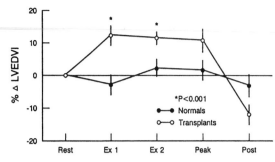

Figure 9.7. The change in left ventricular end-diastolic volume index during progressive supine exercise in patients after orthotopic cardiac transplantation compared with healthy control subjects. (Reprinted with permission from Pflugfelder PW, Purves PD, McKenzie FN, et al: Cardiac dynamics during exercise in cyclosporine treated orthotopic heart transplant recipients: assessment by radionuclide angiography. J Am Coll Cardiol 1987;10:336–341.)

trols. However, at rest and during exercise the cardiac index is lower for transplant patients than for normals, as seen in Figure 9.8.

Skeletal muscle structural abnormalities that develop with chronic heart failure include the following:

Reduced aerobic enzyme activity.
Less capillary development.
Impaired vasodilatory capacity during exercise.
Conversion of slow twitch motor units to fast twitch motor units.
Greater reliance on anaerobic metabolic energy production.

These abnormalities appear to persist after transplantation, with partial improvement after several months (196–198).

Most transplant patients have a normal arterial oxygen saturation and oxygen content at rest and during graded exercise testing. However, patients with pretransplant pulmonary diffusion at rest of less than 70% of normal may experience mild arterial desaturation ($SaO_2\%$ of approximately 90%) with exercise (199). Azathioprine treatment may result in anemia in some patients, which may reduce arterial oxygen content (172).

The efficiency of ventilation during exercise is lower than normal during the first several months after transplantation (172). This is demonstrated by an elevation in the ratio of minute ventilation to carbon dioxide production (the ventilatory equivalent for carbon dioxide,

$\dot{V}E/\dot{V}CO_2$). This excess ventilation results in a heightened sensation of shortness of breath during exercise for many transplant patients.

Extraction of oxygen by body tissues, as indicated by the arterial–mixed venous oxygen difference, is normal for most transplant patients at rest. However, during exercise the arterial–mixed venous oxygen difference does not increase normally and reflects the problems of both delivery of capillary blood to the exercising skeletal muscle as well as the impairment in muscle oxidative capacity (194).

As a result of the impaired increase in both the cardiac output and arterial–mixed venous oxygen difference, during graded exercise the rate of increase in oxygen uptake ($\dot{V}O_2$ kinetics) is slower for transplant recipients than normals (200). Figure 9.9 gives oxygen uptake versus cycle ergometer power output during graded exercise for the same patient, measured 1 year before and 3 months after orthotopic cardiac transplantation. For any given submaximal power output, oxygen uptake was consistently less after transplantation, indicating slower $\dot{V}O_2$ kinetics. Peak $\dot{V}O_2$ was 18% higher for this patient after transplantation, however.

Because of the abnormalities in the cardiac output response and in the extraction and utilization of oxygen by the skeletal muscle during exercise described above, peak oxygen uptake is usually less than average for transplant patients. Typical age- and gender-adjusted average peak $\dot{V}O_2$ is 60% to 70% of normal (172, 192). Even several years after transplantation, average aerobic

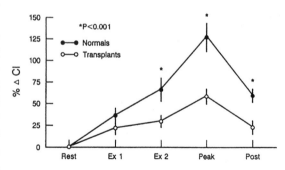

Figure 9.8. The change in cardiac index during progressive supine exercise in orthotopic cardiac transplant patients compared with healthy control subjects. (Reprinted with permission from Pflugfelder PW, Purves PD, McKenzie FN, et al: Cardiac dynamics during exercise in cyclosporine treated orthotopic heart transplant recipients: assessment by radionuclide angiography. J Am Coll Cardiol 1987;10:336–341.)

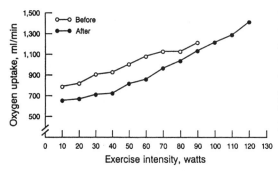

Figure 9.9. Oxygen uptake versus cycle ergometer power output in the same patient measured 1 year before and 3 months after orthotopic cardiac transplantation. (Reprinted with permission from Squires RW: Cardiac rehabilitation issues for heart transplantation patients. J Cardpulm Rehabil 1990;10:159–168.)

capacity is less than that of healthy persons (201, 202). The ventilatory anaerobic threshold is usually impaired (192). There is diversity in peak $\dot{V}O_2$ among transplant patients with some individuals exhibiting above-average cardiorespiratory fitness and some with severely impaired capacities (203, 204). Athletic performance after transplant is possible as evidenced by the return of a 20-year-old elite soccer player to competition after transplantation for treatment of idiopathic dilated cardiomyopathy. Maximal oxygen uptake for this individual was 12.9 METs (205).

In summary, cardiac transplant patients as a group have lower than normal exercise capacities but are capable of performing usual daily activities (many occupations, household tasks, school attendance, some sporting activities). Table 9.7 lists abnormal exercise physiology findings for typical cardiac transplant patients. These patients may benefit from exercise training to improve aerobic capacity, and because of their relatively low fitness, are excellent candidates for supervised cardiac rehabilitation exercise programs.

PARTIAL CARDIAC REINNERVATION

The occasional cardiac transplant patient with accelerated graft coronary artery disease and associated myocardial ischemia will report symptoms of angina pectoris, suggesting partial cardiac afferent reinnervation (206). It also appears that partial sympathetic efferent reinnervation occurs in many transplant patients during the first several months to years after surgery. The evidence for this phenomenon is based on neu-

rochemical evaluation of the heart and on the improved heart rate responsiveness to exercise observed in many patients (207, 208). The heart rate reserve measured during graded exercise testing increases during the 6 weeks after transplantation in most patients. In a subset of patients, there is a further improvement in the heart rate reserve over the next 6 to 12 months. In addition, a faster return of heart rate to baseline after exercise testing, 1 to 2 years after transplantation, has been described.

RESULTS AND BENEFITS OF EXERCISE TRAINING

Cardiac transplant patients are similar to the typical patient after cardiothoracic surgery in that they present the clinical problem of deconditioning and a low physical work capacity. However, the fact that these patients have all suffered from chronic heart failure with the associated pathophysiologic problems before transplantation, coupled with their denervated cardiac status and requirement for immunosuppressants postoperatively, makes them interesting and unusual.

Transplant recipients may be more anxious than other cardiac surgery patients and may have

Table 9.7. Abnormal Exercise Physiology Findings in Cardiac Transplant Patients

Increased resting heart rate
Delayed heart rate increase at onset of exercise
Blunted maximal heart rate
Delayed return of heart rate to resting level after cessation of exercise
Reduced heart rate reserve
Increased exercise left ventricular end-diastolic pressure (diastolic dysfunction)
Increased exercise pulmonary artery pressure, PCWP, right atrial pressure
Increased left ventricular end-systolic and end-diastolic volume indices
Impaired stroke volume increase during exercise
Reduced exercise cardiac output
Decreased exercise arterial–mixed venous oxygen difference
Slower oxygen uptake kinetics during exercise
Decreased maximal oxygen uptake
Reduced maximal power output during exercise testing
Decreased ventilatory anaerobic threshold
Increased ventilatory equivalents for oxygen and carbon dioxide
Potential mild arterial desaturation during exercise

PCWP, pulmonary capillary wedge pressure.

more difficulty in achieving preillness competencies (209). Exercise training may improve psychological function and restore confidence in returning to a more traditional lifestyle. Structured cardiac rehabilitation programs may assist patients in preparing for return to work, school, or other activities.

Several investigations have demonstrated that cardiac transplant patients respond favorably to an aerobic exercise program. The first study was by Squires and colleagues and was published in 1983 (210). These authors presented two case reports of orthotopic cardiac transplant recipients who participated in 7 to 8 weeks of standard cardiac rehabilitation outpatient exercise that began approximately 6 weeks after surgery (1 week after hospital dismissal). The two patients exercised for up to 30 minutes at Borg perceived exertion scale ratings of 12 or 13 ("somewhat hard") using a combination of treadmill walking and cycle ergometry on a three-session-per-week basis. Unlimited unsupervised ambulation was recommended for days of the week that did not include supervised exercise sessions. The patients tolerated the exercise training well, and during graded exercise testing ratings of perceived exertion and systolic blood pressure were consistently lower for all submaximal exercise intensities after training.

A landmark study of exercise training for patients after orthotopic cardiac transplantation was performed by Kavanagh and associates (211). Thiry-six male transplant recipients, average age 47 years, completed a 1.5-year walk/jog exercise training program that began approximately 7 months after surgery. None of the patients took β-blockers or corticosteroids. Compared with age-matched healthy control subjects, pretraining mean maximal oxygen uptake and ventilatory anaerobic threshold were 35% and 42% lower, respectively, in the transplant group. Transplant patients' mean lean body mass was 6 kg less than that of the healthy subjects.

The exercise program consisted of five sessions per week, and included 45 minutes of walking or jogging at an intensity of approximately 65% to 70% of maximal oxygen uptake, as prescribed by Borg perceived exertion scale scores of 14 ("somewhat hard"). During the course of the study, lean body mass increased by an average of 2.4 kg. Training lowered mean resting values for heart rate (-4 beats per minute), systolic blood pressure (-13 mm Hg), and diastolic blood pressure (-9 mm Hg).

After training, maximal oxygen uptake increased by an average of 27% ($+4$ mL· kg^{-1}· min^{-1}), and maximal power output on the cycle ergometer during graded exercise testing increased 33% ($+49$ W). The ventilatory anaerobic threshold improved from 1.18 L/min to 1.50 L/min on average. Minute ventilation and heart rate at maximal exercise were greater after training ($+20$ L/min and $+13$ beats per minute, respectively). For eight extremely motivated patients who performed an average of 32 km/wk of walk/jog, compared with 24 km/wk for the entire group, a greater increase in maximal oxygen uptake was observed ($+11$ mL·kg^{-1} · min^{-1}). No serious complications occurred during the exercise sessions or the graded exercise tests.

A randomized trial of exercise training after cardiac transplantation was performed by Kobashigawa and colleagues (212). Eleven patients participated in approximately 20 supervised treadmill-walking exercise sessions. Control subjects performed unsupervised walking exercise at home. The patients in the supervised cardiac rehabilitation program demonstrated significantly better improvement, compared with controls, in peak oxygen uptake ($+6.4$ versus $+2.6$ mL·kg^{-1}·min^{-1}), peak exercise test workload ($+40$ versus $+12$ W), and in ventilatory efficiency as measured by a reduction in the ventilatory equivalent for carbon dioxide (-14 versus -5).

Other investigations of exercise training in patients after orthotopic cardiac transplantation have reported improvements of 17% to 50% in peak exercise oxygen uptake, small increases in maximal heart rate, decreases in submaximal exercise blood pressure, and reductions in minute ventilation for a given oxygen uptake (213–215).

Two investigations have evaluated the effects of exercise training on patients with heterotopic cardiac transplants (216, 217). Peak cycle ergometer power output and peak oxygen uptake increased by 26% and 23%, respectively, with training. Compared with orthotopic transplant patients, heterotopic recipients apparently have more medical complications, such as acute rejection, gout, arthritis, and respiratory infections, which make exercise training more difficult for this population.

Both supervised exercise programs (traditional cardiac rehabilitation exercise programs) and at-home patient-directed programs have been demonstrated to improve aerobic capacity in transplant patients. However, more structured, supervised programs generally result in greater improvements in fitness than less supervised approaches (212).

Daida and associates (218) made an important observation regarding similarities and differences in the response to exercise training between patients who have undergone orthotopic cardiac transplant or CABG surgery. They studied 17 transplant patients and a similar number of age- and gender-matched CABG surgery patients for 1 year of cardiac rehabilitation. All of the patients enrolled in an outpatient cardiac rehabilitation exercise program. The first 2 to 3 months of the program were supervised in the cardiac rehabilitation exercise center. All patients were then provided a home exercise prescription. Exercise testing was performed at the completion of the supervised portion of the program and repeated at 1 year after surgery. At the completion of the supervised training, average peak exercise oxygen uptake was similar for the transplant and CABG surgery patients (20 versus 22 mL·kg^{-1}·min^{-1}). However, between the end of the supervised exercise program and 1 year after surgery, the CABG patients experienced a substantial further in-

crease in peak oxygen uptake (27 mL·kg^{-1}·min^{-1}) compared with only a modest further increase for the transplant patients (21 mL·kg^{-1}·min^{-1}). Transplant patients do not apparently respond to traditional long-term exercise training as well as do patients after CABG surgery. Novel approaches to training in transplant patients, such as higher volume training, interval high-intensity training, or skeletal muscle strengthening, need further evaluation in these unique patients.

Most cardiac transplant patients require prednisone for immunosuppression, which usually results in skeletal muscle atrophy and weakness. Resistance exercise training improves skeletal muscle strength and partially reverses corticosteroid-related myopathy. Horber and associates (219) found a 20% lower midthigh muscle area, a 36% higher midthigh fat-to-muscle ratio, and a 20% lower peak torque and total work output during isokinetic strength testing in a group of renal transplant patients taking prednisone, compared with normal controls. Fifty days of isokinetic strength training increased the muscle size at midthigh, decreased the fat-to-muscle ratio, and normalized the mean torque and total work output during strength testing. In addition, strength training has been shown to improve bone mineral density and reduce the potential development of steroid-related osteoporosis in transplant recipients (220). Resistance exercise should become a component of the exercise prescription for these patients. Table 9.8 summarizes the potential benefits of exercise training for patients after cardiac transplantation. No data exist to suggest that exercise training alters the typical clinical picture of acute rejection, susceptibility to infection, accelerated graft coronary artery disease, or mortality.

Table 9.8.   Benefits of Exercise Training for Cardiac Transplant Recipients

Increased maximal oxygen uptake
Improved submaximal exercise endurance
Increased peak cycle power output or peak treadmill exercise workload
Increased maximal heart rate
Decreased submaximal exercise heart rate
Increased ventilatory anaerobic threshold
Increased maximal minute ventilation
Decreased submaximal exercise minute ventilation
Reduced exercise ventilatory equivalents
Improved symptoms of dyspnea and fatigue
Reduced rest and submaximal exercise systolic and diastolic blood pressure
Decreased peak exercise diastolic blood pressure
Reduced submaximal exercise perceived exertion
Improved psychosocial function
Increased lean body mass
Increased skeletal muscle strength
Improved bone mineral content
Reduced body fat stores

CARDIAC REHABILITATION INTERVENTIONS FOR CARDIAC TRANSPLANT PATIENTS

Patient/Family Education

Specific topics for transplant patient and family education include the following:

Medications—actions/purposes of the various drugs, potential side-effects, and importance of strict compliance with recommended dosing and schedule for taking medications.

Risk of acute rejection, infection, accelerated graft coronary artery disease, symptom recognition, and appropriate response.

Postoperative management schedule—appointments, biopsies, blood tests, and other periodic tests.

Low fat/cholesterol/sodium diet—prevent body fat gain associated with corticosteroid use and reduce blood pressure and blood lipids.

Importance of regular exercise in promoting functional capacity and feeling of well-being, and counseling regarding return to work, school, avocational activities, and sexual activity.

Psychosocial Intervention

As discussed previously, most patients and loved ones experience a degree of difficulty in making the adjustment to posttransplant living. Patients, in general, will need to rebuild family relationships and reestablish friendships and business and professional contacts. Cardiac rehabilitation professionals can provide ongoing emotional support and encouragement. Group discussion or support sessions including patients, families or significant others, and group leaders are particularly helpful in assisting patients and their loved ones in developing coping skills, stress management techniques, and the practical skills to deal with the multiple issues involved in posttransplant management.

An occasional patient may experience severe anxiety or other symptoms of emotional distress. Cardiac rehabilitation professionals can assist the transplant team or primary physician in identification of patients who may require referral to a psychiatrist.

Traditional Coronary Risk Factor Management

The relationship between classic coronary risk factors, such as cigarette smoking, dyslipidemia, hypertension, and a sedentary lifestyle, and accelerated graft coronary artery disease or longevity in cardiac transplant patients is not well established. However, most transplant programs strongly encourage optimal control of all modifiable coronary risk factors. In particular, transplant patients should receive all the necessary help required to stop all tobacco use, should they resume the habit after surgery.

As discussed previously, the use of statin medications after transplantation has been demonstrated to reduce the incidence of acute rejection and graft vasculopathy and to improve 1-year survival. Whether these beneficial effects are related to the lipid-lowering capability or some other attribute of these drugs is not clear. However, a goal for low-density lipoprotein cholesterol of less than 100 mg/dL (2.59 mmol/L) is common among various transplant programs. Control of blood pressure is also a major concern, given the high prevalence of hypertension after transplantation. The combination of a prudent diet and regular physical activity are critical for the maintenance of an acceptable body weight.

Exercise Training

Specific suggestions for exercise programming for cardiac transplantation patients are presented in chapter 8.

References

1. American Heart Association. 1997 Heart and stroke statistical update. Dallas, TX: American Heart Association, 1997.
2. McDonagh TA, Morrison CE, Lawrence A, et al. Symptomatic and asymptomatic left-ventricular systolic dysfunction in an urban population. Lancet 1997;350: 829–833.
3. Feldman AM, Bristow MR, Parmley WW, et al. Effects of vesnarinone on morbidity and mortality in patients with heart failure. N Engl J Med 1993;329:149–155.
4. Massie BM, Berk MR, Brozena SC, et al. Can further benefit be achieved by adding flosequinan to patients with congestive heart failure who remain symptomatic on diuretic, digoxin, and an angiotensin converting enzyme inhibitor? Results of the flosequinan-ACE inhibitor trial (FACET). Circulation 1993;88:492–501.
5. Cowley AJ, McEntegart DJ, Hampton JR, et al. Long-term evaluation of treatment for chronic heart failure: a 1 year comparative trial of flosequinan and captopril. Cardiovasc Drug Ther 1994;8:829–836.
6. Eichhorn EJ, Bristow MR. Practical guidelines for initiation of beta-adrenergic blockade in patients with chronic heart failure. Am J Cardiol 1997;79:794–798.
7. Bristow MR, O'Connell JB, Gilbert EM, et al. Dose-response of chronic beta-blocker treatment in heart failure from either idiopathic dilated or ischemic cardiomyopathy. Bucindolol Investigators. Circulation 1994;89:1632–1642.
8. Packer M, Bristow MR, Cohn JN, et al. The effect of carvedilol on morbidity and mortality in patients with chronic heart failure. U.S. Carvedilol Heart Failure Study Group. N Engl J Med 1996;334:1349–1355.
9. Young JB. Carvedilol for heart failure: renewed interest in beta blockers. Cleve Clin J Med 1997;64:415–422.
10. Waagstein F, Bristow MR, Wedberg K, et al. Beneficial

effects of metoprolol in idiopathic dilated cardiomyopathy. Lancet 1993;342:1441–1446.

11. Anderson JL, Gilbert EM, O'Connell JB, et al. Long-term (2 year) beneficial effects of (β-adrenergic blockade with bucindolol in patients with idiopathic dilated cardiomyopathy. J Am Coll Cardiol 1991;17:1373–1381.

12. Fothergill JM. The heart and its diseases: with their treatment. London: HK Lewis, 1872:205.

13. Burch GE, Ansari AU. Bed rest, diet, nursing and environment. Am Heart J 1969;77:1–4.

14. Burch GE, Giles TD. Prolonged bed rest in the management of patients with cardiomyopathy. Cardiovasc Clin 1972;4:375–387.

15. Anonymous. On bedresting in heart failure. Lancet 1990;336:975–976.

16. Convertino VA, Goldwater DJ, Sandler H. Bedrest-induced peak $\dot{V}O_2$ reduction associated with age, gender, and aerobic capacity. Aviat Space Environ Med 1986;57:17–22.

17. Saltin B, Blomqvist G, Mitchell JH, et al. Response to exercise after bed rest and after training: a longitudinal study of adaptive changes in oxygen transport and body composition. Circulation 1968;38(Suppl 5):VII1–VII78.

18. Kavanaugh T, Shephard RJ, Pandit V. Marathon running after myocardial infarction. JAMA 1974;229:1602–1605.

19. Maskin CS, Reedy HK, Gulanick M, et al. Exercise training in chronic heart failure: improvement in cardiac performance and maximum oxygen uptake [abstract]. Circulation 1986;74:II-310.

20. Sullivan MJ, Higginbotham MB, Cobb FR. Exercise training in patients with severe left ventricular dysfunction. Hemodynamic and metabolic effects. Circulation 1988;78:506–515.

21. Balady G, Fletcher B, Froelicher E, et al. Cardiac rehabilitation programs. A statement for healthcare professionals from the American Heart Association. Circulation 1994;90:1602–1610.

22. Konstam MA, Dracup K, Baker DW, et al. Heart failure: evaluation and care of patients with left-ventricular systolic dysfunction. Clinical Practice Guideline No. 11. Rockville, MD: US Department of Health and Human Services, Public Health Service, Agency for Health Care Policy and Research. AHCPR Publication #94–0612, June 1994.

23. Wenger NK, Froelicher ES, Smith LK, et al. Cardiac rehabilitation as secondary prevention. Clinical Practice Guideline No. 17. Rockville, MD: US Department of Health and Human Services, Public Health Service, Agency for Health Care Policy and Research and the National Heart, Lung, and Blood Institute. AHCPR Publication #96–0673, October 1995.

24. Weber KT, Wilson JR, Janicki JS, et al. Exercise testing in the evaluation of patients with chronic cardiac failure. Am Rev Respir Dis 1984;129:S60–S62.

25. Wilson JR, Martin JL, Schwartz D, et al. Exercise intolerance in patients with chronic heart failure: role of impaired nutritive flow to skeletal muscle. Circulation 1984;69:1079–1087.

26. Mancini DM. Pulmonary factors limiting exercise capacity in patients with heart failure. Prog Cardiovasc Dis 1995;37:347–370.

27. Lipkin DB, Canepa-Anson R, Stephens MR, et al. Factors determining symptoms in heart failure: comparison of fast and slow exercise tests. Br Heart J 1986;55:439–445.

28. Clark AL, Poole-Wilson PA, Coats AJS. Exercise limitation in chronic heart failure: central role of the periphery. J Am Coll Cardiol 1996;28:1092–1102.

29. Zelis R, Sinoway LI, Musch TI. Why do patients with congestive heart failure stop exercising? J Am Coll Cardiol 1988;12:359–361.

30. Feild BJ, Baxley WA, Russell RO Jr, et al. Left ventricular function and hypertrophy in cardiomyopathy with depressed ejection fraction. Circulation 1973;47:1022–1031.

31. McKay RG, Pfeffer MA, Pasternak RC, et al. Left ventricular remodeling after myocardial infarction: a corollary to infarct expansion. Circulation 1986;74:693–702.

32. Meyer M, Schillinger W, Pieske B, et al. Alterations of sarcoplasmic reticulum proteins in failing human dilated cardiomyopathy. Circulation 1995;92:778–784.

33. Vatner DE, Sato N, Kiuchi K, et al. Decrease in myocardial ryanodine receptors and altered excitation-contraction coupling early in the development of heart failure. Circulation 1994;90:1423–1430.

34. Feldman MD, Copelas L, Gwathmey JK, et al. Deficient production of cyclic AMP: pharmacologic evidence of an important cause of contractile dysfunction in patients with end-stage heart failure. Circulation 1987;75:331–339.

35. Bristow MR, Ginsburg R, Minobe W, et al. Decreased catecholamine sensitivity and beta-adrenergic-receptor density in failing human hearts. N Engl J Med 1982;307:205–211.

36. Franciosa JA, Park M, Levine TB. Lack of correlation between exercise capacity and indexes of resting left ventricular performance in heart failure. Am J Cardiol 1981;47:33–38.

37. Higginbotham MB, Morris KG, Conn EH, et al. Determinants of variable exercise performance among patients with severe left ventricular dysfunction. Am J Cardiol 1983;51:52–60.

38. Benge W, Lichfield RL, Marcus ML. Exercise capacity in patients with severe left ventricular dysfunction. Circulation 1980;61:955–959.

39. Bocchi EA, Bacal F, Auler JOC, et al. Inhaled nitric oxide leading to pulmonary edema in stable severe heart failure. Am J Cardiol 1994;74:70–72.

40. Fink LI, Wilson JR, Ferraro N. Exercise ventilation and pulmonary artery wedge pressure in chronic stable congestive heart failure. Am J Cardiol 1986;57:249–253.

41. Szlachcic J, Massie BM, Kramer BL, et al. Correlates and prognostic implication of exercise capacity in congestive heart failure. Am J Cardiol 1985;55:1037–1042.

42. Wilson JR, Rayos G, Yeoh T, et al. Dissociation between peak exercise oxygen consumption and hemodynamic dysfunction in potential heart transplant candidates. J Am Coll Cardiol 1995;26:429–435.

43. Wilson JR, Rayos G, Yeoh TK, et al. Dissociation between exertional symptoms and circulatory function in patients with heart failure. Circulation 1995;92:47–53.

44. Liang C, Stewart DK, LeJemtel TH, et al. Characteris-

tics of peak aerobic capacity in symptomatic and asymptomatic subjects with left ventricular dysfunction. Am J Cardiol 1992;69:1207–1211.

45. Chomsky DB, Lang CC, Rayos G, et al. Treatment of subclinical fluid retention in patients with symptomatic heart failure: effect on exercise performance. J Heart Lung Transplant 1997;16:846–853.

46. Wilson JR, Martin JL, Ferraro N, et al. Effect of hydralazine on perfusion and metabolism in the leg during upright bicycle exercise in patients with heart failure. Circulation 1983;68:425–432.

47. Cohn JN. Current therapy of the failing heart. Circulation 1988;78:1099–1107.

48. Sullivan MJ, Knight JD, Higginbotham MB, et al. Relation between central and peripheral hemodynamics during exercise in patients with chronic heart failure. Circulation 1989;80:769–781.

49. Wilson JR, Mancini DM. Factors contributing to the exercise limitation of heart failure. J Am Coll Cardiol 1993;22(Suppl A):93A–98A.

50. Sullivan MJ, Higginbotham MB, Cobb FR. Increased exercise ventilation in patients with chronic heart failure: intact ventilatory control despite hemodynamic and pulmonary abnormalities. Circulation 1988;77:552–559.

51. Davies SW, Emery TM, Watling MI, et al. A critical threshold of exercise capacity in the ventilatory response to exercise in heart failure. Br Heart J 1991;65:179–183.

52. Chua TP, Ponikowski P, Harrington D, et al. Clinical correlates and prognostic significance of the ventilatory response to exercise in chronic heart failure. J Am Coll Cardiol 1997;29:1585–1590.

53. Lucas C, Johnson W, Hartley LH, et al. Excessive ventilation evident during low-level exertion in heart failure [abstract]. Circulation 1996;94:I-192.

54. Metra M, Raddino R, Dei Cas L, et al. Assessment of peak oxygen consumption, lactate and ventilatory threshold and correlation with the resting and exercise hemodynamic data in chronic congestive heart failure. Am J Cardiol 1990;65:1127–1133.

55. Al-Rawas OA, Carter R, Richens D. Ventilatory and gas exchange abnormalities on exercise in chronic heart failure. Eur Respir J 1995;8:2022–2028.

56. Davies SW, Emery TM, Watling MI, et al. A critical threshold of exercise capacity in the ventilatory response to exercise in heart failure. Br Heart J 1991;65:179–183.

57. Buller NP, Poole-Wilson PA. Mechanism of the increased ventilatory response to exercise in patients with chronic heart failure. Br Heart J 1990;63:281–283.

58. Chua TP, Clark AL, Amadi AA, et al. Relation between chemosensitivity and the ventilatory response to exercise in chronic heart failure. J Am Coll Cardiol 1996;27:650–657.

59. Hammond MD, Bauer KA, Sharp JT, et al. Respiratory muscle strength in congestive heart failure. Chest 1990;98:1091–1094.

60. McParland C, Krishnan B, Wang Y, et al. Inspiratory muscle weakness and dyspnea in heart failure. Am Rev Respir Dis 1992;146:467–472.

61. Mancini DM, Henson D, LaManca J, et al. Respiratory muscle function and dyspnea in patients with chronic congestive heart failure. Circulation 1992;86:909–918.

62. Lindsay D, Lovegrove C, Dunn M, et al. Histological abnormalities of diaphragmatic muscle may contribute to dyspnoea in heart failure [abstract]. Circulation 1992;86:I-515.

63. Tikunov B, Levine S, Mancini D. Chronic congestive heart failure elicits adaptations of endurance exercise in diaphragmatic muscle. Circulation 1997;95:910–916.

64. Wasserman K. Dyspnea on exertion: is it the heart or the lungs? JAMA 1982;248:2039–2043.

65. Franciosa JA, Leddy CL, Wilen M, et al. Relation between hemodynamic and ventilatory responses in determining exercise capacity in severe congestive heart failure. Am J Cardiol 1984;53:127–134.

66. McCloskey DI, Mitchell JH. Reflex cardiovascular and respiratory responses originating in exercising muscle. J Physiol (Lond) 1972;224:173–187.

67. Rowell LB. The nature of the exercise stimulus. Acta Physiol Scand 1986;556:7–14.

68. Brunier M, Brunner HR. Neurohormonal consequences of diuretics in different cardiovascular syndromes. Eur Heart J 1992;13(Suppl G):28–33.

69. Kaye DM, Lefkovits J, Gennings GL, et al. Adverse consequences of high sympathetic nervous activity in the failing human heart. J Am Coll Cardiol 1995;26:1257–1263.

70. Kirlin PC, Grekin R, Das S, et al. Neurohumoral activation during exercise in congestive heart failure. Am J Med 1986;81:623–629.

71. Bayliss J, Norell M, Canepa-Anson R, et al. Neuroendocrine and hemodynamic interactions at rest and during exercise in chronic heart failure: double-blind comparison of captopril and prazosin [abstract]. Circulation 1984;70:II-1673.

72. Chidsey CA, Harrison DC, Braunwald E. Augmentation of the plasma norepinephrine response to exercise in patients with congestive heart failure. N Engl J Med 1962;267:650–654.

73. Francis GS, Goldsmith SR, Ziesche SM, et al. Response of plasma norepinephrine and epinephrine to dynamic exercise in patients with congestive heart failure. Am J Cardiol 1982;49:1152–1156.

74. Matsumoto A, Hirata Y, Momomura S, et al. Effects of exercise on plasma level of brain natriuretic peptide in congestive heart failure with and without left ventricular dysfunction. Am Heart J 1995;129:139–145.

75. Steele IC, McDowell G, Moore A, et al. Responses of atrial natriuretic peptide and brain natriuretic peptide to exercise in patients with chronic heart failure and normal control subjects. Eur J Clin Invest 1997;27:270–276.

76. deGroote P, Millaire A, Pigny P, et al. Plasma levels of atrial natriuretic peptide at peak exercise: a prognostic marker of cardiovascular-related death and heart transplantation in patients with moderate congestive heart failure. J Heart Lung Transplant 1997;16:956–963.

77. Mancini DM, Davis L, Wexler JP, et al. Dependence of enhanced maximal exercise performance on increased peak skeletal muscle perfusion during long-term captopril therapy in heart failure. J Am Coll Cardiol 1987;10:845–850.

78. Anonymous. Comparative effects of therapy with captopril and digoxin in patients with mild to moderate heart failure. The Captopril-Digoxin Multicenter Research Group. JAMA 1988;259:539–544.

79. Olsen SL, Gilbert EM, Renlund DG, et al. Carvedilol improves left ventricular function and symptoms in chronic heart failure: a double-blind randomized study. J Am Coll Cardiol 1995;25:1225–1231.

80. Anonymous. Randomized, placebo-controlled trial of carvedilol in patients with congestive heart failure due to ischaemic heart disease. Australia/New Zealand Heart Failure Research Collaborative Group. Lancet 1997;349:375–380.

81. Packer M, Colucci WS, Sackner-Bernstein JD, et al. Double-blind, placebo-controlled study of the effects of carvedilol in patients with moderate to severe heart failure. The PRECISE Trial. Prospective Randomized Evaluation of Carvedilol on Symptoms and Exercise. Circulation 1996;94:2793–2799.

82. Colucci WS, Packer M, Bristow MR, et al. Carvedilol inhibits clinical progression in patients with mild symptoms of heart failure. US Carvedilol Heart Failure Study Group. Circulation 1996;94:2800–2806.

83. Meyer TE, Casadei B, Coats AJ, et al. Angiotensin-converting enzyme inhibition and physical training in heart failure. J Intern Med 1991;230:407–413.

84. Nakamura M, Ishikawa M, Funakoshi T, et al. Attenuated endothelium-dependent peripheral vasodilation and clinical characteristics in patients with chronic heart failure. Am Heart J 1994;128:1164–1169.

85. McMurray JM, Ray SG, Abdullah I, et al. Plasma endothelin levels in chronic heart failure. Circulation 1992;85:1374–1379.

86. Gilligan DM, Panza JA, Kilcoyne CM, et al. Contribution of endothelium-derived nitric oxide to exercise-induced vasodilation. Circulation 1994;90:2853–2858.

87. Elis R, Claim SF. Alterations in vasomotor tone in congestive heart failure. Prog Cardiovasc Dis 1982;24:437–459.

88. Zelis R, Mason DT. Diminished forearm arteriolar dilator capacity produced by mineralocorticoid-induced salt retention in man. Circulation 1970;41:589–592.

89. Wilson JR, Chomsky DB. Skeletal muscle and the role of exercise training in chronic heart failure. In: Balady GJ, Piña IL, eds. Exercise and heart failure. Armonk, NY: Futura, 1997:277–284.

90. Massie BM, Simonini A, Sahgal P, et al. Relation of systemic and local muscle exercise capacity to skeletal muscle characteristics in men with congestive heart failure. J Am Coll Cardiol 1996;27:140–145.

91. Weber K, Kinasewitz G, Janicki J, et al. Oxygen utilization and ventilation during exercise in patients with chronic heart failure. Circulation 1982;65:1213–1223.

92. Wilson JR, Martin JL, Ferraro N. Impaired skeletal muscle nutritive flow during exercise in patients with heart failure: role of cardiac pump dysfunction as determined by effect of dobutamine. Am J Cardiol 1984;54:1308–1315.

93. Wilson JR, Ferraro N. Effect of the renin-angiotensin system on limb circulation and metabolism during exercise in heart failure. J Am Coll Cardiol 1985;6:556–563.

94. Wilson JR, Martin JL, Ferraro N, et al. Effect of hydralazine on perfusion and metabolism in the leg during upright bicycle exercise in patients with heart failure. Circulation 1983;68:425–432.

95. Maskin CS, Kugler J, Sonnenblick EH, et al. Acute inotropic stimulation with dopamine in severe congestive heart failure: beneficial hemodynamic effect at rest but not during maximal exercise. Am J Cardiol 1983;52:1028–1032.

96. Massie BM, Kramer BL, Haughom F. Acute and long-term effects of vasodilators on rest and exercise hemodynamics and on exercise capacity. Circulation 1981;64:1218–1226.

97. Mancini DM, Walter G, Reichek N, et al. Contribution of skeletal muscle atrophy to exercise intolerance and altered muscle metabolism in heart failure. Circulation 1992;85:1364–1373.

98. Volterrani M, Clark AL, Ludman PF, et al. Determinants of exercise capacity in chronic heart failure. Eur Heart J 1994;15:801–809.

99. Swan JW, Walton C, Godsland IF, et al. Insulin resistance in chronic heart failure. Eur Heart J 1994;15:1528–1532.

100. Minotti JR, Pillay P, Oka R, et al. Skeletal muscle size: relationship to muscle function in heart failure. J Appl Physiol 1993;75:373–381.

101. Drexler H, Riede U, Munzel T, et al. Alterations of skeletal muscle in chronic heart failure. Circulation 1992;85:1751–1759.

102. Sullivan MJ, Green HJ, Cobb FR. Skeletal muscle biochemistry and histology in ambulatory patients with long-term heart failure. Circulation 1990;81:518–527.

103. Ralston MA, Merola AJ, Leier CV. Depressed aerobic enzyme activity of skeletal muscle in sever chronic congestive heart failure. J Lab Clin Med 1991;117:370–372.

104. Clark AL, Piepoli M, Coats AJ. Skeletal muscle and the control of ventilation on exercise: evidence for metabolic receptors. Eur J Clin Invest 1995;25:299–305.

105. Hall-Angeras M, Angeras U, Zamir O, et al. Interaction between corticosterone and tumor necrosis factor stimulated protein breakdown in rat skeletal muscle, similar to sepsis. Surgery 1990;108:460–466.

106. Goodman JC, Roberson CS, Grossman RG, et al. Elevation of tumor necrosis factor in head injury. J Neuroimmunol 1990;30:213–217.

107. Tracey KJ, Morgello S, Koplin B, et al. Metabolic effects of cachectin/tumor necrosis factor are modified by site of production. Cachectin/tumor necrosis factor-secreting tumor in skeletal muscle induces chronic cachexia, while implantation in brain induced predominantly acute anorexia. J Clin Invest 1990;86:2014–2024.

108. Espat NJ, Copeland EM, Moldawer LL. Tumor necrosis factor and cachexia: a current perspective. Surg Oncol 1994;3:255–262.

109. Chevalier L, Lacoste C, Douard H, et al. Rééducation segmentaire chex les insuffisants cardiaques: résultats à court terme. Arch Mal Couer 1996;89:819–824.

110. Cohn JN, Rector T, Olivari MT, et al. Plasma norepinephrine, ejection fraction and maximal oxygen consumption as prognostic variables in congestive heart failure [abstract]. Circulation 1985;72:III-285.

111. Likoff MJ, Chandler SL, Kay HR. Clinical determinants of mortality in chronic congestive heart failure secondary to idiopathic dilated or to ischemic cardiomyopathy. Am J Cardiol 1987;59:634–638.

112. Coats AJS, Adamopoulos S, Radaelli A, et al. Controlled trial of physical training in chronic heart failure. Exercise performance, hemodynamics, ventilation, and autonomic function. Circulation 1992;85:2119–2131.

113. Sullivan MJ, Cobb FR. The anaerobic threshold in chronic heart failure. Relation to blood lactate, ventilatory basis, reproducibility, and response to exercise training. Circulation 1990;81(Suppl 1): 1147–1158.

114. Dubach P, Myers J, Dziekan G, et al. Effect of high intensity exercise training on central hemodynamic responses to exercise in men with reduced left ventricular function. J Am Coll Cardiol 1997;29:1591–1598.

115. Giannuzzi P, Temporelli PL, Corra U, et al. Attenuation of unfavorable remodeling by exercise training in postinfarction patients with left ventricular dysfunction. Circulation 1997;96:1790–1797.

116. Coats AJ, Adamopoulos S, Meyer TE, et al. Effects of physical training in chronic heart failure. Lancet 1990;335:63–66.

117. Oh BH, Ono S, Gilpin E, et al. Altered left ventricular remodeling with beta-adrenergic blockade and exercise after coronary reperfusion in rats. Circulation 1993;87:608–616.

118. Gaudron P, Hu K, Schamberger R, et al. Effect of endurance training early or late after coronary artery occlusion on left ventricular remodeling, hemodynamics, and survival in rats with chronic transmural myocardial infarction. Circulation 1994;89:402–412.

119. Jugdutt BI, Michororski BL, Kappagoda CT. Exercise training after anterior Q wave myocardial infarction: importance of regional left ventricular function and topography. J Am Coll Cardiol 1988;12:362–372.

120. Dubach P, Myers J, Dzickan G, et al. Effect of exercise training on myocardial remodeling in patients with reduced left ventricular function after myocardial infarction. Circulation 1997;95:2060–2067.

121. Sullivan MJ, Higginbotham MB, Cobb FR. Exercise training in patients with severe left ventricular dysfunction. Hemodynamic and metabolic effects. Circulation 1988;78:506–515.

122. Tomita T, Murakami T, Iwase T, et al. Chronic dynamic exercise improves functional abnormality of the G stimulatory protein in cardiomyopathic BIO 53.58 Syrian hamsters. Circulation 1994;89:836–845.

123. Kiilavuori K, Sovijarvi A, Naveri H, et al. Effect of physical training on exercise capacity and gas exchange in patients with chronic heart failure. Chest 1996;110: 985–991.

124. Davey P, Meyer T, Coats A, et al. Ventilation in chronic heart failure: effects of physical training. Br Heart J 1992;68:473–477.

125. Sullivan M, Higginbotham M, Cobb F. Exercise training in patients with chronic heart failure delays ventilatory anaerobic threshold and improves submaximal exercise performance. Circulation 1989;79:324–329.

126. Clark AL, Skypala I, Coats AJ. Ventilatory efficiency is unchanged after physical training in healthy persons despite an increase exercise tolerance. J Cardiovasc Risk 1994;1:347–351.

127. Mancini D, Donchez L, Levine S. Acute unloading of the work of breathing extends exercise duration in patients with heart failure. J Am Coll Cardiol 1997;29: 590–596.

128. McGowan GA, Murali S, Loftus S, et al. Comparison of metabolic, ventilatory and neurohumoral responses during light forearm isometric exercise and isotonic exercise in congestive heart failure. Am J Cardiol 1996;77:391–396.

129. Radaelli A, Coats AJ, Leuzzi S, et al. Physical training enhances sympathetic and parasympathetic control of heart rate and peripheral vessels in chronic heart failure. Clin Sci 1996;91:92–94.

130. Kiilavuori K, Toivonen L, Naveri H, et al. Reversal of autonomic derangements by physical training in chronic heart failure assessed by heart rate variability. Eur Heart J 1995;16:490–495.

131. Cohn JN, Levine TB, Olivari MT, et al. Plasma norepinephrine as a guide to prognosis in patients with chronic congestive heart failure. N Engl J Med 1984; 311:819–823.

132. Kleiger RE, Miller PJ, Bigger TJ, et al. Decreased heart rate variability and its association with increased mortality after acute myocardial infarction. Am J Cardiol 1987;59:256–262.

133. Blomqvist CG, Saltin B. Cardiovascular adaptations to physical training. Annu Rev Physiol 1983;45:169–189.

134. Braith RW, Feigenbaum MS, Welsch MA, et al. Neuroendocrine hyperactivity in heart failure is buffered by endurance exercise [abstract]. Circulation 1996;94: I-192.

135. Levine B, Kalman J, Mayer L, et al. Elevated circulating levels of tumor necrosis factor in severe chronic heart failure. N Engl J Med 1990;323:236–241.

136. Maskin CS, Reddy HK, Gulanick M, et al. Exercise training in chronic heart failure: improvements in cardiac performance and maximum oxygen uptake [abstract]. Circulation 1986;74:II-310.

137. Hornig B, Maier V, Drexler H. Physical training improves endothelial function in patients with chronic heart failure. Circulation 1996;93:210–214.

138. Yuen JL, Bijou R, Galvao M, et al. Intense forearm training improves vascular endothelium function in patients with congestive heart failure [abstract]. J Am Coll Cardiol 1993;21:316A.

139. Shen W, Hintze TH, Wolin MS. Nitric oxide. An important signaling mechanism between vascular endothelium and parenchymal cells in the regulation of oxygen consumption. Circulation 1995;92:3505–3512.

140. Hambrecht R, Niebauer J, Fiehn E, et al. Physical training in patients with stable chronic heart failure: effects on cardiorespiratory fitness and ultrastructural abnormalities of leg muscle. J Am Coll Cardiol 1995; 25:1239–1249.

141. Adamopoulos S, Coats AJ, Brunotte F, et al. Physical training in skeletal muscle metabolism in patients with chronic heart failure. J Am Coll Cardiol 1993;21: 1101–1106.

142. Kluess HA, Welsch MA, Properzio AM, et al. Accelerated skeletal muscle metabolic recovery following ex-

ercise training in heart failure [abstract]. Circulation 1996;94:I-192.

143. Hambrecht R, Fiehn E, Yu J, et al. Altered peripheral perfusion and skeletal muscle metabolic response to exercise in patients with chronic heart failure: chronic effect of endurance training [abstract]. Circulation 1996;94:I-192.

144. Stratton JR, Dunn JF, Adamopoulos S, et al. Training partially reverses skeletal muscle metabolic abnormalities during exercise in heart failure. J Appl Physiol 1994;76:1575–1582.

145. Minotti JR, Johnson EC, Hudson TL, et al. Skeletal muscle response to exercise training in congestive heart failure. J Clin Invest 1990;86:751–758.

146. Piepoli M, Clark AL, Volterrani M, et al. Contribution of muscle afferents to the hemodynamic, autonomic, and ventilatory responses to exercise in patients with chronic heart failure. Circulation 1996;93:940–952.

147. Young JB, Farmer JA. The diagnostic evaluation of patients with heart failure. In: Hosenpud JD, Greenberg BH, eds. Congestive heart failure; pathophysiology, diagnosis, and comprehensive approach to management. New York: Springer-Verlag, 1994:597–621.

148. Fletcher GF, Balady G, Froelicher VF, et al. Exercise standards. A statement for healthcare professionals from the American Heart Association. Circulation 1995;91:580–615.

149. Piña IL. Exercise testing protocols for use in heart failure. In: Balady GJ, Piña IL, eds. Exercise and heart failure. Armonk, NY: Futura, 1997:213–220.

150. American College of Sports Medicine. Guidelines for exercise testing and prescription. 5th ed. Baltimore: Williams & Wilkins, 1995.

151. Health and Public Policy Committee, American College of Physicians. Cardiac rehabilitation services. Ann Intern Med 1988;109:671–673.

152. McKelvie RS, Teo KK, McCartney N, et al. Effects of exercise training in patients with congestive heart failure: a critical review. J Am Coll Cardiol 1995;25:789–796.

153. Meyer K, Lehmann M, Sünder G, et al. Interval versus continuous exercise training after coronary bypass surgery: a comparison of training-induced acute reactions with respect to the effectiveness of the exercise methods. Clin Cardiol 1990;13:851–861.

154. Meyer K, Schwaibold M, Westbrook S, et al. Effects of physical training and activity restriction on functional capacity in patients with severe chronic heart failure. Am J Cardiol 1996;78:1017–1022.

155. Meyer K, Samek L, Schwaibold M, et al. Interval training in patients with severe chronic heart failure: analysis and recommendations for exercise procedures. Med Sci Sports Exerc 1997;29:306–312.

156. Mangieri E, Tanzilli G, Barilla F, et al. Isometric handgrip exercise increases endothelin-1 plasma levels in patients with chronic congestive heart failure. Am J Cardiol 1997;79:1261–1263.

157. Hare DL, Ryan TM, Selig SE, et al. Effects of resistance weight training in patients with chronic heart failure [abstract]. Circulation 1996;94:I-192.

158. Douard H, Thiaudiere E, Broustet JP. Value of segmental rehabilitation in patients with chronic heart failure. Heart Failure 1997;13:77–82, 96.

159. Mancini DM, Henson D, La Manca J, et al. Benefit of selective respiratory muscle training on exercise capacity in patients with chronic congestive heart failure. Circulation 1995;91:320–329.

160. Gordon A, Tynilenne R, Persson H, et al. Markedly improved skeletal muscle function with local muscle training in patients with chronic heart failure. Clin Cardiol 1996;19:568–574.

161. Magnusson G, Gordon A, Kaijser L, et al. High intensity knee extensor training, in patients with chronic heart failure: major skeletal muscle improvement. Eur Heart J 1996;17:1048–1055.

162. Meyer K, Samek L, Schwaibold M, et al. Physical responses to different modes of interval exercise in patients with chronic heart failure—application to exercise training. Eur Heart J 1996;17:1040–1047.

163. Demopoulos L, Bijous R, Fergus I, et al. Exercise training in patients with severe congestive heart failure: enhancing peak aerobic capacity while minimizing the increase in ventricular wall stress. J Am Coll Cardiol 1997;29:597–603.

164. Belardinelli R, Georgiou D, Scocco V, et al. Low intensity exercise training in patients with chronic heart failure. J Am Coll Cardiol 1995;26:975–982.

165. Physical activity and cardiovascular health. NIH Consensus Statement 1995 Dec 18–20;13:1–33.

166. Dubach P, Froelicher VF. Cardiac rehabilitation for heart failure patients. Cardiology 1989;76:368–373.

167. Giannuzi P, Tavazzi L, Temporelli PL, et al. Long-term physical training and left ventricular remodeling after anterior myocardial infarction: results of the Exercise and Anterior Myocardial Infarction (EAMI) trial. J Am Coll Cardiol 1993;22:1821–1829.

168. Arvan S. Exercise performance of the high risk acute myocardial infarction patient after cardiac rehabilitation. Am J Cardiol 1988;62:197–201.

169. Specchia G, DeServi S, Scire A, et al. Interaction between exercise training and ejection fraction in predicting prognosis after a first myocardial infarction. Circulation 1996;94:978–982.

170. Barnard CN. The operation: a human cardiac transplant: an interim report of a successful operation performed at Groote Schuur Hospital, Cape Town. S Afr Med J 1967;41:1271–1274.

171. Rodeheffer RJ, Naftel DC, Warner Stevenson L, et al. Secular trends in cardiac transplant recipient and donor management in the United States, 1990 to 1994: a multi-institutional study. Circulation 1996;94: 2883–2889.

172. Squires RW. Cardiac rehabilitation issues for heart transplantation patients. J Cardpulm Rehabil 1990;10: 159–168.

173. Perlroth MG, Reitz BA. Heart and heart-lung transplantation. In: Braunwald E, ed. Heart disease: a textbook of cardiovascular medicine. 5th ed. Philadelphia: WB Saunders, 1997; 515–533.

174. Uretsky BF. Physiology of the transplanted heart. Cardiovasc Clin 1990;20:23–56.

175. Scott JP, Higenbottam TW, Large S, et al. Cyclosporine in heart transplant recipients: an exercise study of vasopressor effects. Eur Heart J 1992;13:531–534.

176. Gao SZ, Hunt SA, Schroeder JS, et al. Early develop-

ment of accelerated graft coronary artery disease: risk factors and course. J Am Coll Cardiol 1996;28:673–679.

177. Vassalli G, Gallino A, Kiowski W, et al. Reduced coronary flow reserve during exercise in cardiac transplant recipients. Circulation 1997;95:607–613.

178. Berger PB, Jones JD, Olson LJ, et al. Increase in total plasma homocysteine concentration after cardiac transplantation. Mayo Clin Proc 1995;70:125–131.

179. Halle AA, DiSciascio G, Massin EK, et al. Coronary angioplasty, atherectomy and bypass surgery in cardiac transplant recipients. J Am Coll Cardiol 1995;26: 120–128.

180. Kobashigawa JA, Katznelson S, Laks H, et al. Effect of pravastatin on outcomes after cardiac transplantation. N Engl J Med 1995;333:621–627.

181. Kuhn WF, Davis MH, Lippmann SB. Emotional adjustment to cardiac transplantation. Gen Hosp Psychiatry 1988;10:108–113.

182. McGregor CGA. Cardiac transplantation: surgical considerations and early postoperative management. Mayo Clin Proc 1992;67:577–585.

183. Mai FM. Graft and donor denial in heart transplant recipients. Am J Psychiatry 1986;143:1159–1161.

184. Mai FM, McKenzie FN, Kostuk WJ. Psychiatric aspects of heart transplantation: preoperative evaluation and postoperative sequelae. Br Med J 1986;292:311–313.

185. Jones BM, Chang VP, Esmore D, et al. Psychological adjustment after cardiac transplantation Med J Aust 1988;149:118–122.

186. McAleer MJ, Copeland J, Fuller J, et al. Psychological aspects of heart transplantation. Heart Transplant 1985;4:232–233.

187. Jose AD, Collison D. The normal range and determinants of the intrinsic heart rate in man. Cardiovasc Res 1970;4:160–167.

188. Savin WM, Haskell WL, Schroeder JS, et al. Cardiorespiratory response of cardiac transplant patients to graded, symptom-limited exercise. Circulation 1980; 62:55–60.

189. Nixon JV, Rosenburg H, Romhilt D, et al. Response to dynamic exercise of the orthotopically transplanted human heart in men immunosuppressed with cyclosporine. Am J Cardiol 1989;64:401–403.

190. Quigg RJ, Rocco MB, Gauthier DF, et al. Mechanism of the attenuated peak heart rate response to exercise after orthotopic cardiac transplantation. J Am Coll Cardiol 1989;14:338–344.

191. Yusuf S, Mitchell A, Yacoub MH. Interrelation between donor and recipient heart rates during exercise after heterotopic cardiac transplantation. Br Heart J 1985; 54:173–178.

192. Keteyian SJ, Brawner C. Cardiac transplant. In: American College of Sports Medicine. ACSM's exercise management of persons with chronic diseases and disabilities. Champaign, IL: Human Kinetics, 1997;54–58.

193. Kobashigawa JA. The transplanted heart. In: Balady GJ, Piña IL, eds. Exercise and heart failure. Armonk, NY: Futura, 1997;97–112.

194. Kao AC, Van Trigt P, Shaeffer-McCall GS, et al. Central and peripheral limitations to upright exercise in un-trained cardiac transplant recipients. Circulation 1994;89:2605–2615.

195. Pope SE, Stinson EB, Daughters GT, et al. Exercise response of the denervated heart in long-term cardiac transplant recipients. Am J Cardiol 1980;46:213–218.

196. Stratton JR, Kemp GJ, Daly RC, et al. Effects of cardiac transplantation on bioenergetic abnormalities of skeletal muscle in congestive heart failure. Circulation 1994;89:1624–1631.

197. Lampert E, Mettauer B, Hoppeler H, et al. Structure of skeletal muscle in heart transplant recipients. J Am Coll Cardiol 1996;28:980–984.

198. Hanson P, Slane PR, Lillis DL, et al. Limited oxygen uptake post heart transplant is associated with impairment of calf vasodilatory capacity. Med Sci Sports Exerc 1995;27:S49.

199. Braith RW, Limacher MC, Mills RM, et al. Exercise-induced hypoxemia in heart transplant recipients. J Am Coll Cardiol 1993;22:768–776.

200. Paterson DH, Cunningham DA, Pickering JG, et al. Oxygen uptake kinetics in cardiac transplant recipients. J Appl Physiol 1994;77:1935–1940.

201. Kao AC, Van Trigt P, Shaeffer-McCall GS, et al. Allograft diastolic dysfunction and chronotropic incompetence limit cardiac output response to exercise two to six years after heart transplantation. J Heart Lung Transplant 1995;14:11–22.

202. Bussieres LM, Pflugfelder PW, Menkis AH, et al. Basis for aerobic impairment in patients after heart tranplantation. J Heart Lung Transplant 1995;14:1073–1080.

203. Stevenson LW, Sietsema K, Tillisch JH, et al. Exercise capacity for survivors of cardiac transplantation or sustained medical therapy for stable heart failure. Circulation 1990;81:78–85.

204. Labovitz AJ, Dimmer AM, McBride LR, et al. Exercise capacity during the first year after cardiac transplantation. Am J Cardiol 1989;64:642–645.

205. Golding LA, Mangus BC. Competing in varsity athletics after cardiac transplantation. J Cardpulm Rehabil 1989;9:486–491.

206. Kavanagh T. Physical training in heart transplant recipients. J Cardiovasc Risk 1996;3:154–159.

207. Kaye DM, Esler M, Kingwell B, et al. Functional and neurochemical evidence for partial cardiac sympathetic reinnervation after cardiac transplantation in humans. Circulation 1993;88:1110–1118.

208. Scott CD, Dark JH, McComb JM. Evolution of the chronotropic response to exercise after cardiac transplantation. Am J Cardiol 1995;76:1292–1296.

209. Christopherson LK. Cardiac transplantation: a psychological perspective. Circulation 1987;75:57–62.

210. Squires RW, Arthur PR, Gau GT, et al. Exercise after cardiac transplantation: a report of two cases. J Cardpulm Rehabil 1983;3:570–574.

211. Kavanagh T, Yacoub MH, Mertens DJ, et al. Cardiorespiratory responses to exercise training after orthotopic cardiac transplantation. Circulation 1988; 77:162–171.

212. Kobashigawa JA, Leaf DA, Gleeson JP, et al. Benefit of cardiac rehabilitation in heart transplant patients: a

randomized trial. J Heart Lung Transplant 1994;13: S77.

213. Degré S, Niset GL, Desmet JM, et al. Effets de l'entraînement physique sur le coeur humain dénervé après transplantation cardiaques orthotopique. Ann Cardiol Angeol (Paris) 1986;35:147–149.

214. Niset G, Cousty-Degre C, Degre S. Psychological and physical rehabilitation after heart transplantation: 1 year follow-up. Cardiology 1988;75:311–317.

215. Keteyian S, Shepard R, Ehrman J, et al. Cardiovascular responses of heart transplant patients to exercise training. J Appl Physiol 1991;70:2627–2631.

216. Sieurat P, Roquebrune JP, Grinneiser D, et al. Surveillance et réadaptation des transplantés cardiaques hétérotopiques à la période de convalescence. Arch Mal Coeur 1986;79:210–216.

217. Kavanagh T, Yacoub MH, Mertens DJ, et al. Exercise rehabilitation after heterotopic cardiac transplantation. J Cardpulm Rehabil 1989;9:303–310.

218. Daida H, Squires RW, Allison TG, et al. Sequential assessment of exercise tolerance in heart transplantation compared with coronary artery bypass surgery after phase II cardiac rehabilitation. Am J Cardiol 1996; 77:696–700.

219. Horber FF, Scheidegger JR, Grunig BF, et al. Evidence that prednisone-induced myopathy is reversed by physical training. J Clin Endocrinol Metab 1985;61: 83–88.

220. Braith RW, Mills RM, Welsch MA, et al. Resistance exercise training restores bone mineral density in heart transplant recipients. J Am Coll Cardiol 1996;28: 1471–1477.

Rehabilitation of Patients with Arrhythmias, Pacemakers, and Defibrillators

Robert A. Schweikert, Fredric J. Pashkow, and Bruce L. Wilkoff

INTRODUCTION

Rehabilitation programs are now more likely to encounter patients with more advanced cardiac disease, including those with a history of arrhythmias or disease of the sinus node or conduction system. Improvements in the use of antiarrhythmic medications, including an awareness of the potential toxicities, has led to better control of arrhythmias and a return of a great number of these patients to a more active lifestyle. Advances in the field of cardiac pacemakers have led to smaller, more complex pacemakers with a much greater ability to simulate the normal physiologic response to exercise. An increasing number of these patients may have other implanted devices, such as the implantable cardioverter/defibrillator (ICD).

In this section, we will review the relevant issues regarding the cardiac rehabilitation of patients with arrhythmias and patients with cardiac pacemakers or ICDs. In addition, we will outline the potential problems that may arise in the rehabilitation of such complex patients and offer guidelines regarding the management of these events.

CARDIAC ARRHYTHMIA

Exercise exposes patients with a history of arrhythmias to a period of risk for arrhythmia recurrence owing to the complex interaction among the myocardial substrate, the autonomic nervous system, and circulating catecholamines. In addition, transient metabolic changes during exercise, such as ischemia, may also play a role

(1). However, exercise testing and training can be safely performed in such patients. Overall, there has been a dramatic improvement in the history of cardiac arrest in rehabilitation. From 1960 to 1977, one cardiac arrest per 33,000 patient-hours of exercise was reported (2). From 1980 to 1984, the odds improved to one arrest during 112,000 patient-hours (3). Kelly reported one center's experience with 135 patients hospitalized for malignant ventricular arrhythmias. There was one cardiac arrest per 1,214 patient-hours of activity during inpatient cardiac rehabilitation. The rate of urgent complications, defined as events requiring immediate medical intervention, termination of exercise, or transportation of the patient back to the ward, was one per 173 patient-hours of exercise. A follow-up study of 42 patients enrolled in an outpatient cardiac rehabilitation program after hospitalization for malignant ventricular arrhythmias at the same center examined complications during a 9-year period of 1,246 patient-exercise sessions. Ventricular arrhythmias occurred during exercise in more than 90% of these patients, and ventricular tachycardia occurred in approximately 30%. There were no deaths, and the rate of urgent complications was one per 138 patient-hours of activity (4). Table 10.1 summarizes some of the published data regarding the complications of exercise stress testing for patients with a history of malignant ventricular arrhythmias. The occurrence of sustained ventricular tachyarrhythmias in these groups ranged from 0% to 8%, compared with 0.2% to 0.8% reported for patients with structural heart disease (10).

The safe administration of exercise training for

Table 10.1   Complications of Exercise Stress Testing in Populations with a History of Malignant Arrhythmia

Study	Number of Tests	VT-NS (%)	VT-S (%)	VF (%)	Mortality (%)
Allen, et al. (5)	64	22 (34)	5 (8)	0	0
Fintel, et al. (6)	103	23 (22)	0	0	0
Graboys, et al. (7)	60	39 (65)	0	0	0
Weaver, et al. (8)	86	7 (8)	0	0	0
Young, et al. (9)	1,377	NR	22 (1.6)	9 (0.65)	0

VT-NS = nonsustained ventricular tachycardia; VT-S = sustained ventricular tachycardia; VF = ventricular fibrillation; NR = not reported. Modified from Kelly TM. Exercise testing and training of patients with malignant ventricular arrhythmias. Med Sci Sports Exerc 1995; 28:53–61.

a patient with a history of arrhythmias requires special attention to the emergency and resuscitative equipment that should be available in every exercise facility. Particularly important is maintenance of the proper medications and emergency equipment, including a cardioverter/defibrillator with R-wave synchronizing capability. This equipment and medications should be immediately accessible in case of an arrest before, during, and after exercise. An emergency protocol should be posted and reviewed with the exercise laboratory personnel at least quarterly. There should be a clear, preconceived plan for the transfer of unstable patients to an appropriate hospital for emergency evaluation and treatment (11). More detailed guidelines for cardiac rehabilitation of high-risk patients are available in a recent publication from the American Association of Cardiovascular and Pulmonary Rehabilitation (12).

Medical supervision of the outpatient cardiac rehabilitation patient has generally been dictated by the patient's risk status. Table 10.2 summarizes the guidelines provided by the American College of Cardiology identifying patients at high risk for cardiovascular complications during exercise training who warrant electrocardiogram (ECG) monitoring during the session (13). Patients at very high risk for sudden ventricular fibrillation or cardiac arrest, which includes patients with a history of cardiac arrest without myocardial infarction, exercise-induced ventricular tachycardia, or complex ventricular arrhythmias with significant left ventricular dysfunction, should have on-site medical supervision with continuous ECG monitoring (14, 15). Patients with uncontrolled cardiac arrhythmias, particularly those patients with severely symptomatic or hemodynamically unstable arrhythmias, should not undergo exercise stress testing or training. Recent recommendations

Table 10.2   American College of Cardiology Criteria Identifying Patients in Whom ECG Monitoring Should Be Included During Exercise

Criteria for ECG Monitoring
Severely depressed left ventricular function (ejection fraction less than 30)
Resting complex ventricular arrhythmia (Lown type 4 or 5)
Ventricular arrhythmias appearing or increasing with exercise
Decrease in systolic blood pressure with exercise
Survivors of sudden cardiac death
Patients after myocardial infarction complicated by congestive heart failure, cardiogenic shock, or serious ventricular arrhythmias
Patients with severe coronary artery disease and marked exercise-induced ischemia
Inability to self-monitor heart rate owing to physical or intellectual impairment

Reproduced with permission from American College of Cardiology. Position report on cardiac rehabilitation. J Am Coll Cardiol 1986; 7:451–453.

from the American Heart Association suggest that patients at moderate to high risk for cardiac complications during exercise be monitored and supervised for at least 6 to 12 sessions (16).

Diagnosis and Treatment of Arrhythmias During Cardiac Rehabilitation

When an arrhythmia occurs in the setting of cardiac rehabilitation, especially one that results in severe symptoms or hemodynamic compromise, the staff must act quickly and efficiently to manage the problem. A detailed review of the diagnosis and treatment of specific arrhythmias is available elsewhere (17); however, several important points need to be made here. Most importantly, any tachyarrhythmia resulting in hemodynamic instability with serious signs or symptoms requires consideration for immediate cardioversion. However, especially in the setting of an event during exercise, one must be certain that the patient is not having sinus tachycardia in response to an acute myocardial infarction, a situation for which cardioversion would not be indicated. If the clinical situation permits, a rapid assessment of the cause of the tachyarrhythmia can be made. The tachyarrhythmia should be initially classified as narrow or wide complex (QRS duration greater than 120 msec). Narrow-complex tachycardias are usually supraventricular. The cause of wide-complex tachycardias is more difficult to determine, as these rhythm disorders may include ventricular tachycardia or supraventricular tachycardia with conduction aberrancy. Generally, a wide-complex tachycardia in a patient with a history of myocardial infarction or malignant ventricular arrhythmias without preexisting or rate-dependent bundle branch block, an accessory pathway, or ventricular-paced rhythm is ventricular tachycardia until proven otherwise. The clinical status and hemodynamic stability of a patient is not a reliable means of discriminating the cause of the tachyarrhythmia, as a significant number of patients with ventricular tachycardia may have only minimal signs and symptoms. A more detailed review of the differentiation between supraventricular and ventricular tachycardias can be found elsewhere (17, 18).

Role of Exercise in the Evaluation and Management of Arrhythmia

Exercise may be useful as an adjunctive technique to other methods in the assessment of the risk of arrhythmia recurrence and particularly in the evaluation of the efficacy and safety of arrhythmia therapy. Exercise stress testing can be complementary to other techniques used for the diagnosis and management of arrhythmias, such as electrophysiology studies, ambulatory Holter monitoring/event recorders, and signal-averaged electrocardiography. These tests have important limitations when compared with exercise testing. Ambulatory monitoring may not detect an arrhythmia in a patient who has infrequent episodes. Lown and colleagues (19) reported that up to 10% of patients with a history of sustained ventricular tachycardia had nonsustained or sustained ventricular tachycardia documented by exercise testing and not by ambulatory monitor-

ing. The electrophysiology laboratory may not reproduce the precise physiologic conditions that may be required for the exposure of an arrhythmia, as arrhythmias in some patients may require certain triggers to be uncovered.

Furthermore, exercise testing may provide information about the safety and efficacy of antiarrhythmic drugs, because exercise may counteract or enhance the effects of these agents. Membrane-active antiarrhythmic drugs result in decreased velocity of membrane conduction (phase 0), prolongation of myocardial refractory period (phase 3), decreased excitability, and decreased automaticity (phase 4). These effects are opposed to the physiologic effects of catecholamines. Continued efficacy of antiarrhythmic medications during exercise may therefore provide a degree of reassurance to the patient and physician. However, the complex physiologic changes that occur during and after exercise may also result in enhancement of antiarrhythmic drug action. The sodium-channel blocking (class I) antiarrhythmic drugs have a property called "use dependence." This refers to the enhancement of drug action at higher heart rates. The class IC antiarrhythmic agents, in particular, may have a more enhanced effect at faster heart rates than other class I agents and may be more prone to proarrhythmia during exercise (20). For this reason some authorities have recommended routine exercise testing to assess the proarrhythmic potential of patients initially treated with flecainide (21).

Effect of Antiarrhythmic Drug Therapy on Exercise Parameters

Further consideration for the arrhythmic patient includes the issue of heart rate as a parameter for monitoring exercise intensity. A number of patients with a history of arrhythmia are currently treated with antiarrhythmic agents that have significant negative chronotropic effects, such as sotalol, amiodarone, calcium-channel blockers, or β-blockers. Because these drugs may have significant impact on the maximum heart rate achieved during exercise, we strongly suggest these patients undergo formal exercise testing while taking the drug before starting an exercise training program. In this age of tightening health care budgets, clinicians are loathe to repeat tests, but stress studies in these patients performed for the determination of active ischemia generally are done with the patient off the drug because the reduced maximum heart rate achieved significantly reduces test sensitivity. They should be retested while taking the drug so that the appropriate rate and rating of perceived exertion (RPE) for therapeutic exercise can be determined.

The issue of activity recommendations is common to all patients with a history of arrhythmia. Critical to any recommendation regarding this sensitive and significant issue to patients are the individual characteristics of the patient's arrhythmia problem. When the patient is subject to sudden loss of consciousness or cognitive control related to the onset or offset of their arrhythmia (even when controlled by drug therapy), then they should be advised to restrict themselves from exercise activities in which they may be a potential risk to themselves or others.

CARDIAC PACEMAKERS

Cardiac pacing is a rapidly expanding field of electrophysiology. It is estimated that more than 300,000 pacemakers are now implanted each year, attesting to the prominence of newer technologies in pacing therapy today. As many as 25% of patients in cardiac rehabilitation programs have pacemakers. The use of devices for the treatment of bradycardia is likely to be higher in programs with a large proportion of patients who have undergone valvular surgery because of the high incidence of surgically induced atrioventricular block. With the changes in pacemaker technology, the cardiac rehabilitation prescription for these patients has also been revolutionized. At one time, the rehabilitation of a patient with an implanted pacemaker simply involved reassurance and education about the device. The patient was cautioned to avoid high-level physical activity because the pacemaker's fixed rate could not respond to exertion (22).

Since that time, and particularly during the past decade, there has been enormous progress in the design and manufacture of cardiac pacing devices. The changes relevant to the rehabilitation of severely disabled patients are a result of the development of integrated circuitry and the miniaturization of electronic components, allowing for the emulation of normal rate and rhythm responses under varying physiologic conditions and levels of metabolic demand (23).

Bradycardia Pacing: Understanding the Technology

Pacemakers are now capable of providing atrioventricular synchrony as well as dynamic adjustment of the heart rate to match varying levels of metabolic demand (24–26). Cardiac synchrony may be maintained by the placement of two pacing leads, one in the atrium and a second in the ventricle. A rate-adaptive pacer uses a parameter or physiologic variable other than the natural ones to control the pacing rate (27, 28). A more detailed discussion of pacemaker sensor characteristics is discussed below. In light of the rapidly expanding technology, the North American Society of Pacing and Electrophysiology (NASPE)/British Pacing and Electrophysiology Group (BPEG) generic pacemaker code was proposed in 1987 to provide a universal description of pacemaker characteristics (Table 10.3).

Physiology of Pacing

The physiologic aspects of exercise relevant to these patients is identical to any other (30). What is unique is the way in which their physiology integrates with the implanted technology. Although the relative contribution of chronotropism to cardiac output generally is appreciated, the preeminent relationship of rate to atrioventricular synchrony during progressive levels of exercise needs to be emphasized. The ability to develop an appropriate heart rate response during exercise accounts for about two-thirds of the cardiac output required. Stroke volume, the constituents of which are preload and afterload, accounts for the other third of cardiac output (30). As heart rate increases, the relative contribution from atrioventricular synchrony decreases (31).

The impact of these devices on functional capacity is potentially significant (23). Patients who are limited to a sedentary lifestyle (activity tolerance of 1 to 2 metabolic equivalents [METs]) may achieve the cardiac output necessary to accomplish most activities of daily living (ADL) (3 to 5 METs), given the ability to develop appropriate rate (26, 32). This increase in work capacity allows for the performance of such essential activities as shopping and food preparation, light housework, or care of an invalid spouse—and may sometimes make the difference between institutionalization and independence (26).

Chronotropic competence is the ability to

Table 10.3   NASPE/BPEG Generic (NBG) Pacemaker Code

Position	I	II	III	IV	V
Category	Chamber(s) paced	Chamber(s) sensed	Response to sensing	Programmability, rate modulation	Antitachy-arrhythmia function(s)
Letters:	O = none A = atrium	O = none A = atrium	O = none T = triggered	O = none P = simple programmable	O = none P = pacing (antitachy-arrhythmia)
	V = ventricle	V = ventricle	I = inhibited	M = multi-programmable	
	D = dual (A + V)	D = dual (A + V)	D = dual (T + I) sensor	C = communicating R = rate-adaptive	S = shock D = dual (P + S)
Manufacturers' designation only	S = Single (A or V)	S = Single (A or V)			

Reproduced with permission from Bernstein AD, Parson V. Pacemaker and defibrillator codes. In: Ellenbogen KA, Kay GN, Wilkoff BL, eds. Clinical cardiac pacing. Philadelphia: WB Saunders, 1995:279–283.

produce a heart rate appropriate for a given level of metabolic activity, such as for exercise or for performing heavy physical work (33). For practical purposes, the lack of chronotropic competence appears to be of two types: absolute and relative (26). Those patients with absolute chronotropic incompetence have a low, rigidly fixed rate, so that when paced, the pacemaker rate is the virtual rate. This often is the primary indication for pacemaker implantation. There are people, however, who can increase their heart rate somewhat, but the developed rate is inappropriate for a given level of metabolic demand. These persons have relative chronotropic incompetence, and its presence often is a secondary consideration in pacemaker selection.

Rate-adaptive Pacing

The primary goal of rate-adaptive pacing is to emulate the function of the sinus node for patients with chronotropic incompetence or atrial arrhythmias that preclude reliable sensing of native sinoatrial rhythm. A rate-adaptive pacemaker consists of three primary components: 1) a sensor located in the pacing lead or pacemaker itself that detects a physical or physiologic parameter that is directly or indirectly related to metabolic demand; 2) rate-modulating circuitry within the pacemaker that contains an algorithm that translates a change in the sensed parameter to a change in pacing rate; and 3) algorithm programmability such that a physician can make adjustments to accommodate the heart rate requirements of the individual patient. The ideal rate-adaptive pacemaker system would provide a change in pacing rate proportional to the level of metabolic demand ("proportionality") with a speed of response and recovery ("kinetics") similar to that of the sinus node. In addition, the sensor of an ideal system would be reliable, technically feasible, and sufficiently sensitive to detect both exercise and nonexercise requirements for a change in heart rate, but sufficiently specific such that false signals are not detected (27).

Pacemaker sensors fall into four basic technical categories and have relative advantages and disadvantages (Table 10.4) (27, 34). Motion sensors are the most widely used, partly because of their simplicity, speed of response, and compatibility with standard unipolar and bipolar pacing leads. Other sensors are more physiologic, yet some require technically complex pacing leads. Additionally, a sensor may work better for one person than for another because of activity preferences or lifestyle. Some sensors require more programming to fit the individual patient properly, or they consume more of the battery energy than other sensors do. Of the physiologic sensors, only the minute ventilation variety is widely available.

Sensor technology continues to evolve rapidly. Some pacemakers now have the capability to allow independent programming of the atrial tracking and sensor-indicated upper pacing rates. This provides the physician with the flexibility to limit the maximum intrinsic atrial rate that the device will track, yet allow the sensor to drive the heart

Table 10.4   Sensors in Rate-responsive Pacing

Mathods	Physiologic Parameters	How It Works	Advantages	Disadvantages
Impedance sensing	Respiratory rate Minute ventilation Stroke volume	Impedance plethysmography	Highly physiologic Highly proportional to metabolic demand	Delayed response Susceptible to electrode motion artifact
Ventricular evoked response	Evoked QT interval (stim-T interval)	Reflects catecholamines	More physiological	Requires ventricular pacing
Output pulse sensing				
Vibration, acceleration, gravitation, motion sensing	Body movement	Piezoelectric element	Rapid response No special lead needed	Nonphysiologic and nonspecific Late plateau response
Special sensors on pacing electrode	Central venous temperature[a] dP/dt[b]	Thermistor Piezoelectric element	More physiologic	Complex lead
	Mixed venous oxygen saturation	Optical sensor		

[a]No longer produced, although still in use in Japan.
[b]Presently available only in clinical trials.
Modified from Lau C, Camm AJ. Overview of ideal sensor characteristics. In: Ellenbogen KA, Kay GN, Wilkoff BL, eds.

rate to appropriate levels during exercise. With such a system, patients with episodic atrial tachyarrhythmias would be protected from tracking of inappropriate rapid atrial rates while still having the ability to achieve an appropriate heart rate response to exercise. Another advance in sensor technology designed to avoid tracking of nonphysiologic atrial rates is "cross-checking," whereby the sensor is used to determine whether an increase in the intrinsic atrial rate is appropriate. If the sensor does not confirm activity, but the pacemaker senses an increased atrial rate, the pacemaker will use the sensor to dictate the appropriate heart rate.

Recently, combinations of sensors have been incorporated into pacemakers in an attempt to more closely match the physiologic response to exercise. For example, a desirable sensor combination has been an activity sensor, which typically has a more rapid response, and another sensor such as minute ventilation, which typically has a more delayed but workload-proportional response. The term "sensor blending" refers to the relative contribution of each sensor during each phase of activity, and may be programmable. Some pacemakers with multiple sensors also have the ability to detect intersensor disagreement and thereby avoid inappropriately rapid pacing caused by a false-positive response of one sensor (35, 36).

Automatic Mode Switching

Another feature of modern pacemakers is the capability to automatically convert to another pacing mode under certain circumstances. One example of this feature that would be most commonly encountered is "automatic mode switching" or AMS, which refers to a programmable response of a dual-chamber pacemaker during an atrial tachyarrhythmia designed to avoid nonphysiologic ventricular pacing caused by atrial tracking. Generally the device switches from DDD mode to a VVI mode, usually with a gradual reduction of the pacing rate. The device switches back to the DDD mode after the atrial tachyarrhythmia resolves.

Evaluation Before and After Implantation

Evaluation before (37) and after implantation of a rate-adaptive pacemaker is important for its successful application. Exercise stress testing (28) and 24-hour Holter monitoring are the main tools, but telemetry monitoring (during, for example, exercise training), and other technologies, such as Doppler ultrasound, may be helpful (38).

The pacemaker may be programmed initially on the basis of age and estimated activity, but exercise testing of some type, even "informal," allows for the accurate adjustment of the device and proves the efficacy of the sensor at its current settings. Exercise provides important information for the optimal programming of rate-adaptive pacemaker systems, including proportionality and kinetics as discussed above. If necessary, metabolic stress testing can be especially useful in the evaluation of sensor proportionality to correlate the sensor-indicated pacing rate and oxygen consumption during exercise. In any event, the selection of the proper exercise protocol is important, because the typical protocol for the assessment of myocardial ischemia is designed to rapidly achieve maximum heart rate. However, the focus of protocols for the evaluation of rate-adaptive pacemaker systems should be at the lower workloads (1 to 5 METs) that fall within the range of ADL for most pacemaker patients. A protocol with a gradual increase in workload, such as the chronotropic assessment exercise protocol (CAEP), would be more appropriate for these patients (39).

In addition to consideration of the appropriate exercise test protocol, the selection of the proper mode of exercise is important. Certain sensors have significant disadvantages when evaluated by a particular mode of exercise. For example, the activity-sensing devices respond sluggishly to smoother activities such as bicycle riding or climbing a steeper incline at a steady speed. They also do not reflect the increasing metabolic workloads associated with carrying added weight, such as a suitcase, and during walking, when patients must move their arms for the sensor to function reliably. The temperature sensor may be confused by the loss of body heat during activities such as swimming or prolonged cold exposure.

Once optimal programming has been achieved with a rate-responsive device, the sensing characteristics seem to have long-term stability. An annual exercise test can be used to document the stability of the sensor and the patient's tolerance of currently programmed values of upper rate and sensor response. If 24-hour Holter monitoring is used, the importance of patient diaries needs to be impressed. Transtelephonic exercise monitoring also has been used for this purpose (40).

Potential Problems During Exercise Training

Patients with pacemakers may present with several problems during exercise. Some of the limitations with sensors have already been discussed above. It is imperative that the rehabilitation staff know the type of pacemaker (e.g., single- or dual-chamber) and how the device is programmed, including lower and upper rate limits, maximum tracking limit, and especially the presence of such features as rate adaptation and automatic mode switching.

One potential problem during exercise involves the behavior of the dual-chamber pacemaker when the upper rate limit of the device is reached. Early generations of DDD pacemakers would produce an abrupt, fixed block (commonly 2:1 or 3:1) in which the pacemaker only sensed every other or every third P wave. The hemodynamic effects of a change in heart rate (HR) from 120 to 60 beats per minute or less, for example, during peak exercise can be quite significant. Modern DDD pacemakers have incorporated advanced technologies into their design to minimize heart block at heart rates near the upper rate limit, such as 1) additional timing periods (e.g., maximum tracking rate) that lead to Wenckebach-like behavior, 2) rate-smoothing programs, and 3) rate-adaptive AV delay. However, 2:1 block is still common at the upper rate limit and may be seen if the pacemaker is suboptimally programmed.

Another problem that may be encountered during exercise is pacemaker syndrome, which can be loosely defined as the signs and symptoms that occur in the pacemaker patient because of inadequate timing of atrial and ventricular contractions (41). A common cause of pacemaker syndrome is retrograde ventriculoatrial (VA) conduction, which causes atrial contraction against closed mitral and tricuspid valves. Exercise may result in new or enhanced VA conduction not present at rest. Pacemaker syndrome may also occur during an exercise-induced atrial arrhythmia because of loss of AV synchrony when a device with an automatic mode switching feature converts to VVI pacing.

Atrial arrhythmias that occur during exercise in a patient with a dual-chamber pacemaker without mode switching capability could result in rapid ventricular pacing as the pacemaker attempts to track the atrial rate (a form of pacemaker-mediated tachycardia). The resultant wide-complex (paced) tachycardia may appear, at first glance, to be ventricular tachycardia, especially for pacemakers with bipolar leads in which the pacing artifact may be difficult to discern on the ECG tracing.

Attention to the more common potential problems that may occur during exercise training of patients with a pacemaker, as well as knowledge of the type of pacemaker and its programmed parameters, will reduce the likelihood of a significant complication during exercise. Patients with pacemakers may then participate in cardiac rehabilitation in a safe, well-controlled environment.

IMPLANTABLE CARDIOVERTER/DEFIBRILLATORS

Patients with an ICD pose a special challenge during exercise stress testing and training. Since the introduction of ICDs in 1980 for clinical use in patients with cardiac arrest (42), thousands of these devices have been implanted worldwide. The early devices were relatively simple "shock box" units capable only of detecting ventricular fibrillation and delivering a high-energy defibrillation shock. Implantation of these ICD systems required a thoracotomy for placement of the epicardial patch electrodes, and a subcutaneous pocket in the abdomen for the generator. Over the past decade, technological advances have led to a nonthoracotomy transvenous lead system and the development of smaller generators, which permits implantation into the prepectoral site.

As surgical techniques continue to advance, the technology of the ICD has also evolved. Implantable cardioverter/defibrillators have become complex, multiprogrammable, tiered-therapy systems capable of a wide range of low- and high-energy shocks, antitachycardia pacing, and backup ventricular pacing for bradyarrhythmias (43). Current ICDs can be programmed to provide progressive therapy dictated by the rate of the tachyarrhythmia and the failure of the previous therapy ("tiered" therapy). Thus, these devices may be programmed to deliver antitachycardia pacing, followed by low-energy shock if unsuccessful, then high-energy shocks if necessary. After charging in preparation for therapy delivery, ICDs reconfirm the continued presence of a tachyarrhythmia before delivering the therapy. This is referred to as "noncommitted" shocks, and it is designed to help avoid delivery of therapy for nonsustained arrhythmia (44). Table 10.5 outlines the generic defibrillator code system for the description of the various capabilities of the ICD, as adopted by the North American Society of Pacing and Electrophysiology, together with the British Pacing and Electrophysiology Group (NASPE/BPEG).

Recent advances have produced ICDs that incorporate dual-chamber pacing technology because many patients who receive an ICD also require a pacemaker owing to conduction system disease or the negative chronotropic effects of some antiarrhythmic drugs. This development would virtually eliminate the problem of adverse interaction between an ICD and pacemaker, as well as improve the specificity of ventricular tachycardia detection. An ICD with a sensor-driven, dual-chamber pacing feature was recently approved by the Food and Drug Administration. Another recent innovation is the atrial defibrillator for patients with atrial fibrillation, and future developments may result in combined atrial and ventricular ICDs.

Safety of Exercise Testing and Training for Patients with an ICD

Exercise stress testing and training for a patient with an ICD poses more risk than for the average patient. As discussed above, the history of malignant arrhythmias that led to implantation of the device increases the risk of untoward events during exercise. However, there are also potential problems with the ICD during exercise that may be circumvented with proper precautions. Important considerations before these patients begin an exercise rehabilitation program include knowledge of the type and frequency of the patient's arrhythmias, including any history of precipitation by exercise or catecholamines. Additionally, it is helpful to know the characteristics of the previous arrhythmia, such as rate, hemodynamic stability, and response to cough or vagal maneuvers, and various therapies, such as antiarrhythmic drugs and cardiac medications, antitachycardia pacing, and cardioversion.

Again, as emphasized for pacemakers above, rehabilitation staff need to know how the ICD is programmed. Especially important is knowledge of the detection interval, that is, the interval in milliseconds or heart rate in beats per minute at which the device recognizes a tachyarrhythmia and delivers therapy. One must be aware that, in general, ICDs recognize rate, not specific arrhythmia patterns. Any rhythm that becomes sufficiently rapid to reach or exceed the detection interval of the ICD for sufficient duration, in-

Table 10.5   North American Society of Pacing and Electrophysiology/British Pacing and Electrophysiology Group (NASPE/BPEG) Defibrillator Code (NBD Code)

I:Shock Chamber	II: Antitachycardia Pacing Chamber	III: Tachycardia Detection	IV: Antibradycardia Pacing Chamber
O = none	O = none	E = electrogram	O = none
A = atrium	A = atrium	H = hemodynamic	A = atrium
V = ventricle	V = ventricle		V = ventricle
D = dual (A + V)	D = dual (A + V)		D = dual (A + V)

Reproduced with permission from Bernstein AD, Parsonnet V. Pacemaker and defibrillator codes. In: Ellenbogen KA, Kay GN, Wilkoff BL, eds. Clinical cardiac pacing. Philadelphia: WB Saunders, 1995:279–283.

cluding sinus tachycardia, may be recognized as a tachyarrhythmia and treated accordingly. Although there are now programmable features that attempt to improve the specificity of ventricular tachycardia detection, including distinction between regular and irregular tachycardias, as well as evaluation of tachycardia initiation (gradual versus rapid onset of the rhythm disturbance), these features are imperfect. Therefore, one must assume that any rhythm rapid enough to meet the detection criteria of the ICD may result in activation of the device to deliver therapy. The new dual-chamber pacemaker ICDs include features to improve this situation.

As outlined above, before exercise stress testing and training it is imperative to determine the programmed detection interval of the device to avoid rate crossover during exercise and subsequent inappropriate therapies (particularly shocks) from the ICD for sinus tachycardia or a supraventricular arrhythmia. Inappropriate therapies from an ICD are not only uncomfortable for the patient but also may precipitate arrhythmias (45, 46). Because the average patient receiving an ICD is older than 60 years of age, a training heart rate of 120 beats per minute will likely exceed the rate criterion in only less than 3% of patients implanted with these devices. However, a patient 35 years of age may have a training rate of 140 beats per minute, a value exceeding the rate criterion of about 15% of the patients programmed, so the likelihood of rate crossover is somewhat greater in younger patients (47).

There are several methods of managing the potential for rate crossover and inappropriate ICD therapies during exercise testing and training. The appropriate method should be individualized from one patient to another, and consultation with the patient's physician is recommended. It may be prudent in some complex patients to also consult with the patient's cardiologist or electrophysiologist before exercise training. When the patient has a history of rapid ventricular tachycardia or ventricular fibrillation, the detection interval will most likely be programmed to such a level that sinus tachycardia during exercise will not be detected. In this situation, one need only carefully monitor the heart rate during exercise and terminate the test when the heart rate approaches the detection interval of the device. If the test is being performed only for the assessment of chronotropic response to exercise, particularly to determine the risk of sinus rate crossover, then this approach is suitable for any patient, regardless of the programmed detection interval.

However, when a maximal stress test is required, such as an evaluation for exercise-induced ischemia, then this approach may not be suitable for those patients with slower tachycardias and, therefore, slower programmed detection rates. One approach to managing these patients involves inactivation of the ICD immediately before the test. This method may result in the patient's being unprotected from malignant arrhythmias during the period the test is conducted; therefore, one must be prepared to rapidly reactivate the ICD or use external cardioversion or defibrillation in the event of an emergency. An alternative approach would be to reprogram the detection interval to a level beyond that expected for sinus tachycardia during exercise. This method may be safer for some patients than inactivating the device because they would remain protected from faster ventricular tachycardias and ventricular fibrillation, a situation in which rapid defibrillation is crucial. However, these patients would not be protected from slower ventricular tachycardias, which, in some patients, may result in injury secondary to syncope. Also, both methods require the appropriate programming equipment for the device and someone trained in its use to be present.

Perhaps more convenient is the method of temporarily inactivating or blinding the device with a magnet during exercise. All ICDs have an internal reed switch that closes when a magnetic field of sufficient strength is applied. The response to this maneuver is somewhat variable between ICD models and manufacturers (48); however, they all have in common the capability to be disabled from delivering therapies or shocks with application of the magnet. The magnet used must be of sufficient strength. The most common is a standard ring or donut-shaped magnet. In some cases, particularly for those patients with excess tissue between the skin surface and ICD generator, a second donut magnet stacked on top of the first may be necessary. A note of caution: devices manufactured by Guidant Cardiac Pacemakers, Inc. (St. Paul, MN) are unique in that the application of a magnetic field for a sufficient period (30 seconds) can be used to permanently inactivate the ICD (turning it off) without the use of programming equipment.

Role of Exercise Testing for the Patient with an ICD

Exercise testing can be quite useful to determine the patient's chronotropic response to exercise, particularly for those patients with slower tachyarrhythmias in whom sinus rate crossover during routine daily activities is more likely to occur. Knowledge of the patient's heart rate response during exercise can provide valuable information for appropriate programming of the ICD. Thus, we again advocate that patients be formally exercise tested to be sure that the patient's intrinsic heart rate will not exceed the threshold rate of the device and fire inadvertently during physical activity. In many defibrillator clinics, the patient is ambulated on an informal basis on the assumption that the patient's most strenuous physical activity is walking and that the device only needs to accommodate the heart rate achieved with this activity. Although such informal ambulation will often suffice for follow-up purposes, initial programming for a patient entering or returning to cardiac rehabilitation should be done in conjunction with formal testing. This is especially useful when the patient's detection interval is close to the heart rate achieved at MET levels that approximate realistic

activity for the patient. Precise measures of the heart rate required for an adequate margin of safety can have a significant impact on the patient functionally and psychologically.

Other Considerations for Cardiac Rehabilitation of the ICD Patient

Patients with ICDs are excellent candidates for rehabilitation programs that have supervision by medical professionals and telemetry monitoring capability, at least until the likelihood of inadvertent defibrillation has been ruled out with sufficient experience (49). They also benefit from group support and socialization (50, 51). The implantation of such a potent device into an individual can have significant psychological ramifications (49, 52). The opportunity to share experiences and to be regarded by others as normal is, for many, a significant relief. Formal group psychotherapy can be offered to those who are identified as having significant adjustment problems (50, 52). Most patients employed before ICD implantation are able to return to work after the procedure (53).

SUMMARY

Patients with potentially malignant arrhythmias are a challenge when they present for exercise testing and training. The complex metabolic and electrophysiologic changes that occur during and after exercise may suppress or potentiate arrhythmias and alter the efficacy and safety of antiarrhythmic agents. Exercise testing and training are valuable methods for the evaluation and management of patients with arrhythmia, especially those patients with implanted devices. The presence of an implantable device such as a pacemaker or ICD adds a level of complexity to the patient; however, a general understanding of how these devices function and a review of the programmed parameters before exercise will reduce the likelihood of a complication and allow more efficient and appropriate action should a complication occur.

These patients are excellent candidates for rehabilitation and exercise training programs, which may result in increased functional capacity and improved quality of life. With this knowledge and adherence to the appropriate guidelines for patient selection and testing, exercise testing and training of patients with potentially problematic arrhythmias can be prescribed and conducted in a safe, controlled manner in an atmosphere of confidence and professionalism.

References

1. Podrid PJ, Fuchs T, Candinas R. Role of the sympathetic nervous system in the genesis of ventricular arrhythmias. Circulation 1990;82(Suppl 1):I-103–I-113.
2. Haskell W. Cardiovascular complications during exercise training of cardiac patients. Circulation 1978; 57:920–924.
3. Van Camp S, Peterson RA. Cardiovascular complications of outpatient cardiac rehabilitation programs. JAMA 1986;256:1160–1163.
4. Kelly TM. Exercise testing and training of patients with malignant ventricular arrhythmias. Med Sci Sports Exerc 1995;28:53–61.
5. Allen BJ, Casey TP, Brodsky MA, et al. Exercise testing in patients with life-threatening ventricular tachyarrhythmias: results and correlation with clinical and arrhythmia factors. Am Heart J 1988;116:997–1002.
6. Fintel D, Griffith L, Platia E, et al. Exercise-induced ventricular tachycardia does not predict outcome in patients with recurrent ventricular tachycardia or fibrillation. Pacing Clin Electrophysiol 1984;7:459–462.
7. Graboys TB, Lown B, Podrid PJ, et al. Long-term survival of patients with malignant ventricular arrhythmia treated with antiarrhythmic drugs. Am J Cardiol 1982;50:437–443.
8. Weaver WD, Cobb LA, Hallstrom AP. Characteristics of survivors of exertion- and nonexertion-related cardiac arrest: value of subsequent exercise testing. Am J Cardiol 1982;50:671–676.
9. Young DZ, Lampert S, Graboys TB, et al. Safety of maximal exercise testing in patients at high risk for ventricular arrhythmia. Circulation 1984;70:184–191.
10. Podrid PJ, Bumio F, Fogel RI. Evaluating patients with ventricular arrhythmia. Role of the signal-averaged electrocardiogram, exercise test, ambulatory electrocardiogram, and electrophysiologic studies. Cardiol Clin 1992;10:371–395.
11. Pina IL, Balady GJ, Hanson P, et al. Guidelines for clinical exercise testing laboratories. A statement for healthcare professionals from the Committee on Exercise and Cardiac Rehabilitation, American Heart Association. Circulation 1995;91:912–921.
12. American Association of Cardiovascular and Pulmonary Rehabilitation. Guidelines for cardiac rehabilitation programs. 2nd ed. Champaign, IL: Human Kinetics, 1995.
13. American College of Cardiology. Position report on cardiac rehabilitation. J Am Coll Cardiol 1986;7:451–453.
14. Haskell WL. The efficacy and safety of exercise programs in cardiac rehabilitation. Med Sci Sports Exerc 1994;26:815–823.
15. Dennis C. Rehabilitation of patients with coronary artery disease. In: Braunwald E, ed. Heart disease: a textbook of cardiovascular medicine. 5th ed. Philadelphia: WB Saunders, 1997:1392–1403.
16. Fletcher GF, Balady G, Froelicher VF, et al. Exercise standards: a statement for healthcare professionals from the American Heart Association. Circulation 1995;91:580–615.
17. Zipes DP. Specific arrhythmias: diagnosis and treatment. In: Braunwald E, ed. Heart disease: a textbook of cardiovascular medicine. 5th ed. Philadelphia: WB Saunders, 1997:640–704.
18. Miller JP. Recognition of ventricular tachycardia. In: Zipes DP, Jalife J, eds. Cardiac electrophysiology: from cell to bedside. 2nd ed. Philadelphia: WB Saunders, 1995:990–1008.
19. Lown B, Podrid PJ, DeSilva RA, et al. Sudden cardiac death: management of the patient at risk. Curr Probl Cardiol 1980;4:1–62.
20. Ranger S, Talajic M, Lemery R, et al. Kinetics of use-dependent ventricular conduction slowing by antiarrhythmic drugs in humans. Circulation 1991;83:1987–1994.
21. Anastasiou-Nana MI, Anderson JL, Stewart JR, et al. Occurrence of exercise-induced and spontaneous wide complex tachycardia during therapy with flecainide for complex ventricular arrhythmias: a probable proarrhythmic effect. Am Heart J 1987;113:1071–1077.
22. Wenger NK. Future directions in cardiovascular rehabilitation. J Cardpulm Rehabil 1987;7:168–174.
23. Pashkow F. Patients with implanted pacemakers or implanted cardioverter-defibrillators. In: Wenger N, Hellerstein H, eds. Rehabilitation of the coronary patient. 3rd ed. New York: Churchill Livingstone, 1992:431–438.
24. Nordlander R, Hedman A, Pehrsson SK. Rate responsive pacing and exercise capacity—a comment [editorial]. Pacing Clin Electrophysiol 1989;12:749–751.
25. Humen DP, Kostuk WJ, Klein GJ. Activity-sensing, rate-responsive pacing: improvement in myocardial performance with exercise. Pacing Clin Electrophysiol 1985;8:52–59.
26. Pashkow F. Rate responsive pacing: practical application. Cardiology 1989;6:89–99.
27. Lau C, Camm AJ. Overview of ideal sensor characteristics. In: Ellenbogen KA, Kay GN, Wilkoff BL, eds. Clinical cardiac pacing. Philadelphia: WB Saunders, 1995:141–166.
28. Faerestrand S, Breivik K, Ohm OJ. Assessment of the work capacity and relationship between rate response and exercise tolerance associated with activity-sensing rate-responsive ventricular pacing. Pacing Clin Electrophysiol 1987;10:1277–1290.
29. Bernstein AD, Parsonnet V. Pacemaker and defibrillator codes. In: Ellenbogen KA, Kay GN, Wilkoff BL, eds. Clinical cardiac pacing. Philadelphia: WB Saunders, 1995:279–283.
30. Kristensson BE, Arnman K, Ryden L. Atrial synchronous ventricular pacing in ischaemic heart disease. Eur Heart J 1983;4:668–673.
31. Benditt DG, Mianulli M, Fetter J, et al. Single-chamber cardiac pacing with activity-initiated chronotropic response: evaluation by cardiopulmonary exercise testing. Circulation 1987;75:184–191.
32. Rickards AF, Donaldson RM. Rate responsive pacing. Clin Prog Pacing Electrophysiol 1983;1:12–18.
33. Wilkoff B, Corey J, Blackburn G. A mathematical

model of the cardiac chronotropic response to exercise. J Electrophysiol 1989;3:176–180.

34. Lau CP, Butrous GS, Ward DE, et al. Comparison of exercise performance of six rate-adaptive right ventricular cardiac pacemakers. Am J Cardiol 1989;63:833–838.

35. Benditt DG, Mianulli M, Lurie K, et al. Multiple-sensor systems for physiologic cardiac pacing. Ann Intern Med 1994;121:960–968.

36. Barold SS, Barold HS. Contemporary issues in rate-adaptive pacing. Clin Cardiol 1997;20:726–729.

37. Benditt DG, Mianulli M, Fetter J, et al. An office-based exercise protocol for predicting chronotropic response of activity-triggered, rate-variable pacemakers. Am J Cardiol 1989;64:27–32.

38. Lau CP, Camm AJ. Role of left ventricular function and Doppler-derived variables in predicting hemodynamic benefits of rate-responsive pacing. Am J Cardiol 1988;62:906–911.

39. Wilkoff BL. Cardiac chronotropic responsiveness. In: Ellenbogen KA, Kay GN, Wilkoff BL, eds. Clinical cardiac pacing. Philadelphia, PA: WB Saunders, 1995: 432–446.

40. Hayes DL, Christiansen JR, Vlietstra RE, et al. Follow-up of an activity-sensing, rate-modulated pacing device, including transtelephonic exercise assessment. Mayo Clin Proc 1989;64:503–508.

41. Barold S. The fourth decade of cardiac pacing: hemodynamic, electrophysiological, and clinical considerations in the selection of the optimal pacemaker. In: Zipes DP, ed. Cardiac electrophysiology: from cell to bedside. 2nd ed. Philadelphia, PA: WB Saunders, 1995:1366–1392.

42. Mirowski M, Reid PR, Mower MM, et al. Termination of malignant ventricular arrhythmias with an implanted automatic defibrillator in human beings. N Engl J Med 1980;303:322–324.

43. Pinski SL, Trohman RG. Implantable cardioverter-defibrillators: implications for the nonelectrophysiologist. Ann Intern Med 1995;122:770–777.

44. Estes NAM III. Overview of the implantable cardioverter-defibrillator. In: Estes NAM III, Manolis AS, Wang PJ, eds. Implantable cardioverter-defibrillators: a comprehensive textbook. New York: Marcel Dekker, 1994:635–653.

45. Pinski SL, Fahy GJ. The proarrhythmic potential of implantable cardioverter-defibrillators. Circulation 1995;92:1651–1664.

46. Schmitt C, Montero M, Melichercik J. Significance of supraventricular tachyarrhythmias in patients with implanted pacing cardioverter defibrillators. Pacing Clin Electrophysiol 1994;17(3 Pt 1):295–302.

47. Pashkow FJ. Populations with special needs for exercise rehabilitation: patients with implanted pacemakers or implanted cardioverter-defibrillators. In: Wenger NK, Hellerstein H, eds. Rehabilitation of the coronary patient. 3rd ed. New York: Churchill Livingstone, 1992:431–438.

48. Pashkow FJ, Schweikert RA, Wilkoff BL. Exercise testing and training in patients with malignant arrhythmias. Exerc Sport Sci Rev 1997;25:235–269.

49. Badger JM, Morris PL. Observations of a support group for automatic implantable cardioverter-defibrillator recipients and their spouses. Heart Lung 1989;18: 238–243.

50. Pycha C, Gulledge AD, Hutzler J, et al. Psychological responses to the implantable defibrillator. Psychosomatics 1986;27:841–845.

51. Teplitz L, Egenes KJ, Brask L. Life after sudden death: the development of a support group for automatic implantable cardioverter-defibrillator patients. J Cardiovasc Nurs 1990;4:20–32.

52. Keren R, Aarons D, Veltri EP. Anxiety and depression in patients with life-threatening ventricular arrhythmias: impact of the implantable cardioverter-defibrillator. Pacing Clin Electrophysiol 1991;14: 181–187.

53. Kalbfleisch KR, Lehmann MH, Steinman RT, et al. Reemployment following implantation of the automatic cardioverter defibrillator. Am J Cardiol 1989;64: 199–202.

Associated Medical Conditions

Neil F. Gordon, Byron J. Hoogwerf, Jeffrey W. Olin,
William R. Hiatt, and Fredric J. Pashkow

There are certain medical conditions that occur with extraordinary frequency in patients who have coronary heart disease. Some of these entities, for example, hypertension and diabetes, abet the development and progression of the cardiac disorder as well as complicate the management of these patients, particularly in the rehabilitation setting. These important common concurrent conditions are discussed in the sections that follow.

Part A. Hypertension
Neil F. Gordon

Atherosclerotic coronary heart disease (CHD) is the major cardiovascular sequel of hypertension. In contrast to other cardiovascular sequelae, such as stroke, cardiac failure, and renal failure, no convincing evidence exists to show that CHD morbidity and mortality are substantially attenuated by the pharmacologic treatment of mild to moderate hypertension (1–3). Although the precise reasons for this surprising finding have still to be elucidated, it has led to a reexamination of previously held beliefs about the management of hypertensive patients. In particular, increased emphasis recently has been placed on the prevention of a shift toward a more atherogenic lipid profile during antihypertensive drug therapy and the use of nonpharmacologic interventions, such as regular exercise (4–6).

ANTIHYPERTENSIVE EFFICACY OF EXERCISE TRAINING

Recently, several large epidemiologic studies have examined the relationship between participation in physical activity, cardiorespiratory fitness, and blood pressure (BP) (7–9). These studies strongly suggest not only that regular exercise is associated with a reduced risk of developing hypertension but that it also be used as a therapeutic regimen. The results of such studies are supported by Hagberg's (10) meta-analysis of 25 longitudinal studies on the BP-lowering effects of aerobic exercise training in hypertensive persons. This meta-analysis revealed impressive sample size–weighted reductions in resting systolic and diastolic BP with exercise training of 10.8 and 8.2 mm Hg, respectively.

Existing studies indicate that exercise training can be expected to lower an elevated BP in hypertensive patients. Moreover, as has been emphasized in previous reviews of the topic (7, 8), the magnitude of the reduction in BP compares favorably with that evoked by weight reduction, which is widely regarded as the most effective nonpharmacologic antihypertensive intervention (10, 11). It should be noted, however, that the fall in BP with exercise training was not sufficiently large to normalize BP in many studies. Furthermore, not all trials support the conclusion that regular exercise is a clinically effective antihypertensive intervention (12). Such observations raise the possibility that certain subsets of hypertensive patients are more responsive to the BP-lowering effects of exercise training than others.

Mechanisms for Antihypertensive Efficacy of Exercise Training

Ultimately, for BP to be lowered with exercise training, the cardiac output or total peripheral resistance must be reduced. Proposed mechanisms for alterations in cardiac output or total peripheral resistance with exercise training include resetting of baroreceptors, altered blood volume distribution, changes in the renin-angiotensin axis, increased insulin sensitivity, and reduced sympathetic activity (10, 11, 13). Although the findings of available studies are not very consistent, the hypothesis that a reduction in sympathetic activity with exercise training is the responsible mechanism has gained the most support to date (14–17).

Recently, it has become apparent that a single bout of aerobic exercise may alter CHD risk factors (serum high-density lipoprotein cholesterol levels, serum triglycerides, and glucose tolerance) favorably (18, 19). Likewise, several studies have now confirmed that BP may be reduced for 1 to 3 hours after exercise (20, 21). In these studies, a single workout (30 to 45 minutes) of aerobic exercise elicited systolic and diastolic BP reductions of similar magnitude to those evoked by chronic exercise conditioning. In view of this, the possibility exists that a reduction in BP with aerobic exercise could be related to the cumulative effects of single-exercise workouts rather than by actual chronic adaptation to exercise training.

Interaction with Pharmacologic Therapy

Both the Joint National Committee on Prevention, Detection, Evaluation, and Treatment of High Blood Pressure (JNC V1) and the American College of Sports Medicine (ACSM) advocate regular aerobic exercise as a preventive strategy to reduce the incidence of high BP and indicate that exercise training can be effectively used as definitive or adjunctive therapy for hypertension (4, 22).

Lifestyle modification and drug therapy decisions should be based not only on the level of BP but also on the presence or absence of target organ damage and other risk factors (such as smoking, dyslipidemia, diabetes mellitus, age, sex, and family history of cardiovascular disease). In this respect, risk stratification and treatment guidelines of JNC V1 are shown in Table 11.1.

It is important to emphasize that exercise training is not a panacea and, like other nonpharmacologic interventions, does not normalize BP completely in many hypertensive patients. In such instances, it may be necessary to combine exercise training with drug therapy.

Our research and other studies have shown that certain antihypertensive agents may be inappropriate for patients with uncomplicated essential hypertension who participate in an exercise program (23). Specifically, nonselective β-blockers and, to a lesser degree, selective β_1-blockers are known to impair exercise tolerance in hypertensive patients without CHD. Unless β-blocker therapy is specifically indicated, then physicians should consider using alternative antihypertensive agents for their patients with uncomplicated essential hypertension who participate in exercise programs. It must be emphasized, however, that should β-blocker therapy be prescribed, patients are still able to derive a physiologic cardiorespiratory training effect. Moreover, exercise training may help offset the deleterious effect of β-blocker therapy on high-density lipoprotein cholesterol levels (23).

Unlike hypertensive patients who do not have effort-induced myocardial ischemia, those who do can expect to experience an increase in their exercise tolerance with β-blocker therapy (23). This enhancement of functional capability is achieved largely by the combination of negative chronotropic and inotropic effects, both of which serve to lessen myocardial oxygen requirements. Our observations and those of other investigators further indicate that, irrespective of any specific ancillary pharmacologic properties, β-blockers do not prevent the expected enhancement of cardiorespiratory fitness with exercise training in CHD patients (23).

Antihypertensive agents that reduce total peripheral resistance may predispose to postexercise hypotension. This potential adverse effect can usually be prevented by avoidance of abrupt cessation of exercise and use of a longer cooldown period. Diuretics may result in serum potassium derangements and thereby accentuate the risk for exercise-induced arrhythmias.

EFFECT OF EXERCISE TRAINING ON ACCENTUATED RISK FOR MORTALITY IN HYPERTENSIVE PATIENTS

To date, no studies have investigated the effect of exercise training on mortality in hypertensive patients. In their study of 16,936 Harvard alumni, 9% of whom had physician-diagnosed hypertension, Paffenbarger et al. (24) documented death rates of 173, 117, and 79 per 10,000 person-years of observation in the hyper-

Table 11.1.   Risk Stratification and Treatment[a]

Blood Pressure Stages (mm Hg)	Risk Group A (No Risk Factors; No TOD/CCD)	Risk Group B (At Least 1 Risk Factor, Not Including Diabetes; No TOD/CCD)	Risk Group C (TOD/CCD and/or Diabetes, With or Without Other Risk Factors)
High-normal (130–139/85–89)	Lifestyle modification	Lifestyle modification	Drug therapy[c]
Stage 1 (140–159/90–99)	Lifestyle modification (up to 12 mo)	Lifestyle modification (up to 6 mo)[b]	Drug therapy
Stage 2 and 3 (≥160/≥100)	Drug therapy	Drug therapy	Drug therapy

TOD/CCD = target-organ disease/clinical cardiovascular disease.
[a]For example, a patient with diabetes and a blood pressure of 142/94 mm Hg plus left ventricular hypertrophy should be classified as having stage 2 hypertension with target-organ disease (left ventricular hypertrophy) and with another major risk factor (diabetes). This patient would be categorized as "Stage 1, Risk Group C" and recommended for immediate initiation of pharmacologic treatment. Lifestyle modification should be adjunctive therapy for all patients recommended for pharmacologic therapy.
[b]For patients with multiple risk factors, clinicians should consider drugs as initial therapy plus lifestyle modifications.
[c]For those with heart failure, renal insufficiency, or diabetes.
Reprinted with permission from the Joint National Committee on Prevention, Detection, Evaluation, and Treatment of High Blood Pressure. The sixth report of the Joint National Committee on Prevention, Detection, Evaluation, and Treatment of High Blood Pressure. Arch Intern Med 1997;157:2413–2446.

tensive men who expended fewer than 500, 500 to 1999, and more than 1999 kcal/wk during exercise, respectively. Similarly, in a study by Blair et al. (25) of 1832 men who reported a history of hypertension, age-adjusted, all-cause mortality rates per 10,000 person-years of follow-up ranged from 110.5 in men who fell into the least-fit quintile during baseline treadmill testing to 24.8 in those in the most-fit quintile. These preliminary studies suggest a profound beneficial impact of regular exercise and cardiorespiratory fitness on the risk of mortality in hypertensive patients.

No data are currently available for hypertensive patients with CHD. Two recent meta-analyses of randomized clinical trials that involved more than 4000 post–myocardial infarction patients have documented a 20% to 25% reduction in all-cause and cardiovascular disease mortality in those patients who participated in cardiac rehabilitation exercise training (26, 27). Given the fact that elevated BP is a major risk factor for CHD, it is likely that a sizable number of participants in these studies were hypertensive.

SAFETY ASPECTS OF AEROBIC EXERCISE FOR HYPERTENSIVE PATIENTS

In unmedicated hypertensive patients, dynamic exercise generally elicits a normal rise in systolic BP from baseline levels, although the response may be exaggerated or diminished in certain subsets of patients (28, 29). Because of their elevated baseline values, however, the absolute systolic BP during exercise usually is higher in hypertensive persons. Furthermore, in contrast to normotensive persons, hypertensives may display no change or even a slight increase in diastolic BP as a result of an impaired vasodilatory response (28).

In view of the higher BP experienced by hypertensive persons during dynamic exercise, it often is assumed that they are at greater risk of an acute morbid event, such as sudden cardiac death or hemorrhagic stroke. Contrary to this postulate, no evidence presently exists to support an accentuated immediate risk of participation in an acute bout of dynamic exercise for hypertensive patients (28, 30). Nonetheless, it seems prudent to avoid an excessive rise in BP during exercise training. In this respect, the ACSM considers a resting diastolic BP of more than 115 mm Hg or a systolic BP greater than 200 mm Hg to represent a relative contraindication to exercise testing; a systolic BP in excess of 260 mm Hg or diastolic BP more than 120 mm Hg as an indication for terminating an exercise test; a resting systolic BP greater than 200 mm Hg or a diastolic BP more than 110 mm Hg as a relative contraindication to entry into inpatient and outpatient cardiac rehabilitation exercise programs; and a systolic BP equal to 240 mm Hg or a diastolic BP equal to 110 mm Hg as the safe upper limit for cardiac rehabilitation exercise sessions (31).

Although most antihypertensive drugs do not

substantially alter the change in systolic BP that accompanies dynamic exercise, they do lower the resting systolic BP and, thus, the absolute value attained (28, 32). β-Blockers, however, can attenuate the magnitude of the rise in systolic BP during dynamic exercise as well as lower the resting BP. Consequently, they are the class of antihypertensive agents that represent the greatest potential benefit to hypertensive persons who experience an excessive rise in systolic BP during dynamic exercise. Irrespective of the precise drugs prescribed, the physician and patient should be aware of how they interact with exercise and whether any special precautions are needed (23, 30, 31).

Patients with high BP traditionally have been discouraged from participating in resistance training for fear of precipitating a cerebrovascular event or imposing an excessive demand on a myocardium that may already display a compromised left ventricular (LV) function. Such fears have arisen largely as a result of the marked pressor response elicited during an acute bout of heavy resistance exercise (33).

Studies that investigated the impact of chronic resistance training on resting BP, in fact, have not documented an adverse effect. On the contrary, although considerable additional research is needed to clarify the situation fully, the results of existing, appropriately designed longitudinal training studies suggest that long-term resistance training may modify resting diastolic BP favorably (34–36).

Experimental evidence on the effects of acute and chronic resistance training on the risk for cerebrovascular complications in humans with high BP is currently unavailable. In stroke-prone hypertensive rats, Tipton et al. (37) recently failed to observe an increased risk for cerebrovascular lesions with long-term resistance exercise training. Although much research is required before these findings can be extrapolated to humans with high BP, they do indicate that resistance training may not necessarily increase the risk for cerebrovascular complications.

In hypertensive patients, concentric hypertrophy of the left ventricle has been shown to be associated with an accentuated risk of major cardiovascular events, even in the absence of any conventional cardiovascular disease risk factors (38). Theoretically, resistance training that induces pressure overloading of the left ventricle could be expected to contribute further to concentric hypertrophy in hypertensive patients. Although resistance training may indeed increase LV wall thickness, generally, little or no change occurs in LV internal dimensions, with no effect or even a slight enhancement of systolic function at rest (39, 40). Furthermore, whereas the pathologic concentric hypertrophy caused by high BP produces abnormalities in LV diastolic function, resistance training is typically characterized by normal diastolic function (39, 40). Although the eccentric hypertrophy that may result from volume overloading induced by endurance training is seemingly more desirable than the concentric hypertrophy that may result from resistance training, neither seems to produce any untoward changes in LV function (11).

Resistance training can be performed with a high level of safety by select CHD patients (41). The ACSM considers a diastolic BP less than 105 mm Hg to be one of the indications for resistance exercise training in outpatient cardiac rehabilitation programs.

BASIC EXERCISE PRESCRIPTION GUIDELINES FOR PATIENTS WITH HYPERTENSION

The goal of prevention and management of hypertension is to reduce morbidity and mortality by the least intrusive means possible (4). Because CHD is the most important complication of hypertension, exercise training programs for hypertensive patients should focus primarily on this aspect of hypertension-related morbidity and mortality.

When compiling an exercise prescription with these purposes in mind, several factors must be considered to optimize the likelihood of a safe and effective response. These factors include specific safety aspects, the type of exercise to be performed, and the frequency, intensity, and duration of exercise training. For those patients who require medication, the interaction between the antihypertensive drug in question and exercise training also must be considered.

Like the general population, adult patients with hypertension face the same potential health hazards of exercise training—orthopedic injury and sudden cardiac death. To reduce the risk of orthopedic injury, patients should be cautioned against attempting to perform too much exercise too soon, and they should adhere to other standard injury-prevention guidelines applicable to anyone who participates in exercise programs (42).

To minimize the risk of exercise-related sudden cardiac death, the following three-step approach is recommended. First, certain subsets of hypertensive patients should undergo medical evaluation, including maximal graded exercise testing with electrocardiogram (ECG) and BP monitoring, before beginning a program of vigorous exercise: men 40 years or older; women 50 years or older; and (irrespective of age and sex) all persons with an additional major CHD risk factor or cardiopulmonary or metabolic disease, or symptoms suggestive of such disease (31). For patients who participate in moderate (40% to 60% of maximal oxygen uptake) rather than vigorous (more than 60% of maximal oxygen uptake) exercise and do not have known cardiopulmonary or metabolic disease or symptoms of such disease, exercise testing probably is not necessary, provided that

training is undertaken gradually and with appropriate guidance (31). Second, patients should be educated about the many factors that are necessary for safe exercise, especially the premonitory symptoms and signs of an impending cardiac complication. Third, all patients with documented CHD should exercise under medical direction in accordance with standard guidelines (31, 41).

The type, frequency, intensity, and duration of exercise should be similar to that recommended for healthy persons and, in the case of hypertensive patients with CHD, cardiac patients (31, 41, 43, 44).

Interestingly, exercise training at somewhat lower intensities (40% to 70% of maximal oxygen consumption) appears to lower BP as much as, if not more than, exercise at higher intensities. This is of particular relevance for certain specific populations of persons with hypertension, such as the elderly or those who have chronic diseases in addition to hypertension. The ACSM recommendations for exercise programming for hypertensive patients are summarized in Table 11.2.

Table 11.2. Hypertension: Exercise Programming

Modes	Goals	Intensity/Frequency/Duration	Time to Goal
Aerobic			
Large muscle activities	Increase $\dot{V}O_2$max and ventilatory threshold.	50–85% peak HR.	4–6 months
	Increase peak work and endurance.	RPE of 11–13.	
	Increase caloric expenditure.	3–7 days/week.	
	Control blood pressure.	30–60 min/session. 700–2000 kcal/week.	
Strength			
Circuit training	Increase strength.	High repetitions, low resistance.	

Medications	Special Considerations
β-Blockers: attenuate HR by about 30 contractions per minute	Do not exercise if resting systolic BP > 200 mm Hg or diastolic BP > 115 mm Hg.
α-Blockers, α_2-Blockers, calcium-channel blockers, and vasodilators: may cause postexertional hypotension.	Exercise when pressor response is best controlled by medications. Exercise at 40%–70% $\dot{V}O_2$max appears to lower resting blood pressure as much as, if not more than, exercise at higher intensities. 700 kcal/week should be the initial goal; 2000 kcal/week should be the long-term goal.

Reprinted with permission from Gordon NF. Hypertension. In: ACSM's exercise management for persons with chronic diseases and disabilities. Champaign, IL: Human Kinetics, 1997:59–63.
HR = heart rate; RPE = rating of perceived exertion; BP = blood pressure; $\dot{V}O_2$max = maximal oxygen uptake.

Part B. Diabetes

Byron J. Hoogwerf

Management of the diabetic patient with coronary heart disease (CHD) requires an understanding of the following key areas:

1. The impact of diabetes mellitus (DM) on the risk for CHD.
2. How other complications of diabetes mellitus may affect the management of CHD, especially in the process of cardiac rehabilitation.
3. The effects of diet, exercise, and medication used during the various stages in the rehabilitation process on glycemic control, including differences in the management of type 1 diabetes mellitus compared with type 2 diabetes mellitus.
4. Special considerations of medications used to treat problems associated with CHD in the diabetic patient.

This section addresses these problems by giving an overview of diabetes mellitus and the relationship of hyperglycemia to CHD followed by special considerations for cardiac rehabilitation in the diabetic patient.

CLASSIFICATION OF DIABETES MELLITUS

There are two major types of DM (1), and the discussion of cardiac rehabilitation will be limited to them. Type 1 DM (2), or insulin-dependent diabetes mellitus (IDDM) (ketosis-prone, formerly called juvenile onset), usually has its onset before the age of twenty, although there is clear evidence that it may occur at any time throughout adult life. This is an immunologic disease in which progressive destruction of islet cells results in a loss of the ability to produce insulin. All such patients require an exogenous source of insulin, usually administered by subcutaneous insulin injections. Type 1 DM comprises about 10% of all diabetic patients in the United States. Type 2 DM (3), or non–insulin-dependent diabetes mellitus (NIDDM) (formerly called adult-onset), usually has its onset after age forty. The defects that predispose to hyperglycemia are a combination of insulin resistance (as a result of impaired glucose disposal and in-creased hepatic glucose production) and impaired insulin secretion.

For obese type 2 diabetic patients, the initial treatment is weight loss, and all patients may benefit from proper dietary prescription (4). Exercise is associated with improved glycemic control (5–8). When diet and exercise do not control blood glucose satisfactorily, then drug therapy is initiated. Until recently, sulfonylureas were the mainstay of oral-agent therapy in the United States (9). Sulfonylureas work by stimulating insulin secretion and by improving insulin action. They reduce glycohemoglobin concentrations by approximately 1% to 2%. Metformin, a biguanide, is the second major medication used to improve glycemic control. Metformin lowers glucose by decreasing hepatic glucose production and improving glucose disposal (through nonoxidative metabolic pathways). Glycohemoglobin reduction is usually 1% to 2% (10). Metformin should be used cautiously in patients with renal or hepatic dysfunction. It should also be used cautiously in patients who are at significant risk for hypoxemia—including patients with low cardiac output. When metformin is used in such patients there is increased risk for lactic acidosis. Furthermore, clearance of the drug is affected by radiocontrast agents; for patients who may need coronary angiography, temporarily withholding metformin is advisable. Acarbose, an α-glucosidase inhibitor ("starch blocker") is safe to use in cardiac patients because the drug is essentially nonabsorbable. This agent works by slowing carbohydrate absorption in the gut and reduces glycohemoglobin by about 0.5% to 1% (11–13). Gastrointestinal side effects such as bloating, flatulence, and diarrhea limit the use of acarbose in some patients. Each of the above agents may be used as monotherapy or in combination with each of the other agents because they have additive efficacy.

Troglitazone, a thiazolidinedione (14, 15), improves insulin sensitivity in peripheral tissues. It lowers glycohemoglobin by about 1% to 2%. It may be used as monotherapy, with sulfonylureas or with insulin. (Current data on use with metformin are limited, but there does appear to be improved glycemic control with this combination.) There do not appear to be significant contraindications to use with renal or cardiac disease.

When oral glucose-lowering agents fail to work or renal or hepatic dysfunction limit their use, then insulin therapy usually is initiated in patients with type 2 DM. There generally is a progression, with time, to worsening glycemic control, and, by 20 years of known DM, approximately 40% of all patients take insulin. Approximately 6.6% of all persons between the ages of 20 and 74 years have type 2 DM (16), with a progressive incidence from 2.0% between the ages of 20 and 44 years to 17.7% between the ages of 65 and 74 years. The National Health and Nutrition Examination Study (NHANES II) results indicate that about one-half of all persons with type 2 DM do not know that they have the disease (16).

Whereas the nature of cardiac disease is not apparently different between these 2 types of DM, there may be differences in the cardiac rehabilitation programs in terms of how to deal with caloric intake—especially in conjunction with exercise—and medication administration programs. These issues are discussed next.

RISK OF CORONARY HEART DISEASE IN DIABETES MELLITUS

Diabetes mellitus doubles the risk for CHD events (17–20). The impact of DM on the risk for CHD is particularly evident in young to middle-aged diabetic women in whom the risk for CHD is five to six times greater than their nondiabetic counterparts. The CHD risk in such women is approximately the same as in their male counterparts. Although it is clear that diabetes is an independent risk factor for CHD and is associated with accelerated atherosclerosis, it is not entirely clear whether DM can initiate the atherosclerotic process or whether it accelerates atherosclerosis initiated by other mechanisms (21). There are accumulating data to demonstrate that CHD risk factors are more commonly found (i.e., "cluster") in diabetic patients. Patients with diabetes are more likely to be obese, but, even when obesity is factored out, they are more likely to be hypertensive or have abnormal lipid profiles. Hypertriglyceridemia with an associated low high-density lipoprotein cholesterol (HDL-C) concentration is a common dyslipidemia associated with DM. This lipid profile is associated with a small, dense low-density lipoprotein cholesterol (LDL-C). Furthermore, part of the CHD risk may be associated with an increased risk for coronary thrombosis as a result of increased platelet aggregation or altered fibrinolysis because of elevated plasminogen activator inhibitor-1 (PAI-1) levels (22–24). This combination of risk factors (25–28) and their management play a role in the cardiac rehabilitation process as described next.

Finally, the mortality associated with myocardial infarctions (MIs) in diabetic patients is higher than that in patients without DM. The Minnesota Heart Survey (29) showed that this was true for in-hospital mortality and reported a 40% increased risk of death 6 years after an MI. This increased mortality occurs in both sexes, although overall it appears to be greater in women (29, 30). The mortality risk may be disproportionately higher in diabetic patients after MI when they have fewer preinfarction risk factors (31).

Angiographic studies comparing diabetic patients with nondiabetic patients have shown greater frequency of major stenoses in intermediate segments of major vessels (32) and more diffuse disease (33). In addition, diabetic patients show a greater frequency of interventricular conduction defects and manifestations of left ventricular (LV) dysfunction (32). These differences are not always associated with greater severity of CHD. There is some evidence that there may be "small-vessel" disease in the myocardium and that this may exist in conjunction with atherosclerotic heart disease. It is difficult to distinguish any contribution of this small-vessel disease to diabetes-related heart disease. Because there is no clear evidence that any small-vessel disease has a major impact on the nature of cardiac rehabilitation in the diabetic patient, this subject is not addressed in this chapter.

Coronary heart disease risk reduction in diabetic patients is an important consideration. Observational studies suggest that incremental increases in mean blood glucose are associated with an increased risk for CHD events (34–36). Whether reduction in CHD risk will be associated with glucose lowering has yet to be established. Analyses of data in diabetic patients who have participated in randomized trials of cholesterol lowering clearly demonstrate that the benefits of cholesterol lowering to reduce the risk for CHD events are the same or greater in diabetic patients compared with nondiabetic subjects in the same trial (37–40). Finally, benefits of aspirin (which is commonly used in patients in cardiac rehabilitation programs) have been demonstrated to reduce the risk for CHD events in diabetic patients (41, 42).

COMPLICATIONS OF DIABETES MELLITUS THAT AFFECT CORONARY HEART DISEASE AND REHABILITATION

Diabetes is associated with numerous chronic complications (43) that may affect the management of patients with diabetes, especially during the cardiac rehabilitation period (Table 11.3). These complications include the following:

1. Neuropathy—autonomic and peripheral
2. Retinopathy
3. Nephropathy
4. Atherosclerotic vascular disease

Surgical intervention related to CHD has specific implications in patients with DM, probably as a direct result of the dysmetabolism that occurs. Both saphenous vein coronary artery bypass grafts and vessels opened by percutaneous transluminal coronary angioplasty (PTCA) are at greater risk for occlusion in patients with DM. There is also a greater risk of sternal wound infections after coronary artery bypass grafts—especially with one or two internal thoracic artery grafts in diabetic patients. The effect of these complications of diabetes is discussed next.

Neuropathy is one of the major complications of DM, and problems associated with autonomic neuropathy (44, 45) may have a significant impact on the management of CHD. Autonomic neuropathy is commonly associated with a resting tachycardia and orthostatic hypotension. Patients are not always symptomatic. Autonomic neuropathy may be associated with an increased risk for "silent" myocardial ischemia as assessed by stress thallium testing (46), although this has not been demonstrated with all types of exercise testing (47). Diabetic patients show a delayed anginal perception threshold compared with nondiabetic subjects. The risk for silent myocardial disease is associated with increased duration of DM as well as with microvascular complications (i.e., diabetic retinopathy and nephropathy). Finally, in many patients with longstanding type 1 diabetes, autonomic neuropathy is associated with an impaired counterregulatory response to hypoglycemia—hypoglycemic unawareness. Both glucagon secretion and the adrenergic response to hypoglycemia are impaired. Because most patients rely on adrenergic symptoms, patients who lose the adrenergic response have difficulty detecting hypoglycemia. Loss of these hormones in response to hypo-

TABLE 11.3.   Complications of Diabetes Mellitus and Variables That Affect Cardiac Rehabilitation

Complication	Possible Impact on Rehabilitation
Neuropathy	
Autonomic	Resting tachycardia
	Orthostatic blood pressure changes
	"Silent" myocardial ischemia
	Unrecognized hypoglycemia/impaired glucose counterregulation
Peripheral	Lower extremity ulcer or callus
	Lower extremity amputations
	Loss of kinesthetic sense leading to gait problems
Retinopathy	Decreased visual acuity; may limit use of anticoagulant/antiplatelet therapy (proliferative retinopathy)
Nephropathy	Associated hypertension; may affect selection of antihypertensive agents
	Hemodialysis, CAPD, S/P renal transplant (associated reduced mobility, dietary restrictions, concerns for drug interactions)
	Affects selection of glucose-lowering agents
Atherosclerotic vascular disease	Increased risk of vein graft or PTCA-associated occlusion
	Increased risk of stroke
	Increased risk of lower extremity ischemia
	Increased risk of postoperative wound infections
	Consideration for aggressive cholesterol lowering

CAPD = chronic ambulatory peritoneal dialysis; PTCA = percutaneous transluminal coronary angioplasty; S/P = status post.

glycemia also results in impairment of the intrinsic counterregulatory response to correct hypoglycemia; there is a reduced capability to detect hypoglycemia and initiate exogenous caloric intake, as well as reduced glycogenolysis and gluconeogenesis for endogenous correction of hypoglycemia. Changes in diet, exercise, and medication, in conjunction with rehabilitation, must address these problems with autonomic neuropathy.

Peripheral neuropathy is most commonly associated with loss of sensation in the feet. In the most severe cases, neurotrophic foot ulcers or lower extremity amputation as a result of such ulcers may limit activity. Less common problems include significant lower extremity weakness or loss of kinesthetic sense. Both limit ambulatory capabilities. Foot inspection for calluses, blisters, or infection; absolute avoidance of walking barefoot; and in some cases, prescription footwear should be part of the overall management of diabetic patients, especially those participating in a cardiac rehabilitation program.

The microvascular complications of DM include retinopathy and nephropathy. In general, these conditions have only a limited direct effect on the management of cardiovascular disease in diabetic patients. Severe proliferative retinopathy—especially if it has not been treated adequately—is associated with an increased risk for intraocular bleeding. When such a risk exists, the use of anticoagulants, including aspirin, may be inadvisable. Ophthalmologic stabilization of proliferative retinopathy with laser photocoagulation is necessary, and the decision about the use of anticoagulation must be done with overall assessment of benefits for cardiovascular disease versus possible risks for visual loss. For most diabetic patients with retinopathy whose eyes are stable, anticoagulant therapy does not pose an unacceptable risk. Patients with diabetic retinopathy may have decreased visual acuity as a result of macular edema or retinal hemorrhage, or from laser therapy. Retinopathy that involves the macula usually has its greatest effect on reading vision, whereas laser therapy is more likely to affect peripheral vision. Loss of peripheral vision usually is less problematic to patients.

Diabetic nephropathy has been associated with an increased risk for CHD (48). Patients with diabetic nephropathy who have CHD require some special consideration. First, the well-known risks of radiocontrast materials used with angiography must be considered for those patients who need such procedures. Adequate hydration and care in the selection of quantity and type of radiocontrast material reduce the risk of compromised renal function. Second, the presence of nephropathy may play a role in the selection of antihypertensive drug therapy or in the selection of diuretics for patients with congestive heart failure (CHF). Accumulating evidence suggests that hypertension is associated with the rate of loss of renal function in diabetic patients. Aggressive management of hypertension is indicated in such patients, and data suggest that angiotensin-converting enzyme (ACE) inhibitors may have particularly beneficial effects on slowing the loss of renal function (49–54). Angiotensin II receptor antagonists and calcium-channel blockers may also be beneficial in protecting renal function. Currently these agents are selected when hyperkalemia, cough, or other considerations limit the use of ACE inhibitors. Furthermore, the degree of renal functional impairment may affect the selection of diuretic therapy in patients with diabetic nephropathy. Thiazide diuretics may not only be less effective under these circumstances, they also may have an adverse effect on blood glucose and lipid profiles (55).

In diabetic patients who require surgical intervention for their CHD, some particular considerations must be addressed. First, for both coronary artery bypass graft procedures and PTCA, insulin-requiring DM is a significant risk factor for early occlusion (56–58). Whether this is a function of glycemic control or some other effect of the dysmetabolism of diabetes is still unknown. There is limited information on how early this occlusion may occur, but it may well be in the early postoperative period. Second, the presence of diabetes is associated with an increased risk for sternal wound infections. This is especially true when two internal thoracic artery grafts are used (59). Because this risk may exceed 7%, this complication must be considered in the early postoperative period. Overall postoperative mortality—both in-hospital and long-term—has been higher in diabetic patients in some series (60), but this is not a consistent finding (61).

CARDIAC REHABILITATION IN THE DIABETIC PATIENT

Management of Early Stages

Cardiac rehabilitation in the diabetic patient may be divided into two major stages. The early stage includes the period of hospitalization after an MI or the period immediately after a surgical procedure. The later stage usually consists of the first several months after discharge. Each stage is associated with several risk factors for elevated blood glucose levels. The "stress" of an MI is associated with release of hormones that have potent counterregulatory effects on insulin. This increased insulin resistance is associated with worsening of hyperglycemia. The hormones involved include epinephrine, growth hormone, and cortisol. Hyperglycemia is particularly common in patients undergoing coronary artery bypass graft procedures. This elevation of blood glucose (62) begins during rewarming (perhaps as a result of insulin binding to pump oxygenator membranes) and persists into the postoperative state. Furthermore, complicated medical and surgical patients frequently require the administration of pressor agents, resulting in increased glucose concentrations through the mechanisms of insulin resistance. This immediate post-MI or surgical period usually is best handled by aggressive insulin administration given by continuous intravenous infusion or frequent administration of subcutaneous insulin. Insulin infusions with blood glucose targeted to a mildly hyperglycemic range (120 to 150 mg/dL) can often be achieved without difficulty by experienced nurses in the intensive care unit. After this immediate stage, which usually lasts less than 72 hours, there is a transition into routine management of blood glucose. This management may involve diet only, or it may include oral glucose-lowering agents or insulin for glycemic control. The approach to glycemic control in this stage is governed by a number of variables (Table 11.4), including the following:

1. The nature of the preoperative therapy and associated level of glycemic control.
2. The nature of the nutrient intake.
3. Level of activity or exercise.
4. Blood glucose levels in the hospital.

Each of these will be discussed in turn.

The prehospitalization treatment regimens and level of glycemic control are good predictors of future therapy. For type 1 DM continued use of insulin is absolutely necessary, and prehospitalization doses will be good predictors of insulin needs in many patients. For type 2 diabetic patients, the typical progression from dietary therapy to oral agents to an insulin-requiring state as a result of a progressive loss of insulin production by the pancreas with time helps to determine therapy in the rehabilitation period. As noted previously, with 20 years of known type 2 DM, approximately 50% of all such patients require insulin for satisfactory glycemic control. The recent addition of more oral agents to the pharmacologic armamentarium for glucose control will undoubtedly reduce the number of people on insulin and delay the need for insulin by several years in many patients. Without significant weight loss, it is unusual for patients on oral agents to have their blood glucose levels controlled adequately by diet alone or for insulin-requiring patients to be able to revert back to oral-agent therapy. Furthermore, the preoperative dose of oral agents or insulin is likely to be a good predictor of future doses. For patients with poorly controlled diabetes in the prehospitalization period, the rehabilitation period may be an opportune time to advance the pharmacotherapy by adding an additional oral agent (taking into account the contraindications noted above) or making a change to insulin. Some patients who were on diet only or diet plus oral agents may require short-term use of insulin for adequate glycemic control, either because of marked hyperglycemia or inability to take oral glucose-lowering agents.

Nutritional intake is perhaps the single most important variable in the management of blood glucose in the early cardiac rehabilitation period. In very ill patients who may be malnourished, blood glucose levels actually may be low as a result of poor intake, depleted glycogen stores, and protein malnutrition, leading to low hepatic gluconeogenesis. This is most likely to occur in patients with severe renal disease in conjunction with DM. This group of patients and those with poor oral intake usually require parenteral or enteral feeding. Such feeding usually is associated with a relatively high caloric intake in the range

Table 11.4.   Variables That Affect Glycemic Control During Cardiac Rehabilitation

Prior need for glucose-lowering drugs
Prehospitalization level of glycemic control
Variability in nutrient intake during rehabilitation
Variability in activity/exercise regimens
Studies and procedures that interfere with diet and medication administration
Effects of other medications
Change in renal function

of 35 kcal/kg per 24 hours and associated relatively high insulin requirements, either from endogenous or exogenous sources. For parenteral feeding the insulin can be administered as a component of the feeding solution or as a separate intravenous drip. Insulin infusion rates should be targeted to keep blood glucose levels in the range of 120 to 150 mg/dL. This range minimizes the risk of hypoglycemia and prevents caloric losses in the urine. Occasionally, the combination of parenteral feeding with other intravenous fluids results in marked hyperglycemia that looks like insulin resistance. This usually is the result of a total caloric load in excess of 40 to 50 kcal/kg per 24 hours. This caloric load exceeds the limits of nutrient disposal for most people. The problem must be treated with a reduction in nutrient administration. For enteral feeding with constant infusion rates, subcutaneous insulin given as a mixture of intermediate-acting and regular insulin on a 6- or 8-hour schedule provides a stable reservoir of insulin. Premixed buffered insulins work well for this purpose, e.g., giving 70/30 insulin every 8 hours and targeting blood glucose values into the 150-mg/dL range (80 to 180 mg/dL). It is often necessary to start with coverage R insulin on an every 4-hour dosing schedule for blood sugar values more than 180 mg/dL. Every 24 hours the total dose of R used during that time period is added in equally divided doses to the 70/30 insulin regimen. There is a risk of hypoglycemia if such enteral feeding is stopped inadvertently or deliberately.

For patients who progress through usual oral feeding schedules from liquids to a full diabetic diet, progressive adjustment must be made in the pharmacotherapy. Some of this adjustment needs to anticipate the patient's oral intake to maintain satisfactory glycemic control. For example, patients who have taken a full liquid diet without much hyperglycemia may need to be given oral glucose-lowering agents or insulin on the first day that they take increased calories in the form of a typical diabetic diet. Starting drug therapy—even at low doses—before oral caloric intake increases may avoid unnecessary hyperglycemia. Although the oral intake is limited, oral glucose-lowering agents may be started at lower doses than those needed in the prehospitalization period.

Insulin regimens need to be tailored on the basis of the general principals shown in Table 11.5, section A. First, approximately 50% of all insulin needs are for metabolic reasons independent of nutrient intake. Second, insulin administration should be timed to correspond to nutrient intake. This means that for insulin-requiring patients, intermediate- or long-acting (e.g., NPH, Lente, Ultralente) insulins can be initiated before full nutrient intake. It also means that shorter-acting insulins (e.g., regular, semilente, or short-acting insulin analogs) may be initiated in the preprandial state as patients begin to eat. The common practice of using "coverage" insulin schedules always means that insulin is given several hours after it was needed. Such coverage schedules should be used only to deal with marked hyperglycemia, and then appropriate adjustments must be made in the insulin regimen on subsequent days. For example, if a patient is consistently hyperglycemic late in the afternoon, appropriate increases in the prebreakfast intermediate-acting insulin or the prelunch regular insulin should be made on subsequent days.

Initial exercise regimens in the hospital do not play a major role in pharmacotherapy because the amount of exercise generates relatively low caloric expenditure and also is unlikely to have a major effect on insulin absorption in contrast to the more vigorous regimens.

One common problem that affects the management of diabetes in the hospitalized patient is the impact of studies and procedures—including

Table 11.5.   Insulin Use During Cardiac Rehabilitation

A. General Principles of Insulin Use
   50% of insulin is needed for basal metabolic needs
   50% of insulin is needed for cover nutrient intake
   Insulin administration should "anticipate" nutrient intake
   Insulin concentration should correspond to nutrient intake (e.g., peaks for postprandial glycemic excursion;
      stable levels for continuous nutrient intake)
      "Coverage" schedules have limited use
         Use only for marked hyperglycemia
         Insulin administration is always too late
B. Principles of Insulin Use in Type 1 Diabetes Mellitus
   Necessary for survival
   Usual doses are about 0.5–1.0 units/kg/24 hours
   Multiple-dose regimens are always necessary
      Anticipate insulin needs based on
      Change in diet
         Progression with rehabilitation
         Missed or delayed meals for studies or procedure
      Change in activity/exercise
   Quantity of exercise
   Timing of exercise
   Type of exercise
C. Principles of Insulin Use in Type 2 Diabetes Mellitus
   Not necessary for survival
   Total dose more variable that type 1 DM
      Residual β-cell function may lower dose requirements
      Insulin resistance increases dose requirements
   Weight loss (in obese patients) usually associated with reduced requirements
   Anticipate needs based on diet and activity (see section B)

radiographs, education, and physical or occupational therapy—carried out as a part of routine care. Many times such procedures interfere with the timing of meals and administration of medication, including insulin. Patients who have had their insulin given earlier are at risk for hypoglycemia when meals are delayed. Sometimes studies require NPO (nothing per mouth) status, and appropriate reductions in oral glucose-lowering agents or insulin should be made under these circumstances. Usually oral glucose-lowering agents can be held until the patient is eating again. In insulin-requiring patients, a reduction to about 50% of the usual insulin dose is appropriate for the morning of the procedure. This generally should be given as intermediate-acting insulin. If patients return early enough to avoid a major reduction in caloric intake, then some or all of the remaining dose of insulin can be given before resumption of nutrient intake.

Management of Late Stages

By the time patients have been discharged, they usually are close to total caloric needs and appropriate caloric distribution. If appropriate adjustments in pharmacologic agents to lower glucose have been made during the hospitalization, then only minor changes usually are necessary in the early posthospitalization period. It is during this time that other variables may have greater impact on glycemic control. Regular exercise may have acute and chronic effects on glycemic control. This is a particularly important variable in insulin-requiring patients. The issues are slightly different for type 1 diabetic patients (see Table 11.5, section B) than for type 2 diabetic patients (see Table 11.5, section C)—except for the subset who are quite sensitive to insulin and may be characterized as "brittle."

In type 1 diabetic patients the first consideration is the overall effect of diet and exercise. Multiple-dose insulin regimens (time- and dose-adjusted to caloric intake and based on glucose determinations) are the best way to achieve good glycemic control. A major consideration for exercise adjustments is whether the patient is in reasonably good glycemic control. Poorly controlled type 1 diabetic patients who are not at proper insulin levels may become more hyperglycemic during the course of exercise (63, 64). This is associated with a predisposition to ketosis; therefore, every attempt should be made to improve glycemic control before initiating a regular exercise program. In patients who have normal or nearly normal glycemic control, there are two approaches to the management of blood glucose during exercise—decreasing the dose of insulin or increasing the caloric intake to compensate for energy expenditure. In general it is easier to increase caloric intake with the intention of maintaining blood glucose levels approximately the same after exercise as in the preexercise period. As a starting adjustment, approximately 50% of the total caloric expenditure from the exercise can be administered before exercise. For example, for 30 minutes of jogging with a projected caloric expenditure of 300 kcal, approximately 150 kcal in the form of carbohydrate can be used as an initial caloric replacement. This quantity of food can then be adjusted from the relationship of preexercise and postexercise blood glucose levels.

The nature of drug therapy in type 2 diabetes is determined by blood glucose levels measured on the proper diet. Oral agent doses and insulin doses may be adjusted in either direction. For patients with central obesity (a clinical marker of insulin resistance), metformin use is associated with improved glycemic control and some weight loss. As noted above it must be used cautiously in patients with renal compromise or hypoxemic risk. Troglitazone also lowers blood glucose by reducing insulin resistance. Weight loss is not uniformly seen with troglitazone use. The principles of insulin therapy are different for type 2 diabetic patients. Because this disease is characterized by insulin resistance, many patients may require higher doses of insulin than are typically used in type 1 DM. Some patients with residual β-cell function may have satisfactory control of blood sugars with a single injection of insulin per day; however, most patients on insulin require a multiple-dose regimen. In type 2 DM part of the role of an exercise program is to facilitate weight reduction and to help lower glucose levels (3, 5–8) and, in many cases, corresponding lipid abnormalities. In obese type 2 diabetic patients, it usually is better to reduce insulin (or oral agents) rather than increase calories when blood glucose levels decrease to facilitate weight reduction.

There is one more consideration of insulin use with exercise regimens. Exercise may affect the absorption of insulin as a result of changes in skin temperature and blood flow to tissues surrounding the exercising muscle (65). Because most exercise regimens involve lower extremity muscles, there may be less variability in insulin absorption if it is given routinely into the subcutaneous tissue in the abdomen. There may be delayed effects of exercise on glucose levels. Type 1 diabetic patients, especially, may be at risk for hypoglycemic reactions up to 12 hours after exercise, including nocturnal hypoglycemia (66). If this is a problem, caloric intake may need to be increased later in the day or an appropriate reduction in insulin dose must be initiated.

Finally, patients with peripheral neuropathy that predisposes to loss of sensation in the lower extremities deserve some special consideration when they participate in regular exercise regimens. Poorly fitting shoes may result in unrecognized blister or callus formation, which increases the risk for disruption in the integrity of the skin and, in turn, the risk for infection. Patients and health care professionals must check the feet of diabetic patients on a regular basis. Many manufacturers of athletic footwear make variable width shoes and shoes into which specially designed orthotics may be inserted to redistribute the weight-bearing surfaces of the feet. This reduces the risk for blister or callus formation. In circumstances in which there may be foot deformities, including Charcot changes in the joint, ideally, exercise regimens should minimize or eliminate impact on the feet. These patients also usually require specially designed shoes that can be fitted by properly trained orthoticists.

EFFECT OF OTHER MEDICATIONS ON THE MANAGEMENT OF DIABETES MELLITUS

Because polypharmacy is common in diabetic patients, especially those with CHD, the effect of other drugs on the management of diabetic patients needs to be considered (Table 11.6). The major considerations include the adverse or beneficial effects on glycemic control of commonly

Table 11.6. Effects on Blood Glucose and Lipoproteins of Drugs Commonly Used in Diabetes Mellitus

Drug	Possible Effects
Antihypertensive agents	
Thiazides	Increase glucose, TC, LDL-C, and TG
β-Blockers	Increase TG
	Impair detection of hypoglycemic reactions
ACE inhibitors	Facilitate glucose disposal
	Slow progression of nephropathy
α-Adrenergic blockers	Decrease TG; raise HDL-C
Lipid-lowering agents	
Nicotinic acid	Increase glucose (insulin resistance)
Fibric acid derivatives	Improve glucose disposal
Bile acid-binding resins	Increase TG; impair absorption of other drugs

TC = total cholesterol; LDL-C = low-density lipoprotein cholesterol; TG = triglycerides; HDL-C = high-density lipoprotein cholesterol; ACE = angiotensin-converting enzyme.

used medications as well as the possible effects on dyslipidemias commonly seen in diabetic patients (67–70). These things are particularly true for type 2 diabetic patients who are more likely to have dyslipidemia—especially elevations of very low-density lipoproteins and triglycerides—and have hypertension (21, 25–27).

Several antihypertensive agents have possible adverse effects on the management of diabetic patients. Thiazide diuretics have been associated with worse glycemic control (51, 67–70) as a result of suppressing insulin secretion and increasing insulin resistance. (Associated hypokalemia may also worsen glycemic control.) They also have a tendency to increase LDL-C and triglycerides, at least during a period of weeks to months. The concerns of increased mortality in patients with abnormal electrocardiograms (ECGs) in conjunction with thiazide use (71) may be of particular consideration in diabetic patients. β-Blockers have a number of possible adverse effects. There may be some associated worsening of hyperglycemia and hypertriglyceridemia. In insulin-dependent diabetic patients these agents may limit the ability of patients who are prone to insulin reactions to detect such reactions. There may be beneficial effects from ACE inhibitors that seem to facilitate glucose disposal and α-adrenergic agents (72) which have a beneficial effect to lower triglycerides and raise HDL-C. Calcium-channel blockers appear to be glucose and lipid neutral. In patients with evidence of diabetic nephropathy, there is clear evidence that rigorous blood pressure control may slow the loss of renal function (49–51). There are good animal and human data to support the beneficial effects of ACE inhibitors and calcium-channel blockers in the protection of residual renal function in patients with diabetic nephropathy.

Lipid-lowering agents also may have effects on glycemic control. Niacin may be associated with worsening of glycemic control, presumably because it increases insulin resistance. It should be used only in diabetic patients who are in good glycemic control and in whom hyperinsulinemia is not a major concern. The fibric acid derivatives do not have any adverse effect on glycemic control and there is evidence to suggest that they may have beneficial effects by reducing CHD risk (37). Consequently, these agents generally are the first choice for diabetic patients with hypertriglyceridemia. In patients with elevations of LDL-C, either 3-hydroxy-3-methylglutaryl coenzyme A (HMG-CoA) reductase inhibitors or bile acid-binding resins may be used. The HMG-CoA reductase inhibitors are generally safer and there are data to support their efficacy in CHD risk reduction (38–40). Resins tend to elevate triglycerides and may interfere with the absorption of other drugs.

Anticoagulant therapy in diabetic patients requires some special considerations, including the effects of other drugs used in diabetes and concerns in patients with proliferative retinopathy. Compounds that contain warfarin may be affected by the use of sulfonylureas in diabetic patients. First-generation sulfonylureas (tolbutamide, tolazamide, chlorpropamide) tend to be bound to plasma proteins (9). Initiating therapy with such agents may increase the effect of warfarin compounds, and changing from these to second-generation agents or insulin may produce the opposite effect. In general, patients on such anti-coagulation regimens who require sulfonylurea treatment should take a second-generation agent (glipizide, glyburide). For diabetic patients who take bile acid-binding resins to control elevations of LDL-C, the possible impaired absorption of warfarin needs to be kept in mind. All patients with proliferative retinopathy may be at increased risk for retinal bleeding in the face of anticoagulation. This risk can be minimized by proper referral for routine ophthalmologic examinations, which ensures that any retinopathy that requires photocoagulation can be initiated in a timely fashion. It does not appear that routine use of compounds that contain warfarin or anti–platelet aggregation agents (e.g., aspirin, persantine) poses any adverse risk in patients with earlier stages of retinopathy.

Diabetic patients are at increased risk for impotence; antihypertensive and antianginal agents may aggravate this problem. Because all antihypertensive agents may contribute to the risk for impotence in male diabetic patients, sometimes a trial of several agents is valuable to minimize this side effect. If no antihypertensive can be found to eliminate the problem, then referral for consideration of penile injection therapy, intraurethral medication administration, vacuum devices, or even penile implants should be considered. Newer oral therapy may be considered for patients who are not on nitrate therapy.

SUMMARY

The diabetic patient is at increased risk for CHD and related events; therefore, DM is common among participants in cardiac rehabilitation programs. The other complications of DM, the impact of diet, exercise, and drugs on glycemic control, and the impact of drug therapy for related problems all pose particular challenges in the management of the diabetic patient who is involved in cardiac rehabilitation.

Part C. Peripheral Arterial Disease

Jeffrey W. Olin and William R. Hiatt

Atherosclerosis that affects the abdominal aorta or lower extremity arteries is referred to as peripheral arterial disease (PAD). Patients with PAD most commonly present with intermittent claudication and less often with ischemic rest pain or gangrene. More importantly, PAD is a marker for generalized atherosclerosis; most patients with PAD die of myocardial infarction or stroke.

Data from the Framingham study (1) reveal an annual age-adjusted incidence of intermittent claudication of 0.3% in men and 0.1% in women. Other investigators have shown that approximately 1.8% of patients younger than 60 years, 3.7% of those 60 to 70 years of age, and 5.2% older than 70 years had intermittent claudication (2). If diabetes mellitus is present, the incidence of claudication increases two- to threefold (3).

The incidence of asymptomatic arterial disease is much higher than the numbers cited above (4, 5). Data from the Systolic Hypertension in the Elderly Study (4) showed that the ankle/brachial systolic blood pressure index (ABI) was less than or equal to 0.90 in 25.5% of the 1537 participants. In the Multicenter Study of Osteoporotic Fractures (5), the ABI was less than or equal to 0.90 in 5.5% of 1492 women entered into this study. This has important prognostic implications because a decreased ABI—even in the absence of claudication—directly correlates with increased cardiovascular mortality.

NATURAL HISTORY OF PERIPHERAL ARTERIAL DISEASE

Limb-related Complications

It is important to recognize that some patients with PAD may be entirely asymptomatic (4, 5). Patients who have disease in a single segment (i.e., superficial femoral artery) often have adequate collaterals, and their limb is not jeopardized (6). Most individuals require tandem lesions or multisegment disease to experience severe limb-threatening ischemia.

Most studies involving large numbers of patients have shown that progression to severe ischemia or amputation is unusual in patients with intermittent claudication. Figure 11.1 shows that only 16% of patients progress to worsening claudication, 7% to lower extremity revascularization, and 4% to major amputation. Many studies support a rate of progression of approximately 1.4% per year. This progression rate is much higher in the diabetic population and in those patients who continued to smoke (7).

These data demonstrate that the limb is not in

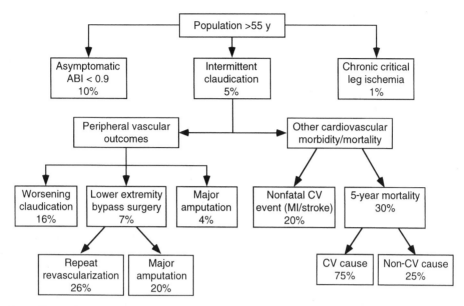

Figure 11.1. Epidemiology of lower extremity arterial disease. (Reprinted with permission from Weitz JI, Byrne J, Clagett GP, et al. Diagnosis and treatment of chronic arterial insufficiency of the lower extremities: a critical review. Circulation 1996;94:3026–3049.)

jeopardy in the majority of individuals with PAD. However it should not be forgotten that intermittent claudication causes a significant walking impairment that profoundly interferes with the patients' activities of daily living. Many patients are so disabled from claudication that they require public assistance (8).

Long-term Survival

Intermittent claudication is a marker for atherosclerosis elsewhere. As previously mentioned, decreases in ABI correlate with long-term cardiovascular mortality (4, 5). Population-based studies and follow-up studies of surgically treated patients indicate that for those individuals with lower extremity occlusive vascular disease, the mortality rate at 5 years is approximately 30%, at 10 years 50%, and at 15 years 70% to 75% (9). Hertzer et al. (10) have demonstrated a very high likelihood of significant asymptomatic coronary artery disease in patients with PAD, abdominal aortic aneurysm, or extracranial cerebrovascular disease.

Criqui and associates (11) showed that the 10-year mortality was 61.7% in men and 33.3% in women with large vessel PAD compared with 16.9% of men and 11.6% of women without evidence of PAD. The relative risk (RR) of dying among subjects with PAD compared to those

without was 3.1 for deaths from all causes, 5.9 for all deaths from cardiovascular disease, and 6.6 for deaths from coronary heart disease.

CLINICAL MANIFESTATION OF PERIPHERAL ARTERIAL DISEASE

The primary symptom of PAD is intermittent claudication. Its onset is usually gradual and often unrecognized by many older adults who may attribute their symptoms to arthritis or simply to aging. Intermittent claudication is usually described as an aching, tiredness, cramping, or discomfort associated with walking. It occurs when the arterial blood supply does not meet the metabolic demand of the muscles in the legs, resulting in muscle ischemia. The discomfort occurs in a muscle group distal to an arterial obstruction. Most characteristically, it occurs in the calf as a result of stenosis or occlusion of the superficial femoral artery or any other proximal vessel. Claudication may also occur in the thigh, hip, and buttock if the obstruction involves the aortoiliac segment or internal iliac arteries. Walking up a grade or at increased speed brings on the discomfort more quickly. In most patients the symptoms are consistent and reproducible. There are three major clinical features in patients with intermittent claudication (6). Depending on variables such as the grade of the terrain and the pace of walking, claudication is reproducible with consistent level of exercise from day to day. Second, it completely resolves within 2 to 5 minutes after exercise has been stopped unless the patient has walked to the point of severe leg pain; then it may take longer for the discomfort to go away. Lastly, the discomfort occurs again at approximately the same distance once walking has been resumed.

Progression to critical limb ischemia is evidenced by the onset of rest pain. Pain at rest characteristically occurs at night when the patient lies supine. Usually described as a dull aching sensation in the toes or forefoot, this sensation may awaken the patient from sleep. The patient may hang the foot over the side of the bed or get up and walk around for relief. As the symptom persists, the individual may start to sleep in a chair with the legs dependent. This often results in a moderate degree of lower extremity edema.

If an individual is able to tolerate ischemic pain at rest, eventually ischemic necrosis between two toes ("kissing ulcer") may occur. Dry gangrene or ulcerations may also begin at the tips of the toes or over pressure points and is common after minor trauma such as nail trimming. By the time tissue necrosis occurs, the individual's ability to walk is usually severely limited.

A careful history and physical examination should be performed on all patients with PAD. A systematic approach should be used to examine the relative strength and quality of the arterial pulsation. Initial examination of the blood pressure in both upper extremities and the palpation of both radial pulses will generally provide a baseline evaluation for comparison with lower extremity pulses. Lower extremity pulsation should be compared in a stepwise fashion beginning with the femoral pulses bilaterally. The popliteal, posterior tibial, and dorsalis pedis pulses of both limbs should be compared with each other, and both of these should be compared with the quality of the radial pulsation. The pulses should be graded as normal, diminished, or absent. Occasionally, patients with typical complaints of intermittent claudication may have palpable pedal pulses at rest. A brief period of walking exercise and reexamination may be required to determine whether the pulses disappear and also whether ankle blood pressure decreases with exercise.

VASCULAR LABORATORY

Although the recording of ABI provides some information at the bedside, segmental Doppler systolic blood pressures and pulse waveform analysis by plethysmography provide more objective information about the level and severity of occlusive disease. Arteriography is the definitive examination and should be reserved for the patient undergoing a revascularization procedure.

Doppler Ankle/Brachial Index

The simplest vascular laboratory test to assess the lower extremity circulation is the ABI. The equipment is inexpensive and consists of an ordinary blood pressure cuff and a Doppler ultrasonic velocity detector. The blood pressure cuff is placed over both brachial areas and inflated to a reading in excess of systolic pressure. Resumption of blood flow is detected with the Doppler probe over the brachial artery. If there is a discrepancy in the readings of the two arms, the higher of the two arm systolic blood pressures is used. Next, the blood pressure cuff is moved to the ankle and inflated to a reading in excess of systolic blood pressure. The Doppler detector is then placed over the posterior tibial artery at the ankle and a separate reading is also made at the dorsalis pedis artery. The higher of the two readings should be used in the calculation of the ABI. The ABI is obtained by dividing the ankle systolic blood pressure by the brachial systolic pressure. Under most circumstances the ABI correlates well with functional symptoms (12). In a normal individual at rest, the index will range from 0.90 to 1.30. Patients with intermittent claudication will have an index that generally ranges from 0.40 to 0.90. Patients experiencing ischemic rest pain will usually have an index of less than 0.40. The absolute ankle pressure may be erroneous in diabetic patients with calcified, noncompressible arteries. In this situation pulse waveform analysis or toe/brachial index is needed to accurately evaluate the circulation. Segmental pressures and pulse-volume recordings can be measured by placing blood pressure cuffs at the thigh, calf, and ankle level to determine the level of occlusive disease. A combination of segmental limb pressure measurements and pulse-volume recording waveform analysis has been accurate to the 97th percentile in predicting the level and extent of occlusive disease (13).

Discussion of other noninvasive tests, such as transcutaneous oximetry, duplex ultrasound, and magnetic resonance angiography, are beyond the scope of this chapter.

MEDICAL MANAGEMENT

Medical management is indicated for all patients with PAD. Some patients will undergo medical management alone whereas others will undergo surgical treatment or endovascular therapy (percutaneous balloon angioplasty or stent) in addition to medical management. Traditionally, intervention has been reserved for patients who experience limb-threatening ischemia (ischemic rest pain or tissue necrosis) or lifestyle-disabling claudication.

There are four main goals in treating patients with PAD: improve functional status, preserve the limb, prevent the progression of atherosclerosis, and reduce cardiac and cerebrovascular morbidity and mortality (Fig. 11.2). Table 11.7 outlines the important components of a medical program for patients with PAD.

Discontinue Cigarette Smoking

Because cigarette smoking is highly correlated with the presence of PAD and its progression, cessation of smoking is mandatory. It is the single most important measure that may prevent the progression of atherosclerosis, improve limb salvage rates, and decrease cardiovascular morbidity and mortality. In the Framingham study (14), cigarette smoking doubled to tripled the risk of intermittent claudication for both men and women. There was a dose-related response between the number of cigarettes smoked and the rate of intermittent claudication for all age groups.

Cigarette smoking is also strongly associated with severe PAD in patients younger than 50 years. Jonason and Ringquist (15) found that in patients who quit smoking after they experienced intermittent claudication, none progressed to rest pain, whereas 16% of patients who continued to smoke had rest pain. Patients who stopped smoking had fewer amputations, fewer myocardial infarctions, and less rest pain, and lived twice as long as those who continued to smoke. In addition, smoking after vascular surgery significantly decreases the patency rate of prosthetic bypass grafts and autologous saphenous vein bypass grafts (16–18). Excluding patients with diabetes, nonsmokers comprise only 1% of all patients with intermittent claudication (19).

Patients who are able to stop smoking successfully may improve their treadmill walking distance, compared with those who continued to smoke (20). The evidence is conclusive that smoking cessation is associated with fewer adverse events related to lower extremity atherosclerosis (21). Every effort should be made to offer assistance to individual patients in their efforts to stop smoking completely. Numerous programs are available for guidance and assistance in stopping this addictive behavior.

Treating Other Risk Factors

It is important to aggressively treat hypertension, hyperlipidemia, glucose intolerance, and diabetes mellitus in patients with PAD. The same principles should be applied to treating these disorders in patients with PAD as with patients who have atherosclerosis elsewhere. Further details regarding risk factor modification are discussed in Chapters 18–20.

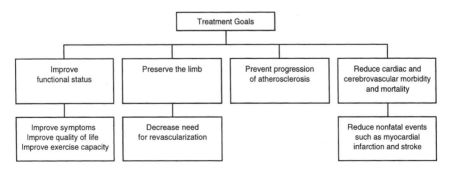

Figure 11.2. Treatment goals in patients with peripheral arterial disease.

Table 11.7.   Factors Important in Affecting the Natural History of Peripheral Arterial Disease

Stop smoking
Exercise
Control blood pressure
Control lipids
Control diabetes
Antiplatelet therapy

Exercise Rehabilitation for Claudication

BACKGROUND

After discontinuation of cigarette smoking, exercise rehabilitation is the next most important step in treating patients with PAD. Exercise has been shown to increase walking distance, improve quality of life, and decrease cardiovascular and all-cause mortality. During the past 35 years, walking exercise has been recommended as a nonsurgical treatment for claudication (22). Subsequent studies of exercise training were conducted in a supervised (usually hospital) setting, with the walking exercise performed on a treadmill (23) or under the direction of a physical therapist (24–26). This allowed a specific exercise intensity to be prescribed that was usually sufficient to bring on at least mild to moderate claudication pain.

TRAINING METHODS

The beginning training workload is determined from the symptom-limited maximal treadmill test on entry, such that the intensity of the treadmill exercise is set to the workload that initially brings on claudication pain in the patient. In subsequent visits, the speed or grade is increased if the patient is able to walk for 10 minutes or longer at the lower workload without reaching moderate claudication pain. Either speed or grade can be increased, but an increase in grade is recommended first if the patient can already walk at 2 mph. An additional goal of the program is to increase patient walking speed up to the "normal" 3.0 mph, from a walking speed of 1.5 to 2.0 mph for the average PAD patient. In addition to treadmill walking exercise, other activities, such as isotonic exercise of specific muscle groups, bicycle exercise, gymnastic exercise, stair climbing, and unsupervised walking in the community, have been incorporated into the training sessions of some programs. However, the value of these other training methods is less well established.

The initial training session is 35 minutes long with subsequent increases of 5 minutes each session until a 50-minute session is possible. During the exercise sessions, the patient walks on the treadmill until a mild or moderate level of pain is reached, followed by a rest period until the pain abates. After the pain is gone, the patient resumes walking until a moderate level of claudication pain is reached again, followed by another rest period. This process is repeated until the 50-minute exercise period has elapsed. In our experience, actual treadmill exercise comprises about 35 minutes, and rest periods total about 15 minutes of the 50-minute exercise time.

Because the morbidity and mortality from coronary artery disease and cerebrovascular disease is so high in patients with PAD (11), it is recommended that a 12-lead electrocardiogram be performed during the initial maximal treadmill test. Some investigators would even perform a full cardiac stress test (dobutamine echocardiogram, dipyridamole thallium scan, positron emission tomographic scan) to uncover occult coronary disease before initiating an exercise rehabilitation program (10, 28). The cost-effectiveness of such an approach has not been clearly demonstrated.

IMPROVEMENTS IN EXERCISE PERFORMANCE

A review of the literature has identified 28 trials of exercise conditioning in the PAD population, of which 13 employed a controlled (sometimes randomized) design (25–27, 29–38). Table 11.8 summarizes the results of the supervised training programs. In most of these studies, the change in walking ability with treatment was evaluated with a constant-load (fixed) treadmill protocol. The improvement in pain-free walking time ranged from 44% to 290%, with an average increase of 134%. The peak walking time increased from 25% to 183%, with an average increase of 96%. Thus, the ability to sustain walking exercise for a longer duration with less claudication pain was improved by training. Studies that employ a graded treadmill protocol have shown improvements in peak exercise performance and peak oxygen consumption (33). The improvement in peak oxygen consumption indicates that patients can perform activities requiring higher work intensities, such as climbing stairs, gardening, and dancing—activities that were not possible on entry into the study. These same studies have also

Table 11.8.   Randomized Controlled Trials of Exercise Therapy in the Treatment of Claudication

Author (year)	Group	n	Duration (months)	Exercise Program[a]	Treadmill[b]	Change in ACD (%)
A. Supervised Exercise Program						
Dahllof	T	23	6	Supervised	Fixed	+117[c,d]
(1974)	C	11		Placebo pill		NC
Dahllof	T	10	4	Supervised	Fixed	+135[c,d]
(1976)	C	6		Placebo pill		+75[c]
Mannarino	T	8	6	Supervised	Fixed	+67[c,d]
(1989)	C	8		Control		+14
Mannarino	T_1	10	6	Supervised + Aspirin	Fixed	−105[c,d]
(1991)	T_2	10		Supervised		+86[c,d]
	T_3	10		Aspirin		+38[c]
Scheffler	T_1	15	1	Supervised	Fixed	+99[c]
(1994)	T_2	15		Supervised + Pentoxifylline		+119[c]
	T_3	14		Supervised + Prostaglandin E_1		+371[c,d]
Regensteiner	T_1	10	3	Supervised	Graded	+137[c,d]
(1997)	T_2	10		Home		+5
Patterson	T_1	19	6	Supervised	Fixed	+195[c,d]
(1997)	T_2	19		Home		+83[c]
B. Treadmill-Based Exercise Training						
Hiatt	T	10	3	Treadmill exercise training	Graded	+123[c,d]
(1990)	C	9		Control		+20
Hiatt	T_1	10	3	Treadmill exercise training	Graded	+74[c,d]
(1994)	T_2			Strength training		+36[c]
	C	8		Control		−1
Holm	T	6	4	Dynamic		+133[c,d]
(1973)	C	6		Placebo pill		NC
Lundgren	T_1	25	6	Surgery + Dynamic	Fixed	+263[c,d]
(1989)	T_2	25		Surgery		+173[c,d]
	T_3	25		Dynamic		+151[c]
Creasy	T_1	20	6	Dynamic	Fixed	+442[c,d]
(1990)	T_2	13		Angioplasty		+57

[a]Exercise programs: Home = unsupervised exercise performed at home consisting of daily walks; Supervised = exercise training performed in a hospital or outpatient facility under the direction of a physical therapist or nurse; Dynamic = jumping, dancing, heel raises.
[b]Type of treadmill test that was performed to determine whether improvement occurred: ACD = Absolute claudication distance.
[c]End of treatment significantly improved compared to baseline value ($P < .05$).
[d]Different between groups ($P < .05$).
T = Treated group, C = Control group, NC = Results reported as no change.

shown that at a given submaximal workload, exercise training decreases heart rate (25, 33), ventilation, and oxygen consumption (33, 36). These changes may contribute to the ability to sustain walking exercise for longer times before claudication pain limits the activity. In addition, there is virtually no morbidity or mortality from exercise rehabilitation.

IMPROVEMENTS IN FUNCTIONAL STATUS

The functional benefits of the training were further assessed by a series of questionnaires (39, 40). This analysis demonstrated that in the community, treated subjects could walk a greater distance, at a faster speed, and thus perform activities that were considered difficult or impossible before

the treatment (e.g., return to work, dancing, outdoor activities, shopping). Control subjects had no change in their level of disability (from questionnaire evaluations) during the course of the study. Thus, a progressive walking exercise program improved exercise performance, relieved the pain of intermittent claudication, and facilitated the ability to perform personal, social, and occupational activities.

MECHANISM OF THE TRAINING EFFECT

The mechanisms by which exercise training improves exercise performance are not well understood. Initially it was believed that an exercise program would increase skeletal muscle blood flow, thereby improving muscle function and walking ability (41). However, we and others have shown that changes in blood flow with training are modest and not correlated to changes in exercise performance (24, 33, 41–43). Another peripheral adaptation with training in PAD is an improvement in muscle metabolism, as evidenced by an increase in the extraction of oxygen across the leg during exercise despite no change in total blood flow (44). Some studies have shown that with exercise training, patients with PAD have increases in muscle enzyme activities, but to a lesser degree as compared to the response of normal subjects (45, 46). Studies in our laboratory have not confirmed these observations, and furthermore, we have not shown a relationship between changes in muscle enzyme activity and improvement in exercise performance. However, we have previously shown that patients with PAD accumulate acylcarnitines (intermediates in oxidative metabolism) in plasma and ischemic muscle (47, 48). Further, this accumulation has functional significance in that patients with the highest levels of acylcarnitines have the worst exercise performance (47). We have previously observed that exercise training reduced the plasma concentration of short-chain acylcarnitines, and treated subjects who had the greatest response to training also had the greatest reduction in the plasma short-chain acylcarnitine concentration (33). In our most recent training studies, similar improvements in muscle carnitine metabolism were observed with exercise training, suggesting that there was an improvement in intermediary metabolism in skeletal muscle. The importance of these findings is that PAD is not simply a disease of abnormal hemodynamics. Therefore, treatment strategies that focus only on improving blood flow (such as surgery) do not necessarily normalize exercise performance.

Drug Therapy for Claudication

VASODILATORS

Arteriolar vasodilators were an early class of agents used to treat claudication. In general, these drugs have not been shown to have clinical efficacy in randomized, controlled trials (49–51). However, in a recent report, verapamil was shown to increase treadmill walking distance in patients with claudication, but only after individual dose titration (52). Despite these findings, as a class of drugs, vasodilators are not recommended for claudication.

ANTIPLATELET DRUGS

The use of aspirin and other antiplatelet agents are important in the long-term treatment of peripheral atherosclerosis. However, there are no studies that have shown benefit of aspirin in the treatment of claudication. The Physician's Health Study (22,071 healthy U.S. males randomized to receive either placebo or 325 mg of aspirin every other day) did show a decrease in the need for peripheral arterial surgery in the aspirin group (RR, 0.54; $P = .03$). In addition, it has been previously demonstrated that aspirin also decreases cardiovascular morbidity and mortality in these patients.

In contrast, ticlopidine is a potent inhibitor of platelet aggregation that also has hemorheologic effects. In two randomized, placebo-controlled trials, ticlopidine was shown to improve claudication symptoms and exercise performance (54, 55). In the Swedish Ticlopidine Multicenter Study (56), when ticlopidine was used in patients with intermittent claudication, sudden death, fatal or nonfatal myocardial infarction, fatal or nonfatal stroke, cardiovascular intervention, and overall mortality were significantly decreased.

The CAPRIE Trial (57) was a randomized, double-blind trial comparing clopidogrel (75 mg once daily) with aspirin (325 mg once daily). Nineteen thousand one hundred eighty-five patients with recent ischemic stroke, recent myocardial infarction, or symptomatic PAD were entered into the study and followed up for 1 to 3 years. The study found that 5.83% of the aspirin group and 5.32% of the clopidogrel group (RR reduction in favor of clopidogrel 8.7%, $P = .043$) experienced a myocardial infarction, stroke, or other vascular death. Therefore, although many trials have not shown that antiplatelet therapy improves the symptoms of PAD, antiplatelet agents should be used in patients with PAD to prevent myocardial infarction, stroke, and vascular death.

HEMORHEOLOGIC AGENTS

Patients with PAD have been shown to have elevated fibrinogen levels, increased blood viscosity, and white cell activation that are all correlated with the severity of disease as defined by the ABI (58). The extent to which these phenomena reduce large vessel blood flow, or flow in the microcirculation, is unknown. Pentoxifylline improves red cell deformability, lowers fibrinogen levels, and decreases platelet aggregation, and has been shown to increase walking distance in patients with PAD. In early controlled trials, the drug produced a 22% improvement compared with placebo in walking distance before the onset of claudication and a 12% improvement in the maximal walking distance (59). A recent meta-analysis has been performed on randomized, controlled trials of pentoxifylline (60). The authors concluded that the drug resulted in a 29.4-m increase in initial claudication distance and a 48.4-m improvement in absolute claudication distance (compared with placebo). They also concluded that additional properly conducted trials were needed to assess the benefits of this drug. Importantly, patient-based questionnaires to assess efficacy have not been used in the clinical trials of pentoxifylline, so the actual clinical benefit of the drug has not been fully defined.

METABOLIC AGENTS

Although the exact mechanism is unknown, it has thus been hypothesized that supplementation of patients with carnitine would improve ischemic muscle metabolism and exercise performance. Carnitine and an acyl form of carnitine, propionyl-L-carnitine, are drugs that have been shown to increase exercise performance and improve claudication symptoms in small phase II trials (61, 62). In addition, propionyl-L-carnitine has been shown to improve quality of life in patients with claudication (63). Larger phase II trials have also shown benefit of propionyl-L-carnitine, with the optimal dose of 2 g/day (64). In a multi-center trial in Europe, 485 patients were randomized to placebo or propionyl-L-carnitine 2 g/day. After 12 months of treatment, the drug resulted in a significant improvement compared with placebo in maximal walking distance on a fixed treadmill protocol. Patients on propionyl-L-carnitine also reported improvements in walking ability in the community setting. Thus, propionyl-L-carnitine was found to be safe and effective in improving treadmill exercise performance and community-assessed functional status.

PROSTAGLANDINS

Beraprost is a PGI_2 analog that is orally active. In a phase II dose-ranging study, 164 patients were randomized to receive either placebo or three doses of drug (65). The improvement in absolute claudication distance compared with placebo was as follows: 60 μg/day produced a 48% increase, 120 μg/day a 51% increase, and 180 μg/day a 31% increase. None of these changes were statistically significant. A concern was that at the highest dose, 62% of the patients reported side effects of headache, flushing, and gastrointestinal intolerance.

CILOSTAZOL

Cilostazol is a phosphodiesterase inhibitor that has vasodilator and antiplatelet activity (66). This agent has been evaluated in several phase III trials. In a large phase III trial (unpublished data from company files), 516 patients with claudication were randomized to receive either placebo or cilostazol 100 or 200 mg/day. Compared to placebo, 100 mg/day resulted in a 39% increase in maximal walking distance, and 200 mg/day a 91% increase (both highly significant). The higher dose of cilostazol also resulted in improvements in walking-defined distances and speeds, vitality, and bodily pain perceptions. Side effects included headache, diarrhea, and dizziness, but there were no more dropouts in the active drug group compared to the placebo group. Thus, cilostazol should prove to be a very effective agent for patients with claudication.

ANGIOGENIC GROWTH FACTORS

Vascular endothelial growth factor (VEGF) and basic fibroblast growth factor (bFGF) are mitogenic agents for the development of new collateral channels in models of peripheral ischemia. In a rabbit model using femoral artery ligation, VEGF has been shown to augment collateral vessel development and increase capillary density in skeletal muscle (67). This effect has been observed when the VEGF protein is administered by intra-arterial infusion and when the DNA encoding for VEGF is given by intramuscular injection (67, 68). Early phase I and phase II trials are now in progress to determine whether this novel therapy has clinical application in patients with claudication and critical leg ischemia.

Randomized, prospective trials have demonstrated ketanserin (a serotonin antagonist) (69), suloctidil, fish oil supplementation, naftidrofuryl, and EDTA chelation therapy (70) are not effective in the treatment of intermittent claudication.

Part D. Chronic Lung Disease
Fredric J. Pashkow

Patients with concurrent chronic obstructive pulmonary disease (COPD) and coronary heart disease are familiar problem patients for most clinicians. The frequency with which this concurrence is seen does not approach that of peripheral vascular disease, for example, but it is common enough that it presents significant challenges in the rehabilitative management of these patients. Certainly these two entities share a major risk factor—cigarette smoking (1)—and smoking cessation is crucial to the therapy of each (2, 3).

PULMONARY REHABILITATION: A MAJOR MODALITY OF THERAPY

Rehabilitation for patients with chronic lung disease is similar conceptually to the rehabilitation of patients with cardiac disease (4–6), though the population of patients appears somewhat different (7). Pulmonary rehabilitation has become an accepted part of pulmonary medical practice (8–10). It too consists of exercise (11), education (12), and psychosocial support (13–15). Respiratory and chest physical therapy, including bronchial hygiene and breathing training, and the application of collateral technologies, such as nasally administered continuous positive airway pressure, are important additional elements in pulmonary rehabilitation (16, 17). The availability of this service and the recognition of its value as a modality of therapy has increased substantially during the last 10 years (9, 17), and it has become a standard component of pulmonary care (18).

RESTRICTIONS TO EXERCISE IN CHRONIC LUNG DISEASE

Patients with concurrent cardiac and lung disease, in addition to having significant exercise limitation from dyspnea, have little or no ventilatory reserve at peak exercise (19, 20). They may desaturate with exercise or have erythrocytosis, lowering their ischemia threshold (21). They are prone to cardiac arrhythmias secondary to hypoxia and hypercarbia (22) and to medications such as bronchodilators that increase the likelihood of arrhythmia (23). They frequently are taking systemic steroids that potentially affect their peripheral conditioning response (24).

EXERCISE AND CHRONIC OBSTRUCTIVE PULMONARY DISEASE

Patients with severe COPD do not improve pulmonary function (6), hemodynamic parameters (25), or peripheral muscle indices with exercise therapy (24). They are rarely able to reach a maximal oxygen uptake or achieve the necessary threshold of exercise level, duration, and frequency required for cardiopulmonary conditioning (24). However, these patients do improve mechanical skills in the trained muscles (26), enjoy improvement in dyspnea (27, 28), and benefit psychologically (5, 15). Elderly patients show comparable benefits to younger patients with similar lung function abnormalities (29, 30). The application of such training, however, has been questioned before lung reduction or lung transplant surgery, and further research has been suggested (31).

ASSESSMENT OF FUNCTION IN PATIENTS WITH COMBINED DISEASE

Similar to patients with peripheral vascular disease, routine techniques of exercise evaluation may produce misleading results. To better characterize functional measures in patients with chronic heart failure and chronic lung disease, Guyatt and colleagues (32) administered functional status questionnaires, a 6-minute walk test, and a cycle ergometer exercise test to patients severely limited in their day-to-day activities as a result of their underlying heart and lung disease. The walk test correlated well with the cycle ergometer, and almost as well with the functional status questionnaires. The results suggest that exercise capacity in the laboratory can be differentiated from the ability to undertake physically demanding activities of daily living and that the walk test provides a good measure of function in patients with combined heart and lung disease (32).

Exercise testing may be helpful in the calculation of a target heart rate for exercise training (21), determining other reasons for dyspnea and potentially important measures of function such as anaerobic threshold using gas analysis (33), assessing the arrhythmic potential of exercise, determining whether oxygen supplementation may be necessary during exercise (34), evaluating often unexpected changes in arterial blood gases, and screening for exercise-induced bronchospasm (35). The appropriate test to use depends on several considerations, including patient and program goals, questions identified in the initial patient evaluation, the specific exercise training program, available laboratory expertise, and cost (35).

CONSIDERATIONS IN THE EXERCISE PRESCRIPTION

All of these measured parameters have important implications with respect to the exercise regimen prescribed—intensity, duration, intermittency, and supervision. Activities that use the upper extremities, such as rowing, may not be appropriate because of the high ventilation required for a given power output (21). Walking, cycling, or swimming may be activities that will be better tolerated. For patients with near normal spirometry and coronary disease who are symptomatic only during heavy exertion, the heart rate method may be used to prescribe exercise intensity (21). Patients with mild-to-moderate ventilatory impairment (forced vital capacity [FVC] and forced expiratory volume in 1 second [FEV_1] 60% to 80% of predicted), should have their exercise intensity maintained at a level at which the ventilatory rate is less than 75% of the patient's maximal exercise ventilation. Those more severely impaired (FVC and FEV_1 less than 60% predicted, or desaturation of O_2 at rest or with exercise), should be regulated with the use of a dyspnea scale (21).

Patients who demonstrate O_2 desaturation with exercise will benefit from oxygen supplementation during exercise (36, 37). Transtracheal oxygen therapy (38) has been demonstrated to improve exercise tolerance (39), and in our experience has allowed pulmonary rehabilitation in patients who otherwise would not have been able to participate. Patients will often require modification of the duration and frequency of the exercise regimen. For example, an intermittent regimen of two 10-minute sessions may be preferable to one 20-minute continuous session (21). A patient with very severe disease-limitation to exercise may better tolerate four 5-minute sessions. As the patient progresses, the duration of the exercise intervals can be increased while the rest intervals are short-ened (21). Our experience has been that even patients with very severe combined disease will derive enough benefit from the program that they will report greater subjective functional capacity and self-efficacy (40) and less anxiety and depression (15, 18). The impact of the education and improved pulmonary toilet are important potential benefits as well (12).

HOME-BASED PROGRAMS OF POTENTIAL BENEFIT

Analogous to the movement for at-home therapy in cardiac patients, and in an effort to overcome similar obstacles to participation that occur in pulmonary rehabilitation (41), several papers have looked at the issue of home-based programs for pulmonary patients (42–45). Wijkstra et al. (45) found that 12 weeks of rehabilitation at home under supervision by general practitioners, physiotherapists, and home nurses for patients with moderate to severe COPD had a beneficial effect on lactate production, metabolic gas exchange data, and dyspnea during exercise. Compliance with such home-based programs is high, complications are infrequent, and those performing the therapy report that it appears feasible to provide the service (43). Equal improvement was reported in exercise capacity and perceived dyspnea in patients who underwent rehabilitation in a hospital-based program versus a group randomized to a home program, but those in the home program continued to improve with time. Improvements in cycle ergometer workload and the dyspnea score were significantly better maintained after home training as compared with hospital-based patients (42).

References

Part A.
1. Helgeland A. Treatment of mild hypertension: a five-year controlled drug trial. The Oslo study. Am J Med 1980;69:725–732.
2. Medical Research Council Working Party MRC trial of treatment of mild hypertension: principal results. Br Med J 1985;291:97–104.
3. Houston MC. New insights and new approaches for the treatment of essential hypertension: selection of therapy based on coronary heart disease risk factor analysis, hemodynamic profiles, quality of life, and subsets of hypertension. Am Heart J 1989;117:911–951.
4. Joint National Committee on Prevention, Detection, Evaluation, and Treatment of High Blood Pressure. The sixth report of the Joint National Committee on

Prevention, Detection, Evaluation, and Treatment of High Blood Pressure. Arch Intern Med 1997;157: 2413–2446.

5. Kaplan NM. Importance of coronary heart disease risk factors in the management of hypertension. Am J Med 1989;86(Suppl 1B):1–4.

6. Wilhelmsen L. Risks of untreated hypertension. Hypertension 1989;13(Suppl 1):133–135.

7. Paffenbarger RS, Wing AL, Hyde RT, et al. Physical activity and incidence of hypertension in college alumni. Am J Epidemiol 1983;117:245–257.

8. Blair SN, Goodyear NN, Gibbons LW, et al. Physical fitness and incidence of hypertension in healthy normotensive men and women. JAMA 1984;252:487–490.

9. Darga LL, Lucas CP, Spafford TR, et al. Endurance training in middle-aged male physicians. Physician Sportsmed 1989;17:85–101.

10. Hagberg JM. Exercise, fitness, and hypertension. In: Bouchard C, ed. Exercise, fitness, and health: a consensus of current knowledge. Champaign, IL: Human Kinetics, 1990:455–466.

11. Gordon NF, Scott CB, Wilkinson JW, et al. Exercise and mild hypertension. Recommendations for adults. Sports Med 1990;10:390–404.

12. Gilders RM, Voner C, Dudley GA. Endurance training and blood pressure in normotensive and hypertensive adults. Med Sci Sports Exerc 1989;21:629–636.

13. Tipton CM. Exercise, training and hypertension: an update. Exerc Sport Sci Rev 1991;19:447–505.

14. Duncan JJ, Farr JE, Upton SJ, et al. The effects of aerobic exercise on plasma catecholamines and blood pressure in patients with mild essential hypertension. JAMA 1985;254:2609–2613.

15. Kiyonaga A, Arakawa K, Tanaka H, et al. Blood pressure and hormonal responses to aerobic exercise. Hypertension 1985;7:125–131.

16. Urata H, Tanabe Y, Kiyonaga A, et al. Antihypertensive and volume-depleting effects of mild exercise on essential hypertension. Hypertension 1987;9:245–252.

17. Jennings GL, Deakin G, Dewar E, et al. Exercise, cardiovascular disease and blood pressure. Clin Exp Hypertens 1989;A11:1035–1052.

18. Gordon NF, Cooper KH. Controlling cholesterol levels through exercise. Compr Ther 1988;14:52–57.

19. Vranic M, Wasserman D. Exercise, fitness, and diabetes. In: Bouchard C, ed. Exercise, fitness, and health: a consensus of current knowledge. Champaign, IL: Human Kinetics, 1990:467–490.

20. Bennett T, Wilcox RG, MacDonald IA. Post-exercise reduction of blood pressure in hypertensive men is not due to acute impairment of baroreflex function. Clin Sci 1984;67:97–103.

21. Hagberg JM, Montain SJ, Martin WH. Blood pressure and hemodynamic responses after exercise in older hypertensives. J Appl Physiol 1987;63:270–276.

22. American College of Sports Medicine. Position stand. Physical activity, physical fitness, and hypertension. Med Sci Sports Exerc 1993;25:i–x.

23. Gordon NF, Duncan JJ. Effect of beta-blockers on exercise physiology: implications for exercise training. Med Sci Sports Exerc 1991;23:668–676.

24. Paffenbarger RS, Hyde RT, Wing AL, et al. Physical activity, all-cause mortality, and longevity of college alumni. N Engl J Med 1986;314:605–613.

25. Blair SN, Kohl HW, Barlow CE, et al. Physical fitness and all-cause mortality in hypertensive men. Ann Med 1991;23:307–312.

26. Oldridge NB, Guyatt GH, Fischer ME, et al. Cardiac rehabilitation after myocardial infarction. Combined experience of randomized clinical trials. JAMA 1988;260: 945–950.

27. O'Connor GT, Buring JE, Yusaf S, et al. An overview of randomized trials of rehabilitation with exercise after myocardial infarction. Circulation 1989;80:234–244.

28. Pickering TG. Pathophysiology of exercise hypertension. Herz 1987;12:119–124.

29. Wong HE, Dasser IS, Bruce RA. Impaired maximal exercise performance with hypertensive cardiovascular disease. Circulation 1969;39:633–638.

30. Frohlich ED, Lowenthal DT, Miller HS, et al. Task Force IV: systemic arterial hypertension. J Am Coll Cardiol 1985;6:1218–1221.

31. American College of Sports Medicine. Guidelines for exercise testing and prescription. Baltimore: Williams & Wilkins, 1995.

32. Chick TW, Halperin AK, Gacek EM. The effect of antihypertensive medications on exercise performance: a review. Med Sci Sports Exerc 1988;20:447–454.

33. MacDougall JD, Tuxen D, Sale DG, et al. Arterial blood pressure response to heavy resistance exercise. J Appl Physiol 1985;58:785–790.

34. Hagberg JM, Goldring D, Ehsani AA, et al. Effect of exercise training on the blood pressure and hemodynamic features of hypertensive adolescents. Am J Physiol 1983;63:270–276.

35. Harris KA, Holly RG. Physiological responses to circuit weight training in borderline hypertensive subjects. Med Sci Sports Exerc 1987;19:246–252.

36. Hurley BE, Hagberg JM, Goldberg AP, et al. Resistive training can reduce coronary risk factors without altering $\dot{V}O_2$max or percent body fat. Med Sci Sports Exerc 1988;20:150–154.

37. Tipton CM, McMahon S, Youmans EM, et al. Response of hypertensive rats to acute and chronic conditions of static exercise. Am J Physiol 1988;254:H592–H598.

38. DiPette DJ, Frohlich ED. Cardiac involvement in hypertension. Am J Cardiol 1988;61:67H–72H.

39. Fleck SJ. Cardiovascular adaptations to resistance training. Med Sci Sports Exerc 1988;20:S146–S151.

40. Effron MB. Effects of resistive training on left ventricular function. Med Sci Sports Exerc 1989;21:694–697.

41. American Association of Cardiovascular and Pulmonary Rehabilitation. Guidelines for cardiac rehabilitation programs. Champaign, IL: Human Kinetics, 1995.

42. Jones BH, Rock PB, Moore MP. Musculoskeletal injury: risks, prevention, and first aid. In: Blair S, ed. Resource manual for guidelines for exercise testing and prescription. American College of Sports Medicine, Philadelphia: Lea & Febiger, 1988:285–294.

43. American College of Sports Medicine. Position stand. The recommended quantity and quality of exercise for developing and maintaining cardiorespiratory and muscular fitness in healthy adults. Med Sci Sports Exerc 1990;22:265–274.

44. Gordon NF. Hypertension. In: ACSM's exercise management for persons with chronic diseases and disabilities. Champaign, IL: Human Kinetics, 1997: 59–63.

Part B.

1. National Diabetes Data Group. Classification and diagnosis of diabetes mellitus and other categories of glucose intolerance. Diabetes 1979;28:1019–1157.
2. American Diabetes Association. Physicians guide to insulin dependent (type I) diabetes: diagnosis and treatment. 2nd ed. Alexandria, VA: ADA, 1988.
3. American Diabetes Association. Physicians guide to non–insulin-dependent (type II) diabetes: diagnosis and treatment. 2nd ed. Alexandria, VA: ADA, 1988.
4. Franz MJ, Horton ES, Hoogwerf BJ, et al. Technical review: nutrition principles for management of diabetes and related complications. Diabetes Care 1994;17: 490–518.
5. Koivisto VA, DeFronzo RA. Exercise in the treatment of type II diabetes. Acta Endocrinol 1984;262 (Suppl): 107–111.
6. Schneider SH, Amorosa LF, Khachadurian AK, et al. Studies on the mechanism of improved glucose control during regular exercise in type 2 (non–insulin-dependent) diabetes. Diabetologia 1984;26:355–360.
7. American Diabetes Association. Diabetes mellitus and exercise (position statement). Diabetes Care 1991;14 (Suppl 2):36–37.
8. Schneider SH, Ruderman NB. Exercise and NIDDM (American Diabetes Association technical review). Diabetes Care 1991;14(Suppl 2):52–56.
9. Gerich JE. Drug therapy—oral hypoglycemic agents. N Engl J Med 1989;321:1231–1245.
10. DeFronzo RA, Goodman AM. Multicenter Metformin Study Group. Efficacy of metformin in patients with non–insulin dependent diabetes mellitus. N Engl J Med 1995;333:541–545.
11. Coniff R, Shapiro JA, Seaton TB, et al. Multicenter, placebo-controlled trial comparing acarbose (BAY g 5421) with placebo, tolbutamide and tolbutamide-plus-acarbose in non–insulin-dependent diabetes mellitus. Am J Med 1995;98:443–451.
12. Coniff RJ, Shapiro JA, Seaton, TB, et al. A double-blind placebo-controlled trial evaluating the safety and efficacy of acarbose for the treatment of patients with insulin-requiring type II diabetes. Diabetes Care 1995; 18:928–932.
13. Chiasson JL, Josse RG, Hunt JA, et al. The efficacy of acarbose in the treatment of patients with non–insulin-dependent diabetes mellitus. Ann Intern Med 1994;121:928–935.
14. Whitcomb RW, Saltiel AR. Thiazolidinediones. Exp Opin Invest Drugs 1995;4:1299–1309.
15. Saltiel AR, Olefsky JM. Thiazolidinediones in the treatment of insulin resistance and type II diabetes mellitus. Diabetes 1996;45:1661–1669.
16. Harris MI, Hadden WE, Knowler WC, et al. Prevalence of diabetes and impaired glucose levels in US population age 20–74 years. Diabetes 1988;36:523–534.
17. Kannel WB, McGee DL. Diabetes and glucose tolerance as risk factors for cardiovascular disease: the Framingham study. Diabetes Care 1979;2:120–126.
18. Kannel WB, McGee DL. Diabetes and cardiovascular disease, the Framingham study. JAMA 1979;241: 2035–2039.
19. Fuller JH, Shipley MJ, Rose G, et al. Coronary heart disease risk and impaired glucose tolerance: the Whitehall study. Lancet 1980;1:1373–1376.
20. Fuller JH, Shipley MJ, Rose G, et al. Mortality from coronary heart disease and stroke in relation to the degree of hyperglycaemia: the Whitehall Study. Br Med J 1983;287:867–870.
21. Krolewski AS, Warram JH, Salvania P, et al. Evolving natural history or coronary artery disease in diabetes mellitus. Am J Med 1991;90:56S–61S.
22. Davi G, Violi F, Giammarresi C, et al. Increased plasminogen activator inhibitor antigen levels in diabetic patients with stable angina. Blood Coagul Fibrinolysis 1991;2:41–45.
23. Kwaan HC. Changes in blood coagulation, platelet function, and plasminogen-plasmin system in diabetes (review). Diabetes 1992;41(Suppl 2):32–35.
24. Matsuda T, Morishita E, Jokaji H, et al. Mechanism on disorders of coagulation and fibrinolysis in diabetes. Diabetes 1996;45(Suppl 3):S109–S110.
25. Wingard DL, Barrett-Connor E, Crugui M, et al. Clustering of heart disease risk factors in diabetic compared to non-diabetic adults. Am J Epidemiol 1983; 117:19–26.
26. Reaven GM. Role of insulin resistance in human disease, Banting lecture 1988. Diabetes 1988;37:1595–1607.
27. Reaven FM, Hoffman BB. Hypertension as a disease of carbohydrate and lipoprotein metabolism. Am J Med 1989;87(Suppl):2S–6S.
28. American Diabetes Association (Consensus Statement). Role of cardiovascular risk factors in prevention and treatment of macrovascular disease in diabetes. Diabetes Care 1991;14(Suppl 2):69–75.
29. Sprafka JM, Burke GL, Folsom AR, et al. Trends in prevalence of diabetes mellitus, in patients with myocardial infarction and effect of diabetes on survival: the Minnesota Heart Survey. Diabetes Care 1991;14: 537–543.
30. Abbott RD, Donahue RP, Kannel WB, et al. The impact of diabetes on survival following myocardial infarction in men vs. women: the Framingham study. JAMA 1988;260:3456–3460.
31. Singer DE, Moulton AW, Nathan DM. Diabetic myocardial infarction: interaction of diabetes with other preinfarction risk factors. Diabetes 1989;38:350–357.
32. Wilson CS, Gau GT, Fulton RE, et al. Coronary artery disease in diabetic and nondiabetic patients: a clinical and angiographic comparison. Clin Cardiol 1983;9: 440–446.
33. Salomon NW, Page US, Okies JE, et al. Diabetes mellitus and coronary artery bypass. Short-term risk and long-term prognosis. J Thorac Cardiovasc Surg 1983; 85:264–271.
34. Wilson PW, Cupples LA, Kannel WB. Is hyperglycemia associated with cardiovascular disease? The Framingham study. Am Heart J 1991;121:586–590.
35. Laakso M. Glycemic control and the risk for coronary

heart disease in patients with non–insulin-dependent diabetes mellitus. Ann Intern Med 1996;124:127–130.

36. Klein R. Hyperglycemia and microvascular and macrovascular disease in diabetes. Diabetes Care 1995; 18:258–268.

37. Koskinen P, Mänttäri M, Manninen V, et al. Coronary heart disease incidence in NIDDM patients in the Helsinki Heart Study. Diabetes Care 1992;15:820–825.

38. Pyörälä K, Pedersen TR, Kjekshus J, et al. Cholesterol lowering with simvastatin improves prognosis of diabetic patients with coronary heart disease: a subgroup analysis of the Scandinavian Simvastatin Survival Study (4S). Diabetes Care 1997;20:614–620.

39. Sacks FM, Pfeffer MA, Moye LA, et al. The effect of pravastatin on coronary events after myocardial infarction in patients with average cholesterol levels. N Engl J Med 1996;335:1001–1009.

40. Hoogwerf B, Hunninghake D, Campeau L, et al. LDL cholesterol lowering shows angiographic and clinical benefit in diabetic patients in the Post CABG trial (abstract). Circulation 1997;96(Suppl 1):I-414.

41. ETDRS Investigators. Aspirin effects on mortality and morbidity in patients with diabetes mellitus. JAMA 1992;268:1292–1300.

42. Colwell J. Aspirin therapy in diabetes. Diabetes Care 1997;20:1767–1771.

43. Watkins PJ, ed. Long-term complications of diabetes. Clin Endocrinol Metab 1986;15:1–87.

44. Ewing DJ, Clarke BF. Diabetic autonomic neuropathy: present insights and future prospects. Diabetes Care 1986;9:648–665.

45. Krolewski AS, Warram JH, Cupples A, et al. Hypertension, orthostatic hypotension and microvascular complications of diabetes. J Chronic Dis 1985;38:319–326.

46. Nesto RW, Watson FS, Kowalchuk GJ, et al. Silent myocardial ischemia and infarction in diabetics with peripheral vascular disease: assessment by dipyridamole thallium-201 scintigraphy. Am Heart J 1990;120: 1073–1077.

47. Chipkin SR, Frid D, Alpert JS, et al. Frequency of painless myocardial ischemia during exercise tolerance testing in patients with and without diabetes mellitus. Am J Cardiol 1987;59:61–65.

48. Deckert R, Feldt-Rasmussen B, Borch-Johnsen K, et al. Albuminuria reflects widespread vascular damage: the Steno hypothesis. Diabetologia 1989;29:282–286.

49. Mogensen CE. Long term antihypertensive treatment inhibiting progression of diabetic nephropathy. Br Med J 1982;285:685–688.

50. Bjorck S, Nyberg G, Mulec H, et al. Beneficial effects of angiotensin converting enzyme inhibition on renal function in patients with diabetic nephropathy. Br Med J 1987;293:471–474.

51. Tolins JP, Raij L. Concerns about diabetic nephropathy in the treatment of diabetic hypertensive patients. Am J Med 1989;87(Suppl 6A):29S–33S.

52. Lewis EJ, Hunsicker LG, Bain RP, et al. The effect of angiotensin-converting enzyme inhibition on diabetic nephropathy. N Engl J Med 1993;329:1456–1462.

53. Ravid M, Sarin RSN, Jutrin I, et al. Long-term stabilizing effect of angiotensin-converting enzyme inhibi-

tion on plasma creatinine and on proteinuria in normotensive type II diabetic patients. Ann Intern Med 1993;118:577–581.

54. Salem JK, Hoogwerf BJ. Diabetic nephropathy: strategies for preventing renal failure. Cleve Clin J Med 1996;63:331–338.

55. Ames RP. Coronary heart disease and the treatment of hypertension: impact of diuretics on serum lipids and glucose. J Cardiovasc Pharmacol 1984;6(Suppl 3): S466–S473.

56. Levine GN, Jacobs AK, Keeler GP, et al. for the CAVEAT-I Investigators. Impact of diabetes mellitus on percutaneous revascularization (CAVEAT-I) Coronary Angioplasty Versus Excisional Atherectomy Trial. Am J Cardiol 1997;79:748–758.

57. Vandormael MG, Deligonul U, Kern MJ, et al. Multilesion coronary angioplasty: clinical and angiographic follow-up. J Am Coll Cardiol 1987;10:246–252.

58. Lytle B, Loop FD, Cosgrove DM, et al. Long-term (5 to 12 years) serial studies of internal mammary artery and saphenous vein coronary bypass grafts. J Thorac Cardiovasc Surg 1985;80:248–258.

59. Loop FD, Lytle BW, Cosgrove DM, et al. Sternal wound complications after isolated coronary artery bypass grafting: early and late mortality, morbidity, and cost of care. Ann Thorac Surg 1990;49:179–187.

60. Lawrie GM, Morris GC, Glaeser CH. Influence of diabetes mellitus on the results of coronary bypass surgery. Follow-up of 212 diabetic patients ten to 15 years after surgery. JAMA 1986;256:2967–2971.

61. Deveineni R, McKenzie FN. Surgery for coronary artery disease in patients with diabetes mellitus. Can J Surg 1985;28:367–370.

62. Hoogwerf BJ, Sheeler LR, Licata AA. Endocrine management of the open heart surgical patient. Sem Thorac Cardiovasc Surg 1991;3:75–80.

63. Mitchell TH, Abraham G, Schiffrin A, et al. Hyperglycemia after intense exercise in IDDM subjects during continuous subcutaneous insulin infusion. Diabetes Care 1988;11:311–317.

64. Richter EA, Ruderman NB, Schneider SH. Diabetes and exercise. Am J Med 1981;79:201–209.

65. Koivisto VA, Felig P. Effects of leg exercise on insulin absorption in diabetic patients. N Engl J Med 1978;298:77–83.

66. Caron D, Poussier P, Marliss EB, et al. The effect of postprandial exercise on meal-related glucose intolerance in insulin-dependent diabetic individuals. Diabetes Care 1982;5:364–369.

67. Weinberger MH. Antihypertensive therapy and lipids: paradoxical influences on cardiovascular disease risk. Am J Med 1986;80(Suppl 2A):64–70.

68. Zawada ET. Metabolic considerations in the approach to diabetic hypertensive patients. Am J Med 1989;87 (Suppl 6A):34S–38S.

69. Andren L. General considerations in selecting antihypertensive agents in patients with type II diabetes mellitus and hypertension. Am J Med 1989;87(Suppl 6A):39S–41S.

70. Pollare T, Lithell H, Berne C. A comparison of the effects of hydrochlorothiazide and captopril on glucose

and lipid metabolism in patients with hypertension. N Engl J Med 1989;321:868–873.

71. The Multiple Risk Factor Intervention Trial Research Group. Multiple Risk Factor Intervention Trial: risk factor change and mortality results. JAMA 1982;248:1465–1477.

72. Pool JL. Plasma lipid lowering effects of doxazosin, a new selective alpha$_1$ adrenergic inhibitor for systemic hypertension. Am J Cardiol 1987;59:46G–50G.

Part C.

1. Kannel WB, McGee DL. Diabetes and cardiovascular disease: the Framingham Study. JAMA 1979;241:2035–2038.

2. McDaniel MD, Cronenwett JL. Basic data related to the natural history of intermittent claudication. Ann Vasc Surg 1989;3:273–277.

3. Brand FN, Abbott RD, Kannel WB. Diabetes, intermittent claudication, and risk of cardiovascular disease. The Framingham Study. Diabetes 1989;38:504–509.

4. Newman AB, Sutton-Tyrrell K, Vogt MT, et al. Morbidity and mortality in hypertensive adults with a low ankle/arm blood pressure index. JAMA 1993;270:487–489.

5. Vogt MT, Cauley JA, Newman AB, et al. Decreased ankle/arm blood pressure index and mortality in elderly women. JAMA 1993;270:465–469.

6. Hertzer NR. The natural history of peripheral vascular disease. Implications for its management. Circulation 1991;83(Suppl 1):I-12–I-19.

7. Jonason T, Ringqvist I. Diabetes mellitus and intermittent claudication. Relation between peripheral vascular complications and location of occlusive atherosclerosis in the legs. Acta Med Scand 1985;218: 217–221.

8. Olsen PS, Gustafsen J, Rasmussen L, et al. Long-term results after arterial surgery for arteriosclerosis of the lower limbs in young adults. Eur J Vasc Surg 1988;2:15–18.

9. Coffman JD. Intermittent claudication: not so benign. Am Heart J 1986;112:1127–1128.

10. Hertzer NR, Young JR, Beven EG, et al. Late results of coronary bypass in patients presenting with lower extremity ischemia: the Cleveland Clinic Study. Ann Vasc Surg 1987;1:411–419.

11. Criqui MH, Lawyer RD, Fronek A, et al. Mortality over a period of 10 years in patients with peripheral arterial disease. N Engl J Med 1992;326:381–386.

12. Yao JST. Pressure measurement in the extremity. In: Bernstein EF, ed. Vascular diagnosis. 4th ed. St. Louis: Mosby, 1993:169–175.

13. Rutherford RB, Lowenstein DH, Klein MF. Combining segmental systolic pressures and plethysmography to diagnose arterial disease of the legs. Am J Surg 1979;38:211–18.

14. Kannel WB, McGee DL. Update on some epidemiologic features of intermittent claudication: the Framingham study. J Am Geriatr Soc 1985;33:13–18.

15. Jonason T, Ringquist I. Factors of prognostic importance for subsequent rest pain in patients with intermittent claudication. Acta Med Scand 1985;218:27–33.

16. Myers KA, King RB, Scott DF, et al. The effect of smoking on the late patency of arterial reconstruction in the legs. Br J Surg 1978;65:267–271.

17. Greenhalgh RM, Laing SP, Cole PV, et al. Smoking and arterial reconstruction. Br J Surg 1981;68:605–607.

18. Herring M, Gardner A, Glover J. Seeding human arterial prostheses with mechanically derived endothelium. The detrimental effect of smoking. J Vasc Surg 1984;1:279–289.

19. Thomas M. Smoking and vascular surgery. Br J Surg 1981;68:601–604.

20. Quick CRG, Cotton LT. The measured effect of stopping smoking on claudication. Br J Surg 1982;69 (Suppl):24–26.

21. Radack K, Wyderski RJ. Conservative management of intermittent claudication. Ann Intern Med 1990;113: 135–146.

22. Foley WT. Treatment of gangrene of the feet and legs by walking. Circulation 1957;15:689–700.

23. Skinner JS, Strandness DE. Exercise and intermittent claudication. II. Effect of physical training. Circulation 1967;36:23–29.

24. Ericsson B, Haeger K, Lindell SE. Effect of physical training on intermittent claudication. Angiology 1970;21:188–192.

25. Dahllof A, Holm J, Schersten T, et al. Peripheral arterial insufficiency. Effect of physical training on walking tolerance, calf blood flow, and blood flow resistance. Scand J Rehabil Med 1976;8:19–26.

26. Ekroth R, Dahllof A, Gundevall B, et al. Physical training of patients with intermittent claudication: indications, methods, and results. Surgery 1978;84:640–643.

27. Larsen OA, Lassen NA. Effect of daily muscular exercise in patients with intermittent claudication. Lancet 1966;2:1093–1096.

28. Krajewski LP, Olin JW. Atherosclerosis of the aorta and lower extremity arteries. In: Young JR, Olin JW, Bartholomew JR, eds. Peripheral vascular diseases. 2nd ed. St. Louis: CV Mosby, 1996:208–233.

29. Holm J, Dahllof A, Bjorntorp P, et al. Enzyme studies in muscles of patients with intermittent claudication. Effect of training. Scand J Clin Lab Invest 1973;31 (Suppl 128):201–205.

30. Dahllof A, Bjorntorp P, Holm J, et al. Metabolic activity of skeletal muscle in patients with peripheral arterial insufficiency. Effect of physical training. Eur J Clin Invest 1974;4:9–15.

31. Mannarino E, Pasqualini L, Menna M, et al. Effects of physical training on peripheral vascular disease: a controlled study. Angiology 1989;40:5–10.

32. Creasy TS, McMillan PJ, Fletcher EWL, et al. Is percutaneous transluminal angioplasty better than exercise for claudication?—Preliminary results from a prospective randomized trial. Eur J Vasc Surg 1990;4: 135–140.

33. Hiatt WR, Regensteiner JG, Hargarten ME, et al. Benefit of exercise conditioning for patients with peripheral arterial disease. Circulation 1990;81:602–609.

34. Mannarino E, Pasqualini L, Innocente S, et al. Physical training and antiplatelet treatment in stage II peripheral arterial occlusive disease: alone or combined? Angiology 1991;42:513–521.

35. Scheffler P, de la Hamette D, Gross J, et al. Intensive vascular training in stage IIb of peripheral arterial occlusive disease. The additive effects of intravenous prostaglandin E1 or intravenous pentoxifylline during training. Circulation 1994;90:818–822.

36. Hiatt WR, Wolfel EE, Meier RH, et al. Superiority of treadmill walking exercise vs. strength training for patients with peripheral arterial disease. Implications for the mechanism of the training response. Circulation 1994;90:1866–1874.

37. Regensteiner JG, Meyer TJ, Krupski WC, et al. Hospital vs home-based exercise rehabilitation for patients with peripheral arterial occlusive disease. Angiology 1997;48:291–300.

38. Patterson RB, Pinto B, Marcus B, et al. Value of a supervised exercise program for the therapy of arterial claudication. J Vasc Surg 1997;25:312–318.

39. Regensteiner JG, Steiner JF, Panzer RJ, et al. Evaluation of walking impairment by questionnaire in patients with peripheral arterial disease. J Vasc Med Biol 1990;2:142–152.

40. Regensteiner JG, Steiner JF, Hiatt WR. Exercise training improves functional status in patients with peripheral arterial disease. J Vasc Surg 1996;23:104–115.

41. Alpert JS, Larsen OA, Lassen NA. Exercise and intermittent claudication. Blood flow in the calf muscle during walking studied by the xenon-133 clearance method. Circulation 1969;39:353–359.

42. Andriessen MPHM, Barendsen GJ, Wouda AA, et al. The effect of six months intensive physical training on the circulation in the legs of patients with intermittent claudication. Vasa 1989;18:56–62.

43. Lundgren F, Dahllof A, Lundholm K, et al. Intermittent claudication—surgical reconstruction or physical training? A prospective randomized trial of treatment efficiency. Ann Surg 1989;209:346–355.

44. Zetterquist S. The effect of active training on the nutritive blood flow in exercising ischemic legs. Scand J Clin Lab Invest 1970;25:101–111.

45. Lundgren F, Dahllof AG, Schersten T, et al. Muscle enzyme adaptation in patients with peripheral arterial insufficiency: spontaneous adaptation, effect of different treatments and consequences on walking performance. Clin Sci 1989;77:485–493.

46. Holloszy JO, Coyle EF. Adaptations of skeletal muscle to endurance exercise and their metabolic consequences. J Appl Physiol 1984;56:831–838.

47. Hiatt WR, Nawaz D, Brass EP. Carnitine metabolism during exercise in patients with peripheral vascular disease. J Appl Physiol 1987;62:2383–2387.

48. Hiatt WR, Wolfel EE, Regensteiner JG, et al. Skeletal muscle carnitine metabolism in patients with unilateral peripheral arterial disease. J Appl Physiol 1992;73:346–353.

49. Solomon SA, Ramsay LE, Yeo WW, et al. β-Blockade and intermittent claudication: placebo controlled trial of atenolol and nifedipine and their combination. Br Med J 1991;303:1100–1104.

50. Coffman JD. Vasodilator drugs in peripheral vascular disease. N Engl J Med 1979;300:713–717.

51. Spence JD, Arnold JMO, Munoz CE, et al. Angiotensin-converting enzyme inhibition with cliazapril does not improve blood flow, walking time, or plasma lipids in patients with intermittent claudication. J Vasc Med Biol 1993;4:23–28.

52. Bagger JP, Helligsoe P, Randsbaek F, et al. Effect of verapamil in intermittent claudication. A randomized, double-blind, placebo-controlled, cross-over study after individual dose-response assessment. Circulation 1997;95:411–414.

53. Goldhaber SZ, Manson JE, Stampfer MJ, et al. Low-dose aspirin and subsequent peripheral arterial surgery in the Physicians' Health Study. Lancet 1992;340:143–145.

54. Balsano F, Coccheri S, Libretti A, et al. Ticlopidine in the treatment of intermittent claudication: a 21-month double-blind trial. J Lab Clin Med 1989;114:84–91.

55. Arcan JC, Blanchard J, Boissel JP, et al. Multicenter double-blind study of ticlopidine in the treatment of intermittent claudication and the prevention of its complications. Angiology 1988;39:802–811.

56. Janzon L, Bergqvist D, Boberg J, et al. Prevention of myocardial infarction and stroke in patients with intermittent claudication; effects of Ticlopidine. Results from STIMS, the Swedish Ticlopidine Multicentre Study. J Intern Med 1990;227:301–308.

57. CAPRIE Steering Committee. A randomized blinded trial of Clopidogrel versus aspirin in patients at risk of ischemic events (CAPRIE). Lancet 1996;348:1329–1339.

58. Lowe GDO, Fowkes FGR, Dawes J, et al. Blood viscosity, fibrinogen, and activation of coagulation and leukocytes in peripheral arterial disease and the normal population in the Edinburgh Artery Study. Circulation 1993;87:1915–1920.

59. Porter JM, Cutler BS, Lee BY, et al. Pentoxifylline efficacy in the treatment of intermittent claudication: multicenter controlled double-blind trial with objective assessment of chronic occlusive arterial disease patients. Am Heart J 1982;104:66–72.

60. Hood SC, Moher D, Barber GG. Management of intermittent claudication with pentoxifylline: meta-analysis of randomized controlled trials. Can Med Assoc J 1996;155:1053–1059.

61. Brevetti G, Chiariello M, Ferulano G, et al. Increases in walking distance in patients with peripheral vascular disease treated with l-carnitine: a double-blind, cross-over study. Circulation 1988;77:767–773.

62. Brevetti G, Perna S, Sabba C, et al. Superiority of L-propionyl carnitine vs L-carnitine in improving walking capacity in patients with peripheral vascular disease: an acute, intravenous, double-blind, cross-over study. Eur Heart J 1992;13:251–255.

63. Brevetti G, Perna S, Sabba C, et al. Effect of propionyl-L-carnitine on quality of life in intermittent claudication. Am J Cardiol 1997;79:777–780.

64. Brevetti G, Perna S, Sabba C, et al. Propionyl-L-carnitine in intermittent claudication. Double-blind, placebo-controlled, dose titration, multicenter study. J Am Coll Cardiol 1995;26:1411–1416.

65. Lievre M, Azoulay S, Lion L, et al. A dose-effect study of beraprost sodium in intermittent claudication. J Cardiovasc Pharmacol 1996;27:788–793.

66. Okuda Y, Kimura Y, Yamashita K. Cilostazol. Cardiovasc Drug Rev 1993;11:451–465.

67. Takeshita S, Zheng LP, Brogi E, et al. Therapeutic angiogenesis. A single intraarterial bolus of vascular endothelial growth factor augments revascularization in a rabbit ischemic hind limb model. J Clin Invest 1994;93:662–670.

68. Tsurumi Y, Takeshita S, Chen D, et al. Direct intramuscular gene transfer of naked DNA encoding vascular endothelial growth factor augments collateral development and tissue perfusion. Circulation 1996;94: 3281–3290.

69. Prevention of Atherosclerotic Complications with Ketanserin Trial Group. Prevention of atherosclerotic complications: controlled trial of Ketanserin. Br Med J 1989;298:424–430.

70. Ernst E. Chelation therapy for peripheral arterial occlusive disease: a systematic review. Circulation 1997; 96:1031–1033.

Part D.

1. Weintraub WS. Cigarette smoking as a risk factor for coronary artery disease. Adv Exp Med Biol 1990;273: 27–37.

2. McIntosh HD. Risk factors for cardiovascular disease and death: a clinical perspective. J Am Coll Cardiol 1989;14:24–30.

3. Colditz GA. Cigarette smoking and coronary artery disease. Adv Exp Med Biol 1990;273:311–326.

4. Petty T, Branscomb B, Farrington J, et al. Community resources for rehabilitation of patients with chronic obstructive pulmonary disease and cor pulmonale. Circulation 1974;49:A1–A19.

5. Ries AL. Pulmonary rehabilitation: rationale, components and results. J Cardpulm Rehabil 1991;11:23–28.

6. Niederman MS, Clemente PH, Fein AM, et al. Benefits of a multidisciplinary pulmonary rehabilitation program. Improvements are independent of lung function. Chest 1991;99:798–804.

7. Reardon JZ, Levine S, Peske G, et al. A comparison of outpatient cardiac and pulmonary rehabilitation patients. J Cardpulm Rehabil 1995;15:277–282.

8. Sahn S, Nett L, Petty T. Ten year follow-up of a comprehensive rehabilitation program for severe COPD. Chest 1980;77(Suppl):311–314.

9. Hodgkin JE. Pulmonary rehabilitation. Clin Chest Med 1990;11:447–460.

10. Petty TL. Pulmonary rehabilitation in chronic respiratory insufficiency. 1. Pulmonary rehabilitation in perspective: historical roots, present status, and future projections. Thorax 1993;48:855–862.

11. Toshima M, Kaplan R, Ries A. Experimental evaluation of rehabilitation in chronic obstructive pulmonary disease: short-term effects on exercise endurance and health status. Health Psychol 1990;9: 237–252.

12. Neish C, Hopp T. The role of education in pulmonary rehabilitation. J Cardpulm Rehabil 1988;11:439–441.

13. Kersten L. Changes in self-concept during pulmonary rehabilitation, part 1. Heart Lung 1990;19(5 Pt 1): 456–462.

14. Kersten L. Changes in self-concept during pulmonary rehabilitation, part 2. Heart Lung 1990;19(5 Pt 1): 463–470.

15. Emery CF, Leatherman NE, Burker EJ, et al. Psychological outcomes of a pulmonary rehabilitation program. Chest 1991;100:613–617.

16. Ries AL. Scientific basis of pulmonary rehabilitation: position paper of the American Association of Cardiovascular and Pulmonary Rehabilitation. J Cardpulm Rehabil 1990;10:418–441.

17. Olopade CO, Beck KC, Viggiano RW, et al. Exercise limitation and pulmonary rehabilitation in chronic obstructive pulmonary disease. Mayo Clin Proc 1992; 67:144–157.

18. Ries AL, Kaplan RM, Limberg TM, et al. Effects of pulmonary rehabilitation on physiologic and psychosocial outcomes in patients with chronic obstructive pulmonary disease. Ann Intern Med 1995;122:823–832.

19. Carter R, Linsenbardt S, Blevins W, et al. Exercise gas exchange in patients with moderately severe to severe chronic obstructive pulmonary disease. J Cardpulm Rehabil 1989;9:243–249.

20. Casaburi R, Porszasz J, Burns MR, et al. Physiologic benefits of exercise training in rehabilitation of patients with severe chronic obstructive pulmonary disease. Am J Respir Crit Care Med 1997;155:1541–1551.

21. American College of Sports Medicine. Guidelines for exercise testing and prescription. 5th ed. Philadelphia: Lea & Febiger, 1995.

22. Shih HT, Webb CR, Conway WA, et al. Frequency and significance of cardiac arrhythmias in chronic obstructive lung disease. Chest 1988;94:44–88.

23. Conradson TB, Eklundh G, Olofsson B, et al. Cardiac arrhythmias in patients with mild-to-moderate obstructive lung disease. Comparison of beta-agonist therapy alone and in combination with a xanthine derivative, enprofylline or theophylline. Chest 1985;88:537–542.

24. Weg JG. Therapeutic exercise in patients with chronic obstructive pulmonary disease. Cardiovasc Clin 1985;15:261–275.

25. Casaburi R, Wasserman K. Exercise training in pulmonary rehabilitation. N Engl J Med 1986;314: 1509–1511.

26. Holle RH, Williams DV, Vandree JC, et al. Increased muscle efficiency and sustained benefits in an outpatient community hospital-based pulmonary rehabilitation program. Chest 1988;94:1161–1168.

27. Reardon J, Awad E, Normandin E, et al. The effect of comprehensive outpatient pulmonary rehabilitation on dyspnea. Chest 1994;105:1046–1052.

28. Sassi-Dambron DE, Eakin EG, Ries AL, et al. Treatment of dyspnea in COPD. A controlled clinical trial of dyspnea management strategies. Chest 1995;107: 724–729.

29. Rodrigues JC, Ilowite JS. Pulmonary rehabilitation in the elderly patient. Clin Chest Med 1993;14:429–436.

30. Couser JI Jr, Guthmann R, Hamadeh MA, et al. Pulmonary rehabilitation improves exercise capacity in

older elderly patients with COPD. Chest 1995;107: 730–734.

31. Kesten S. Pulmonary rehabilitation and surgery for end-stage lung disease. Clin Chest Med 1997;18:173–181.

32. Guyatt G, Thompson P, Berman L, et al. How should we measure function in patients with chronic heart and lung disease? J Chronic Dis 1985;38:517–524.

33. Casaburi R, Wasserman K, Patessio A, et al. A new perspective in pulmonary rehabilitation: anaerobic threshold as a discriminant in training. Eur Respir J 1989;2(Suppl 7):618S–623S.

34. Ries AL, Farrow JT, Clausen JL. Pulmonary function tests cannot predict exercise-induced hypoxemia in chronic obstructive pulmonary disease. Chest 1988; 93:454–459.

35. Ries AL. The importance of exercise in pulmonary rehabilitation. Clin Chest Med 1994;15:327–337.

36. Zack MB, Palange AV. Oxygen supplemented exercise of ventilatory and nonventilatory muscles in pulmonary rehabilitation. Chest 1985;88:669–675.

37. Davidson AC, Leach R, George RJ, et al. Supplemental oxygen and exercise ability in chronic obstructive airways disease. Thorax 1988;43:965–971.

38. Christopher KL, Spofford BT, Petrun MD, et al. A program for transtracheal oxygen delivery. Assessment of safety and efficacy. Ann Intern Med 1987;107:802–808.

39. Bell C, O'Donohue W, Dewan N, et al. Effects of transtracheal oxygen therapy on exercise capacity. J Cardpulm Rehabil 1988;11:449–452.

40. Scherer YK, Schmieder LE. The effect of a pulmonary rehabilitation program on self-efficacy, perception of dyspnea, and physical endurance. Heart Lung 1997;26:15–22.

41. Emery CF. Adherence in cardiac and pulmonary rehabilitation. J Cardpulm Rehabil 1995;15:420–423.

42. Strijbos JH, Postma DS, van Altena R, et al. A comparison between an outpatient hospital-based pulmonary rehabilitation program and a home-care pulmonary rehabilitation program in patients with COPD. A follow-up of 18 months. Chest 1996;109:366–372.

43. Strijbos JH, Postma DS, van Altena R, et al. Feasibility and effects of a home-care rehabilitation program in patients with chronic obstructive pulmonary disease. J Cardpulm Rehabil 1996;16:386–393.

44. Wijkstra PJ, van der Mark TW, Kraan J, et al. Long-term effects of home rehabilitation on physical performance in chronic obstructive pulmonary disease. Am J Respir Crit Care Med 1996;153(4 Pt 1): 1234–1241.

45. Wijkstra PJ, van der Mark TW, Kraan J, et al. Effects of home rehabilitation on physical performance in patients with chronic obstructive pulmonary disease (COPD). Eur Respir J 1996;9:104–110.

Noncardiologic Complications of Coronary Bypass Surgery and Common Patient Concerns

William A. Dafoe and Arvind Koshal

This chapter outlines the common problems that the practicing physician is asked to evaluate in outpatients who have had coronary artery bypass graft (CABG) surgery. Medical issues prevalent during hospitalization are addressed in surgical texts (1). It should be appreciated that numerous problems result from the surgical procedure superimposed on existing medical conditions. Most areas of concern are self-limiting and pose no long-term difficulties; however, a small number of complications may result in protracted problems. The total list of potential problems after open heart surgery is exhaustive and could occupy a separate text. The problems discussed here are those that often are provoked by the techniques before, during, and after surgery—the angiogram, anesthetic procedures, sternal retraction, cardiopulmonary bypass, and vein harvesting. Table 12.1 lists the probability of complications in the postoperative period and at 6 months. Common issues and patient concerns are also addressed. These issues need to be discussed as part of the total cardiac rehabilitation continuum. Patients have difficulty attending to risk factor reduction or exercise programs if their concerns are focused on physical problems.

HEAD AND NECK

Headaches and Cervical Pain

Cervical pain and headaches may be a source of discomfort after bypass surgery. Although axiomatic, it is important to document a history of headaches or cervical disorders before surgery. Preexisting conditions, such as tension headaches, may become more prevalent in the postoperative period because drugs previously used have been discontinued. Cervical degenerative disease may be aggravated as a result of intubation procedures that require cervical extension. Hypertension is an uncommon cause of headaches in the early postoperative period because patients are monitored closely and treated while in the hospital.

Headaches can be caused by drugs used postoperatively, such as nitroglycerin, dipyrimadole, and, occasionally, heparin. These three drugs induce headaches by vasodilation. Occipital headaches may arise from irritation of the greater occipital nerve secondary to cervical degenerative joint disease or spasm of the trapezius muscle. Decreased visual acuity may present as headaches because of excessive visual strain. Headaches may be an accompanying complaint of neurologic problems, such as a cerebral vascular accident (CVA) and anoxia. Classic tension headaches may result in headaches in the temporal or occipital region. Fibromyalgic pain with trigger points in the sternocleidomastoid or the upper trapezius may present as a dull pain with proximal radiation (10).

Trauma secondary to misplaced anesthetic monitoring lines may result in anterior neck pain. These lines are placed in the jugular vein and may cause local trauma, perforation of the carotid artery, or dissection of the jugular vein. The facial nerve has been reported to be damaged presumably because of mechanical compression forces during intubation (11).

Infections of the paranasal sinuses occurred in 1.3% of patients in one series post-CABG. Risk factors identified were prolonged tracheal intubation, airway colonization with nosocomial bacteria, inability to clear nasal secretions, sinus ostial obstruction, and critical organ system dysfunction (12).

Table 12.1. Early Postoperative Complications After Coronary Artery Bypass Surgery

Complication	Probability of Initial Occurrence (% Total Population)	Probability of Persistent Deficit (% Total Population)	Ref.
Vocal cord paralysis	1.1%[a]	0%	2
	0.4%	Not reported	3
Ophthalmologic	32%[b]	3.4%[d]	4
	13%[c]	Not reported	5
	26%[a]	Not reported	5
Brachial plexopathy	8.0%[b]	2.3%[d]	4
	5.5%[a]		2
Peripheral neuropathy—general	2.7[a]	0.2%[d]	3
	6.4%[a]	Not reported	2
	6.5%[b]	2.3%[d]	4
	36%[a]	Not reported	6
Upper extremity—Peripheral neuropathy			
Ulnar nerve	40%[a]	Not reported	7
Phrenic neuropathy	1.4%[a]	0%	2
	9.3%[a]	2.3%	8
Lower extremity—peripheral neuropathy			
Saphenous nerve	3%	Not reported	2
Peroneal nerve	2%	1.0%[d]	2
Cerebrovascular accident			
Definite stroke	5.7%[b]	2.7%[d]	4
	3.1%[a]	Not reported	9
Minor stroke	3.0%[b]	0.35[d]	4
	3.0%[a]	Not reported	9

[a] Postoperative.
[b] At 1 month.
[c] Preoperative.
[d] At 6 months.

Horner's syndrome (exophthalmos, ptosis, miosis, and anhidrosis on the side of the lesion indicating cervical plexus sympathetic involvement) was reported in one series to have an incidence of 7.7% postoperatively and 4% at 6 months. It was believed that hypertensive and diabetic patients were at highest risk for developing such a syndrome (13).

Visual Changes

The reported occurrence of ophthalmologic abnormalities after CABG surgery varies from 25% (4, 5, 14) to 100% (15) depending on the mechanism and criteria used for detection. It should be noted that approximately 13% of bypass patients have ophthalmologic abnormalities preoperatively (5). Any studies that report the incidence of visual changes should record the preoperative visual status. The most sensitive method for detecting abnormalities uses retinal fluorescein angiography during surgery. One hundred percent of patients on a bubble oxygenator and 56% of those on membrane oxygenators had abnormalities (15) when this method was used. Significant visual problems (field defects, cortical blindness) may be sequelae to central nervous system (CNS) disorders.

The postulated mechanism for these changes is that microemboli migrate to the retinal vessels during the surgery. It should be noted that control populations who do not require bypass surgery do not develop these changes. Williams (16) observed white plugs in the retinal circulation that developed during surgery. Postmortem studies showed that these plugs were composed of platelets and fibrin with red cells and leukocytes. Some of the emboli lodged at sites of bifurcation caused microinfarctions.

In one series, the postoperative ophthalmologic abnormalities included areas of retinal infarction (17%), retinal emboli (3%), visual field defects (3%), and a reduction in visual acuity (4.5%) (5). Most documented neuro-ophthalmologic changes are asymptomatic or short in duration. Of all those patients who have defects in the postoperative period, approximately 10% will have problems that persist at the 6-month follow-up. Persistent deficits occur primarily in patients who have visual field infarctions with resultant field deficits. In general, patients should be advised that visual acuity may change after surgery, but they should not make any changes in their eyeglasses until at least 6 months. Significant visual impairment deserves an ophthalmologic assessment to determine prognosis and to rule out any other disorders.

Vocal Changes

A change in vocal quality is normal in the first few days after surgery. There may be a change in both the quality of the voice and forcefulness of speech. One possible mechanism includes irritation to the vocal cords during intubation (17). In general, a prolonged intubation results in a greater incidence of vocal cord pathology. There is a higher likelihood of laryngeal problems with hypotension and mucosal hypoperfusion. Even apparently minimal laryngeal complications may cause marked edema of the laryngeal mucosa, leading to hematoma formation and ulceration. Finally, granuloma formation may result from infection of the ulcerative tissue. One series of 270 cases reported a 1.9% incidence of vocal cord dysfunction. All of these cases developed respiratory insufficiency and required reintubation (17). Another frequent cause includes damage to the recurrent laryngeal nerve, with an incidence of 0.4% (3) to 1.1% (2). Nasogastric tubes and nasopharyngeal leads can lead to increased mouth breathing, nasal drying, and resultant irritation of the laryngeal membranes. Patients with a prolonged intubation may require tracheostomy. The tracheostomy seldom is a cause of permanent voice difficulties, although tracheal stenosis may cause voice abnormalities.

Other surgeries more likely to damage the recurrent laryngeal nerve would include coarctation repair, surgery on the aortic arch and upper thoracic aorta, or carotid endarterectomy. The presumed mechanism is traction or direct trauma to the nerve. In most cases, the symptoms are secondary vocal cord edema or neurapraxia of the recurrent laryngeal nerve, both of which tend to improve with time.

Persistence of laryngeal problems beyond 1 month should lead to consultation with an otolaryngologist to assess vocal cord appearance and mobility. A speech pathologist can help with appropriate voice hygiene. Such recommendations could include voice rest, adequate hydration, elimination of throat clearing, lozenges to stimulate swallowing, no whispering, avoidance of medications that dry the laryngeal mucosa, and cessation of smoking. Patients have a number of practical questions that may include clearance for singing in a choir or use of a wind instrument. Problems for these activities usually relate to a reduced vital capacity and are independent of vocal cord pathology. If vocal cord immobility still persists, further speech pathology treatments can result in a compensatory glottic closure, in which the remaining mobile vocal cord overcompensates. Finally, surgical procedures may be required to augment the immobile cord with an injection of an absorbable gelatin sponge (Gelfoam), collagen, or polytetrafluoroethylene (Teflon). Another surgical procedure involves medialization of the vocal cords with laryngoplasty using the thyroid cartilages. These surgical procedures should not take place until after at least 1 year, when there is little possibility of spontaneous resolution.

UPPER EXTREMITY

Brachial Plexopathies

The probability of brachial plexus problems is about 8% at 1 month postoperatively, with only 2.3% of patients having persistent deficits at 6 months (4). There appears to be a male predilection that may relate to the preponderance of male patients or anatomic differences. Kirsch et al. (18) reported in 1971 on five patients who had nerve injury after having an operation that included a median sternotomy. There were varying degrees of partial or complete paralysis apparent in the immediate postoperative period. Motor function was affected more than sensory function. Normal function returned to all five patients after several months.

Graham et al. (19) reported on five patients who developed brachial plexus injuries. The medial cord of the plexus (the lower roots) was the most affected, with slightly less involvement in the lateral cord. Motor symptoms were more prominent than sensory symptoms. There was an asymmetrical involvement in patients who have bilateral lesions. Honet et al. (6) found that the medial cord of the brachial plexus was involved in all 11 patients referred to an electromyographic (EMG) clinic. Two patients had involvement of the lateral cord, and one with the posterior cord.

The mechanism for brachial plexopathies (18) can be attributed to mechanical stresses that occur during surgery. The median sternotomy incision and retraction (20) results in numerous pathophysiologic changes (Fig. 12.1).

Abnormal tension and stretching forces may occur when the unconscious patient is positioned so that the arm is hyperabducted. The usual muscular restraints to such positioning are not present when the person is under anesthesia. The anatomic reasons for stretching of the brachial plexus derive from the fixed positions of the plexus (from the prevertebral fascia to the axillary fascia). During surgery, the following factors may play a role on impingement of the brachial plexus:

1. Clavicular depression into the retroclavicular space.
2. Compression of the plexus between the clavicle and the first rib.
3. Lateral deviation or extension of the patient's head.
4. Stretching of the plexus over the humeral head with the arm in external rotation.
5. Stretching of the nerves over the arch formed by the attachment of the pectoralis minor to the coracoid process of the scapula (Fig. 12.2).

Cadaver studies have shown that when the retractor is opened fully, the clavicles are pushed

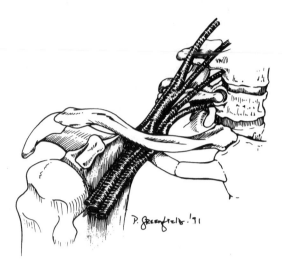

Figure 12.2. Impingement of brachial plexus during sternal retraction.

into the retroclavicular space and rotation of the first ribs occurs. These actions produce tension on the brachial plexus. Any structural abnormality, such as a cervical rib, would predispose to brachial plexus injury. Another potential cause includes inappropriately situated shoulder braces. In cases of left ventricular hypertrophy or internal thoracic artery dissection, wider retraction of the sternum may be needed to visualize the heart properly. In these situations, there is a greater likelihood of brachial plexus injury. Trauma from jugular vein cannulation also may lead to brachial plexus injury. Lederman et al. (2) found that in 74% of cases of brachial plexopathy, the jugular vein cannulation was on the same side.

Peripheral Neuropathies

Peripheral nervous system complications have been found to occur in 6% to 13% of patients after CABG surgery (2, 3, 14, 21). In general, upper extremity nerves are more affected than lower extremity nerves. Isolated peripheral nerves affected include the posterior interosseous nerve, ulnar nerve, circumflex nerve, and lateral cutaneous nerve (3). Graham et al. (19) found the ulnar nerve to be affected most frequently, with less involvement of the median or radial nerve. The frequent occurrence of ulnar nerve problems may be explained by the "double crush" syndrome. This syndrome postulates two areas of compression of the same nerve. In this case, the nerve is compressed in the ulnar groove

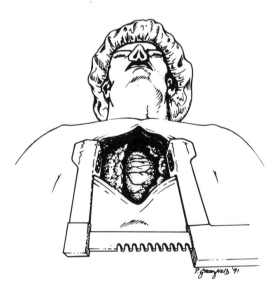

Figure 12.1. Median sternotomy and retraction.

from local pressure during bed rest, and more proximal involvement of the brachial plexus arises from compression during surgery.

If peripheral nerve problems exist in the postoperative period, the probability of a residual deficit at 6 months is low and ranges from 0% (18) to 2.3% (4, 19).

It is important to document preoperative neurologic abnormalities. Lederman et al. (2) found that 33% of patients scheduled for bypass surgery had some neurologic abnormality. Any conditions predisposing to nerve injuries, such as diabetes, should be documented. If peripheral nerve problems are determined after surgery, an EMG can determine the extent of abnormalities and help with prognostication. Nerve conduction studies can help determine whether the damage is to the nerve itself (axonal) or to the myelin sheath. To determine whether proximal damage has occurred to the nerve, specific EMG techniques such as F or H waves are necessary. In addition, somatosensory evoked potentials may help localize the area of proximal damage (22, 23). Proximal involvement after CABG surgery usually involves the brachial plexus.

The radial artery can be used as a coronary artery bypass graft with the advantages of an arterial conduit. Although the technique requires meticulous harvesting, the complications have been minimal. Reyes et al. (24) described local complications caused by hematoma formation, and paresthesia of the thumb. Symptoms resolved by 2 months postoperatively.

THORAX

Altered Structure

After CABG surgery (especially procedures that involve one or both internal thoracic arteries, which require extra retraction), it is not unusual to have some prominence of one side of the chest compared to the other. This appearance may be the result of asymmetric healing of the sternum. From a cosmetic perspective, this condition may be of concern; however, there is no need for corrective surgery. Occasionally, there is a fullness in the upper part of the incision above the manubrium. This condition usually reflects mild edema around the suture line. No specific treatment is required if there are no other signs of inflammation.

The mediastinal shadow on a postoperative chest radiograph may be widened from the collection of clots around the aorta and the heart. Subsequent radiographs should ensure that there is no progressive enlargement.

Unstable Sternum

Minor degrees of instability of the sternum are not uncommon in the early postoperative stage and are usually described as a click or movement of the two edges of the bone in certain positions. If there is no associated infection or drainage from the incision, reassurance and, at times, a chest binder to support the chest may be all that are required.

An unstable sternum, especially associated with purulent drainage of the incision, usually requires a referral for detailed investigation, as well as surgical debridement and subsequent reclosure of the sternum. Some of these patients may require musculocutaneous flaps to cover defects of the sternum that result from widespread infection and necrosis of the bone.

Occasionally, patients continue to have an unstable sternum for months after surgery. If there is considerable discomfort and no infection, reapproximation of the sternal edges is required.

Chest Wall Pain: Local Origin

Costochondritis is a relatively frequent cause of postoperative anterior chest pain, although an occult rib fracture may present in a similar way. The pain involves the costochondral and chondrosternal regions, and multiple lesions are present in most cases (25). The second to fifth costal cartilages are the usual sites. The principal physical sign is diffuse tenderness over the involved costal cartilages without swelling or inflammation. Certain movements of the chest and body may provoke the pain. Although most of these conditions are self-limiting, they may impede a smooth postoperative recovery. Although radiographs are not usually helpful, a bone scan may help to define further the areas involved. Patients are often concerned that the pain is cardiac in origin, and appropriate reassurance is required. In most cases, nonsteroidal anti-inflammatory drugs (NSAIDs) provide sufficient analgesia. In some refractory cases, indomethacin may be required. Intra-articular injections may be beneficial but should be done only by an experienced practitioner. Physical therapy modalities and techniques can lessen localized pain and address concomitant problems (decreased thoracic spine mobility).

With the now common use of the internal thoracic artery (ITA) as the preferred conduit for bypass surgery, a distinct entity of chest wall pain has been described (26). Symptomatology may include numbness to pinprick in the T1 through T6 dermatomal distributions; severe tenderness over the manubriosternal junction; pain elicited with minimal stimuli (allodynia); and constant pain across the anterior chest wall. The quality of the pain has been described as "burning, dull, or pricking." The mechanism for this painful condition has been postulated as severance of the anterior branches of the intercostal nerves or interference of the blood supply to the sternum. This may establish a "sympathetically" driven pain syndrome. Another potential mechanism for pain includes the prolonged chest retraction required to harvest the ITA (Fig. 12.3).

Treatment has included trials of transcutaneous electrical nerve stimulation (TENS), thoracic sympathetic ganglia blocks, desensitization techniques, and amitriptyline. The use of the ITA also has resulted in more musculoskeletal complaints in the arms, shoulders, and back (21).

A "trigger zone" has been identified in the pectoralis major muscle after an acute myocardial infarction (MI) or open heart surgery. These tender areas can refer pain in a similar manner

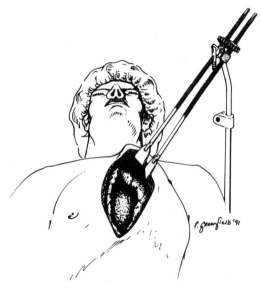

Figure 12.3. Prolonged chest retraction to harvest internal thoracic artery.

and distribution as angina. Travell and Simons (10) have identified specific distributions of referral, depending on the location of the trigger point. Such trigger points can be treated with vapocoolant spray (a mixture of fluorocarbons) and stretch technique, local injections, and mobilization techniques (10).

Incisional Problems

The most common problem related to the incision is pain, which can be localized or generalized. Generalized pain usually presents in the early stages and is related to musculoskeletal discomfort that arises from the sternotomy closure. Most cases respond to analgesics and reassurance. It is important to rule out a postpericardiotomy syndrome, which may require nonsteroidal analgesics.

Localized pain, especially that associated with signs of inflammation (erythema, swelling), may reflect infection at that site. Treatment consists of appropriate antibiotics, hot compresses, or dry heat, or, if there is a fluctuant area, local incision and drainage. A not infrequent cause of localized discomfort a few months after surgery is protrusion of sternal wires. This can be identified easily by palpation of the offending sternal wires and associated local tenderness. An infrequent cause of chest pain is a hypersensitivity reaction to the metal wires. Cases that have been described involved sensitivity to nickel, cobalt, or chromium (27). If the pain is significant, surgical removal of the wire under local anesthesia is recommended.

Muscular pain is more common in the early postoperative period. At times, this persists for many weeks after surgery. The pain is in the intercostal and accessory thoracic muscles and is made worse by maneuvers that tend to stretch or tense these muscles. The treatment is similar to that for rib pain. Local injection of a steroid or lidocaine is required for refractory cases.

Occasionally, an incisional hernia presents at the lower part of the incision through the linea alba. This may or may not be associated with pain or discomfort. Often, it gives a feeling of fullness in the epigastrium. If the hernia is causing discomfort or is of significant size, it should be attended to surgically. Before surgery, any conditions that may adversely affect adequate repair of the hernia, such as a chronic cough or wound infection, should be treated.

The incidence of sternal wound infections

varies according to the institution, the type of patient, and surgery. In general, the incidence is less than 2%. In one series of 4124 patients, the incidence was 1.8% (28). Uncomplicated conditions include those patients with a serosanguineous drainage or a stable sternum with a superficial infection. More serious conditions would include a purulent draining infection, unstable sternum, a deep sinus tract, or a retrosternal space infection. Risk factors for infection include the following (29):

1. Host conditions—older patients, obesity, malnutrition, preoperative infection, concomitant steroid use, and diabetes mellitus.
2. Operative conditions—more than one surgery during the same admission, prolonged surgery (longer than 6 hours), use of ITA grafts, difficulty in closure of the sternum, tracheostomy, prolonged ventilatory assistance, respiratory infection, septicemia, and low cardiac output.

Persistent draining sinuses through the incision should be assessed carefully, and bacterial culture and sensitivity should be obtained from the draining material. If the sinus tract is suggestive of deeper extension, a sinogram is recommended. Subsequent treatment would depend on the extent and rate of healing of the area. Often a localized excision of the sinus tract and immediate or delayed closure may be required in conjunction with systemic antibiotics. A persistent sinus drainage suggests an underlying infected sternal wire or osteomyelitis. This would require appropriate surgical treatment to remove the focus of infection.

Localized abscess formation usually presents early rather than late and requires local incision and drainage. Subsequent care by means of irrigation with a red rubber catheter (using normal saline or povidone-iodine solution two to three times a day) is useful in eliminating the underlying infection.

A painful, itchy, swollen incision can be distressing to a patient. Local application of various forms of ointments and creams by the patient is not an uncommon accompaniment of these problems. These treatments are ineffective and can be discouraged. For a keloid, local application of a topical steroid may relieve some of the itching. Vitamin E creams are often used, although no evidence exists to show that such a modality is effi-

cacious. Those patients who are refractory to this form of therapy should be referred for intradermal injection of corticosteroids. Surgical excision of the keloids is not generally recommended because there is a high incidence of recurrence of the keloid in the new scar. Local pressure is often beneficial and is done most effectively with a custom-fitted elastic garment and a pliable stent made by an occupational therapist. Surgery combined with postoperative radiation is done rarely but is effective in selective cases.

Most centers use subcuticular sutures for skin closure. It is not uncommon to see a small piece of suture material sticking out at the end of the incision. This represents the knot at the end of a continuous suture. Removal of this is simple and relieves considerable anxiety. Sutures that show at the site of infection should always be removed because a persistent foreign body impairs wound healing.

Rib Trauma

Trauma to the rib cage, with or without a fracture, is a common cause of chest wall pain, especially in the early postoperative period. This pain is usually made worse by deep breathing and movement. There is localized tenderness and sometimes swelling. Baisden et al. (30) found that 66% of patients had rib fractures after open heart surgery through a median sternotomy incision. None of these fractures was apparent on routine radiograph and thus required bone scans for the diagnosis. A healing callus may appear some weeks later. The fractures involved the first rib (94%), second rib (81%), third rib (25%), fourth rib (38%), and fifth and sixth ribs (18%). There was an average of 3.6 fractures per patient. It was shown that by removing the uppermost pair of retracting blades, the number of fractures decreased significantly (31).

A less widely known cause of rib pain is the slipping rib syndrome, which is characterized by pain at the lower costal margin, associated with increased mobility of the anterior end of costocartilage, usually in the area of the tenth and, occasionally, the eighth or ninth rib. The involved costocartilage is tender, and the pain may be duplicated by hooking the fingers under the costal margin and pulling the rib cage anteriorly.

Treatment of this condition usually requires recognition of the problem, reassurance, and analgesics. Local warmth application is often rewarding. The patient should be taught to avoid movements and positions that provoke the pain. Strapping is not generally recommended; however, local infiltration of lidocaine, intercostal nerve block, or surgical excision of the affected rib cartilages is reserved for refractory cases.

Respiratory Problems

Respiratory problems of noncardiac origin can arise from numerous causes. Shortness of breath and decreased exercise tolerance may be related to deconditioning from prolonged immobilization, atelectasis, or pleural effusion. Any previous pulmonary problems may worsen with the additional stress of surgery.

Increased age and a history of smoking are not unusual in patients who have CABG surgery, and one should exclude a possible case of pulmonary neoplasm. This may be visualized by a chest radiograph and found by a subsequent needle aspiration biopsy of a suspicious nodule, or by computed tomographic scanning.

Small degrees of pleural effusion can be treated effectively with diuretics. Early pleural effusions, especially left-sided ones, are seen more with the ITA dissection, which may require opening of the pleura. Some effusions may diminish spontaneously. Occasionally, a large pleural effusion requires confirmation by chest radiograph and, possibly, a thoracentesis. It is important to send the fluid for culture and sensitivity and for cytology.

An early patient complaint is the severe discomfort associated with sneezing or coughing. This can be alleviated partially by counterpressure against the sternum with a pillow.

The incidence of phrenic nerve palsy varies from 1.4% to 10%. By 1 year, 25% of affected patients have residual problems (2, 8). Howard and Panayiotopoulos (32) prospectively studied 59 subjects and found that 15% of patients had changes in the amplitude and area of the phrenic nerve response indicating that some of the fibers were not conducting. Postulated mechanisms for damage to the phrenic nerve include intraoperative traction, the use of cold "slush" for hypothermia, and surgical trauma.

The phrenic nerves have a close relationship to the ITA, and some cases of paralysis of the diaphragm can result from surgical trauma. The ITAs cross the phrenic nerve at a distance varying from 0.5 to 4.5 cm from its origin from the subclavian artery. Inadvertent damage can occur with the electrocautery when less care is taken in dissecting these arteries. Damage to the pericardiophrenic arterial branches of the internal mammary artery can also cause ischemia to the phrenic nerve and subsequent paralysis of the diaphragm (33).

LOWER EXTREMITY

Nerve Injuries

The femoral nerve, lateral femoral cutaneous nerve (meralgia paresthetica), or obdurator nerve may be affected as a result of complications secondary to cardiac catheterization. The cause usually is a bleed or damage to the femoral artery. Although the swelling may look threatening, conservative management is required. If the mass is pulsatile, an ultrasound is required to rule out a false aneurysm. Surgical intervention is required in the presence of infection or expansion. With more extensive bleeds into the retroperitoneal space, the lumbosacral plexus or the femoral and obturator nerves may be compromised. Sciatic nerve compression may result from prolonged immobilization associated with extended use of the intra-aortic balloon pump (34). The incidence of saphenous nerve dysfunction is 3% (2). Numbness and paresthesia are common in smaller segments because of incisional trauma. Possible mechanisms include inadvertent incision, ligation, or stretching of the saphenous nerve during the removal of the saphenous vein. Saphenous neuropathy may be alleviated with local injections of steroids or anesthetic, transcutaneous nerve stimulation, and neurolysis for refractory cases.

Peroneal nerve mononeuropathies can occur with a probability of about 2%. Patients with bilateral involvement had previous aortoiliac disease, and 50% of the involved patients had preexisting polyneuropathy. In the series by Lederman et al. (2), about 50% of the patients had continuing problems at 6 months.

Incision Problems

Saphenous vein incision problems are similar to those seen for the sternal incision. The usual site for problems includes the knee joint (increased swelling and tenderness) because of constant flexion and extension. Patients who have diabetes and peripheral vascular disease require scrupulous attention to surgical detail. Lower leg ischemia can result in impaired healing of the vein harvest sites. Gandhi et al. (35) described a patient who required infrainguinal revascularization for wound necrosis at the harvest site. Aggressive wound care, antibiotics, and infrainguinal reconstruction was required. Control of diabetes is important, especially in the presence of infection. Infection in the early postoperative period is easily treated. More serious, however, is the occurrence of cellulitis. One series reported an incidence of 2% for 700 patients (36). The mechanism of entry is unknown but may include previous skin lesions (for instance, fungal infection of toes). Recurrent cellulitis may occur if lymphatic drainage is impaired.

If patients have peripheral vascular disease, ischemic problems may occur after saphenous vein harvesting. Patients who have intermittent claudication should have a vascular work-up before bypass surgery. If there is bilateral aortoiliac disease, using upper extremity veins and ITAs may be preferable (36).

Swollen Leg

A common problem after bypass surgery is a swollen leg on the side of vein harvesting. This is an expected phenomenon because the normal venous return from the distal legs is diminished with removal of the saphenous vein. If there is a high index of suspicion for a deep vein thrombosis (DVT), then further diagnostic procedures, such as Doppler, plethysmography, or venography, are required.

Conservative methods (leg elevation and compression stockings) should suffice in the majority of cases. If the swelling is persistent (more than 3 months), the edema may become fixed in the extravascular tissue. In these cases, compression stockings are important. Such stockings can include "off-the-shelf" stockings or specialized custom-fitted stockings with graduated pressures (with the maximal pressures at the distal extremity). Distal pressures of 20 to 40 mm Hg are required. It is important not to wrinkle knee-length stockings in the popliteal space, because this can cause further compression.

If there is persistent swelling, certain activities should be avoided, including the Valsalva maneuver, heavy weight lifting, or tightening of the abdominal muscles, all of which impede venous return. Activities that involve a pounding motion (jogging or skipping) impart an additional moment of inertia to the already present hydrostatic pressure. Passive leg dependency, such as prolonged standing, should be avoided.

GENITOURINARY PROBLEMS

Patients who undergo bypass surgery have an indwelling catheter during the perioperative period. Men and women often experience transient dysuria after catheter removal, secondary to catheter-induced prostate and urethral congestion. This may require a short course of antibiotics for persistent symptoms and bacteriuria.

Persisting symptoms of benign prostatic hypertrophy can be aggravated by catheterization, and transurethral resection may be necessary. It can be performed safely 6 to 8 weeks after surgery. The urologist should be aware of the use of any antiplatelet medication or anticoagulants.

Occasionally, anticoagulation precipitates hematuria from a preexisting lesion in the genitourinary tract. Such patients should be referred to a urologist for cystoscopy and intravenous pyelography.

A 12% incidence of urethral strictures occurred in men catheterized with a latex catheter (37). These problems were diminished markedly with a change from latex to silicone. A Canadian study showed an incidence of strictures of 7.5% when urethral catheters were used, with none present when suprapubic catheters were used. It was suggested that ischemia during bypass surgery was involved with stricture development (38).

Symptoms usually are noticed immediately after removal of the catheter. Some patients, however, may present as long as 12 months after cardiac surgery (39). Treatment may require urethral dilatation, visual urethrectomy, and, in some cases, urethroplasty.

Fever with chills and rigors and increased frequency of urination are strongly suggestive of a urinary tract infection (UTI). Midstream urine samples should be obtained as well as blood cultures. Appropriate antibiotic therapy can be determined. Predisposing causes include prostatic enlargement with residual urine or previous history of calculi.

Renal failure occurs in about 1% of all CABG patients and in greater than 3% of elderly CABG patients (40). A later presentation of renal failure can occur presumably because of enteric-coated aspirin or any other NSAID. The putative mechanism is a toxic reaction to aspirin presumably mediated through prostaglandin inhibition with loss of vasodilator effect. Resolution occurs with discontinuation of these medications (41).

Hemoglobinuria may be an indication of hemolysis secondary to valvular insufficiency and may require detailed investigation.

Erectile function may be improved or adversely affected by alterations in circulatory homeostasis. Heaton and colleagues (42), in a retrospective analysis of 30 patients, found that 11 men reported an improvement, whereas 10 men reported a deterioration of functioning.

NERVOUS SYSTEM PROBLEMS

It has been estimated that cerebral disorders of any kind are seen in at least 35% of patients (43). Major neurologic abnormalities have been reported in 1% to 2% of patients (14, 44, 45). A large prospective study of 24 U.S. institutions documented type I neurologic outcomes (focal injury, stupor, or coma) in 3.1% of patients, and type II outcomes (deterioration in intellectual function, memory deficit, or seizures) in 3.0% (9). Numerous potential mechanisms may cause CNS disorders (5). Microemboli may be gaseous in origin because of inadequate defoaming in the oxygenator (46). Platelet and fibrin clots may form during extracorporeal circulation despite presumed adequate levels of heparin. Fat microemboli may occur from sternal splitting; atheromatous debris can occur from the aorta either during cannulation or from cross-clamping; and mediastinal fat globules can migrate into the perfusion circuit. Components of the extracorporeal circulation, such as silicone or polyvinyl tubing fragments, may also generate microemboli.

Other factors during surgery relate to decreased or altered flow. These include alteration in the normal pulsatile flow and complement activation, resulting in vasoconstriction (47). Hypotension may be a causative agent (48), but the findings are inconsistent (49).

The mechanism for peripheral nerve injuries may be attributed to compression or ischemia to the nerves. Malpositioning during surgery is the primary cause for compression neuropathies. Preexisting conditions that affect the nerves (i.e., diabetes) may predispose to peripheral nerve damage. Microemboli during surgery have been postulated as a causative mechanism. The concept of the double crush syndrome postulates that mild damage to two or more distinct areas of the nerve (at the ulnar groove and the brachial plexus) may produce a symptomatic lesion. Intra-arterial catheters (in the radial or femoral artery) may produce thrombotic complications. Hypothermia could be a contributory factor by altering the metabolic processes of the Schwann cell or impairing the circulation of the vasa nervorum. Risk factor analyses have shown conflicting results. A risk factor analysis that evaluates preoperative, intraoperative, and postoperative factors found that the use of systemic hypothermia was the only statistically significant risk factor (2). Seyfer et al. (7) found that previous neuropathies, wide retraction of the sternum, and prolonged duration for cardiopulmonary bypass all predispose to injury. Most peripheral nervous system deficits clear within a 6- to 8-week period, suggesting that the pathogenic mechanism was a conduction block.

The incidence of CVA is approximately 5% for definite strokes and 3% for possible minor strokes (4). At 6 months, 58% of those patients with a definite stroke still had a deficit, whereas only 13% of patients with a minor stroke continued to have problems. Of patients who have had a previous stroke, about 13% had new strokes or worsening of prior deficits; however, only 3% of these events were moderate to severe (50). The degree of resultant functional impairment from a stroke depends on many factors, including the extent of the neurologic deficit, the amount of resolution, and the course of a formalized rehabilitation program.

Intellectual dysfunction (as determined by deterioration on at least one test) has been found by psychometric methods in as many as 80% of bypass patients (51) at 1 week after surgery. The cognitive abilities that deteriorated most were psychomotor speed, attention and concentration, new learning ability, and auditory short-term memory. Importantly, only 48% of patients were aware of any deterioration in their intellectual abilities. Those who were aware complained of memory impairment, difficulty in concentrating, or mental slowness. It has been theorized that neuropsychologic deterioration could be caused by physical factors (tiredness, depression, lack of motivation) that lessened the performance on the psychological tests; however, such intellectual deterioration has not been seen with other types of surgery. It should be noted that most studies that assess cognitive changes failed to evaluate the patients prospectively before surgery. Klonoff et al. (52) assessed 135 patients 2 weeks before operation and 3, 12, and 24 months after surgery. Evaluations included tests to measure cognitive, neuropsychologic, and personality functions. Results showed the anticipation of the operation resulted in increased emotional arousal and distress that lessened after surgery. Interestingly, three of the seven tests for the Halstead Impairment Index were below limits for brain dysfunction, but these levels returned to normal after surgery. No adverse effects on intellectual functioning were seen after surgery. It is important to note that all these patients had successful outcomes with revascularization.

Another indicator of brain damage after bypass surgery included an elevated adenylate kinase in the cerebral spinal fluid. This enzyme is normally intracellular (53). Another proposed mechanism includes a reduction in mean cerebral blood flow during cardiopulmonary bypass operations (54), although no correlation was seen between measured cerebral flows and cognitive scores (55).

TIME COURSE OF SYMPTOMS AND GENDER ISSUES

Approximately 27% to 30% of CABG operations are now done on women (56). Thus, it is important to be aware of gender issues for recovery. Moore (57) studied 20 women and 20 men after bypass surgery at three time points: discharge, 48 hours after discharge, and 3 weeks after discharge. The time course of physical symptoms is shown in Table 12.2. Although the numbers were small, Moore concluded that women and men have different symptom complexes during this period. Breast discomfort was reported by 20% of women at discharge. Men reported more chest incisional pain, fatigue, and emotional symptoms.

SYSTEMIC ISSUES

Hypertension

Hypertension after bypass surgery has an incidence of from 24% to 50% (58, 59) in the early postoperative period. The proposed mechanism is a high peripheral resistance secondary to elevated plasma epinephrine and norepinephrine levels. Conversely, some hypertensive patients are adequately controlled during their hospitalization without medications. After discharge, some of these patients may be hypertensive if they do not resume their preoperative medications.

Fatigue

Fatigue may be secondary to altered sleep patterns, physical deconditioning, or a physiologic anemia. Such an anemia is produced by hemodilution for cardiopulmonary bypass. Because of the possibility of contracting acquired immunodeficiency syndrome from blood products, most centers use blood and blood products only if absolutely necessary. It is therefore not unusual for patients to be discharged with a hemoglobin around 9 mg/dL with resultant fatigue. Anemias can be treated with iron supplementation. Pick et al. (60) evaluated 74 patients for depression, fatigue, and circulating catecholamines. They found that postoperative fatigue was not amenable to psychological counseling. It was greatest in patients whose norepinephrine levels were highest preoperatively. Fatigue at 30 days correlated with levels of depression and anxiety.

Nausea

Nausea is a universal phenomenon in the first few days after surgery, but in some cases, it may persist after discharge. Nausea, if present, is generally related to medications; however, other conditions, such as hepatitis or gastrointestinal problems, should be excluded.

Fever

Fever is always abnormal. A careful history and examination are required to rule out an infective source such as a wound or bladder infection. Appropriate cultures and blood smears should be performed and the cause should be ascertained. There should be a special concern for those patients who have had concomitant valve surgery or any synthetic graft. Any fever that lasts more than

Table 12.2. Physical Symptoms Reported By Women and Men (40)

Symptoms	Discharge		48 hours after discharge		3 weeks after discharge	
	Women n (%)	Men n (%)	Women n (%)	Men n (%)	Women n (%)	Men n (%)
Chest incision	15(75)	12(60)	2(10)	19(95)	5(25)	12(60)
Energy level	5(25)	16(80)	3(15)	17(85)	4(20)	18(90)
Breathing	7(35)	6(30)	3(15)	4(20)	3(15)	4(20)
Eating	7(35)	4(20)	3(15)	3(15)	2(10)	2(10)
Sleeping	5(25)	10(50)	3(15)	11(55)	2(10)	9(45)
Breast	4(20)	0(0)	2(10)	0(0)	1(5)	0(0)
Back, neck, shoulder	3(15)	9(45)	5(25)	10(50)	2(10)	8(40)
Leg incision	3(15)	9(45)	5(25)	8(40)	2(10)	8(40)

48 hours in cardiac patients should be considered as endocarditis until proved otherwise.

COMMON PATIENT CONCERNS

Noncardiac Surgical Procedures (Including Dental Work)

For patients with bypass grafting, no prophylactic antibiotics are required because no artificial material is used. Patients with valvular problems should be treated appropriately. The only concern is the antiplatelet or anticoagulation medication, which may need to be discontinued if major bleeding is anticipated. The anesthesiologist involved should monitor the patient for arrhythmias, or ischemia for post-CABG patients. The timing of elective surgery is not influenced by the bypass operation. Six weeks is a reasonable time frame to allow the patient to recover from the discomfort of surgery. The urgency of the procedure and the patient's willingness to undergo another surgical procedure determine the timing. Patients who had a recent infarction in the perioperative period should be viewed as post-MI with regard to surgical procedures. Anesthetic and surgical procedures within 6 months of an MI are associated with increased morbidity and mortality (61).

Medications

Cardiac-related medications should be managed by the treating physicians. Noncardiac medications, especially over-the-counter drugs, should be checked for any cardiac stimulants or cross-reaction. This could be done by the pharmacist.

Sexual Relations

In general, many patients find that they are able to resume sexual relations with little difficulty. In particular, those persons who were limited with angina or shortness of breath find significant improvement (62). Assuming that the cardiac status is stable (no perioperative MI), sexual relations can be resumed safely when the patient is able to achieve approximately 4 metabolic equivalents (METs) in terms of exercise capacity. To allow complete healing of the sternum, 4 weeks after discharge can be given as a recommended time.

Risk of Transfusion

The risk of human immunodeficiency virus (HIV) infection after transfusion of 1 unit of blood is 1:420,000. The risk of viral hepatitis infection is 1:5000 (63). Because of these risks, most centers are discharging patients with a relatively low hemoglobin count. This transient anemia affects the general level of energy and the ability to exercise and may require iron supplementation.

Flu Shots

Bypass surgery in itself is not a contraindication to flu shots. Patients with acute respiratory or other active infections or any severe febrile illness should not receive the vaccine until medically stable.

Sleep Disturbances

Sleep disturbances are issues of common concern after bypass surgery. A telephone survey of 49 CABG patients (64) showed that 60% of patients reported sleeping difficulties, even up to 6 months after discharge. There was little difficulty falling asleep, but there were problems staying asleep. The most common reasons identified were incisional pain, nocturia, and difficulty in finding a comfortable position. Such changes may be a result of altered sleep patterns (sleeping in the daytime) or the change from habitual hypnotic medication. Nightmares appear to be most common in the hospital and may resolve with a change in hypnotic sedation. Diaphoretic spells during the night are reported; however, the cause has not been explained.

References

1. Karp RB, Kouchoukos NT. Postoperative care of the cardiovascular surgical patient. In: Baue AE, ed. Glenn's thoracic and cardiovascular surgery. 5th ed. Norwalk, CT: Appleton and Lange, 1990;2:1535–1546.
2. Lederman RJ, Breuer AC, Hanson MR, et al. Peripheral nervous system complications of coronary artery bypass graft surgery. Ann Neurol 1982;12:297–301.
3. Keates JRW, Innocenti DM, Ross DN. Mononeuritis multiplex. J Thorac Cardiovasc Surg 1975;69:816–819.
4. Shaw PJ, Bates D, Cartlidge NEF, et al. Neurological complications of coronary artery bypass graft surgery: six month follow-up study. Br Med J 1986;293:165–167.
5. Shaw PJ, Bates D, Cartlidge NEF, et al. Neuro-ophthalmological complications of coronary artery bypass graft surgery. Acta Neurol Scand 1987;76:1–7.
6. Honet JC, Raikes JA, Kantrowitz A, et al. Neuropathy in the upper extremity after open-heart surgery. Arch Phys Med Rehabil 1976;57:264–267.
7. Seyfer A, Grammer NY, Bogumill GP, et al. Upper extremity neuropathies after cardiac surgery. J Hand Surg 1985;10(A):16–19.
8. Dajee A, Pellegrini J, Cooper G, et al. Phrenic nerve palsy after topical cardiac hypothermia. Int Surg 1983;68:345–348.
9. Roach GW, Kanchuger M, Mangano CM, et al. Adverse cerebral outcomes after coronary bypass surgery. N Engl J Med 1996;335:1857–1863.
10. Travell JG, Simons DG. Myofascial pain and dysfunction. Baltimore: Williams & Wilkins, 1983.
11. Fuller JE, Thomas DV. Facial nerve paralysis after general anesthesia. JAMA 1956;162:645.
12. Picone AL, Baisden CE, Ford EG, et al. Paranasal sinusitis: cryptic sepsis after coronary artery bypass operations. Ann Thorac Surg 1993;55:706–710.
13. Barbut D, Gold J, Heinemann M, et al. Horners syndrome after coronary after bypass surgery. Neurology 1996;46:181–184.
14. Shaw PJ, Bates D, Cartlidge NEF, et al. Early neurological complications of coronary artery bypass surgery. Br Med J 1985;291:1384–1387.
15. Arnold JV, Blauth CI, Smith PL, et al. Demonstration of cerebral microemboli occurring during coronary artery. J Audiov Media Med 1990;13:87–90.
16. Williams IM. Fundus oculi findings associated with cardio-pulmonary bypass procedures. Trans Asia-Pacific Acad Opthalmol, 4th Congress, 1972:72–76.
17. Shafei H, el-Kholy A, Azmy S, et al. Vocal cord dysfunction after cardiac surgery: an overlooked complication. Eur J Cardiothorac Surg 1997;11:564–566.
18. Kirsh MM, Magee KR, Gago O, et al. Brachial plexus injury following median sternotomy incision. Ann Thorac Surg 1971;11:315–319.
19. Graham JG, Pye IF, McQueen IN. Brachial plexus injury after median sternotomy. J Neurol Neurosurg Psychiatry 1981;44:621–625.
20. Julian OC, Lopez-Belio M, Dye WS, et al. The median sternal incision in intracardiac surgery with extracorporeal circulation: a general evaluation of its use in heart surgery. Surgery 1957;42:753–761.
21. Roy RC, Stafford MA, Charlton JE. Nerve injury and musculoskeletal complaints after cardiac surgery: influence of internal mammary artery dissection and left arm position. Anesth Analg 1988;67:277–279.
22. Hallikainen H, Partanen J, Mervaala E. The importance of neurophysiological evaluation of plexus brachialis injury caused by open heart surgery. Electromyogr Clin Neurophysiol 1993;33:67–71.
23. Morin JE, Long R, Elleker MG, et al. Upper extremity neuropathies following median sternotomy. Ann Thorac Surg 1982;34:181–185.
24. Reyes A, Frame R, Brodman R. Technique for harvesting the radial artery as a coronary artery bypass graft. Ann Thorac Surg 1995;59:118–126.
25. Fam AG, Smythe H. Musculoskeletal chest wall pain. Can Med Assoc J 1985;133:379–389.
26. Mailis A, Chan J, Basinski A, et al. Chest wall pain after aortocoronary bypass surgery using internal mammary. Heart Lung 1989;18:553–558.
27. Ancalmo N, Perniciaro C, Ochsner J. Hypersensitivity reaction to sternal wires: a possible cause of postoperative pain. Cardiovasc Surg 1993;1:439–441.
28. Serry C, Bleck PC, Javid H, et al. Sternal wound complications. J Thorac Cardiovasc Surg 1980;80:861–867.
29. Marshall J, Conkey C. Sternal wound complications. Nursing care for coronary surgery patients. AORN J 1985;42:700–706.
30. Baisden CE, Greenwald LV, Symbas PN. Occult rib fractures and brachial plexus injury following median sternotomy for open-heart operations. Ann Thorac Surg 1984;38:192–194.
31. Vander Salm TG, Cereda JM, Cutler BS. Brachial plexus injury following median sternotomy. J Thorac Cardiovasc Surg 1980;80:447–452.
32. Howard R, Panayiotopoulos C. A comprehensive electrophysiological evaluation of phrenic nerve injury related to open-heart surgery. Acta Neurol Scand 1995;91:225–229.
33. Henrique-Pino J, Gomes W, Prates J, et al. Surgical anatomy of the internal thoracic artery. Ann Thorac Surg 1997;64:1041–1045.
34. McManis PG. Sciatic nerve lesions during cardiac surgery. Neurology 1994;44:684–687.
35. Gandhi RH, Katz D, Wheeler JR, et al. Vein harvest ischemia: a peripheral vascular complication of coronary artery bypass grafting. Cardiovasc Surg 1994;2:478–483.
36. Lavee J, Schneiderman J, Yorav S, et al. Complications of saphenous vein harvesting following coronary artery bypass surgery. J Cardiovasc Surg (Torino) 1989;30:989–991.
37. Ruutu M, Alfthan O, Heikkinen L, et al. Unexpected urethral strictures after short-term catheterization in open-heart surgery. Scand J Urol Nephrol 1984;18:9–12.
38. Abdel-Hakim A, Bernstein J, Teijeira J, et al. Urethral stricture after cardiovascular surgery: a retrospective and prospective study. J Urol 1983;130:1100–1101.
39. Sutherland PD, Maddern JP, Jose JS, et al. Urethral

stricture after cardiac surgery. Br J Urol 1983;55: 413–416.

40. Ennabli K, Pelletier L. Morbidity and mortality of coronary artery surgery after the age of 70 years. Ann Thorac Surg 1986;42:197–200.

41. Clive DM, Stoff JS. Renal syndromes associated with nonsteroidal antiinflammatory drugs. N Engl J Med 1984;310:563–572.

42. Heaton JP, Evans H, Adams MA, et al. Coronary artery bypass graft surgery and its impact on erectile function: a preliminary retrospective study. Int J Impot Res 1996;8:35–39.

43. Pedley TA, Emerson RG. Neurological complications of cardiac surgery. In: Mathews WB, Glaser GH, eds. Recent advances in clinical neurology. Edinburgh: Churchill Livingstone, 1984.

44. Bojar RM, Najafi H, Dealria GA, et al. Neurological complications of coronary revascularization. Ann Thorac Surg 1983;36:427–432.

45. Breuer AC, Furlan AJ, Hanson MR, et al. Central nervous system complications of coronary artery bypass graft. Stroke 1983;14:682–687.

46. Solis RT, Kennedy PS, Beall AC, et al. Cardiopulmonary bypass: microembolism and platelet aggregation. Circulation 1975;52:103–108.

47. Chenoweth DR, Cooper SW, Hygli TF. Complement activation during cardiopulmonary bypass. N Engl J Med 1981;304:497–503.

48. Stockard J, Bickford RG, Schauble JF. Pressure-dependent cerebral ischemia during cardiopulmonary bypass. Neurology 1973;23:521–529.

49. Kolkka R, Hilberman M. Neurologic dysfunction following cardiac operation with low-flow, low-pressure cardiopulmonary bypass. J Thorac Cardiovasc Surg 1980;79:432–437.

50. Rorick MB, Furlan AJ. Risk of cardiac surgery in patients with prior stroke. Neurology 1990;40:835–837.

51. Shaw PJ, Bates D, Cartlidge NE, et al. Early intellectual dysfunction following coronary bypass surgery. Q J Med 1986;58:59–68.

52. Klonoff H, Clark C, Kavanagh-Gray D, et al. Two-year follow-up study of coronary bypass surgery. J Thorac Cardiovasc Surg 1989;97:78–85.

53. Aberg T, Tyden H, Ronquist G, et al. Release of adenylate kinase into the cerebro-spinal fluid during open-heart surgery and its relation to post-operative intellectual function. Lancet 1982;1:1139–1142.

54. Henriksen L. Evidence suggestive of diffuse brain damage following cardiac operations. Lancet 1984;1: 816–820.

55. Freeman AM, Folks DG, Sokol RS, et al. Cognitive function after coronary bypass surgery: effect of decreased. Am J Psychiatry 1985;142:110–112.

56. King K, Clark P, Kicks G. Patterns of referral and recovery in women and men undergoing coronary artery bypass grafting. Am J Cardiol 1992;69:179–182.

57. Moore S. A comparison of women's and men's symptoms during home recovery after coronary artery bypass surgery. Heart Lung 1995;24:495–501.

58. Estafanous FG, Tarazi RC. Systemic arterial hypertension associated with cardiac surgery. Am J Cardiol 1980;46:685–694.

59. McIlvaine W, Boulanger M, Maille J, et al. Hypertension following coronary artery bypass graft. Can Anaesth Soc J 1982;29:212–217.

60. Pick B, Molloy A, Hinds C, et al. Post-operative fatigue following coronary artery bypass relationship to emotional state and to the catecholamine response surgery. J Psychosom Res 1994;38:599–607.

61. Raol LK, Jacobs KH, El-Etr AA. Reinfarction following anesthesia in patients with a myocardial infarction. Anesthesiology 1983;59:499–505.

62. Papadopoulos C. Sexual aspects of cardiovascular disease. In: Lief HI, ed. Sexual medicine. New York: Praeger, 1989;10:1–22.

63. Klein H. Allogeneic transfusion risks in the surgical patient. Am J Surg 1995;170:21S–26S.

64. Schaefer KM, Swaverly D, Rothenberger C, et al. Sleep disturbances postcoronary artery bypass surgery. Prog Cardiovasc Nurs 1996;11:5–14.

Common Musculoskeletal Problems in the Exercising Adult

Joseph A. Abate and John A. Bergfeld

GENERAL CONSIDERATIONS

There is limited literature on the epidemiology of sports- or exercise-related injuries in elderly athletes. Most studies have looked at elderly elite marathoners or participants in World Master's Games. These studies were primarily undertaken during these championship events (1). It is hard to use any of these studies to assess the risk of injury for cardiac patients or normal healthy elderly adults undertaking increasing physical activity or rehabilitation programs.

An exercise prescription for patients with cardiac disease normally begins with walking, which is then increased to light calisthenics and weight lifting and eventually progresses to more rigorous activities such as biking, jogging, or swimming (2). Patients with cardiac disease may also participate in other activities or sports during their leisure time for relaxation. Golf, racquet sports, skiing, and hiking may often be enjoyed by many elderly athletes or cardiac rehabilitation patients. There can be acute traumatic or more commonly chronic overuse injuries during any of these activities.

Most elderly individuals are fairly cautious when they exercise, and therefore physical activity is usually safe. Most serious incapacitating injuries occur from falls; therefore, balance training and exercise to strengthen the lower extremities is most important to prevent these types of injuries. Sudden cardiovascular death also seems to be rare in the elderly, but most studies have been carried out in healthy younger or very fit adults; therefore, the risk of sudden cardiac death in patients with coronary disease is harder to quantify. Most studies that have looked at the injury rates in elderly patients mainly relate to walking and jogging. The rates of injury vary from 14% to as much as 57% of the participants (2). The most common injuries were of the knee in the lower extremity, and for upper extremity injuries, the shoulder and arm were often involved. It is also common for patients to sustain injuries during exercise training that are related to previous orthopedic problems. Specific injuries will be discussed in more detail in the next sections.

FRACTURES

Fractures are more common in elderly athletes and patients for two basic reasons. Elderly patients are more prone to falls because of poor balance and decreased muscular strength (3). In addition, the aging skeleton has a decrease in bone mass and in cortical thickness with time that causes weakening of the bone. Therefore, patients with osteoporosis and women in general are at increased risk for sustaining these types of injuries.

ARTHRITIS

Degenerative arthritis of the weight-bearing joints in the lower extremities can make it very difficult for patients to follow an aggressive exercise regimen. Arthritis of hip, knee, and the foot and ankle are commonly encountered in elderly patients. Usually conservative treatment with shoe wear modifications or equipment changes combined with a program that increases both endurance and strength in general yields the best results. Selected surgeries such as arthroscopic or open debridement and realignment procedures may be extremely helpful in patients who have failed conservative management. Total joint arthroplasty usually provides excellent pain relief and increases the patient's functioning (4).

These procedures may prevent many athletes and some elderly patients from continuing very strenuous physical activity.

SOFT TISSUE INJURIES

Soft tissue problems commonly affect all athletes and are frequently seen in the elderly. These injuries can occur from traumatic events or overuse. There are many reasons why elderly patients are more prone to these types of injuries. Muscle strains and tendinitis occur when the soft tissues are stressed beyond their physiologic capacity. Aging connective tissue loses its physiologic capacity (5). Increasing tissue stiffness secondary to dehydration, increased collagen cross-linking, and loss of muscular flexibility and strength contribute to injuries of the soft tissues in the elderly. Muscle strain is reported to be the most typical injury found among older athletes. Achilles tendon injuries are common with increasing age (1). Most ruptures occur in the fourth decade, but become much more infrequent in patients older than 60 years. Also, overuse injuries of the rotator cuff, the quadriceps, and the biceps tendon and epicondylitis of the elbow all seem to occur more frequently with increasing age (6).

Therefore, any exercise program should focus on improving not only strength, but also flexibility. By increasing their flexibility many patients can function at a higher level during their daily activities and they may also make great strides during their exercise and rehabilitation programs. Flexibility exercises should be performed at least three times per week, but can be performed more often if there is severe involvement in certain areas (7).

EFFECTS OF TEMPERATURE

Elderly individuals are usually less able to adapt to changes in temperature. Total body water is also decreased; therefore, elderly patients are prone to dehydration and hyperthermia. Elderly patients should be advised to consume fluid before exercising and have regularly scheduled water breaks while exercising to prevent some of these problems.

Elderly patients are also more susceptible to cold injuries and hypothermia. This may be related to multiple factors including the loss of subcutaneous fat, peripheral vascular disease,

decreased muscle mass, and the effects of various medications and alcohol. Therefore, elderly patients must be instructed to carefully monitor all environmental conditions to avoid injuries during sporting activities and exercise (7).

COMMON SPORTS-SPECIFIC PROBLEMS

Golf

Flexibility is very important for all golfers. As described previously, elderly athletes have less flexibility then their younger counterparts. Most orthopedic problems in golfers are manifestations of overuse syndromes. Low back and neck pain are frequent complaints in golfers of all ages, and therefore flexibility exercises and strengthening of the abdominal, trunk, and paraspinal muscles are important to avoid this problem (8).

Golfers also must worry about injuries to the meniscal cartilage because they often perform squatting activities during golf and this causes increased loads and the possibility of meniscal tears. Also, the twisting motion involved in a normal golf swing may cause injury to degenerative meniscal cartilage. It is unlikely, though, that patients will sustain significant knee ligament injuries during normal golf.

In the upper extremity shoulder pain is frequently associated with rotator cuff overuse syndromes, and these types of shoulder problems are very common in elderly golfers. Instability is usually not a problem except in young athletes. Therefore, most shoulder problems in older golfers involve rotator cuff tears and tendinitis or impingement syndromes from scarring within the subacromial space (1).

Elbow and wrist pain are also common from repeated striking of the ground during the golf swing. Elderly golfers normally complain of lateral epicondylitis ("tennis elbow") in the nondominant elbow, and medial epicondylitis ("golfer's elbow") is seen in the dominant elbow. Wrist pain is usually caused by extensor tendinitis (8).

Because most injuries in golf are overuse syndromes, prevention is the best treatment. Therefore, proper warm-up, flexibility and stretching exercises, and specific muscle strengthening are important to enjoying the game and preventing injuries (5).

Tennis and Other Racquet Sports

Racquet sports such as tennis, squash, and racquetball are enjoyed by many elderly athletes and patients. Chronic overuse injuries are similar to other sports and again include rotator cuff tendinitis, back problems, elbow epicondylitis, and generalized osteoarthritis. Acute injuries normally involve the lower extremities, especially degenerative meniscal tears as described previously and very commonly tears of the medial head of the gastrocnemius, which in the past was thought to be a rupture of the plantaris tendon. These types of medial gastrocnemius head tears usually occur while pushing off with the toes when running for the ball. Also, Achilles tendon ruptures are commonly seen in racquet sports as patients have forced dorsiflexion of the ankle while the gastrocnemius-soleus complex is actively plantar flexing the ankle while reaching for a shot.

Treatment for meniscal tears normally involves arthroscopic meniscectomy and most players return to their previous level of play without difficulty. The treatment of Achilles tendon ruptures is somewhat controversial, but surgery usually allows return to tennis within 6 months after the injury. Chronic injuries and overuse syndromes again respond best to properly directed conditioning and rehabilitation programs (9).

Swimming

Swimming is a sport enjoyed by many elderly patients both for recreation and as part of a cardiac exercise program. There are also many elite elderly athletes who participate in master's swimming competitions. Many older individuals with lower extremity degenerative arthritis do extremely well with swimming because of the decreased weight-bearing status of the sport caused by the buoyancy of the water (5).

A common problem in the older swimmer is called "swimmer's shoulder," which is an overuse phenomenon and impingement syndrome of the subacromial bursa related to multiple years of swimming with the overhead stroke. Tendinitis of the rotator cuff or the biceps tendon with impingement of the subacromial space is common, but complete rupture of the rotator cuff is not unusual. Supraspinatus tendon rupture is much more common in older swimmers than in their younger counterparts (10).

Tendinitis may be treated with a program of exercise, anti-inflammatory medications, and, occasionally, cortisone injection. Treatment of complete rotator cuff ruptures is generally by surgical repair of the tendon and then a progressive rehabilitation program. It may take 4 to 6 months after repair before swimmers are able to get back in the pool. Elderly swimmers may need to modify their training schedule or stroke to avoid the problems commonly associated with impingement. Equipment such as hand paddles, which increase the resistance during the stroke, during training also can increase the impingement syndrome pain and should be avoided in senior swimmers. The use of fins on the lower extremities can help increase the overall leg strength of many elderly swimmers, but these types of devices should be avoided in athletes with chronic patellofemoral pain as this may increase their symptoms (10).

In general, swimming is an excellent exercise for elderly athletes and patients undergoing cardiac rehabilitation, especially if they have degenerative arthritis that makes weight-bearing activities difficult.

Running

As mentioned previously, many patients involved in cardiac rehabilitation are encouraged to progress from walking and light jogging to full running to increase their exercise intensity. Problems associated with osteoarthritis and degenerative articular and meniscal cartilage changes may make this activity difficult for many elderly athletes and patients. There also are multiple overuse problems associated with running. In general, these occur in the lower extremity, especially the knee, ankle, and foot.

Normally appropriate equipment and the correct type of running surface are keys to helping older runners prevent injuries (5). One of the biggest problems is that older athletes often neglect to perform adequate shoe replacement, which should usually occur after 250 to 500 miles if the patient runs on hard surfaces and slightly longer if the patient normally runs on softer surfaces. Running shoe replacement at these regular intervals will increase the cushioning and shock-absorbing capacity and may help to prevent these types of overuse injuries (11).

Cycling and Treadmill

For patients who cannot tolerate fast walking or running, cycling or treadmill is an excellent alternative mode of exercise. Normal outdoor bicycling or stationary indoor cycling or treadmill can be enjoyed by most patients and provides an excellent aerobic activity that may be less stressful on patients with degenerative joint complaints (5). Another advantage of stationary cycling or treadmill is that it still can be performed during poor weather, and it may be enjoyed by patients at home during any time of the day.

To avoid injury, elderly cyclists or treadmill users should be sure they have the proper equipment. Correct frame dimensions and rider positioning on the cycle is of utmost importance. Correct seat height and adequate padding of the handles for both stationary cycles and outdoor bicycles are important to prevent upper extremity compression syndromes of the wrist and hand (12). The treadmill should have impact absorption capacity and a safety kill switch.

Alpine and Cross-Country Skiing

Skiing is an excellent exercise for many elderly athletes and patients undergoing cardiac rehabilitation, but there are certain injuries that occur during skiing caused by the fact that falls are very common during the sport. Older skiers are obviously at higher risk of fracture for any given force than younger skiers because the older skiers have relative or absolute osteopenia in many instances. The most common fractures occur in the hip, tibial plateau, proximal humerus, distal radius, and spine. Upper extremity injuries are also common during skiing, and these mostly include sprains of the wrist and thumb or dislocation of the shoulder during a fall (13).

In contrast to other sports, injuries in elderly skiers commonly involve the knee ligaments. The most common ligament injured is the medial collateral ligament, but anterior cruciate ligament tears are also seen in elderly skiers. Ski binding and boot improvements have not lessened the incidence of these knee ligament injuries. Patellofemoral problems are also common in older skiers because skiing involves being in a bent-knee position for much of the activity.

Treatment of most of these knee complaints initially involves conservative measures, although there are some patients who are so physically active that knee ligament reconstruction, such as of the anterior cruciate ligament, may be considered

in selected cases. Again, increases in strength and flexibility are extremely important for older athletes involved in skiing and may prevent many of these types of injuries by decreasing the risks of falling as patients have improved balance and strength. In addition to these injuries, the common overuse injuries of the shoulder and legs are seen in cross-country skiers (5).

SUMMARY

Exercise training can improve the daily life of cardiac patients and the average sedentary adult. Participation in sporting activities is an excellent way for many patients to continue a prolonged cardiac rehabilitation program after discharge from supervised medical care. It is important that the patient and older athlete understand the principles of correct exercise training to avoid injury and to enjoy the chosen activity. In this way, both musculoskeletal and cardiac complications can hopefully be avoided. Prevention and early treatment of these injuries may help.

References

1. Kallinen M, Markku A. Aging, physical activity and sports injuries. An overview of common sports injuries in the elderly. Sports Med 1995;20:41–52.
2. Kamon E. Exercise prescription for heart disease. In: Torg JS, Shepard RJ, Welsh RP, eds. Current therapy in sports medicine. Philadelphia: BC Decker, Inc., 1994:85–92.
3. Lillegard WA, Terrio JD. Appropriate strength training. Med Clin North Am 1994;78:457–477.
4. Door LD. Arthritis and athletics. Clin Sports Med 1991;10:343–357.
5. Elia EA. Exercise and the elderly. Clin Sports Med 1991;10:141–155.
6. Tidball JG. Myotendinous junction injury in relation to function, structure and molecular composition. Exerc Sports Sci Rev 1991;19:419–445.
7. Barry HC, Eathorne SW. Exercise and aging. Issues for the practitioner. Med Clin North Am 1994;78:357–376.
8. Jobe FW, Schwabb DM. Gold for the mature athlete. Clin Sports Med 1991;10:269–283.
9. Leach RE, Abramowitz A. The senior tennis player. Clin Sports Med 1991;10:284–291.
10. Richardson AB, Miller JW. Swimming and the older athlete. Clin Sport Med 1991;10:301–318.
11. Ting AJ. Running and the older athlete. Clin Sports Med 1991;10:319–325.
12. McLennan JG, McLennan JC. Cycling and the older athlete. Clin Sports Med 1991;10:292–299.
13. Burns TP, Steadman JR, Rodney WG. Alpine skiing and the mature athlete. Clin Sports Med 1991;10:327–342.

SECTION IV.

Psychosocial Considerations in Cardiovascular Rehabilitation

Psychosocial Interventions for Cardiac Patients

Wayne M. Sotile

The advisability of bolstering the psychosocial aspect of cardiopulmonary care has been widely called for (1). This call is justified from both clinical and research perspectives. Between 40% and 50% of patients with myocardial infarction (MI) experience elevated levels of anxiety and fear in the hospital, and approximately one-fifth continue to report anxiety at 1-year follow-up (2). Prevalence rates for depression during the first 6 months after hospitalization vary between 20% and 30%, and up to 33% of patients may remain chronically depressed despite recovery of functional capacity (3). Some evidence suggests that spouses actually experience more severe symptoms of psychological distress than do their recovering mates (4–6). Patients who are given simple psychosocial interventions cope better with the challenges of rehabilitation and adhere more readily to medical advice than do those who receive only ordinary care (7–9).

Unfortunately, the worldwide literature suggests that, in actual practice, relatively few cardiac care facilities provide psychosocial interventions (10–13). Sotile (1) argued that this dearth of psychosocial care is owing to the misguided notion that only professionals trained in a mental health specialty are qualified to deliver psychosocial intervention. Recent research strongly suggests that even a little attention to psychosocial issues at bedside or during office-based consultation, either by a physician or a nurse, can significantly enhance psychosocial functioning (14, 15), decrease lengths of hospital stays (16), and improve morbidity and mortality rates (17).

The purpose of this chapter is to provide a brief overview of the psychosocial adjustment processes faced by cardiac patients and their loved ones and offer practical guidelines for structuring psychosocial interventions in medical settings. As will be seen, a continuum of interventions can be structured in office, hospital, and rehabilitation settings.

PSYCHOSOCIAL ADJUSTMENT TO CARDIAC ILLNESS

Individual and family perceptions, attitudes, stages of life, and coping repertoires all converge to affect adjustment to illness. Rose and Robbins (18) proposed that the patient and the family should be viewed as emotionally healthy individuals who are simply facing a frightening and unusual situation that stirs stress reactions. When perceived demands exceed perceived coping abilities (19), a range of stress responses emerge, varying from transient adjustment disorders to psychotic reactions, even in patients with no prior history of psychiatric maladjustment. Adjustment to illness is a process that is affected by many factors (1, 6, 20).

For many individuals and families cardiac illness complicates problems that precede onset of illness. For example, both longitudinal and cross-sectional studies have found that MI is often predated by depression (21), other psychiatric illnesses (22), or high levels of marital conflict (20) or sexual dysfunction (23).

Recovery may also be complicated by stressors such as vocational, medical, financial, or family difficulties, or by the simple wear-and-tear effects of life's stress (22). In addition, periods of mourning losses associated with the illness are typical of recovering patients and their loved ones (6, 24, 25).

Cassem and Hackett (26) proposed a model of the psychological course of reacting to acute cardiac care that has been expanded to apply to long-range psychosocial adjustment (1):

Stage 1: Anxiety predominates the initial stage of adjustment. During this period, the patient's premorbid personality-based coping tendencies shape the clinical presentation. For example, the type A coper may become excessively competitive or controlling, or the timid may become paralyzed with fear. These exaggerated reactions diminish as the patient gains familiarity with the rehabilitation process, trust in health care providers, and ample social support.

Stage 2: Progress in physical rehabilitation during the first months of recovery typically bolsters the patient's motivation and soothes anxieties. Optimism regarding long-range recovery blossoms during this stage, often to rather unrealistic degrees.

Stage 3: Depression, anxiety, and pessimism surface when the patient fails to continue at the same rate of improvement.

Stage 4: Finally, characterological coping patterns surface, both for the patient and his or her loved ones. Here, the effects of the illness may subtly shape individual and family coping.

It is crucial to remember that the psychosocial adjustment course is cyclical, not linear. This fact may explain the discrepancies in research findings regarding the "typical" frequency and duration of symptoms of psychosocial struggles for recovering patients (27). Patterson (28, 29) proposed that family-based coping paradigms solidify somewhere between 3 months and 1 year after onset of illness and remain resistant to change thereafter. Croog and Levine (30) found that wives' evaluations of their marriage after a husband's MI remain stable from the first to the eighth year. In an ongoing study of relationship patterns after MI, Laerum and associates (31, 32) found that patient assessments of their total life situation and of their family life did not change significantly during evaluations performed 3 to 5 months and 2 to 4 years after MI.

Although many patients enter clinical care already having solidified individual and family coping patterns, others present while still malleable and responsive to input. This fact underscores the tremendous opportunity and obligation that health care providers are given to help shape patients' individual and interpersonal adjustment patterns.

STRUCTURING PSYCHOSOCIAL INTERVENTIONS: GENERAL GUIDELINES

A number of guidelines for structuring psychosocial interventions with cardiac patients have been published (1, 33–36). In clinical practice, the following general guidelines should be kept in mind.

Think Crisis Intervention

Because medical intervention either comes at a time of crisis in a patient's life or constitutes a crisis in and of itself, crisis intervention theory can serve as a helpful backdrop to recognizing and treating patients' psychosocial concerns (37). Crisis theory proposes that patients and their loved ones cope better with a crisis when they are offered a combination of reassurance, advice, challenge to cope cooperatively together, and follow-up. Repeated, brief therapeutic contacts that focus on the crises being caused by hospitalization, medical procedures, or rehabilitation tasks are advised.

The efficacy of crisis intervention is especially evident when patients and loved ones are offered preoperative anticipatory guidance that facilitates postsurgery coping. Simply put, patients who are coached in simple coping strategies, like deep-breathing relaxation, distraction, and the importance of family support strategies, evidence a wealth of positive postoperative outcomes, including the following: increased patient cooperation and satisfaction; lowered requests for pain medications; less reported and observed symptoms of anxiety; lessened incidence of postoperative delirium; and lessened medical need for rehospitalization (7, 38).

Normalize the Intervention

Every effort should be made to normalize receiving psychosocial help. In this regard, Gruen (39) recommended that inpatient psychological consultation might be framed as intervention from the "Department of Patient Care Improvement." The advisability of framing interventions in stress management terminology will be discussed below.

Remember That Education and Support Are Not Enough

In addition to advice and support, effective psychosocial interventions must incorporate skill-building for habit change (36, 40, 41). The tenets of behavior modification and behavior therapy can be helpful here. Behavior modification interventions promote self-control through pairing reinforcement with desired behaviors, disrupting chains of maladaptive behaviors, and contracting. Behavior therapy focuses on skill-building, pattern disruption, and the establishment of new stimulus-response patterns (1).

Set Goals That Are Relevant to the Patient

In dealing with patients with multiple problems, care should be taken to determine the patient's most important rehabilitation goals (42). Prochaska and colleagues (43) have noted five stages of changing and their accompanying psychological frames of reference that should be considered in shaping interventions that match the patient's rehabilitation goals:

- Precontemplation: Here, the patient evidences no intention of changing a problem behavior in the near future (i.e., within the upcoming 6 months).
  Recommended intervention: Offer information that promotes consciousness raising regarding the importance of changing.
- Contemplation: The patient voices a serious intention to change in the near future.
  Recommended intervention: Emphasize the pros of changing and reassure the patient that he will be able to cope with the cons of the process (e.g., discomfort, frustration, lost pleasures).
- Preparation: The patient voices the intention to take action in the next month, but has not had success in taking such action in the past year.
  Recommended intervention: Offer encouragement, advice regarding helpful change strategies, and reinforcement for the small steps toward changing that have been taken.
- Action: The patient is actively modifying behaviors, experiences, or the environment to overcome a targeted problem.
  Recommended intervention: Support change that is in progress, coach in behavioral change strategies, encourage the patient's

support system to participate in and support the change.
- Maintenance: The change has been successfully implemented for approximately 6 months and the patient is seeking to avoid backsliding.
  Recommended intervention: Help the patient see that the advantages of having made the change outweigh the costs of implementing the change. Positively reinforce successes. Express admiration of the patient's courage and offer compassion about the fact that change is difficult to maintain. Encourage the patient to learn from "slip-ups" and to view them as inevitable steps in developing lasting change.

Contracting for change with a patient can be formal or informal, but several components should always be incorporated: operationalize desired behavior changes, specify short-term steps that approximate a long-term rehabilitation goal, and encourage the patient to build in rewards and supports in the process (44). Follow-up is also crucial.

Speak to the Family Team

When possible and appropriate, feedback and goal-setting should be conducted in the presence of both the patient and his or her most significant other (4, 5, 45–47). In this session, the family team should be forewarned of the likelihood of encountering homecoming depression on discharge, increased family tensions as rehabilitation progresses, and other family issues to be outlined below.

STRUCTURING PSYCHOSOCIAL INTERVENTIONS: SPECIFIC GUIDELINES

Psychosocial interventions can be tailored depending on the patient's particular needs. Techniques and concepts from various schools of thought can be integrated in designing both brief and extended interventions.

Cognitive and Behavioral Therapy

Several cognitive factors are especially crucial in determining reactions to cardiac illness: general attitudes regarding the causes or effects of the illness; attitudes toward the anticipated roles of health care providers; and attitudes toward the rehabilitation tasks (48).

Bar-On and Cristal (49) found that patients at high risk of a maladaptive reaction to heart illness can be flagged with two questions: "Why did it happen to you?" and "What will help you cope with it?" Troubled patients tend to attribute their illness to fate, not to any aspects of lifestyle that are under their direct control. Further, patients are more likely to evidence difficult rehabilitation courses if they perceive themselves without resources to help them cope.

Coping is enhanced if patients and their loved ones are helped to adopt the three C's of "healthy stress" reactions (1, 50): seeing illness and rehabilitation as a challenge; committing to mastering rehabilitation tasks; and learning what needs to be done to attain a reasonable sense of control over the adaptive process.

Stress Management Training

"Stress management training" has been used in the literature to refer to a wide range of interventions (1, 51). Fortunately, research suggests that relatively simple stress management interventions can significantly improve outcomes in cardiac populations (17).

Protocols for structuring stress management programs have recently been published (1, 51). In addition to reducing distress during the formal rehabilitation period, stress management interventions should help patients cope with the long-range challenges they face. Ideally, such intervention should incorporate didactic discussion of the physical aspects of the stress response; self-assessment exercises that help patients identify their most prevalent causes of stress and their typical coping reactions; training in a relaxation technique; modeling appropriate methods of communicating and dealing with interpersonal conflict; and coaching regarding ways to disrupt problem coping sequences. Information is best presented in a combination of modalities: video and audio tapes, brief discussions, and brief instructions.

The efficacy of such a stress management program was recently demonstrated by Trzcieniecka-Green and Steptoe (52). Seventy-eight cardiac patients exposed to a 12-week multifaceted stress management program evidenced significant pretreatment to posttreatment reductions in anxiety and depression and improvements in psychological well-being, activities of daily living, social activity, and satisfaction with sexual relationships. Similar responses were noted in MI and coronary artery bypass graft (CABG) patients.

Clinical experience suggests that "stress management" is a palatable frame of reference for introducing a variety of interventions. Individuals who view themselves as being strong, capable copers are likely to discredit their need for psychosocial intervention but respond to the notion that stress management training might be helpful.

Treating Type A Behavior, Anger, and Hostility

Type A behavior pattern (TYABP) is an action–emotion complex that typically combines various of the following coping styles: excessive focus on work and striving for achievement; cynicism and hostility; chronic hurriedness; doing and thinking more than one thing at once; energetic, tense behaviors; perfectionism; competitiveness; and a tendency to try to control others (1). Comprehensive treatment programs for TYABP have been described and have been shown to both reduce TYABP and improve medical outcomes with this population (53).

Brief counseling for TYABP should focus on education and coaching regarding the importance of managing anger (54, 55). Here, intervention should center on education about the health risks and lifestyle consequences that come with uncontrolled hostility (56). It is important to emphasize that behaviors such as aggression or antagonism appear to be more damaging to one's health and relationships than does the subjective experience of angry feelings and thoughts (57). The notion that expressing anger helps relieve tension should be challenged. Rather, appropriate stress management, cognitive control, relaxation, and interpersonal skills must be learned to manage angry reactions. Excellent summaries of anger management protocols are available (58–60).

Relaxation Training

Relaxation training has also been found to reduce heart rate, respiratory rate, and muscle tension (61), and surgical patients who received brief training in relaxation have shown diminished incidence of postsurgical delirium, diminished medical complication, and shorter lengths of hospital stay. A variety of relaxation interventions have been reported with cardiac patients. Positive effects have been noted from yoga, progressive muscular relaxation, autohypnosis, transcendental meditation, and biofeedback training (1).

Training in biofeedback tends to particularly appeal to patients who are fond of gadgetry and those who are skeptical about the usefulness of "talk therapies." Biofeedback is a method for learning to control voluntary and involuntary stress responses with the aid of visual or auditory cues regarding various physiologic functions. The patient is presented with digital displays, auditory feedback, or graphic representations of the effects of arousal on heart rate, blood pressure, skin temperature, or palmar sweating (62). Patients are then taught cognitive strategies for controlling these physiologic functions. Biofeedback has been shown to be effective in treating hypertension (63) and as a treatment for individuals who show exaggerated TYABP (64).

At a minimum, patients can benefit from relaxation training that instructs them to use abdominal breathing and visual imagery to focus attention on soothing stimuli, memories, or fantasies. They can also be encouraged to recall and practice previously learned relaxation techniques, such as training in Lamaze childbirth techniques. Both taped and live instruction in relaxation techniques can be helpful.

Group Therapy

The effectiveness of group interventions in promoting psychosocial adjustments in recovering cardiopulmonary populations and their families has been extensively discussed (65). For example, Rahe et al. (66), in a controlled comparison study, found that patients who attended group therapy aimed at lessening stress, not at altering risk factors such as smoking or excess body weight, experienced significantly fewer cardiac recurrences and coronary heart disease (CHD) deaths after hospitalization in comparison to a control group that received no special intervention. The noteworthy interventions of Ornish and colleagues (67) hinge on group support and stress management training (along with moderate exercise and a reduced fat and calorie diet) and have been shown to improve left ventricular performance, lessen chest pain, and lessen severity of CHD as assessed by angiography.

Group experiences can be structured in various ways. Issues that are often addressed in patient groups include concerns about illness, medication, discharge, and sex, and explorations of family issues, with special emphasis on aggravation about being treated in an overprotective manner (68). Group themes in support programs for spouses of recovering patients might include catharsis, discussion of depression and anger management, dealing with loss, communication within marriage and family, fear of death of spouse, and concerns regarding return to work and other activities (especially sexual fears) (25, 69). Support groups for couples when one or both members have heart illness might focus on the following themes: establishment of a reference group of other cardiac couples; and the various ways in which rehabilitation is a family affair (6, 70).

Bolstering Family Functioning

A broad literature has called attention to the importance of a supportive, intimate relationship in promoting recovery from cardiac illness. The Honolulu Heart Study (71) showed that loving support from wives buffered the effect of anxiety on the incidence of angina. Being stressed and socially isolated and lacking a confidant predicts poor survival for recovering cardiac patients (72–74). Even the perception of support by a caring individual—the feeling of being loved and the belief that others would be available in times of need—predicted the degree of coronary atherosclerosis in a study that investigated coronary angiographic findings (75).

Most protective are relationships that contain healthy elements of solidarity, trust, intimate attachment, and helping behaviors (76–79). However, various types of supportive relationships may provide such protection (80). This fact is especially noteworthy given that older cardiopulmonary patients are likely to depend on their grown children for such support (81). Family support during hospitalization can be a key to recovery. Kulik and Mahler (82) reported that CABG patients who received frequent visitations from their spouse were more quickly discharged from both the intensive care unit (ICU) and hospital and took less pain medications than did those who received low levels of spouse visitation. The patients who seemed to benefit most from such visitation were those with low levels of self-rated marital harmony. In another study, family visits that included the family member touching the patient and orienting the patient frequently to time and place lead to reduction in the incidence of postoperative delirium (83).

Clearly, family members should be encouraged to visit the recovering patient in the hospital. However, care should be taken to prepare the family members for what they will encounter when seeing their loved one in the hospital, and the family should be coached in helpful versus unhelpful support behaviors during their hospital visits (84).

In outpatient settings, family function plays a significant role in risk factor management and overall psychosocial adjustment (46, 47). When handled appropriately, the shock of rehabilitation can actually lead to enhanced family functioning (31, 32, 85). It therefore seems important to provide help regarding marital and family functioning from the outset of the illness. Two forms of family-level intervention are those that provide support for family members of recovering patients and those that coach family members in how to provide effective support for each other.

In hospital settings, patients and their loved ones should be explicitly reassured that the hospital staff is taking nurturing care of the other party. Such support can involve specialized "spouse care plans" in ICUs and rehabilitation care plans that include provision of brief supportive interactions with the loved ones of hospitalized patients (86). Educational classes during post-ICU stays (87) and formal support groups in waiting room areas have also been described in the literature (1).

Extensive guidelines for families, one member of which suffers heart illness, have been published (6, 69). At a minimum, patients and their families should be encouraged to recognize that recovery may stress each of the family members, not only the heart patient. They should especially be cautioned to avoid putting the patient in a "spectator" role. Rather, the family should be encouraged to cooperate in creating a "new normal" that includes viable contributions to family processes from each of its members.

Bolstering Social Support

For some recovering patients, the family may not provide the needed form of support. Here, it may be helpful to intervene to impact the social network that extends beyond the patient's family.

One such intervention is to expose the patient to others who have endured the ordeal being faced. Anderson and Masur (88) reported that patients anticipating angiography who watched a film of another patient describing the experience and how it was dealt with displayed less postsurgical distress in comparison to patients who did not receive this modeling intervention. Even simply having a patient awaiting surgery share a room with a postoperative patient, as opposed to a roommate also awaiting surgery, has been shown to lead to more postsurgical physical activity and shortened hospital stay (82).

In an outpatient setting, Burgess et al. (89) demonstrated the importance of staff support and of directly working with a recovering heart patient's social network to effect adaptive work return. This study promoted work return in 89 acute MI patients by exposing them to a relatively simple, 3-month psychosocial adjustment program run by nurse clinicians who have master's degrees. The intervention incorporated direct consultation with patients and their coworkers or supervisors to address mutual concerns about the patients' planned return to work. Each patient received an average of 6.32 contacts. Follow-up 13 months after hospitalization indicated that, in comparison to the control group, the intervention group evidenced overall enhanced psychological and social functioning, including enhanced vocational adjustment.

Sexual Counseling

Sexual concerns of recovering patients and their loved ones are often overlooked in delivering cardiac care (90–92).

Extensive guidelines for structuring sexual counseling with cardiac patients are available (1, 6). Interventions should provide information, permission, and reassurance to both the patient and his or her significant other. Key factors to bear in mind when offering sexual counseling include the following:

- The issue of sexual adjustment should always be validated as an acceptable aspect of medical care, but if patients indicate no interest in receiving information regarding sexual adjustment, their needs must be respected.
- Care should be taken not to discriminate against aging or unmarried patients. It is too often assumed that patients who are either

aged or single—and especially those who are both aged and single—are not appropriate candidates for sexual counseling.

- Information about an expected time frame for return to sexual functioning should be given, based on the patient's medical condition, functional capacity, medication regimen, and premorbid sexual functioning.
- Patients and their partners should be forewarned that symptoms of sexual arousal may mimic those of cardiovascular illness. Offer reassurance that sexual response is a typically safe form of exercise, and encourage patients to use the same common-sense guidelines for structuring sexual relations as would apply to other forms of physical exercise.
- Patients should be reassured and encouraged that sexual functioning can be enhanced by overall physical conditioning and psychosocial adjustment.
- Finally, it is important to offer follow-up consultation regarding sexual functioning. Clinical experience suggests that sexual concerns do sometimes surface immediately, but they most often develop several months into the rehabilitation process. In addition, sexual performance may be affected by medications, aging, or other medical conditions that progress during the course of the treatment of a cardiac patient. Accordingly, as rehabilitation progresses, it is important to periodically inquire about sexual concerns.

Follow-Up

The importance of offering follow-up psychosocial assessment and intervention cannot be overemphasized. Take time to inquire about overall psychosocial functioning during routine follow-up examinations. Alternatively or adjunctly, structure brief, nurse-delivered telephone follow-up. Brief telephone consultation provided to outpatients has been found to promote a range of positive rehabilitation outcomes (93–96).

Formal Cardiac Rehabilitation

One of the most powerful ways to bolster patients' overall psychosocial functioning is to refer them to a formal cardiac rehabilitation program. In addition to training in exercise and nutrition management, comprehensive cardiac rehabilitation programs typically provide a combination of social support, psychosocial education about the adjustment process, relaxation training, and behavior change classes. Many incorporate consultation from mental health professionals who conduct psychosocial evaluations and provide feedback and brief counseling interventions.

OFFICE MANAGEMENT AND COLLABORATION

Not all psychosocial concerns of patients can be dealt with effectively in a cardiology office-based practice. Whether a primary care physician and the office staff can intervene effectively will depend on factors such as severity and chronicity of the problem; provider skill, time, and resources; and the patient's adaptability (97). Adjustment problems that extend beyond the range of management capability indicate a need for referral for specialized care.

It is generally agreed that brief physician-delivered psychosocial intervention should center on education, prevention, support, and challenge (1, 97, 98). In the reality of a busy medical practice, it is most often the nurse, not the physician, who delivers patient education and counseling. However, patient adherence is significantly enhanced by physician-delivered encouragement to participate in psychosocial counseling. For example, even brief, unequivocal endorsement of the importance of attending to psychosocial concerns, followed by a combination of nurse-delivered interventions, can be tremendously effective in promoting positive psychosocial changes.

Collaboration between health care providers of different disciplines is the intervention of choice in promoting comprehensive biopsychosocial adjustment for cardiac patients. Kallio et al. (99) demonstrated the effectiveness of a collaborative approach in office-based rehabilitation of acute MI patients. Intervention with 150 male and 37 female MI patients began 2 weeks after discharge. Medical examinations were performed monthly for the first 6 months after MI, then at least at 3-month intervals. A treatment team consisting of a social worker, psychologist, dietitian, and physiotherapist provided patients with health education, dietary advice, smoking cessation counseling, discussions of psychosocial problems, and physical exercise recommendations. The counseling was delivered intensively during the first 3 months of rehabilitation and then tapered thereafter.

Compared with 151 male and 37 female patients who received routine cardiac care, the intervention group evidenced significant improvements in blood pressures, serum cholesterol levels, serum triglyceride levels, and body weight. Improvements were maintained at 1-, 2-, and 3-year follow-ups. In addition, the intervention group evidenced significantly lower death rates during follow-up: 35 deaths for the intervention group compared to 55 deaths in the control group.

Whether the patient needs specialized psychosocial care should be determined by several factors. First, if the patient evidences protracted adjustment struggles and does not respond to brief, crisis management interventions, referral should be considered. Several specific issues should also be considered in making this determination.

Does the Patient Need Psychotropic Medication?

As will be discussed in chapter 16, a wealth of psychotropic interventions can be used safely with cardiac patients. The majority of such cases are competently managed by primary care physicians. However, evaluation by a psychiatrist should be considered for any patient who evidences symptoms of ongoing anxiety disorder or clinical depression; a history of the same; or is described by loved ones as having suffered from extended periods of anxiety or depression.

Does the Patient Need Pastoral Counseling?

Spiritual crisis can take various forms during the course of coping with illness (100, 101):

Questioning or anger directed toward one's god.
Urgent appeal to one's higher power for help in coping.
Anxiety over being separated from one's spiritual support system.

Stoll (102) and Shaffer (101) recommend that every patient should be questioned about spiritual issues and resources. Here, as in all aspects of psychosocial intervention, the intervention should be a response to the needs of the patient and remain within the provider's personal comfort zone. At a minimum, an offer to arrange pastoral counseling should be made if the patient so desires.

Is the Patient at High Risk of Psychosocial Struggles?

Patients who present complex psychosocial patterns or histories may benefit from formal evaluation that uses extensive interviews and standardized psychosocial assessment instruments and from extended psychosocial intervention from a mental health professional.

Certain factors characterize patients who are at high risk of suffering prolonged, long-range adjustment struggles (20, 103–107). Special caution should be exercised when treating the following types of individuals:

- Younger patients (younger than 55 years).
- Socially isolated individuals.
- Divorced or widowed patients who live alone.
- Poor or unemployed patients.
- Patients with a history of angina, previous hospitalizations, or repeated bouts with major illnesses.
- Patients with a history of psychiatric treatment before hospitalization.
- Substance abusers.
- Those with pre-MI physical limitations in activity level.
- Those who show high levels of anxiety the night before surgery or medical intervention.
- Those with high pre-MI levels of marital conflict.

Shanefield (107) cautioned that wives of male recovering MI patients who are especially likely to have difficulty adjusting manifest a combination of young age (younger than 65 years), blue-collar socioeconomic status, psychological dependency, and diminished capacity to express feelings. Finally, in outpatient settings, particular attention should be paid to those patients whose distress does not lift within a reasonable period of time after entry into rehabilitation.

CONCLUSIONS

The specific causes and effects of targeted psychosocial factors important in adjusting to cardiac illness remain to be clarified by future researchers. Clinical experience and preliminary research in this area does, however, strongly suggest that—by choice or by default—cardiologists deliver care that impacts on psychosocial adjustment for recovering patients. Comprehensive cardiology care promotes open and active collaboration between patients, their families, and the team of health care providers involved in their treatment.

References

1. Sotile WM. Psychosocial interventions for cardiopulmonary patients: a guide for health professionals. Champaign, IL: Human Kinetics, 1996.
2. Trelawney-Ross C, Russell O. Social and psychological responses to myocardial infarction: multiple determinants of outcome at six months. J Psychosom Res 1987;31:125–130.
3. Stern MJ, Pascale L. Psychosocial adaptation postmyocardial infarction: the spouse's dilemma. J Psychosom Res 1979;23:83–87.
4. Coyne JC, Smith DAF. Couples coping with myocardial infarction: a contextual perspective on wives' distress. J Pers Soc Psychol 1991;61:404–412.
5. Gilliss CL. Reducing family stress during and after coronary artery bypass surgery. Nurs Clin North Am 1984;19:103–112.
6. Sotile WM. Heart illness and intimacy: how caring relationships aid recovery. Baltimore: Johns Hopkins University Press, 1992.
7. Mumford E, Schlesinger HJ, Glass GV. The effects of psychological intervention on recovery from surgery and heart attacks: an analysis of the literature. Am J Public Health 1982;72:141–152.
8. Bennet P, Carroll D. Cognitive-behavioral interventions in cardiac rehabilitation. J Psychosom Res 1994; 38: 169–182.
9. Oldridge NB, Pashkow FJ. Compliance and motivation in cardiac rehabilitation: effects of written agreement and self-monitoring. J Card Rehabil 1993;3:257–262.
10. Sikes WW, Rodenhauser P. Rehabilitation programs for myocardial infarction patients: a national survey. Gen Hosp Psychiatry 1987;9:182–186.
11. Maes S. Psychosocial aspects of cardiac rehabilitation in Europe. Br J Clin Psychol 1992;31;473–483.
12. Berra K. Program design for the 21st century: expanding the cardiopulmonary rehabilitation model to meet the needs of diverse patient populations. Presented at the Sixth Annual Meeting of the American Association of Cardiovascular and Pulmonary Rehabilitation, Long Beach, CA, November 1991.
13. Southard DR, Broyden R. Psychosocial services in cardiac rehabilitation: a status report. J Card Rehabil 1990;10:255–263.
14. Dracup K, Moser DK, Marsden C, et al. Effects of a multidimensional cardiopulmonary rehabilitation program on psychosocial function. Am J Cardiol 1991; 68: 31–34.
15. Lewin B, Robertson IH, Cay EL, et al. Effects of self-help post-myocardial infarction rehabilitation on psychological adjustment and use of health services. Lancet 1992;339:1036–1040.
16. Schindler BA, Shook J, Schwartz GM. Beneficial effects of psychiatric intervention on recovery after coronary artery bypass graft surgery. Gen Hosp Psychiatry 1989;11:358–364.
17. Frasure-Smith N. In-hospital symptoms of psychological stress as predictors of long-term outcome after acute myocardial infarction in men. Am J Cardiol 1991;67:121–127.
18. Rose MI, Robbins B. Psychosocial recovery issues and strategies in cardiac rehabilitation. In: Pashkow FJ, Dafoe WA, eds. Clinical cardiac rehabilitation: a cardiologist's guide. Baltimore: Williams & Wilkins, 1993:248–261.
19. Lazarus A, Folkman S. Stress, appraisal, and coping. New York: Springer, 1984.
20. Havik OE, Maeland JG. Verbal denial and outcome in myocardial infarction patients. J Psychosom Res 1990; 32:145–157.
21. Crisp AH, Desouza M, Queenan M. Myocardial infarction and the emotional climate. Presented at the Sixth World Congress of the International College of Psychosomatic Medicine, Montreal, PQ, September 1981.
22. Lloyd GG, Cawley RM. Distress or illness? A study of psychological symptoms after myocardial infarction. Br J Psychiatry 1983;142:120–125.
23. Wabrek AJ, Burchell RC. Male sexual dysfunction associated with coronary heart disease. Arch Sex Behav 1980;9:69–75.
24. Clark S. Nursing interventions for the depressed cardiovascular patient. J Cardiovasc Nurs 1990;5:54–64.
25. Sotile WM. The intimacy factor in cardiopulmonary rehabilitation: a practical model for structuring interventions. J Card Rehabil 1993;13:237–242.
26. Cassem NH, Hackett TP. Ego infarction: psychological reactions to a heart attack. J Pract Nurses 1979; 29:17–39.
27. Johnson JL, Morse JM. Regaining control: the process of adjustment after myocardial infarction. Heart Lung 1990;19:126–135.
28. Patterson JM. Families experiencing stress: I. The Family Adjustment and Adaptation Response model. II. Applying the FAAR model to heal-related issues for intervention and research. Fam Syst Med 1988;6:202–237.
29. Patterson JM. Illness beliefs as a factor in patient-spouse adaptation to treatment for coronary artery disease. Fam Syst Med 1989;7:428–442.
30. Croog S, Levine S. Life after heart attack: social and psychological factors. New York: Human Science Press, 1982.
31. Laerum E, Johnsen N, Smith P, et al. Can myocardial infarction induce positive changes in family relationships? Fam Pract 1987;4:302–305.
32. Laerum E, Johnsen N, Smith P, et al. Positive psychological and life-style changes after myocardial infarction: a follow-up study after 2–4 years. Fam Pract 1991;8:229–233.
33. American Association of Cardiovascular and Pulmonary Rehabilitation. Guidelines for cardiac rehabilitation programs. Champaign, IL: Human Kinetics, 1995.
34. Orth-Gomer K, Schneiderman N, eds. Behavioral medicine approaches to cardiovascular disease pre-

vention. Mahwah, NJ: Lawrence Erlbaum Associates, Publishers, 1996.

35. Allan R, Scheidt S. Heart and mind: the practice of cardiac psychology. Washington, DC: American Psychological Association, 1996.

36. US Department of Health and Human Services. Cardiac rehabilitation clinical practice guideline. Rockville, MD: Agency for Health Care Policy and Research, 1995.

37. Pimm JB, Feist JR. Psychological risks of coronary artery bypass surgery. New York: Plenum Press, 1984.

38. Kendall PC, Williams L, Pechacek TF, et al. Cognitive-behavioral and patient education interventions in cardiac catheterization procedures: the Palo Alto Medical Psychology Project. J Consult Clin Psychol 1979;47: 49–58.

39. Gruen W. Effects of brief psychotherapy during the hospitalization period on the recovery process in heart attacks. J Consult Clin Psychol 1975;43:252–270.

40. Carmody TP, Fey SG, Pierce DK, et al. Behavioral treatment of hyperlipidemia: techniques, results, and future directions. J Behav Med 1982;5:91–116.

41. Schultz SJ. Educational and behavioral strategies related to knowledge of and participation in an exercise program after cardiac positron emission tomography. Patient Educ Counsel 1993;22:47–57.

42. Oldenburg B, Graham-Clarke P, Shaw J, et al. Modification of health behavior and lifestyle mediated by physicians. In: Orth-Gomer K, Schneiderman N, eds. Behavioral medicine approaches to cardiovascular disease prevention. Mahwah, NJ: Lawrence Erlbaum Associates, Publishers, 1996:203–227.

43. Prochaska JO, DiClimente CC, Norcross JC. In search of how people change: applications to addictive behaviors. Am Psychol 1992;47:1102–1114.

44. Mayou R. Quality of life in cardiovascular disease. Psychother Psychosom 1990;54:99–109.

45. Coyne JC, Smith DAF. Couples coping with a myocardial infarction: a contextual perspective on wives' distress. J Pers Soc Psychol 1991;61:404–412.

46. Sotile WM, Sotile MO, Ewen GS, et al. Marriage and family factors relevant to effective cardiac rehabilitation: a review of the risk factor literature. Sports Med Training Rehabil 1993;4:115–128.

47. Sotile WM, Sotile MO, Sotile LJ, et al. Marriage and family factors relevant to cardiac rehabilitation: an integrative review of the psychosocial literature. Sports Med Training Rehabil 1993;4:217–236.

48. Rejeski WJ, Morley D, Sotile W. Cardiac rehabilitation: a conceptual framework for psychologic assessment. J Card Rehabil 1985;5:172–180.

49. Bar-On D, Cristal N. Causal attributions of patients, their spouses and physicians, and the rehabilitation of the patients after their first myocardial infarction. J Cardpulm Rehabil 1987;7:285–298.

50. Kobasa SC, Maddi SR, Kahn S. Hardiness and health: a prospective study. J Pers Soc Psychol 1982;42:168–172.

51. Sotile WM. Stress management. In: Roitman J, ed. American College of Sports Medicine resource manual for guidelines for exercise testing and prescription. 3rd ed. Baltimore: Williams & Wilkins, 1997.

52. Trzcieniecka-Green A, Steptoe A. Stress management in cardiac patients: a preliminary study of the predictors of improvement in quality of life. J Psychosom Res 1994;38:267–280.

53. Friedman M, Ulmer D. Treating type A behavior and your heart. New York: Knopf, 1984.

54. Williams RB, Barefoot JC, Schekelle RB. The health consequences of hostility. In: Chesney MA, Rosenman RH, eds. Anger and hostility in cardiovascular and behavioral disorders. Washington, DC: Hemisphere, 1985: 173–185.

55. Krantz DS, Contrada RJ, Hill DR, et al. Environmental stress and biobehavioral antecedents of coronary heart disease. J Cons Clin Psychol 1988;56:333–337.

56. Williams RW, Williams V. Anger kills. New York: Harper Collins, 1993.

57. Siegman AW. The role of hostility, neuroticism, and speech style in coronary artery disease. In: Siegman AW, Dembroski TM, eds. In search of coronary-prone behavior. Hillsdale, NJ: Erlbaum, 1989: 65–89.

58. Williams R. The trusting heart: great news about type A behavior. New York: Time Books, 1989.

59. McKay M, Rogers P, McKay J. When anger hurts. San Francisco: New Harbinger Publications, 1989.

60. Smith TW. Hostility and health: current status of a psychosomatic hypothesis. Health Psychol 1992; 11:139–150.

61. Paul GL. Physiological effects of relaxation training and hypnotic suggestion. J Abnorm Psychol 1969;74: 425–437.

62. Schwartz MS. Biofeedback: a practitioner's guide. New York: Guilford Press, 1987.

63. Kaufman PG, Jacob RG, Ewart CK. Hypertension intervention pooling project. Health Psychol 1988;7: 209–215.

64. Stoney CM, Langer AW, Stutterer JR, et al. A comparison of biofeedback assisted cardiodeceleration in type A and B men: modification of stress-associated cardiopulmonary and hemodynamic adjustments. Psychosom Med 1987;49:79–83.

65. Ibrahim M, Feldman J, Sultz H, et al. Management after myocardial infarction: a controlled trial of the effect of group psychotherapy. Int J Psychiatry Med 1974;5:253–268.

66. Rahe RM, Ward HW, Hayes V. Brief group therapy in myocardial infarction rehabilitation: three to four year follow-up of a controlled trial. Psychosom Med 1979; 41:229–242.

67. Ornish D, Brown SE, Scherwitz LW, et al. Can lifestyle changes reverse coronary heart disease? Lancet 1990; 336:129–133.

68. Bilodeau BC, Hackett TP. Issues raised in a group setting by patients recovering from myocardial infarction. Am J Psychiatry 1971:128;73–78.

69. Levin R. Heartmates: a survival guide for the cardiac spouse. New York: Pocket Books, 1987.

70. Dracup K, Meleis A, Baker K, et al. Family-focused cardiac rehabilitation: a role supplementation program for cardiac patients and spouses. Nurs Clin North Am 1984;19:113–124.

71. Medalie JH, Goldbourt U. Angina pectoris among

10,000 men: II. Psychosocial and other risk factors as evidenced by a multivariate analysis of a five-year incidence study. Am J Med 1976;60:910–921.

72. Case RB, Moss AJ, Case N, et al. Living alone after myocardial infarction: impact on prognosis. JAMA 1992;267:515–519.

73. Williams RB, Barefoot JC, Califf RM, et al. Prognostic importance of social and economic resources among medically treated patients with angiographically documented coronary artery disease. JAMA 1992;267: 520–524.

74. Ruberman W, Weinblatt AB, Goldberg JD, et al. Psychosocial influences on mortality after myocardial infarction. N Engl J Med 1984;311:552–559.

75. Seeman TE, Syme SL. Social networks and coronary artery disease: a comparison of the structure and function of social relations as predictors of disease. Psychosom Med 1987;49:340–353.

76. Pearlin LI, Menaghan EG, Lieberman MA, et al. The stress process. J Health Soc Behav 1981;22:337–356.

77. Waltz M. Marital context and post-infarction quality of life: is it social support or something more? Soc Sci Med 1986;22:791–805.

78. Burke R, Weir T. Marital helping relationships: the moderators between stress and well-being. J Psychol 1977;95:121–130.

79. Fontana AF, Kerns RD, Rosenberg RL, et al. Support, stress, and recovery from coronary heart disease: a longitudinal causal model. Health Psychol 1989;8: 175–193.

80. Lowenthal MF, Haven C. Interaction and adaptation: intimacy as a critical variable. Am Soc Rev 1968;33:20–30.

81. Sotile WM, Miller H. Helping older patients to cope with cardiac and pulmonary disease. J Cardpulm Rehabil 1998;18:124–128.

82. Kulik JA, Mahler IM. Social support and recovery from surgery. Health Psychol 1989;8:221–238.

83. Chatham MA. The effect of family involvement on patients' manifestations of postcardiotomy psychosis. Heart Lung 1978;7:995–999.

84. Doerr BC, Jones JW. Effect of family preparation on the state anxiety level of the CCU patient. Nurs Res 1979;28:315–316.

85. Jenkins CD, Stanton BA, Savageau JA, et al. Physical, psychologic, social and economic outcomes after cardiac valve surgery. Arch Intern Med 1983;132: 2107–2113.

86. Dracup K, Breu CS. Using nursing findings to meet the needs of grieving spouses. Nurs Res 1978;27:212–216.

87. Dracup K, Bryan-Brown CW. An open door policy in ICU. Am J Crit Care 1992;1:16–18.

88. Anderson KO, Masur FT. Psychologic preparation for cardiac catheterization. Heart Lung 1989;18:154–163.

89. Burgess AW, Lerner DJ, D'Agostino RB, et al. A randomized control trial of cardiac rehabilitation. Soc Sci Med 1987;24:359–370.

90. Schover LR, Jensen S. Sexuality and chronic illness: a comprehensive approach. New York: Guilford Press, 1988.

91. Papadopoulos C, Larrimore P, Cardin S, et al. Sexual concerns and needs of the postcoronary patient's wife. Arch Intern Med 1980;140:38–41.

92. Boone T, Kelley R. Sexual issues and research in counseling the postmyocardial infarction patient. J Cardiovasc Nurs 1990;4:65–75.

93. Taylor CB, Houston-Miller N, Lilen JD, et al. Smoking cessation after acute myocardial infarction: effects of a nurse-managed intervention. Ann Intern Med 1990; 113:118–123.

94. Follick MJ, Gorkin L, Capone RJ, et al. Psychological distress as a predictor of ventricular arrhythmias in a post-myocardial infarction population. Am Heart J 1988;116:32–36.

95. Daltroy LH. Improving cardiac patient adherence to exercise regiments: a clinical trial of health education. J Card Rehabil 1985;5:40–49.

96. Beckie T. A supportive-educative telephone program: Impact on knowledge and anxiety after coronary artery bypass graft surgery. Heart Lung 1989;18:46–55.

97. Doherty WJ, Baird MA. Family therapy and family medicine: toward the primary care of families. New York: Guilford Press, 1983.

98. Christie-Seely J, ed. Working with the family in primary care. New York: Praeger, 1984.

99. Kallio V, Hamalainen H, Hakkila J, et al. Reduction in sudden deaths by a multifactorial intervention programme after acute myocardial infarction. Lancet 1979;2:1091–1094.

100. American Psychiatric Association. Diagnostic and statistical manual of mental disorders. 4th ed. Washington, DC: American Psychiatric Association, 1994.

101. Shaffer JL. Spiritual distress and critical illness. Crit Care Nurse 1991;11:42–46.

102. Stoll R. Guidelines for spiritual assessment. Am J Nurs 1979;11:1574–1577.

103. Dhooper S. Social networks and support during the crisis of heart attack. Health Soc Work 1984;9: 294–303.

104. Siegrist J, Siegrist K, Weber I. Sociological concepts in the etiology of chronic disease; the case of ischemic heart disease. Soc Sci Med 1986;22:247–253.

105. Shaw R, Cohen F, Doyle B, et al. The impact of denial and repressive style on information gain and rehabilitation outcomes in myocardial infarction patients. Psychosom Med 1985;47:262–273.

106. Swenson JR, Abbey SE. Management of depression and anxiety disorders in the cardiac patient. In: Pashkow FJ, Dafoe WA, eds. Clinical cardiac rehabilitation: a cardiologist's guide. Baltimore: Williams & Wilkins, 1993:263–286.

107. Shanfield SB. Myocardial infarction and patients' wives. Psychosomatics 1990;31:138–145.

Depression and Prognosis in Coronary Disease

Nancy Frasure-Smith and François Lespérance

Heart attack patients and their families have long been convinced of the close ties between their emotions and their hearts. However, it has only been in the last 15 years that a significant body of evidence has emerged suggesting that the brain and the heart interact to influence postmyocardial infarction (MI) prognosis. In the 1980s and early 1990s studies reported that life stress (1), psychological distress (2, 3), depressive symptoms (4), some aspect of type A behavior, hostility, or anger (5), and social support or its absence in the form of social isolation and loneliness (1, 6) were all linked to poor outcomes after MI.

These studies were all consistent in finding links between psychological factors and post-MI prognosis, and led many clinicians working in cardiac rehabilitation to suggest that psychological treatment might improve prognosis. However, the clinical usefulness of the findings was limited. All of the research was based on secondary analysis of data sets originally collected to test other hypotheses. Because secondary analyses that show positive results are much more likely to be published than those that show no relationship between two variables, there is no way of judging the publication bias in this literature. In addition, none of the studies involved a general sample of post-MI patients. Each focused on a special subgroup, for example, patients with significant arrhythmias, males, or patients younger than 65 years. Another difficulty was that despite the risks reported to be associated with the different psychological factors, treatment implications were not clear. There are no recognized interventions for life stress, psychological distress, or social isolation. Finally, none of the studies convincingly ruled out the possibility that psychosocial factors influence prognosis because sicker patients are more likely to be distressed or depressed, as well as more likely to die.

It was within this context that in 1991 to 1992 we collected baseline data for the Emotions and Prognosis Post-Infarction project (EPPI), a prospective study designed to examine the prognostic importance of depression after MI. Clinical experience at the Montreal Heart Institute and some existing research suggested that symptoms of depression, including loss of interest, sadness, and irritability, were particularly common in patients with coronary artery disease, especially after MI. Unlike many of the other psychosocial risks demonstrated in the literature, there are established pharmaceutical and psychotherapeutic treatments for depression, at least in patients without comorbid medical illness. We reasoned that if depression influenced prognosis in post-MI patients, it would be a meaningful new target for post-MI intervention. This chapter will be devoted to outlining the results of the EPPI study and its implications. In particular, we will focus on the following questions:

1. What is the prevalence of depression in patients hospitalized for an acute MI? How does it compare with other groups of hospitalized cardiac and medically ill patients?
2. What is the impact of in-hospital depression on long-term cardiac mortality?
3. Is the impact of depression on prognosis related to cardiac disease severity?
4. Is there evidence that depression acts as a trigger for MI?
5. Are patients with a recurrent depression in the hospital at greater risk?

6. Does in-hospital depression influence other outcomes besides mortality?
7. What is the role of β-blockade in post-MI depression?
8. What mechanisms may explain the links between depression and prognosis?

THE EPPI STUDY

The EPPI study was an ancillary project carried out in conjunction with the Canadian Assessment of Myocardial Infarction (CAMI) study at the Montreal Heart Institute (7). The CAMI study provided us with high-quality measures of cardiac risk for EPPI patients including measures of left ventricular ejection fraction for 99% of subjects. To be eligible patients had to meet research criteria for acute MI (at least two of three standard criteria: typical chest pain lasting at least 20 minutes, elevated creatinine phosphokinase, new Q waves). Patients were excluded if their MI was secondary to a revascularization procedure, they had another life-threatening condition, they were unable to speak English or French, they had major cognitive problems, or they were not medically stable enough to complete an hour-long baseline interview. Of 337 eligible patients, 227 consented to be interviewed. The 222 patients who survived to discharge comprised the sample for EPPI. There were no limits on inclusion in terms of age, sex, or previous cardiac history. The average age was 59.6 years (SD, ±11.7 years), 22% of the patients were women, and 37% had previous MIs.

The baseline psychosocial interview focused primarily on depression, but patients also completed self-report questionnaires assessing anxiety, anger, and satisfaction with social support from friends and family. In addition, patients responded to questions about medical history, smoking behavior, and social and demographic characteristics.

The psychiatric epidemiologic literature includes two approaches to measuring depression: a diagnostic approach based on the presence or absence of key symptoms, along with evaluation of symptom duration and the degree of impairment in daily functioning; and an approach based on the global severity of depressive symptoms without consideration of the pattern of symptoms. We used both approaches to assessing depression. Patients responded to a modified version of the National Institute of Mental Health Diagnostic Interview Schedule (DIS) (8), as well as the 21-item Beck Depression Inventory (BDI) (9). The DIS is a standardized set of questions that allows trained research assistants to assess the diagnostic criteria for current major depression outlined in the Diagnostic and Statistical Manual (DSM) of the American Psychiatric Association (10) (see chapter 15). It also includes questions to assess the history of major depression. A computer algorithm is then used to transform patient responses into psychiatric diagnoses. In our application of the DIS for current major depression, patients were asked only about the occurrence of depression symptoms since admission (on average 7 days and in most cases less than the 2 weeks required by DSM-III-R). In addition, because of difficulties in judging impairment in daily activities while hospitalized, we did not assess impairment from symptoms. The criteria for history of depression, however, used the full psychiatric criteria of symptoms, duration, and impairment.

In contrast to the categorical diagnostic approach of the DIS, the BDI is a self-administered questionnaire with scores ranging from 0 to 63. Increasing scores reflect increasingly severe symptoms of depression. Patients with scores of 10 or greater are usually considered to show at least mild to moderate symptoms of depression. The major difference between the DIS and the BDI approaches is that to be diagnosed as depressed using the DIS patients must report either pervasive ("almost every day") sadness or lack of interest, but with the BDI it is possible to have a score high enough to indicate depression without reporting either of these symptoms. In addition the BDI is a pencil and paper measure, whereas the DIS is interviewer-administered.

Data on patients' medical conditions were obtained from hospital charts and the CAMI database and included Killip class (11), left ventricular ejection fraction (n = 220), and prescription at discharge of β-blockers and angiotensin-converting enzyme (ACE) inhibitors. Holter monitoring for 18 to 24 hours during hospitalization for cardiac arrhythmias was available for 197 patients.

All patients or their family members were contacted at 6, 12, and 18 months after the MI to assess patient survival status. Causes of death were coded as cardiac or noncardiac by three independent cardiologists. Some 97.1% of patients surviving at 6 months, and 88.8% of those surviving at 1 year also completed follow-up psychosocial interviews, including modified questions from the DIS to assess new episodes of depression after discharge, the BDI, and other self-report measures.

PREVALENCE OF IN-HOSPITAL DEPRESSION AFTER MYOCARDIAL INFARCTION

We found that about one in six patients (15.8%) met modified psychiatric (DSM-III R) criteria for major depression at the time of the baseline interview. A similar number (18.5%) reported elevated numbers of depressive symptoms (BDI ≥ 10) without meeting the modified criteria for major depression. This is similar to the results of other studies conducted in the early postinfarction period. For example, Schleifer and colleagues (12) administered the Schedule for Affective Disorders to 283 patients 8 to 10 days after an MI and found that 18% met Research Diagnostic Criteria (RDC) for major depressive disorder, while another 27% had minor depressive disorder. More recently, German researchers evaluated the level of depression 17 to 21 days after an MI in a sample of 560 male patients 65 years or younger (13). They found that 14.5% had extreme depression according to their scale with another 22.3% exhibiting mild depression. Thus, estimates for the percentage of patients affected by some degree of depression while in the hospital after MI range from about 34% to 45% depending on the sample's sex and age composition and the measure of depression used.

Recent work by our team indicates that these levels of depression are not unique to post-MI patients. An ongoing study of 430 patients hospitalized for unstable angina revealed that 19.8% met criteria for major depression and an additional 26.3% had high BDI scores, but did not meet the full criteria for depression. We observed similar degrees of depression the day after elective angioplasty in a sample of 244 patients (11.1% major depression and 24.2% high BDI scores without full criteria). Langeluddecke and colleagues (14), using a different measure of depression (the CES-D), observed a 36% rate of depression in a sample of 89 patients hospitalized for bypass surgery. Thus, depression appears to be a common problem in patients hospitalized for cardiac problems in general, and not specifically a difficulty for heart attack patients. Further, work by other researchers with groups of hospitalized medically ill individuals shows that some 20% to 40% of these patients have significant depressive symptomatology (15, 16).

It is clear that the relatively high levels of depression associated with hospitalizations for cardiac disease and other medical illness have been at least partially responsible for the belief of many physicians that some degree of depressed mood is part of the normal coping process after a serious physical threat like an MI, and that such depression has little lasting effect. However, the results of our long-term follow-up of the patients involved in the EPPI study bring into question the perception that depression is a normal reaction, at least after MI (17–21). We found that post-MI patients who are depressed during hospitalization are at increased risk of both cardiac mortality and chronic depression.

IMPACT OF IN-HOSPITAL DEPRESSION ON LONG-TERM CARDIAC MORTALITY

During the 18-month follow-up 21 patients died (9.5%), including 19 of cardiac causes and 2 of cancer. Twelve of the cardiac deaths took place during the first 6 months after discharge, five between 6 and 12 months, and two between 1 year and 18 months. Figure 15.1 shows the survival curves during 18 months of follow-up for patients with major depression, those with high BDI scores who did not meet criteria for major depression, and those with no evidence of depression while in the hospital. Major depression significantly increased the risk of mortality during the full follow-up period (odds ratio [OR] = 3.64; 95% confidence interval [CI] 1.32, 10.05; P = .018). However, its impact was largely during the first 6 months (OR = 6.24; 95% CI 1.88, 20.67; P = .004). Thereafter, the increase in risk associated with high levels of depressive symptoms began to increase, so that by the end of 18 months the risk for patients with high BDI scores who did not meet the criteria for major depression in contrast to the nondepressed patients was

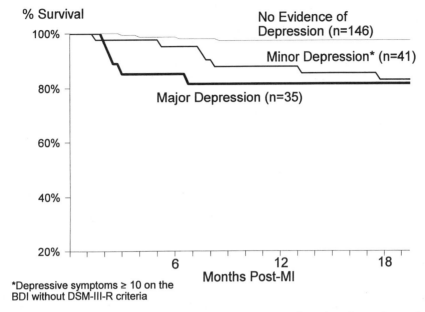

Figure 15.1.   Cumulative 18-month survival for patients with major depression, minor depression, and no evidence of depression in the hospital after myocardial infarction (MI).

similar to the risk associated with major depression (OR = 7.20; 95% CI 1.99, 26.02; P = .0026).

We speculate that patients with elevated BDI scores who did not meet diagnostic criteria for major depression may have been more mildly depressed individuals or individuals with subthreshold or subsyndromal depression. After discharge from hospital, these patients may have gone on to develop full-blown major depression, and died subsequent to this later depression. However, it is also possible that there is a risk associated with more minor forms of depression that is similar to the risk conveyed by major depression, and that it does not depend on the development of major depression to have an impact. Finally, there is the possibility that the modified DIS failed to identify a number of patients with significant depressive symptomatology who would have fulfilled diagnostic criteria for major depression in a different context. Some patients may be willing to disclose symptoms of depression using a self-report questionnaire, but be reluctant to admit them in the context of a face-to-face interview with a research assistant in a hospital room. Thus, the best screening process to identify patients at risk may simply involve the BDI and the cutoff score of 10. In fact, in our sample the odds ratio for 18-month cardiac mortality associated with elevated BDI scores in contrast to lower scores was highly significant (OR=7.82; 95% CI 2.42, 25.26; P = .0002). However, the precise clinical meaning of a high BDI score detected while in the hospital after an MI remains to be established. In the absence of additional research data, the use of the BDI as a screen for post-MI depression requires cross-validation by a skilled mental health professional with appropriate experience with cardiac patients.

DEPRESSION AND CARDIAC DISEASE SEVERITY

As important as depression appears to be in post-MI prognosis, it seems reasonable to argue that sicker patients have every reason to be depressed, and that depression may simply be a proxy measure for disease severity. To assess this possibility we took several steps. First, we compared the patients with positive DIS ratings (meeting psychiatric criteria for major depression) with other patients on measures of disease severity and demographic factors. Similarly, we compared patients with BDI scores of 10 or more with those with lower scores. The results of these analyses appear in Table 15.1.

Table 15.1.   Baseline Characteristics Associated with Major Depression and Depressive Symptoms in the Hospital After MI

Characteristic	Major Depression (DIS)			Depressive Symptoms (BDI)		
	Yes (n = 35)	No (n = 187)	P	≥10 (n = 68)	<10 (n = 150)	P
Age						
Mean	58.3	60.1	.039	60.4	59.3	.49
%≥ 65 years	28.6	34.2	.52	32.4	32.7	.96
% Female	34.3	19.8	.058	33.8	16.0	.003
%≤8 yr education	37.1	28.9	.33	38.2	26.0	.067
% Living alone	20.0	18.7	.86	27.9	13.3	.009
% No close friends	31.4	16.0	.031	25.0	16.0	.12
% Daily smoker	40.0	39.6	.96	33.8	41.3	.29
% Previous MI	45.7	35.3	.24	39.7	34.7	.47
% Left ventricular ejection	37.1	27.6	.25	32.8	27.5	.43
fraction ≤35%		(n = 185)		(n = 67)	(n= 149)	
% Killip class ≥ 2	28.6	19.8	.24	29.4	16.0	.022
% PVCs ≥ 10/hr	14.7	13.4	.84	15.2	12.5	.61
	(n = 34)	(n = 164)		(n = 66)	(n= 128)	
% Prescribed B-Blockers at discharge	60.0	63.6	.68	51.5	67.3	.025
% Prescribed ACE inhibitors at discharge	40.0	26.2	.097	36.8	24.7	.067

MI= myocardial infarction; DIS =Diagnostic Interview Schedule; BDI = Beck Depression Inventory; PVC = premature ventricular contraction; ACE = angiotensin-converting enzyme.

Although women were marginally more likely to meet criteria for major depression than men, patients with major depression did not differ on any measures of disease severity from other patients. In understanding this result it is important to note that the absolute number of patients with positive DIS ratings of depression was relatively small (n = 35), and it is possible that the sample was not large enough to pick up subtle differences in disease severity. In fact, when we examine the results for patients with BDI scores of at least 10 (n = 68) in contrast to patients with BDI scores of less than 10, some differences in disease severity emerge. Patients with high BDI scores were more likely to be women, to have a Killip class of 2 or more, and to not have been prescribed β-blockers at discharge. Their higher Killip class, indicating more complications during the acute phase of the MI, suggests poorer cardiac function in patients with high BDI scores. The less frequent prescription of β-blockade for this group may also indicate that they were sicker patients. However, the impact of BDI score on 18-month cardiac mortality remained significant even after control for these three factors (adjusted OR = 6.42; 95% CI 1.85, 22.19; $P = .0017$).

In addition to controlling for baseline differences in cardiac measures as a way of assessing the importance of cardiac disease severity in explaining the impact of depression, we compared the prognostic importance of other clinical variables with the importance of depression. We first derived a multivariate clinical model to predict 18-month cardiac mortality using backward stepwise multiple regression analysis confirmed by forward stepping. The individual baseline variables significantly related to cardiac mortality included previous MI, Killip class of 2 or more, left ventricular ejection fraction less than or equal to 35%, 10 or more premature ventricular contractions (PVCs) per hour, and prescription of β-blockade and ACE inhibitors at baseline. However, the multivariate stepwise analyses revealed that only previous MI, PVCs, and Killip class had predictive value independent of each other. Depression (BDI ≥ 10) significantly improved the model based on these three clinical factors (likelihood ratio = 9.07; $P = .0026$). The adjusted odds ratios for previous MI, PVCs, Killip class, and the BDI score appear in Table 15.2. In summary, there is little evidence in our data to support the notion that depression was related to cardiac mortality simply because of its relationship to cardiac disease severity.

Further exploration of the interrelationships among previous MI, PVCs, Killip class, and BDI scores revealed a marginally significant ($P = .094$) interaction of PVCs and BDI score (Fig. 15.2). Although there was no evidence that PVCs were any more frequent among the depressed than among the nondepressed, patients who were depressed

Table 15.2.   Significant Multivariate Predictors of 18-Month Cardiac Morality After Myocardial Infarction

Variable	Adjusted Odds Ratio (%95 CI)	P
Killip class ≥ 2	3.92 (1.14. 13.55)	.031
Previous MI	4.78 (1.27, 18.05)	.021
≥ 10 PVCs/hr	7.92 (2.12, 29.57)	.0021
BDI ≥ 10 (at least mild to moderate symptoms)	6.64 (1.76, 25.09)	.0053

CI= confidence interval.

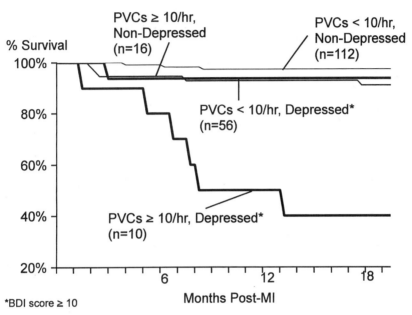

Figure 15.2.   Cumulative 18-month survival in relation to premature ventricular contractions (PVCs) and major depression in the hospital after MI.

and who had significant PVCs were at particularly high risk. Not only was the risk of depression enhanced by the presence of PVCs, but the risk associated with PVCs was almost entirely restricted to patients with elevated numbers of symptoms of depression. These results fit well with the autonomic dysregulation hypothesis of depression, which suggests that depressed patients have increased noradrenergic activity. In patients recovering from MI, who have a susceptible myocardium, such dysregulation related to depression could potentially lead to fatal cardiac events.

OVERLAP OF SYMPTOMS OF DEPRESSION WITH CARDIAC SYMPTOMS

It has often been argued that post-MI depression is not the same as depression in the non-medically ill because some depression symptoms may be attributed to the MI or the hospital setting (22, 23). Therefore, we compared the symptoms reported by patients who met the modified DSM-III-R criteria for major depression in the hospital with those who were not depressed. Three major conclusions emerged from these comparisons. First, although sadness was very frequent and highly specific to the depressed group (80.0% of depressed patients reported sadness versus 7.0% of the nondepressed; $P <$ .0001), only about half of the depressed complained about loss of pleasure or interest (48.6% of the depressed versus 2.1% of the nondepressed; $P <$ .0001). It is possible that the hospital setting makes it difficult for patients to evaluate this aspect of depression. Second, fatigue was mainly a symptom in the depressed group (77.1% of the depressed versus 23.5% of the nondepressed; $P <$ .0001). Further, in our sample, there were no relationships between reports of fatigue and any markers of cardiac disease severity, including left ventricular ejection fraction ($P = .67$), Killip class ($P = .49$), and previous MI ($P = .71$). Third, sleep and appetite disturbances were common in both the depressed and nondepressed groups. Difficulties sleeping were reported by 65.7% of the depressed and 49.6% of the nondepressed patients ($P = .089$). Changes in appetite affected 80.0% of the depressed and 71.1% of the nondepressed ($P = .29$).

The frequency of sleep and appetite problems suggests that they could be attributed, at least in part, to the hospital environment. For this reason, we wondered whether defining depression without these symptoms would change its impact on mortality. We found that when sleep and appetite disturbances were eliminated from the criteria for depression, 31 of the 35 patients originally classified as depressed continued to meet the criteria for depression. All of the depressed patients who died by 18 months met the revised criteria for depression. Thus, the impact of depression in the hospital remained after symptoms that could be related to the hospital environment were removed as a basis for diagnosis. In addition, the depression construct became more specific in predicting mortality when highly prevalent in-hospital complaints were excluded from its definition. This suggests that those patients for whom sleep and appetite disturbances are needed to meet criteria for major depression may not really be depressed, and that in the hospital setting clinicians should focus on the other symptoms of depression in making their diagnosis. In fact, although controversial, this approach has been advocated by some clinicians working with depressed patients with medical illness (24).

LIFETIME PREVALENCE OF DEPRESSION IN POST-MI PATIENTS: IS DEPRESSION A TRIGGER OF MI?

The high percentage of post-MI patients with depression while in the hospital suggests the hypothesis that depression may have preceded and triggered the MI for many patients. However, our data do not support this interpretation. Using information from the DIS conducted while in the hospital, we were able to determine the lifetime prevalence of depression before the MI, as well as the timing of previous depressions. We found that 27.5% of patients had experienced at least one episode of major depression meeting full psychiatric symptom, duration, and impairment criteria (DSM-III-R) at some point in their lives before the infarct. However, the last depression for the majority of these patients had occurred more than 1 year earlier. Only 7.7% had been depressed at some time in the previous year and only 5.4% during the 6 months before the MI. Thus, in our sample of MI survivors there was little evidence that major depression was a precipitating factor for the heart attack in most patients. Although other recent research has suggested that depressive symptomatology and vital exhaustion (a term used in Europe for a condition closely related to depression) may be risk factors for MI (25, 26), our results show that major depression is not that frequent in the year before an MI. However, we do not know the psychiatric status of patients who did not survive their MIs. It is possible that many of those who did not survive to be interviewed while in the hospital were depressed. Clearly, a large-scale, prospective, population-based study would be needed to determine the extent to which depression is involved in triggering MIs.

It is also important to note that the lifetime and 12-month prevalence rates of depression in our sample before the MI were not appreciably different from data collected in community surveys. Although the Epidemiological Catchment Area (ECA) study (27) reported lower current and lifetime prevalences of major depression than we observed, the ECA figures may be underestimates (28, 29). Several community-based studies have found higher lifetime prevalence rates (30–32). For example, Kovess and Fournier (30) used a modified version of the DIS similar to ours in a Montreal community sample and reported a lifetime prevalence of major depression of 27.4%. Kessler et al. (32) recently observed a lifetime prevalence of 14.6% and a 12-month prevalence rate of 8.8% (weighted according to the current study's proportion of female patients) using the Composite International Diagnostic Interview, an approach similar to the DIS. Although these studies used different structured instruments on different populations, limiting their comparability, they suggest that before the MI depression was probably no more common in our sample than in the general population.

We found that patients with a history of depression were more likely to be women ($P = .00055$), less likely to report exercising at least once a week ($P = .0046$), and had higher BDI scores ($P = .0029$). Although they did not differ on two indices of cardiac disease severity, previous MI ($P = .65$) and left ventricular ejection fraction ($P = .28$), patients with a history of depression were more likely to have physical signs of heart dysfunction during the acute phase of their MI, as indicated by their elevated Killip class ($P = .0029$).

In conclusion, the prevalence of major depression before the index MI was not apparently higher than the one observed in the community. However, it remains to be established whether subdromal or subthreshold depressive symptomatology before the MI, not measured in our study, could have led to an MI or a major depressive disorder later.

IMPACT OF PREVIOUS DEPRESSION ON POST-MI DEPRESSION AND PROGNOSIS

The psychiatric literature indicates that a history of depression predicts further recurrences or relapses (33), and our study suggests that this is also true for post-MI patients. We found that MI patients with a previous depression were more than twice as likely to become depressed in the hospital as patients without a history of depression (OR = 2.30; 95% CI 1.09, 4.86; $P = .029$). They also tended to have more severe depressions in terms of BDI scores (mean BDI = 18.5 for patients with a recurrent depression versus 13.8 for those with a first depression; $P = .093$). Also, those with a recurrent depression in the hospital were at increased risk of death. Although the subgroup sizes are small, we found that 40.0% of the 15 patients with a recurrent depression died by 18 months, in comparison to 10.0% of the 20 patients with a first episode of depression. Surprisingly, those patients with a previous depression who did not become depressed in the hospital were the group with the lowest mortality (4.6% of 46 at 18 months). In any case, it seems clear that in settings with limited psychiatric resources, primary attention should be given to recent post-MI patients who experience a recurrent depression.

POST-DISCHARGE DEPRESSION

At the 6- and 12-month interviews, we used questions from the DIS to find out about symptom occurrence, symptom duration, and impairment from these symptoms during the previous 2 weeks as well as since the last interview. As described earlier, we were able to interview 97.1% of surviving patients at 6 months, and 88.8% at 1 year. We found that in addition to the 35 patients (15.8%) with major depression in the hospital, 30 (13.5%) others became depressed between discharge and 6 months, and five (2.3%) more between 6 and 12 months after the MI. Thus, during the first post-MI year 31.5% of patients experienced at least one episode of major depression. The majority of these depressions began in the hospital or during the first 6 months after discharge.

Patients who became depressed after discharge differed from those who remained depression-free in terms of age, history of depression, and severity of depression symptoms measured by BDI scores. However, a predictive model including these variables was able to identify only 5 of the 35 patients who became depressed after returning home. Therefore, the only way to detect depression either in the hospital or after discharge is to systematically screen patients with appropriate psychiatric instruments. However, we believe that without research data clearly documenting the efficacy and safety of treatments for post-MI depression, it is premature to institute routine screening programs. It is also important to point out that a significant proportion of those patients for whom screening measures suggest depression either do not fulfill clinical criteria for major depression when interviewed by a skilled psychiatrist or do not wish to receive treatment with antidepressants or psychotherapy.

Figure 15.3 shows the outcomes at 6 and 12 months after the MI for patients meeting psychiatric criteria for major depression in the hospital, those with elevated BDI scores who did not meet criteria (minor depression), and those with no evidence of depression in the hospital. It is clear that death is not the only consequence of early post-MI depression. Patients with either major depression or elevated BDI scores who survived tended to remain depressed. For example, although 76.8% of the nondepressed patients were alive and depression-free at 6 months,

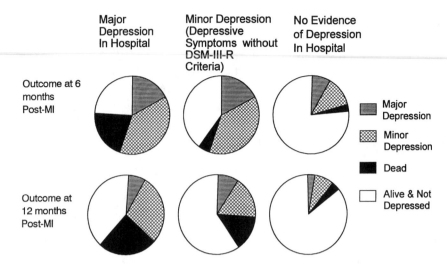

Figure 15.3.   Outcome at 6 and 12 months after MI for patients with major depression, minor depression, and no evidence of depression in the hospital after MI.

and 85.3% were alive and depression-free at 1 year after the MI, only 24.1% of the patients with major depression in the hospital were alive and depression-free at 6 months, with only 39.3% surviving and nondepressed at 1 year. Among the patients with elevated BDI scores in the hospital who did not meet criteria for major depression, 40.0% were alive and depression free at 6 months and 60.0% at 1 year.

If we consider the number of patients with at least one depression in their lifetime before the MI in combination with those who experienced a first depression after the MI, by 1 year after the infarction the lifetime prevalence for depression among those who survived was 45.4%. Psychiatric studies have shown that people who experience one episode of depression are at substantial risk of repeated episodes (33). Thus, in addition to the risk for mortality and continuing depression at 6 months and 1 year after the infarction, patients with post-MI depression who survive and recover from their depression are likely to be at risk of experiencing another depression. However, longer term follow-up would be needed to establish this risk.

β-BLOCKERS AND DEPRESSION

For years, clinicians have speculated that β-blockers can cause depression. Although the limited data available from the β-Blocker Heart Attack Trial showed no difference between treatment and placebo groups in terms of the

percentage of patients who reported "frequent depression that interfered with work, recreation or sleep" for the first 30 months of treatment (34), case reports and some epidemiologic studies have suggested a direct link between β-blockade and depression. For example, Avorn et al. (35) studied the medication records of Medicaid recipients and found that patients receiving the β-blockers commonly used in the early 1980s (propranolol, metoprolol, and nadolol) were more likely to be concurrently prescribed antidepressants than patients not on β-blockers. However, the data were not analyzed in terms of time of prescription so it was impossible to untangle possible cause and effect relationships. Using a more complete and comprehensive database, Thiessen et al. (36) replicated these findings and also reported a temporal relationship between new prescriptions for propranolol and prescriptions for antidepressants in the following month. More recent studies have questioned this relationship. For example, Schleifer et al. (37) did not find any association between the prescription of β-blockers after an admission for an MI and the development of depression 3 to 4 months later in a sample of 190 patients. Carney and colleagues (38) studied 77 patients admitted for elective cardiac catheterization and also found no association between the use of β-blockers and depression. In our own work in the post-MI period, we found that patients not taking β-blockers were more likely to be depressed than other patients (18). However, β-blockade was not randomly assigned and may have been a proxy measure of disease severity. Finally, a large epidemiologic study compared the records of 4302 Medicaid patients with markers for depression with those of randomly selected control patients (39). Although the depressed patients were more likely to have taken β-blockers (propranolol, metoprolol, nadolol), control for confounders, including the frequent use of other medications, eliminated this relationship. The authors concluded that "β-blockers as a group are not causally associated with depression on a population level." Despite this conclusion and the fact that, to our knowledge, there have been no randomized trials of β-blockers that evaluated their impact on depression using a valid and reliable measure of depression, clinicians and patients continue to talk about an association. It is likely that depressed cardiac patients are commonly deprived of the potential survival benefits of β-blockers. Although it is established that central nervous system side effects, including sedation, nightmares, impotence, and fatigue, may develop during time with the use of β-blockers, these side effects are not necessarily equivalent to a psychiatric diagnosis of depression. In addition, given the relatively high rate of depression in patients with cardiac disease, what appear to be the depressive side effects of β-blockade in some patients may in fact be symptoms of depression unrelated to the medication. In the absence of additional research data, we recommend that physicians be cautious before blaming β-blockers for significant symptoms of depression and depriving such patients the protection these drugs afford. Patients might benefit more from antidepressant treatments than from the withdrawal of β-blockade.

POTENTIAL MECHANISMS LINKING DEPRESSION WITH PROGNOSIS

There is little direct research evidence explaining why depression is related to prognosis. However, there is considerable speculation about the potential mechanisms, and studies are underway in a number of centers. Current hypotheses include the possibilities that both behavioral and physiologic factors are involved. There is evidence suggesting that depressed patients are less likely to comply with physician advice than other patients, that they have amplified somatic and pain responses to stimuli, and that they differ in their patterns of health care use. On a physiologic basis, depression may be associated with changes in both autonomic balance and hemostatic factors that could place depressed cardiac patients at increased risk of arrhythmic and thrombotic events.

Potential Behavioral Mechanisms

Although research is lacking in post-MI patients, studies in other illnesses have found depression and anxiety to be related to reduced compliance (40–42). One recent study focused on coronary artery disease patients 65 years of age and older, a group that is probably similar in behavior to post-MI patients, and used pill containers with computer chips that registered the opening and the closing of the container (43). Results showed that patients with major depression took their prescription of aspirin twice a day on only 45% of days in comparison to the nondepressed patients who complied on 69% of days ($P < .02$). Although statistically significant, the clinical implications of this difference in compliance with aspirin are unclear. However, similar levels of noncompliance with other medications could conceivably have an impact on patient outcomes. There is also evidence that depressed post-MI patients may be more likely to drop out of exercise programs (41), so it is possible that they may also be less likely to comply with physicians' recommendations about other lifestyle changes. We also know that depression and anxiety are often associated with multiple physical complaints. Because of its impact on autonomic arousal, depression may cause amplification of pain and other physical symptoms, leading to earlier or more frequent use of medical care (44). In fact, studies of patients without cardiac disease have found higher rates of health care system use and higher health costs among the depressed (45–48). Although it is likely that similar results would be found for post-MI patients, the patterns of health care utilization and costs associated with post-MI depression have not yet been documented. In short, although depressed patients may be less compliant, they may also visit physicians more often and may seek care earlier for relatively minor problems. Links between depression, patient behavior, and outcome are, thus, likely to be quite complex. Although as yet unstudied, it is likely that these complexities are also compounded by changes in the physician's treatment behavior in response to patients with depressed affect and other psychological symptoms. For example, as mentioned earlier, some observational literature has suggested that β-blockers are related to depression (35), although there have been no randomized studies indicating that this is the case. β-Blockade is known to improve post-MI survival (49), but we do not know how often physicians remove β-blockade from post-MI patients who repeatedly complain of depression.

Potential Physiologic Mechanisms

The physiologic mechanisms linking depression with post-MI mortality are likely to be at least as complicated as the behavioral ones. Post-MI cardiac deaths are usually secondary to either ventricular fibrillation or recurrent acute MIs. The two main hypotheses concerning physiologic links between depression and prognosis involve these mechanisms. The first hypothesis is that post-MI patients with high levels of depressive symptomatology or major depression have an increase in sympathetic nervous system activity compared with nondepressed patients, which may make them more prone to lethal arrhythmias. The second hypothesis is that post-MI depression is associated with activation of platelet aggregation, which can lead to acute thrombus formation.

Although direct data are lacking in depressed post-MI patients, indirect evidence from basic animal research, as well as studies in some clinical samples, supports the idea that depressed patients have a chronic increase in sympathetic nervous activity. By itself this increase could increase the risk of a fatal ventricular arrhythmic event. Animal research has demonstrated that when the heart is vulnerable after an MI, increased sympathetic activity significantly increases the risk of ventricular fibrillation (50). In this model, β-blocking medication, left stellate ganglion blockade, and increased vagal tone all act to protect against fatal arrhythmias (51, 52). It has also been demonstrated that increased sympathetic activity has a strong negative impact in post-MI patients with left ventricular dysfunction (53). Although reduced pump function induces an increase in sympathetic activity as an adaptive mechanism to maintain adequate cardiac outflow, patients with more pronounced neurohormonal activation, including norepinephrine activity, have a poorer prognosis. This neurohormonal activation seems to make patients particularly prone to ventricular arrhythmias. Meredith et al. (54) found that patients admitted for sustained ventricular arrhythmias had an increased cardiac production of norepinephrine in comparison to coronary patients without arrhythmias. Finally, heart rate variability, another measure of autonomic tone, is also a predictor of mortality among post-MI patients (55). In conclusion, post-MI patients seem to be at increased risk of mortality if they are exposed to the effect of increased sympathetic nervous activity without receiving treatment to limit its effects (i.e., β-blockers, left stellate ganglion blockade) (56, 57).

An overall increase in sympathetic nervous system activity is well documented in depressed patients. The basal heart rate is increased (58–60). There is an increase in plasma norepinephrine levels (61), and it has been suggested that most of this is secondary to an increase in sympathetic outflow (60). Carney et al. (59) found indirect evidence of this increase in sympathetic activity in depressed cardiac patients. They reported that there is a reduction in heart rate variability associated with depression in patients with established coronary disease.

In addition to the fact that depression seems to influence sympathetic nervous system outflow, patients with left ventricular dysfunction are particularly vulnerable to the negative effect of sympathetic arousal. In fact, our results showed that most of the impact of high BDI scores on mortality was in those patients with low ejection fractions and frequent PVCs (18). In fact, all of the patients with depression, low ejection fraction, and PVCs (n = 6) died by 18 months, five of the six because of fatal arrhythmias. It is possible that these patients were at especially high risk because of the impact of increases in sympathetic activity associated with depression, low ejection fraction, and PVCs. Although to date research indicates that the increases in norepinephrine activity in patients with major depression are restricted to those with melancholic features (62), it is possible that in our study the patients who had high BDI scores, frequent PVCs, and low ejection fractions had particularly high sympathetic drive. Although the hypothesis of increased sympathetic nervous system activity in depressed post-MI patients is supported by existing literature, it remains to be documented in a well-designed study of depression after MI.

It is widely accepted that, in addition to deaths from fatal arrhythmias, post-MI deaths frequently involve recurrent MIs (63). Platelet aggregation is one of the major players in this recurrent thrombogenic process that may be related to depression. Because platelets are assumed to be a peripheral model of the neuroregulation of norepinephrine and serotonin in the brain, they have been extensively studied in relation to emotional states, particularly in relation to major depression (64, 65). Although the clinical impact has not been assessed in coronary patients, recent data suggest that there may be an increase in platelet reactivity to serotonin and epinephrine in patients with major depression. Serotonin is a 5-HT$_2$ receptor agonist that weakly induces platelet aggregation in a direct fashion. However, it also amplifies platelets' reactions to other agonists like ADP and thrombin (66, 67). Many studies have found increased 5-HT$_2$ binding (Bmax) in depressed patients compared to normal controls (65, 68, 69). This increase in 5-HT$_2$ binding in depressed patients has also been documented using measures of receptor function based on phosphoinositide turnover (70), intracellular platelet calcium mobilization (71), and 5-HT$_2$-induced platelet aggregation (72), suggesting an upregulation of the 5-HT$_2$ receptors in depressed patients. Therefore, although none of these measures of platelet serotonin function have been evaluated in depressed patients with cardiac disease, there are some data to suggest more reactive platelet aggregation in major depression. If this is also true in depressed post-MI patients, they would be more likely to have a recurrent thrombogenic event.

In summary, although the literature supports two major physiologic links between depression and post-MI mortality, increased sympathetic nervous system function and changes in platelet aggregability, additional direct data are needed to establish the precise mechanisms.

CONCLUSIONS

The research summarized in this chapter has attracted much attention to the importance of depression in cardiac patients. The epidemiologic data strongly suggest that depression has a major impact on survival for post-MI patients. However, we are far from having clear clinical guidelines on the management of depression in this population. Ongoing clinical trials targeting depression in post-MI patients will certainly help in gauging the risks and benefits of different treatment strategies. Until this data becomes available, the identification and treatment of depression in cardiac patients should be much like the management of any patients with depression. The next chapter provides the reader with guidance on this issue.

References

1. Ruberman W, Weinblatt E, Goldberg JD, et al. Psychosocial influences on mortality after myocardial infarction. N Engl J Med 1984;311:552–559.
2. Follick MJ, Gorkin L, Capone RJ, et al. Psychological distress as predictor of ventricular arrhythmias in a post-myocardial infarction population. Am Heart J 1988;116:32–36.
3. Frasure-Smith N. In-hospital symptoms of psychological stress as predictors of long-term outcome after acute myocardial infarction in men. Am J Cardiol 1991;67:121–127.
4. Ahern DK, Gorkin L, Anderson JL, et al. Biobehavioral variables and mortality or cardiac arrest in the Cardiac Arrhythmia Pilot Study (CAPS). Am J Cardiol 1990; 66:59–62.
5. Booth-Kewley S, Friedman HS. Psychological predictors of heart disease: a quantitative review. Psychol Bull 1987;101:343–362.
6. Case RB, Moss AJ, Case N, et al. Living alone after myocardial infarction: impact on prognosis. JAMA 1992; 267:515–519.
7. Rouleau JL, Talajic M, Sussex B, et al. Myocardial infarction patients in the 1990s—their risk factors, stratification and survival in Canada: the Canadian Assessment of Myocardial Infarction (CAMI) Study. J Am Coll Cardiol 1996;27:1119–1127.
8. Robins LN, Helzer JE, Croughan J, et al. National Institute of Mental Health Diagnostic Interview Schedule: its history, characteristics, and validity. Arch Gen Psychiatry 1981;38:381–389.
9. Beck AT, Ward CH, Mendelson M, et al. An inventory for measuring depression. Arch Gen Psychiatry 1961; 4:561–571.
10. American Psychiatric Association. Diagnostic and statistical manual of mental disorders. 3rd ed. Washington, DC: American Psychiatric Association, 1987.
11. Killip T III, Kimball JT. Treatment of myocardial infarction in a coronary care unit: a two year experience with 250 patients. Am J Cardiol 1967;20:457–464.
12. Schleifer SJ, Macari-Hinson MM, Coyle DA, et al. The nature and course of depression following myocardial infarction. Arch Intern Med 1989;149:1785–1789.
13. Ladwig KH, Kieser M, König M, et al. Affective disorders and survival after acute myocardial infarction: results from the post-infarction late potential study. Eur Heart J 1991;12:959–964.
14. Langeluddecke P, Fulcher G, Baird D, et al. A prospec-

tive evaluation of the psychosocial effects of coronary artery bypass surgery. J Psychosom Res 1989;33:37–45.

15. Cohen-Cole SA, Kaufman KG. Major depression in physical illness: diagnosis, prevalence, and antidepressant treatment (a ten year review: 1982–1992). Depression 1993;1:181–204.

16. Silverstone PH. Prevalence of psychiatric disorders in medical inpatients. J Nerv Ment Dis 1996;184:43–51.

17. Frasure-Smith N, Lespérance F, Talajic M. Depression following myocardial infarction: impact on 6-month survival. JAMA 1993;270:1819–1825.

18. Frasure-Smith N, Lespérance F, Talajic M. Depression and 18-month prognosis following myocardial infarction. Circulation 1995;91:999–1005.

19. Lespérance F, Frasure-Smith N, Talajic M. Major depression before and after myocardial infarction: its nature and consequences. Psychosom Med 1996;58:99–110.

20. Lespérance F, Frasure-Smith N. Negative emotions and coronary heart disease: getting to the heart of the matter. Lancet 1996;347:414.

21. Williams RB, Chesney MA. Psychosocial factors and prognosis in established coronary artery disease: the need for research on interventions. JAMA 1993;270:1860–1861.

22. Fielding R. Depression and acute myocardial infarction: a review and reinterpretation. Soc Sci Med 1991;32:1017–1027.

23. House A. Mood disorders in the physically ill—problems of definition and measurement. J Psychosom Res 1988;32:345–353.

24. Silverstone PH, Lemay T, Elliott J, et al. The prevalence of major depressive disorder and low self-esteem in medical inpatients. Can J Psychiatry 1996;41:67–74.

25. Anda R, Williamson D, Jones D, et al. Depressed affect, hopelessness, and the risk of ischemic heart disease in a cohort of U.S. adults. Epidemiology 1993;4:285–294.

26. Appels A, Mulder P. Excess fatigue as a precursor of myocardial infarction. Eur Heart J 1988;9:758–764.

27. Robins LN, Helzer JE, Weissman MM, et al. Lifetime prevalence of specific psychiatric disorders in three sites. Arch Gen Psychiatry 1984;41:949–958.

28. Helzer JE, Robins LN, McEvoy LT, et al. A comparison of clinical and diagnostic interview schedule diagnoses: physician reexamination of lay-interviewed cases in the general population. Arch Gen Psychiatry 1985;42:657–666.

29. Parker G. Are the lifetime prevalence estimates in the ECA study accurate? Psychol Med 1987;17:275–282.

30. Kovess V, Fournier L. The DISSA: an abridged self-administered version of the DIS approach by episode. Soc Psychiatry Psychiatr Epidemiol 1990;25:179–186.

31. Weissman MM, Myers JK. Affective disorders in a US urban community: the use of research diagnostic criteria in an epidemiological survey. Arch Gen Psychiatry 1978;35:1304–1311.

32. Kessler RC, McGonagle KA, Zhao S, et al. Lifetime and 12-month prevalence of DSM-III-R psychiatric disorders in the United States. Arch Gen Psychiatry 1994;51:8–19.

33. Keller MB, Lavori PW, Lewis CE, et al. Predictors of re-

lapse in major depressive disorder. JAMA 1983;250:3299–3304.

34. Davis BR, Furberg C, Williams CB. Survival analysis of adverse effects data in the Beta-Blocker Heart Attack Trial. Clin Pharmacol Ther 1987;41:611–615.

35. Avorn J, Everitt DE, Weiss S. Increased antidepressant use in patients prescribed β-blockers. JAMA 1986;255:357–360.

36. Thiessen BQ, Wallace SM, Blackburn JL, et al. Increased prescribing of antidepressants subsequent to β-blocker therapy. Arch Intern Med 1990;150:2286–2290.

37. Schleifer SJ, Slater WR, Macari-Hinson MM, et al. Digitalis and β-blocking agents: effects on depression following myocardial infarction. Am Heart J 1991;121:1397–1402.

38. Carney RM, Rich MW, teVelde A, et al. Prevalence of major depressive disorder in patients receiving beta-blocker therapy versus other medications. Am J Med 1987;83:223–226.

39. Bright RA, Everitt DE. β-Blockers and depression: evidence against an association. JAMA 1992;267:1783–1787.

40. Surridge DHC, Williams EDL, Lawson JS, et al. Psychiatric aspects of diabetes mellitus. Br J Psychiatry 1984;145:269–276.

41. Blumenthal JA, Williams RS, Wallace AG, et al. Physiological and psychological variables predict compliance to prescribed exercise therapy in patients recovering from myocardial infarction. Psychosom Med 1982;44:519–527.

42. Richardson JL, Marks G, Johnson CA, et al. Path model of multidimensional compliance with cancer therapy. Health Psychol 1987;6:183–207.

43. Carney RM, Freedland KE, Eisen SA, et al. Major depression and medication adherence in elderly patients with coronary artery disease. Health Psychol 1995;14:88–90.

44. Katon W. Depression: somatization and social factors. J Fam Pract 1988;27:579–580.

45. Coe RM, Wolinsky FD, Miller DK, et al. Complementary and compensatory functions in social network relationships among the elderly. Gerontologist 1984;24:396–400.

46. Katon W, Berg A, Robins AJ, et al. Depression: medical utilization and somatization. West J Med 1986;144:564–568.

47. Simon GE, VonKorff M, Barlow W. Health care costs of primary care patients with recognized depression. Arch Gen Psychiatry 1995;52:850–856.

48. Unützer J, Patrick DL, Simon G, et al. Depression symptoms and the cost of health services in HMO patients aged 65 years and older. JAMA 1997;277:1618–1623.

49. Bassan MM, Shalev O, Eliakim A. Improved prognosis during long-term treatment with beta-blockers after myocardial infarction: analysis of randomized trials and pooling of results. Heart Lung 1984;13:164–168.

50. Schwartz PJ, Billman GE, Stone HL. Autonomic mechanisms in ventricular fibrillation induced by myocardial ischemia during exercise in dogs with healed myocardial infarction: an experimental preparation for sudden cardiac death. Circulation 1984;69:790–800.

51. de Ferrari GM, Schwartz PJ. Autonomic nervous system and arrhythmias. Ann N Y Acad Sci 1990;601: 247–262.

52. Podrid PJ, Fuchs T, Candinas R. Role of the sympathetic nervous system in the genesis of ventricular arrhythmia. Circulation 1990;82(Suppl 1):I-103–I-113.

53. Rouleau J, Packer M, Moyé L, et al. Prognostic value of neurohumoral activation in patients with an acute myocardial infarction: effect of captopril. J Am Coll Cardiol 1994;24:583–591.

54. Meredith IT, Broughton A, Jennings GL, et al. Evidence of selective increase in cardiac sympathetic activity in patients with sustained ventricular arrhythmias. N Engl J Med 1991;325:618–624.

55. Bigger JT Jr, Fleiss JL, Steinman RC, et al. Frequency domain measures of heart period variability and mortality after myocardial infarction. Circulation 1992;85: 164–171.

56. Verrier RL, Calvert A, Lown B. Effect of posterior hypothalamic stimulation on ventricular fibrillation threshold. Am J Physiol 1975;228:923–927.

57. Coats AJS, Radaelli A, McCance A, et al. Controlled trial of physical training in chronic heart failure: exercise performance, hemodynamics, ventilation, and autonomic function. Circulation 1992;85:2119–2131.

58. Lahmeyer HW, Bellur SN. Cardiac regulation and depression. J Psychiatr Res 1987;21:1–6.

59. Carney RM, Rich MW, teVelde A, et al. The relationship between heart rate, heart rate variability and depression in patients with coronary artery disease. J Psychosom Res 1988;32:159–164.

60. Veith RC, Lewis N, Linares OA, et al. Sympathetic nervous system activity in major depression—basal and desipramine-induced alterations in plasma norepinephrine kinetics. Arch Gen Psychiatry 1993;50:1–12.

61. Lake CR, Packar D, Ziegler MG, et al. High plasma norepinephrine levels in patients with major affective disorder. Am J Psychiatry 1982;139:1315–1318.

62. Roy A, Linnoila M, Potter WZ. Plasma norepinephrine level in affective disorders: relationship to melancholia. Arch Gen Psychiatry 1985;42:1181–1185.

63. Cairns JA, Singer J, Gent M, et al. One year mortality outcomes of all coronary and intensive care unit patients with acute myocardial infarction, unstable angina or other chest pain in Hamilton, Ontario, a city of 375,000 people. Can J Cardiol 1989;5:239–245.

64. Garcia-Sevilla JA, Padró D, Giralt T, et al. α_2-Adrenoceptor-mediated inhibition of platelet adenylate cyclase and induction of aggregation in major depression: effect of long-term cyclic antidepressant drug treatment. Arch Gen Psychiatry 1990;47:125–132.

65. Meltzer HY, Arora RC. Platelet serotonin studies in affective disorders: evidence for a serotonergic abnormality? In: Sandler M, Coppen A, Harnett S, eds. 5-Hydroxytryptamine in psychiatry. London: Oxford University Press, 1991:50–89.

66. Badimon L, Lassila R, Badimon J, et al. An acute surge of epinephrine stimulates platelet deposition to severely damaged vascular wall [abstract]. J Am Coll Cardiol 1990;15:181A.

67. Vanhoutte PM. Platelet-derived serotonin, the endothelium, and cardiovascular disease. J Cardiovasc Pharmacol 1991;17(Suppl 5):S6–S12.

68. Meltzer HY, Lowy MT. The serotonin hypothesis of depression. In: Meltzer HY, ed. Psychopharmacology: the third generation of progress. New York: Raven Press, 1987:513–526.

69. Arora RC, Meltzer HY. Increased serotonin$_2$ (5-HT$_2$) receptor binding as measured by ^{3}H-lysergic acid diethylamide (^{3}H-LSD) in the blood platelets of depressed patients. Life Sci 1989;44:725–734.

70. Mikuni M, Kagaya A, Takahashi K, et al. Serotonin but not norepinephrine-induced calcium mobilization of platelets is enhanced in affective disorders. Psychopharmacology 1992;106:311–314.

71. Kusumi I, Koyama T, Yamashita I. Serotonin-stimulated Ca^{2+} response is increased in the blood platelets of depressed patients. Biol Psychiatry 1991;30:310–312.

72. Brusov OS, Beliaev BS, Katasonov AB, et al. Does platelet serotonin receptor supersensitivity accompany endogenous depression? Biol Psychiatry 1989;25: 375–381.

Management of Depression and Anxiety in the Cardiac Patient

J. Robert Swenson and Susan E. Abbey

. . . every affection of the mind that is attended with either pain or pleasure, hope or fear, is the cause of an agitation whose influence extends to the heart.
William Harvey, 1628

In chapter 14, Sotile discusses psychosocial interventions that have been found to benefit most patients in the process of adapting to cardiac disease, including stress management, bolstering family functioning and social support, and sexual counseling. The chapter by Frasure-Smith and Lespérance discusses the significance of major depression in patients who sustain myocardial infarction (MI) with respect to increased risk of cardiac mortality and chronic depression. This chapter focuses on diagnosis and management of depressive and anxiety disorders, which may occur in up to 25% of patients who have cardiovascular disease (1). Results of randomized, controlled trials evaluating treatment of depressive or anxiety disorders in cardiac patients are not yet available, so the clinician must be guided by knowledge of the response to psychiatric treatment of these disorders in patients without medical illness, and studies of psychiatric interventions in small numbers of patients with cardiac disease and comorbid depression or anxiety. The management of patients with other psychiatric conditions, such as bipolar affective disorder (manic-depressive illness), or psychotic disorders is not discussed; the reader is referred to a standard textbook of psychiatry (2). Before reviewing the individual depressive and anxiety disorders, we present a general approach to the diagnosis and management of patients who have possible psychiatric complications, from the perspective of physicians or other professionals involved in their cardiac rehabilitation.

AN APPROACH TO THE PATIENT WHO SHOWS ANXIETY OR DEPRESSION

Different patients develop similar psychiatric disorders for different reasons. Biologic factors such as nutritional, electrolyte, or endocrine abnormalities, drug effects, and the consequences of multisystem or neurologic disease may play major causative roles in the development of anxiety or depressive disorders. Serious medical illness also may represent an intolerable psychological loss, with loss of autonomy, loss of intact body image, and loss of the capacity to work and interact with family and friends. This sense of loss of control over life may lead to overwhelming anxiety or profound depression. Although any person has the potential to develop a psychiatric disorder, the following groups of patients may be especially vulnerable to anxiety or depressive disorders:

1. Patients who have had a previous depressive or anxiety disorder.
2. Patients with a strong family history of psychiatric illness (particularly anxiety or mood disorders and alcoholism).
3. Patients with ongoing alcohol or drug abuse or a history of substance abuse.
4. Patients with a history of unstable interpersonal relationships or social isolation, and pa-

tients who cannot maintain consistent employment.

5. Patients who have sustained repeated major losses such as the death of parents or family members, divorce, estrangement from family, and major illnesses with resultant disability or need to take ongoing medication.

The depressed patient may present with sad or withdrawn appearance, poor motivation or compliance with suggested rehabilitative goals, difficulty with memory or concentration, complaints of insomnia and undue fatigue in excess of what would be expected from knowledge of the patient's medical condition. Patients with anxiety disorders often present with physical symptoms of anxiety such as shortness of breath, shakiness or dizziness, weakness, numbness, and chronic chest pain. Physical complaints associated with anxiety or depression nevertheless require careful evaluation, because the patient's confidence in and rapport with the treating physician and rehabilitation staff are compromised if the patient perceives that complaints are dismissed as "it's all in your head."

Taking a psychiatric history usually is best incorporated with the patient's general medical assessment or assessment at the start of a rehabilitation program. Patients often respond best to nonthreatening open-ended questions that convey interest in their psychological state; such questions might include "How are you coping with the stress of having heart disease?" "How is the family reacting?" "Have you ever become discouraged or depressed with your situation?" If indicated, additional questions can be directed toward obtaining the following information:

1. The history of present symptoms should be obtained, including an assessment of the patient's emotional state, thought processes, memory and concentration, sleep pattern, appetite and weight gain or loss, somatic symptoms of anxiety, and unusual psychiatric symptoms such as hallucinations or delusions.

2. Patients should be asked whether they have thought about wanting to die, and if the answer is positive, the patient should be asked directly whether he or she has had any suicidal thoughts or made actual plans or has actually attempted suicide.

3. The pattern of alcohol use should always be determined, because alcohol abuse can be the basis for many psychiatric symptoms. It also can explain poor compliance with treatment regimens or with the rehabilitation program. The patient should be asked about the use of recreational drugs (e.g., cannabis, cocaine, amphetamines) and an accurate determination of the use of prescribed medication (analgesics and benzodiazepines) is essential.

4. The past history of psychiatric illness and response to treatment should be determined because a positive response to previous treatment is usually the best predictor of future success with treatment.

5. A family history of psychiatric illness may help with diagnosis, because psychiatric conditions such as major depression, certain anxiety disorders, and alcoholism may occur in many family members.

6. A thorough review of the patient's medical status and medications should be taken and a physical examination should be performed; any appropriate investigations of unexplained physical symptoms also should be arranged. Medical conditions and medications that may give rise to secondary anxiety or depressive disorders are discussed in subsequent sections of this chapter.

We encourage the treatment of the cardiac patient who has a depressive or anxiety disorder within the rehabilitation setting if the patient is already involved in a rehabilitation program. Nevertheless, there are some patients who should be referred to a mental health professional, either before being considered for a cardiac rehabilitation program or in conjunction with attendance in an ongoing program. Examples of such patients include the suicidal patient, patients who are severely impulsive (at risk of harming themselves or others), patients with psychosis or bipolar illness, and patients who have responded poorly to a trial of antidepressant or anxiolytic therapy. Overly demanding, "needy" patients may provoke dislike or anger on the part of the treating staff and may sabotage groups in a rehabilitation setting (3). These patients often benefit by psychologic assessment and ongoing psychotherapeutic support, and collaboration with a psychiatrist or psychologist may help the rehabilitation staff better understand the patient's conflicts with dependency and authority. We have found that patients who demonstrate uncontrolled alcoholism or drug abuse benefit most by direct confrontation of this problem and referral to professionals who are expert in addictions. Littman (4) suggests that referral to a mental health professional should also be considered for cardiac patients who have the following problems: patients having problems with memory and concentration, sexual dysfunction, marital conflict, or interpersonal strife; patients unable to modify their cardiovascular risk factors after adequate education; and patients with cardiac disease who are physiologically able to work but have marked work stress or marked reluctance to return to work.

DEPRESSION

The Medical Outcomes Study found that patients who show depressive disorders tend to have worse physical, social, and role functioning, worse perceived current health, and greater bodily pain than patients who have no chronic illness (5). The impairment in functional state associated with major depression was comparable to or worse than the impairment uniquely associated with any of eight major chronic medical conditions, including acute coronary artery disease (CAD). The study also found that the effects of depressive symptoms and medical conditions on functioning were additive; for example, the combination of advanced CAD and depressive symptoms was associated with roughly twice the reduction in social functioning associated with either condition alone. Katon and Sullivan (6) describe the following maladaptive effects of major depression on patients who have chronic medical illness: 1) depression often leads to amplification of somatic symptoms of the chronic medical illness, adding to the patient's disability and possibly confusing the treating physician; 2) depression may decrease the patient's motivation to care for his or her illness; and 3) depression may have direct, adverse physiologic effects on the patient's disease.

The previous chapter by Frasure-Smith and Lespérance highlights the prevalence and prognosis of major depression in patients who have CAD. In seeking to understand and empathize with the patient's loss of health, some physicians may not appreciate the nature of this psychiatric complication and may ascribe the patient's depression as a "normal reaction" to illness. Unfortunately, in this situation, the patient's depression remains untreated with consequent failure at not only psychological but physical rehabilitation. The following section discusses an approach to diagnosis and treatment of major depression in patients who have cardiac disease. It examines the efficacy and safety of antidepressant medication in this group of patients.

Diagnosis of Depressive Disorders

Mood refers to an inner sustained emotional state. *Depression* often is used to refer to a transient mood state that may last from hours to days and often occurs as a predictable response to life's disappointments (often called "normal sadness"). A *depressive disorder,* however, is distinguished from a normal mood state by particular symptom constellations and duration of symptoms that have predictable clinical courses and responses to treatment (e.g., "major depression"). A depressive disorder also must be distinguished from normal bereavement, which is a profound sadness after a severe loss or trauma, and may have acute symptoms indistinguishable from a major depression. With time (often after a few months), the symptoms of bereavement become less intense and the person regains attachment to everyday living and interacting with others. Sometimes depressive symptoms may persist or become more severe, and a major depression develops.

A *primary depressive disorder* occurs when a patient sustains a major depressive episode that is the first appearance of psychiatric illness in the patient's lifetime and is not associated with other psychiatric illnesses or intrinsically related to a physical illness. A primary depressive disorder may be *unipolar* (major depression only) or *bipolar* (manic and depressive episodes). The lifetime prevalence for major depression is about 5% to 7% of the population, with women affected twice as often as men (7). A secondary depressive disorder may occur in a patient who has other psychiatric illness or medical illness. Psychiatric illnesses such as schizophrenia, alcoholism, drug abuse, dementia, and anxiety disorders can give rise to depressive episodes that may require specific treatment. Medical illnesses such as endocrinopathies, neurologic diseases, and malignancies are associated with a high incidence of depressive disorders. In addition, many medications may precipitate a depressive episode, particularly those with central nervous system effects. Table 16.1 lists medical illnesses and specific medications that have been found to be associated with depressive disorders.

An a*djustment disorder* is a maladaptive reaction to what usually is a major life stress; this maladaptive reaction occurs soon after the stressful event and usually takes the form of impairment in the patient's important relationships and the ability to work and interact socially (8). Symptoms include anxious or depressed moods that seem out of proportion to a normal reaction to the stressor, or a disturbance of conduct that may get the patient into trouble. An adjustment disorder, by definition, lasts less than 6 months, and when the acute stress abates, the patient may resume previous adaptive functioning. If symptoms of depression are present, they are less severe and pervasive than those of a major depression. An adjustment reaction may occur in the context of major medical illness, particularly with heart disease. What often is seen is the patient who encounters a sudden or an unexpected cardiac problem and reacts either by ignoring symptoms and denying the possibility of illness or by refusing to resume appropriate activities after the acute event has been treated. Most patients who have adjustment disorders respond to psychotherapy aimed at helping them to express feelings about loss of bodily integrity. Some patients who have an adjustment disorder may not resolve their feelings of loss and go on to develop a major depression, particularly if they have a history of previous depressive episodes.

A patient who experiences a *major depressive episode* must have a depressed mood (commonly described as feeling "sad, blue, down in the dumps, fed up"), a pervasive loss of interest in almost all aspects of living, or lack of pleasure in previously pleasurable activities. This state lasts at least 2 weeks (8). Patients who have major depression have a recognizable pattern of symptoms and demonstrate signs that, if present, allow one to predict that the patient is likely to respond to a combination of psychotherapy and antidepressant medication. Table 16.2 outlines the fourth edition of the Diagnostic and Statistical Manual of Mental

Table 16.1. Common Illnesses and Medications Associated with Depressive Disorders

Neurologic disorders	Cardiovascular disease
Stroke	Congestive heart failure
Alzheimer's disease	Acute myocardial infarction
Multiple sclerosis	Collagen diseases
Parkinson's disease	Lupus erythematosus
Epilepsy	Rheumatoid arthritis
Endocrine disorders	Drugs and poisons
Addison's disease	Alcohol
Cushing's disease	Amphetamines
Diabetes	Barbiturates
Hypothyroidism	Cocaine
Uremia	Digitalis
Infections	Lead poisoning
Encephalitis	Methyldopa
Hepatitis	Opiates
Mononucleosis	Oral Contraceptives
Subacute bacterial endocarditis	Benzodiazepines
Syphilis	Propranolol
Tuberculosis	Steroids
Malignancies	Cimetidine
Gastrointestinal	Metoclopramide
Breast	
Pancreas	
Brain	
Lung	

Table 16.2.   Diagnostic Criteria for Major Depressive Episode

A. Five or more of the following symptoms have been present during the same 2-week period and represent a change from previous functioning; at least one of the symptoms is either (1) depressed mood or (2) loss of interest or pleasure (do not include symptoms that are clearly due to general medical condition or mood-incongruent delusions or hallucinations).

   (1) Depressed mood most of the day, nearly every day, as indicated by either subjective report (e.g., feels sad or empty) or observation made by others (e.g., appears tearful).

   (2) Markedly diminished interest or pleasure in all, or almost all, activities most of the day, nearly every day.

   (3) Significant weight loss when not dieting, or weight gain, or decrease in appetite nearly every day.

   (4) Insomnia or hypersomnia nearly every day.

   (5) Psychomotor agitation or retardation nearly every day (observable by others, not merely subjective feelings of restlessness or being slowed down).

   (6) Fatigue or loss of energy nearly every day.

   (7) Feelings of worthlessness or excessive or inappropriate guilt (which may be delusional) nearly every day (not merely self-reproach or guilt about being sick).

   (8) Diminished ability to think or concentrate, or indecisiveness, nearly every day (either by subjective account or as observed by others).

   (9) Recurrent thoughts of death (not just fear of dying), recurrent suicidal ideation without a specific plan, or a suicide attempt or a specific plan for committing suicide.

B. The symptoms do not meet criteria for a mixed episode (mixed manic and depressive episode).

C. The symptoms cause clinically significant distress or impairment in social, occupational, or other important areas of functioning.

D. The symptoms are not due to the direct physiologic effects of a substance (e.g., drug of abuse, a medication) or a general medical condition (e.g., hypothyroidism).

E. The symptoms are not better accounted for by bereavement, i.e., after the loss of a loved one, the symptoms persist for longer than 2 months, or are characterized by marked functional impairment, morbid preoccupation with worthlessness, suicidal ideation, psychotic symptoms, or psychomotor retardation.

Adapted from the Diagnostic and Statistical Manual of Mental Disorders. 4th ed. Washington, DC: American Psychiatric Association, 1994.

Disorder's (DSM-IV) criteria for major depressive disorder developed by the American Psychiatric Association (8). The patient who presents a major depression can also show a variety of symptoms, ranging from severe anxiety and psychomotor agitation to profound retardation in thought processes, speech, and motor movements, as well as marked social withdrawal.

Some depressed patients, often elderly, do not complain of depressed mood but describe somatic symptoms as their primary problem, particularly fatigue, insomnia, and anxiety-related symptoms (lightheadedness, dyspnea, tachycardia, or nausea). Patients with depressive disorders may also complain of chronic pain. These patients blame their lack of interest in everyday living on their physical problems, but family members often will say "he just doesn't try any more." Certainly, somatic complaints require thorough medical investigation, particularly in the patient who has had previous cardiac disease. Fatigue that seems out of proportion to objective physical findings or unexplained chest pain that has many noncardiac qualities should prompt

consideration that the patient may be suffering from depression.

If a depressive disorder is the direct physiologic consequence of a patient's medical illness, the DSM-IV distinguishes this secondary depressive disorder from a major depression by calling the condition a *mood disorder due to a general medical condition* (8). Examples include depressive disorders caused by degenerative neurologic conditions (e.g., Parkinson's disease), cerebrovascular disease (e.g., stroke), and endocrine disorders (e.g., hypothyroidism). The distinction is important in that if the underlying illness is responsive to treatment or if causative medications can be stopped, the mood disorder often improves without specific treatment (Table 16.1). There also is some evidence that depressive disorders that are intrinsically related to underlying medical illness are less responsive to antidepressant medication (9). In many cases, however, it is difficult to prove a causative role for the underlying medical illness because the patient may have had previous depressions or may have a familial vulnerability toward mood disorders. Certainly, if no improvement in the depressive disorder is seen with optimal medical treatment, consideration should be given to specific treatment of depression.

Although the previous discussion outlines the different types of depressive disorders according to the DSM-IV classification, in practice patients may present with some symptoms or signs of depression but don't meet all criteria for major depression. Recently there has been a focus on the clinical significance of depressive symptoms below the threshold for major depressive disorder, referred to by some as *subsyndromal depression.* A recent study of 3962 outpatients of either mental health clinics or general medical care providers found that subsyndromal depression appeared to be a variant of depressive disorder; those patients who attended mental health clinics received similar treatment to patients with classic depressive illness, but patients with subsyndromal depression attending general medical clinics often were not treated (10). The section that follows describes an approach to treatment of the patient who has cardiac disease and major depression; however, it should be kept in mind that psychiatric treatment, including antidepressant medication, may be effective for patients with subsyndromal depression.

Treatment of Major Depression

Successful treatment of any patient who has a chronic medical illness and a coexisting major depressive disorder requires an integrated biologic, psychological, and social approach familiar to those who work in cardiac rehabilitation. We have found that the integration of the patient's psychiatric and medical care is often essential; many depressed patients are reluctant to be referred for psychiatric care but will accept treatment for major depression if directed by their family physician or cardiac specialist. The development of a therapeutic alliance between patient and physician is an essential first step in the treatment of a major depression. Before discussion of a specific treatment, it is essential that the patient 1) recognize and accept that a problem with a major depressive disorder is causing impairment in everyday life; 2) understand a "disease concept" of depression—that a major depression involves emotional symptoms and physical symptoms (such as sleep disturbance and decreased energy), and that a depressive illness is different from normal and expected emotional ups and downs; and 3) understand that this illness requires treatment that involves "talking about the problem" and often consideration of antidepressant medication. It is obvious, but must be stressed, that a patient who is motivated to participate in treatment of a depressive disorder has a much better chance of success.

Social Support and Cardiac Rehabilitation in Patients with Cardiac Disease and Depression

Social support has been found to play an important role in recovery from and adaptation to cardiac disease as well as to act as an important factor in primary prevention of MI (11). For example, the degree of emotional support was found to be independently related to risk for death in the subsequent 6 months after MI in a prospective study of 195 elderly patients hospitalized for acute MI (12). However, recently reported randomized trials of psychosocial interventions for post-MI patients have not shown benefit in mortality reduction or reduction of anxiety or depression (13, 14). Another study of 187 patients with mild to moderate depressive or anxiety symptoms who were randomly assigned within 6 weeks of acute MI to usual care or brief cardiac rehabilitation lasting 8 weeks, and then followed up for 12 months, did not find any difference in the intervention or control groups, with most patients in both groups showing similar and significant improvement in symptoms of anxiety and depression for the duration of the trial (15). The authors suggest that the lack of difference in the intervention and control groups is explained by the natural course of recovery in psychological status, including mood states, that occurs with time in post-MI patients. In these studies the interventions have not focused on the treatment of patients with moderate to severe symptoms, indicative of full-fledged depressive or anxiety disorders. Major depression is unlikely to resolve on its own and most patients require specific psychiatric treatment.

With respect to participation in cardiac rehabilitation, it should be kept in mind that most patients who have a depressive disorder also have diminished motivation and interest in daily life, along with the overwhelming fatigue that accompanies a major depression. Consequently, the patient's progression with cardiac rehabilitation is often slow or nonexistent. Finnegan and Suler (16) found that depressive symptoms after MI had a negative effect on the maintenance of healthy behavioral changes during cardiac rehabilitation and that they sometimes contribute to problems in returning to a reasonable level of function. Depression also has been associated with poor compliance with medical therapy and follow-up (17). If a patient with major depression is involved in a formal cardiac rehabilitation program and is not meeting specified goals, we suggest that these goals be modified in accordance with anticipated recovery from the depressive disorder, but that the patient be kept in the program. However, severely depressed patients referred for cardiac rehabilitation in most cases should receive treatment for depression before starting the program, or immediately on starting the program.

Psychotherapy for Cardiac Patients with Major Depression

Psychotherapeutic treatment of cardiac patients with major depression has not yet been evaluated in randomized clinical trials. A review of smaller controlled studies of psychosocial interventions with coronary heart disease patients suggests that efficacy is strongest for short-term outcomes and that interventions targeting patients who are at higher risk for psychological distress are more useful than those aimed at the general population of patients with heart disease (18). We find that supportive psychotherapy enabling patients to verbalize their concerns about coping with cardiac disease, along with talking about other life stresses, is helpful to most depressed patients. Treatment with antidepressant medication is rarely successful unless it is prescribed in the context of an ongoing psychotherapeutic relationship. Psychotherapy without antidepressant medication can also be helpful for some patients who have major depression (19). If a patient is reluctant to consider an antidepressant medication, it often is helpful to start out with regular psychotherapy sessions and defer a decision on antidepressant therapy. If there is concern about the potential for the patient to attempt suicide with an antidepressant overdose, the physician should not prescribe medication until this issue is clarified and referral to a psychiatrist is considered.

An approach to psychotherapy should include an agreement with the patient to meet at regular intervals (as often as every 1 or 2 weeks at first) for 30 to 60 minutes. The patient should understand that the focus of these sessions is on the patient's psychological difficulties and not solely on physical status. Central to most patients' psychological reaction to physical illness is dealing with grief about their loss of health—this involves anger, sadness, guilt, and eventual acknowledgment and acceptance to some degree. Psychotherapy might include focusing on any or all of the following issues: 1) the meaning of heart disease and other physical illness and its impact on lifestyle; 2) conflicts in the patient's important interpersonal relationships; and 3) conflicts from the past that may have been reactivated by the patient's present circumstances. For example, onset of cardiac disease can bring to the surface feelings of despair, anger, or guilt stemming from such experiences as major childhood illness or serious illness in a parent or sibling.

Antidepressants in Patients Who Have Cardiovascular Disease

The use of antidepressant agents to treat patients who have cardiovascular disease has expanded remarkably in the past decade as "new generations" of antidepressants have come on the market with decidedly different side effect profiles, such as the selective serotonin-reuptake inhibitors (SSRIs). Treatment with an antidepressant should be considered for the patient who presents with symptoms and signs of a major depression, and particularly for the patient who has had such symptoms for many weeks or months. It has been shown that a combination of psychotherapy and antidepressant medication is, in most cases, more effective in the treatment of patients who have major depression than psychotherapy alone (20). Recently, use of antidepressants in cardiac transplant recipients has been described (21). It is helpful to know the various commonly used antidepressants, as well as their advantages and disadvantages, and to know how to choose a specific type of antidepressant to suit the individual patient. For example, postural hypotension is likely to occur in patients who have congestive heart failure (CHF) if given certain types of antidepressants.

The older tricyclic antidepressants (TCAs), such as amitriptyline (Elavil and others), imipramine (Tofranil and others), desipramine (Norpramin, Pertofrane, and others), nortriptyline (Pamelor, Aventyl, and others), and doxepin (Sinequan and others) were found to cause life-threatening ventricular arrhythmias and conduction blocks in patients who took overdoses. Clinicians were also reluctant to use them in patients with CAD because of side effects such as tachycardia and hypotension seen with therapeutic doses. Patients who are prescribed TCAs often discontinue them because of intolerable dry mouth and sedation. Tricyclic antidepressants were found to suppress arrhythmias and resemble class I antiarrhythmic drugs; these cardiac effects were initially thought to be particularly beneficial to depressed patients with preexisting arrhythmias (22). Unfortunately, in the late 1980s and early 1990s, all randomized trials of class I antiarrhythmic drugs designed to determine whether suppression of ventricular arrhythmias after MI would improve survival have demonstrated excess mortality in the groups of patients treated given these drugs. These findings have led Glassman et al. (23) to reconsider the safety of TCAs in cardiac patients, and they suggest using an SSRI type of antidepressant or bupropion, and to consider a TCA only if the patient fails to respond. We agree with this recommendation; however, at this time there are no published randomized clinical trials of SSRIs in depressed cardiac patients demonstrating efficacy and safety. Table 16.3 outlines commonly used antidepressants, their dosage ranges, side effects, advantages, and disadvantages. The next section of this chapter expands on the use of these antidepressants and attempts to guide the reader to make rational choices about medication to treat patients who have various cardiac diseases. After discussing the profile of different classes of antidepressants, an approach to the use of antidepressant medication will be discussed.

Selective Serotonin Reuptake Inhibitors

The SSRIs have become the first line of antidepressant medication in most patients with major depression who are started on antidepressants for the first time. These medications have established records of greater safety and tolerability compared to TCAs, as well as comparable efficacy. Since the introduction of fluoxetine about 10 years ago, there has been a fourfold increase in the antidepressant market in the United States (24). The SSRIs do not cause the side effects that commonly occur with treatment with TCAs, such as postural hypotension, anticholinergic side effects (e.g., dry mouth, constipation,

blurred vision), sedation, and weight gain. In trials involving depressed but otherwise healthy patients, there were no adverse effects seen on cardiac conduction or contractility. There are no large randomized trials yet reported that document the safety and efficacy of SSRIs in patients with cardiac disease. A case report of 17 patients with complex cardiac disease treated with various types of SSRIs reported that the antidepressants were safe and reasonably effective in most of these patients (25). Fluoxetine, however, was reported in two case reports to have been associated with sinus bradycardia and syncope (26, 27), and an elderly patient developed atrial fibrillation and bradycardia shortly after beginning treatment with fluoxetine (28). Common side effects of SSRIs include nausea (often transient when starting the medication but sometimes persistent and severe), loose stools (actual diarrhea is uncommon), headache, nervousness, drowsiness, sweating, and sexual dysfunction. Sexual dysfunction in women often presents as anorgasmia and in males as delayed ejaculation or inability to ejaculate.

Serotonin syndrome is an uncommon but dangerous reaction to serotonergic antidepressants and usually occurs when SSRI antidepressants are combined with other antidepressants (especially monoamine oxidase inhibitors) or tryptophan, which is a precursor of serotonin (29). The serotonin syndrome presents with severe agitation or frank delirium, shakiness, coarse tremor, hyperreflexia, fever, sweating, hypertension, nausea, vomiting, and diarrhea, and in severe cases can progress to seizures, cardiovascular collapse, and death (30).

A particular concern in patients with cardiac disease who are prescribed SSRIs is the potential for interaction with cardiac drugs. The potential for interaction between a certain antidepressant and another drug depends on both pharmacodynamic factors (e.g., synergistic or additive effects) and pharmacokinetic factors, which affect drug absorption, distribution, metabolism, and elimination. Both the SSRIs and TCAs are substrates or inhibitors of the hepatic cytochrome P450 (CYP) isoenzymes; the different antidepressants affect each of the isoenzymes to a variable extent. The TCAs are substrates of the CYP system but are less likely to act as inhibitors compared with the SSRIs; thus drug–drug interac-

Table 16.3.   Common Antidepressants and Their Side Effects

Drug	Usual Dosage (mg/day)	Hypotension	Tachycardia	Anticholinergic	Conduction Block	Sedation	Sexual Dysfunction	Serotonergic (nausea, diarrhea, headache)	Remarks
Tricyclic antidepressants									
Amitriptyline (Elavil)	100–300	++	++	+++	++	+++	+++	+	Sedation, dry mouth, weight gain
Imipramine (Tofranil)	100–300	++	++	+++	++	+++	+++	+	Dry mouth, weight gain, sometimes shakiness
Doxepin (Sinequan)	100–300	++	++	+++	++	+++	+++	+	Sedation, dry mouth, weight gain
Nortriptyline (Pamelor)	75–100	+	+	++	++	++	++	+	Sedation, dry mouth, weight gain
Desipramine (Pertofrane)	100–300	++	++	+	++	+	++	+	Postural lightheadedness may occur
Specific serotonin-reuptake inhibitors									
Fluoxetine (Prozac)	20–40	0	0	+	0	0	++	++	Anxiety, insomnia in some patients
Fluvoxamine (Luvox)	100–200	0	0	+	0	++	++	+++	Mild sedation in some patients; nausea and diarrhea may occur in some
Sertraline (Zoloft)	100–200	0	0	+	0	+	+++	++	Often well tolerated; sexual dysfunction common
Paroxitine (Paxil)	20–40	0	0	++	0	++	+++	+++	Mild anticholinergic effects may occur; withdraw gradually
Other antidepressants									
Trazodone (Desyrel)	50–500	++	+	+	0	+++	++	++	Often used as nighttime sedation in low doses; priapism reported (rare)
Nefazodone (Serzone)	200–400	0	0	+	0	++	+	+++	Low incidence of sexual dysfunction; may be better to promote normal sleep cycle
Venlafaxine (Effexor)	75–300	0	0	+	0	+	++	++	Watch for hypertension; some may have headache, shakiness; withdraw gradually

[a] 0 = absent; + = uncommon; ++ = occasional; +++ = common.

tions caused by TCAs are often pharmacodynamic in nature rather than the pharmacokinetic interactions that the SSRIs can potentially cause. For more information about antidepressant interactions involving this enzyme system, the reader is referred to other sources (24, 31–33). The CYP enzyme system is also responsible for the metabolism of several cardiac drugs including certain β-blockers (e.g., metoprolol, timolol, propranolol), calcium antagonists (e.g., diltiazem, nifedipine, felodipine, verapamil), angiotensin-converting enzyme inhibitors (e.g., captopril), and antiarrhythmics (e.g., quinidine, propafenone, mexiletine, flecainide).

Table 16.4 shows drugs known to depend to a greater or lesser extent on the CYP system for metabolism or known to inhibit or induce synthesis of certain CYP isoenzymes. Other drugs will likely be added to this list when future studies demonstrate that they interact with the CYP enzyme system. Many interactions between these drugs have been demonstrated in vitro but their clinical significance has yet to be established. In some cases,

however, administration of SSRIs with these medications may result in an increase in incidence or severity of expected dose-dependent adverse effects of either medication; in other cases, efficacy of certain drugs could be reduced. For example, in patients taking warfarin, SSRIs have been reported to increase the international normalized ratio an average of 3.0 points (25). Another interaction involving inhibition of an isoenzyme of the CYP system could occur between certain antidepressants (especially fluvoxamine and nefazodone) and the antihistamines astemizole and terfenadine, or cisapride, a gastrointestinal motility agent. Such an interaction has the risk of increased accumulation of toxic amounts of the antihistamines or cisapride, or their metabolites, resulting in serious cardiac arrhythmias (torsades de pointes). This interaction has been seen between these antihistamines and the ketoconazole-related antifungal agents, and with macrolide antibiotics such as erythromycin (24). Other studies document that concomitant fluvoxamine therapy can elevate the levels of the following medications:

Table 16.4.   Drugs That Interact with the Cytochrome P450 Enzyme System[a]

Drug Class	Representative Drugs
Analgesics	Acetaminophen, alfentanil, codeine, ethylmorphine, hydrocodone
Angiotensin-converting enzyme inhibitors	Captopril
Antiarrhythmics	Flecainide, mexiletine, propafenone, amiodarone, disopyramide, lidocaine, quinidine, perhexiline
Anticonvulsants	Phenytoin, barbiturates, carbamazepine, ethosuximide
Antidepressants	Citalopram, sertraline, paroxetine, fluoxetine, fluvoxamine, venlafaxine, nefazodone, trazodone, tricyclic antidepressants, maprotiline
Antihistamines	Astemizole, loratadine, terfenadine
Anti-inflammatories	Naproxen, ibuprofen, diclofenac, piroxicam, mefenamic acid
Antipsychotics	Clozapine, haloperidol, perphenazine, risperidone, thioridazine, olanzapine, sertindole, chlorpromazine
β-Blockers	Propranolol, alprenolol, metoprolol, timolol, penbutolol, labetalol
Benzodiazepines	Alprazolam, clonazepam, diazepam, midazolam, triazolam
Calcium-channel blockers	Diltiazem, felodipine, nicardipine, nifedipine, nilvadipine, nimodipine, nisoldipine, nitrendipine, verapamil
Chemotherapeutics	Doxetaxel, paclitaxel, tamoxifen
Immunosuppressants	Cyclosporine, tacrolimus
Local anesthetics	Cocaine, lidocaine
Macrolide antibiotics	Clarithromycin, erythromycin, troleandomycin
Steroids	Androstenedione, cortisol, dihydroepiandrosterone, dexamethasone, estradiol, ethinyl estradiol, progesterone, testosterone
Miscellaneous	Caffeine, theophylline, warfarin, debrisoquin, amphetamine, phenformin, benzphetamine, cisapride, dapsone, lovastatin, omeprazole, tolbutamide, ketoconazole, itraconazole, tacrine, fluoroquinolones, sulfaphenazole, dextromethorphan, cimetidine, diphenhydramine, ondansetron, yohimbine, papaverine, rifampin, protease inhibitors

[a] Various drugs may be substrates, inhibitors, or inducers of specific cytochrome isoenzymes (see references 24, 31–33).

theophyllines, phenytoin, propranolol, and the benzodiazepines triazolam and alprazolam (these elevated benzodiazepine levels have also been seen with concomitant nefazodone) (32). Richelson (33) has summarized the likelihood that specific newer antidepressants will cause clinically significant pharmacokinetic drug–drug interactions with drugs metabolized by the CYP enzymes—the most likely antidepressants include fluvoxamine, fluoxetine, paroxetine, and nefazodone; sertraline is less likely and venlafaxine is least likely to cause such interactions.

TRICYCLIC ANTIDEPRESSANTS

Most patients who take TCAs such as amitriptyline, imipramine, or doxepin have few problems with adverse cardiovascular effects; rather, the common anticholinergic side effects (dry mouth, constipation, urinary hesitancy, blurred vision) and the daytime sedative effects (antihistaminic) may cause problems with compliance. Nevertheless, the sedative effects of amitriptyline or doxepin taken at bedtime may be useful in helping the depressed patient who has severe insomnia achieve sleep in the initial phase of treatment, before the onset of the antidepressant effect (which may take up to 4 weeks after the optimal dose is reached). Relative contraindications to the use of a strongly anticholinergic antidepressant include prostatic hypertrophy, narrow-angle glaucoma, and severe constipation. Of major concern in the elderly, in patients with neurologic disease, and in patients who take other drugs with anticholinergic properties is the potential for development of a central anticholinergic syndrome—a delirium characterized by confusion, disorientation, agitation, visual and auditory hallucinations, anxiety, and, possibly, delusions. Peripheral signs of anticholinergic toxicity may include decreased bowel sounds, urinary retention, anhidrosis, mydriasis, increased body temperature, tachycardia, and flushing. If delirium occurs, the antidepressant and any other anticholinergic medication should be stopped immediately, and the patient should receive supportive management.

Desipramine and nortriptyline are TCAs that are active metabolites of imipramine and amitriptyline, respectively. They both have far less anticholinergic activity and are less sedating than their parent compounds, and nortriptyline has the added advantage of a lower incidence of postural hypotension, particularly in patients who have coexisting cardiac disease. Both drugs tend to be "activating" (as opposed to sedating) antidepressants, and some patients complain of anxiety and insomnia when prescribed these medications.

Cardiovascular effects of TCAs are of particular concern when prescribed to depressed patients who have coexisting cardiac disease. A few studies have investigated the use of TCAs in patients who have cardiac disease and have particularly examined the effect of TCAs on blood pressure, heart rate, and rhythm and their use in patients who have CHF. Postural hypotension is the most common and potentially serious cardiovascular side effect in patients treated with TCAs. Psychotropic medications are a common drug-related cause of falls with subsequent fractures, particularly in the elderly. Risk factors that increase the likelihood of patients who have cardiac disease developing clinically significant postural hypotension when treated with antidepressant drugs include pretreatment postural hypotension, impaired cardiac conduction, CHF, and, possibly, higher doses of drug (although some studies have not found a relationship between plasma level and hypotension) (34). Nortriptyline has been found to have less chance of causing postural hypotension compared with other TCAs (35). All patients treated with antidepressant medication, and particularly those who have cardiac disease, should be warned about the symptoms of postural hypotension and should be taught to arise slowly from supine positions, maintain adequate fluid intake, and, if necessary, self-monitor their blood pressure.

Heart rate may increase slightly in patients treated with TCAs for many reasons: 1) anticholinergic activity of the drug; 2) compensation for postural hypotension; and 3) catecholamine effects on the central nervous system and on the heart. In most patients, this effect on heart rate is not clinically significant; however, in the patient who has marginally compensated myocardial ischemia or heart failure, it may be desirable to choose an antidepressant that has no anticholinergic side effects, such as an SSRI type. Concern about the effect of TCAs on cardiac conduction is related to their association with complex and life-threatening ventricular arrhythmias when taken as overdoses. In a study of patients who had taken toxic levels of TCAs, prolonged QRS duration was found to be correlated with risk of ventricular arrhythmias (36), although other investigators did not find it was of value in predicting this risk (37). Tricyclic antidepressants have properties similar to class I antiarrhythmic agents and tend to prolong conduction below the A-V node (i.e., in the His-Purkinje system). In patients who have preexisting atrial or ventricular arrhythmia, TCAs have the potential to suppress the arrhythmia or, like many antiarrhythmic drugs, can exacerbate the arrhythmia, particularly in high doses or in patients who are taking another class I antiarrhythmic drug. With respect to conduction block, a study of depressed patients treated with nortriptyline or imipramine demonstrated that the prevalence of second-degree A-V block was significantly greater in those patients who had preexisting bundle branch block than in patients who showed normal electrocardiograms (34).

Studies have investigated the effects of TCAs on left ventricular performance in small groups of depressed patients who have chronic heart disease (38, 39). Tricyclic antidepressants did not reduce left ventricular ejection fraction in patients with CAD; however, postural hypotension was a major concern in patients with CHF who received them. Nevertheless, worsening of CHF related to taking TCAs was reported in an elderly man with major depression and preexisting cardiovascular disease, indicating that safety of TCAs with respect to use in patients with CHF is not absolute (40).

OTHER ANTIDEPRESSANT MEDICATIONS

Two relatively new antidepressants that have favorable cardiovascular profiles in medically healthy patients are venlafaxine (Effexor) and nefazodone (Serzone). Venlafaxine affects both serotonin and norepinephrine reuptake. Unlike SSRIs, venlafaxine does not significantly inhibit the CYP isoenzymes, which may be advantageous for treatment of depression in patients taking many different cardiac medications (41). It has been found to cause small increases in blood pressure in some patients, and on discontinuation it should be tapered slowly because a "flu-like" syndrome of nausea, vomiting, and malaise can occur if stopped suddenly. Nefazodone blocks type 2A serotonin receptors as well as reuptake of serotonin and norepinephrine. It has been shown to be relatively free of cardiovascular side effects in trials of depressed, but otherwise healthy, patients and may cause fewer problems with sleep disturbance and sexual dysfunction than other antidepressants (42). It does significantly interact with the CYP system, however, and cardiac patients given nefazodone should be monitored for drug interactions.

Trazodone is a very sedating antidepressant that acts on the serotonin system. It is often used in lower doses for nighttime sedation. It may produce postural hypotension and some gastric irritation, and it also has been associated with priapism. Men given this drug should be warned about this uncommon side effect. Trazodone was reported to have been associated with worsening of ventricular ectopy in two patients (43).

Bupropion (Wellbutrin) is a new nontricyclic antidepressant acting on the dopamine and norepinephrine systems. It caused less postural hypotension, compared to imipramine, in a study that involved depressed patients who had CHF (44). A subsequent uncontrolled study found that bupropion did not exacerbate ventricular arrhythmias or conduction blocks in patients who had these conditions (45). This drug is associated with a high incidence of seizures at higher doses, and the maximum dosage should be 450 mg daily in no fewer than three divided doses (46, 47).

Monoamine oxidase inhibitors (MAOIs), such as phenelzine (Nardil), are efficacious antidepressants that have not been commonly used because of their well-described adverse effect of sudden severe hypertension when combined with exogenous pressor substances, such as tyramine-containing foods and numerous medications. Their use in patients who have medical illness is frequently limited by the difficulty with intolerable hypotension that many patients experience, and also with the dangerous interaction that can occur if MAOIs are given to patients taking commonly prescribed medications, such as meperidine, and other antidepressants such as fluoxetine. A new type of MAOI called moclobemide (Manerix) reversibly inhibits monoamine oxidase. It does not require dietary restrictions and also has less potential to interact with other medications. It is not available in the United States, and its use in cardiac patients has not been reported.

Benzodiazepines generally are ineffective for the treatment of major depression; all too often the patient who presents with severe anxiety or insomnia caused by a depressive disorder is prescribed a benzodiazepine without benefit.

An Approach to Treatment with Antidepressant Medication

After deciding that a patient would benefit from treatment with an antidepressant, the immediate goal of therapy is to form a treatment alliance with the patient that enables the patient to accept this treatment with a sense of security and optimism. When a psychotropic medication is suggested, many patients react with fear that the drug "will control my mind" or that they may become dependent on or addicted to the antidepressant. The physician should bring up these issues and find out whether the patient has concerns about dependence on medication before proceeding to an explanation of the actual drug and its side effects.

CHOOSING AN ANTIDEPRESSANT

The choice of antidepressant depends on many factors, including the age and medical status of the patient, the predominant depressive symptoms, and previous response to an antidepressant. If the patient has a past history of major depression and had a good response to a particular antidepressant, that drug should be used again, if no reasons exist to preclude its use, bearing in mind the previously mentioned concern about using TCAs in patients with ischemic heart disease. We generally recommend a trial of an SSRI for cardiac patients being treated with an antidepressant for the first time, and for patients previously treated with TCAs who have not yet been tried on an SSRI for treatment of depression. Nevertheless, there may be valid reasons to use a TCA to treat depression in some cardiac patients, such as for patients who cannot tolerate the side effects of SSRIs or who have previously not responded to SSRIs. Table 16.5 outlines the general advantages and disadvantages of SSRIs and TCAs for treatment of depression in patients with cardiac disease.

DOSAGES

Antidepressants usually can be given in a single daily dose, with sedating antidepressants given at bedtime and the nonsedating ones given in the morning. Patients who are elderly or who have complex medical illness should be started on one-third to one-half the usual initial dose of antidepressant, and dosage increments and final therapeutic dose should likewise be one-third to one-half lower than usual therapeutic doses. In such patients, ongoing clinical evaluations, as well as monitoring electrocardiograms and drug plasma levels, at regular intervals during therapy are important. The patient should be maintained on target therapeutic doses for at least 4 weeks before concluding that the medication is ineffective. Early signs of improvement may be seen as early as 1 or 2 weeks after initiation of therapy; however, early improvement may not yet be obvious to the patient.

PLASMA LEVELS

Plasma levels are used clinically for TCAs, but are not available for SSRIs or the other new antidepressants. Levels are usually available for amitriptyline (a combined level of amitriptyline and nortriptyline is reported), imipramine (a combined level of imipramine and desipramine is reported), nortriptyline, desipramine, and doxepin (a combined level of doxepin and desmethyldoxepin is reported). Research has demonstrated that nortriptyline has maximal efficacy at a plasma level of approximately 50 to 150 ng/mL—the "therapeutic window" above or below which the patient is less likely to respond therapeutically—whereas imipramine has a linear correlation with the maximal efficacy found with levels of imipramine and desipramine greater than 200 ng/mL (46). It is important to keep in mind that toxicity may be present in some patients with levels that fall within the therapeutic range, particularly in patients who have complex medical illness. Indications for monitoring plasma levels include evaluating lack of response to an adequate dose given for at least 4 weeks; treating patients with complex medical illnesses or elderly patients who may develop toxicity at lower doses; monitoring patients who may be noncompliant with taking the drug; and evaluating unusual side effects, toxicity, or possible drug interactions.

MAINTAINING AND DISCONTINUING THERAPY

If the patient responds well to an antidepressant, he or she should continue to take the antidepressant at that dosage for at least 8 to 12 months after full response is seen; the patient then can receive a tapering regimen for the following 3 months. If signs of depressive symptoms recur, then the dose should be increased to the previously effective dose and maintained

Table 16.5.   Advantages and Disadvantages of Selective Serotonin-Reuptake Inhibitors and Tricyclic Antidepressants

	Advantages	Disadvantages
Selective serotonin-reuptake inhibitors (SSRIs)	Lack of cardiovascular side effects (shown in healthy depressed patients only) Nonsedating Few anticholinergic side effects Not lethal in overdose	No studies in patients with cardiac disease Inhibition of the cytochrome P450 system leads to the interactions with other drugs Nausea, loose stool, headache, shakiness, sweating, sexual dysfunction
Tricyclic antidepressants(TCAs)	Small studies in cardiac patients show relative safety Plasma levels available Useful if patient responded before to a TCA Useful for patients who do not respond to SSRIs	Type IA antiarrhythmic effect may increase risk of mortality in patients with ischemic cardiac disease Can be lethal in overdose Postural hypotension Cardiac conduction affected Sedation Anticholinergic side effects Weight gain

again for another few months before trying to taper the medication. We explain to the patient that an antidepressant medication does not "cure" the depressive illness, but rather helps ameliorate symptoms until the underlying illness resolves, and that this process usually takes about 1 year. It should be stressed to the patient that premature discontinuation of the antidepressant involves a sizable risk of recurrence of depression. Antidepressant withdrawal is best done gradually because sudden discontinuation of some antidepressants may cause a syndrome of nausea, vomiting, abdominal cramps and diarrhea, headache, insomnia, and vivid dreams; these symptoms have been attributed to anticholinergic rebound. There have also been recent case reports of cardiac arrhythmia after abrupt TCA withdrawal (48, 49).

If the patient does not respond to the antidepressant after completing a trial of medication at an appropriate dosage for at least 4 weeks, a plasma level should be obtained if the patient is taking a TCA. If noncompliance is a problem, this should be discussed with the patient; often, education with respect to the need to persist with treatment at appropriate doses for a long enough time is needed. If the patient shows no signs of toxicity or undesirable side effects, the drug should be increased slowly to achieve a reasonably high plasma level, and the patient should be maintained at the higher dose for 2 or 3 more weeks before concluding that it is ineffective. For SSRIs and other antidepressants for which plasma levels cannot be measured, we suggest increasing the dose to the higher end of the range suggested in Table 16.3 if the patient does not experience dose-limiting side effects before concluding that the medication is ineffective. If a depressed patient cannot complete a medication trial because of adverse side effects, a switch to another antidepressant with a different profile is recommended. Finally, if the patient who has a major depression has not responded to a valid trial of an antidepressant, consideration of a trial with another antidepressant or consultation with a psychiatrist may be necessary. In the event of an unsuccessful trial of an antidepressant, the diagnosis of major depression should be reconsidered and coexisting medical illnesses or medications that might contribute to depression should be ruled out. For treatment of severe depression that has responded poorly to antidepressants, electroconvulsive therapy can be given with relative safety to patients who have severe cardiac disease (50).

ANXIETY

Although anxiety and fear are common responses to major medical illnesses and often respond to education and reassurance (51), the cardiac rehabilitation process may be disrupted by more severe anxiety disorders that require treatment. These disorders may have existed before the onset of the cardiac disease or may have occurred either concurrently with or after the onset of cardiac disease. In individuals with a premorbid history of an anxiety disorder, cardiac illness may exacerbate the disorder. Traditionally, cardiologists and psychiatrists focused on disorders such as "effort syndrome" or "Da Costa's syndrome" (52), which are somatic presentations of primary anxiety disorders in which the patient focuses on cardiac symptoms of anxiety in the absence of demonstrable cardiac pathology. More recently, attention has turned to the association with and impact of anxiety disorders on documented cardiac disease (53–55).

Diagnostic Categories of Anxiety Disorders

Anxiety has been defined as a subjective experience of dread and foreboding that occurs in association with a variety of autonomic signs and symptoms (56). Anxiety is manifested by a range of symptoms, the characteristic cluster of which varies between diagnostic categories, but typically includes affective (e.g., nervousness, anxiety, irritability), cognitive (e.g., a preoccupation with worries, a sense of impending doom, dread, or foreboding), and somatic (e.g., palpitations, shortness of breath, paresthesias, unsteady feelings, lightheadedness, choking) components. Katon (57) and Wise and Taylor (58) have emphasized that the autonomic and somatic manifestations of anxiety are diverse and are often misdiagnosed.

Psychiatric classification defines a variety of different anxiety disorders, including panic disorder (PD, with and without agoraphobia), agoraphobia without a history of PD, social phobia, simple phobia, obsessive-compulsive disorder, post-traumatic stress disorder, and generalized anxiety disorder (GAD) (8). The most common and clinically significant disorders in a cardiac rehabilitation practice are PD (Table 16.6) and GAD (Table 16.7), which will be discussed at greater length in this chapter. A small number of patients may present with post-traumatic stress disorder secondary to distressing medical events—typically multiple invasive or painful procedures, prolonged intensive care unit stays, and life-threatening illness (59, 60). These patients present with 1) recurrent and intrusive distressing recollections or dreams of the event(s); 2) persistent avoidance of stimuli associated with the trauma or a numbing of general responsiveness (i.e., markedly diminished interest in formerly pleasurable activities, feelings of detachment, and restricted range of affect); and 3) persistent symptoms of increased arousal (e.g., difficulty falling or staying asleep, irritability, hypervigilance, difficulty concentrating) (8).

Panic disorder (Table 16.6) is characterized by the sudden onset of a variety of somatic and affective symptoms. It has been described as occurring in a substantial number of patients presenting in cardiology clinics. In many patients, the somatic symptoms of PD predominate, and patients experience the attacks as evidence of serious underlying illness. The typical age of onset of PD is in the late teens and twenties, although there is a group of people who develop PD at an older age in association with medical illness (57). Patients with PD are at increased risk for major depression, alcohol abuse, and suicidal ideation and suicide attempts (suicidal risk is increased independent of coexistent major depression and substance abuse) (61–63). Limited-symptom panic attacks have been described in which there is a paroxysmal onset of less than four panic symptoms, including a "cardiac cluster" limited-symptom panic attack characterized by sudden onset of palpitations and dyspnea (64). Antipanic pharmacotherapy has been helpful in alleviating limited-symptom panic attacks (64). Katon (57) has reviewed current theories regarding the underlying neurobiology of PD and has summarized the evidence on familial predisposition and the specificity of the response in panic patients to pharmacologically provocative challenges (e.g., lactate, caffeine, yohimbine). A growing body of research implicates the septohippocampal region, the locus caeruleus and noradrenergic system, and the gamma-amino-butyric acid system and the benzodiazepine receptor in PD (57).

Generalized anxiety disorder (Table 16.7) is characterized by uncontrollable worry that is accompanied by a variety of physical symptoms of motor tension and vigilance (8). The cardinal feature is apprehensive expectation or worry that is uncontrollable (65). Abnormal regulation of noradrenergic, serotonergic, and gamma-amino-butyric acid systems has been implicated in GAD (66).

Table 16.6.   Diagnostic Criteria for Panic Attack, Agarophobia, and Panic Disorder

Panic Attack

A discrete period of intense fear or discomfort, in which four (or more) of the following symptoms developed abruptly and reached a peak within 10 minutes:

 1. Palpitations, pounding heart, or accelerated heart rate
 2. Sweating
 3. Trembling or shaking
 4. Sensations of shortness of breath or smothering
 5. Feeling of choking
 6. Chest pain or discomfort
 7. Nausea or abdominal distress
 8. Feeling dizzy, unsteady, lightheaded, or faint
 9. Derealization (feelings of unreality) or depersonalization (being detached from oneself)
10. Fear of losing control or going crazy
11. Fear of dying
12. Paresthesias (numbness or tingling sensations)
13. Chills or hot flushes

Criteria for Agoraphobia

A. Anxiety about being in places or situations from which escape might be difficult (or embarrassing) or in which help may not be available in the event of having an unexpected or situationally predisposed panic attack or paniclike symptoms. Agoraphobic fears typically involve characteristic clusters of situations that include being outside the home alone; being in a crowd or standing in a line; being on a bridge; and traveling in a bus, train, or automobile.

B. The situations are avoided (e.g., travel is restricted) or else are endured with marked distress or with anxiety about having a panic attack or paniclike symptoms, or require the presence of companion.

C. The anxiety or phobic avoidance is not better accounted for by another mental disorder.

Diagnostic Criteria for Panic Disorder Without/With Agoraphobia

A. Both (1) and (2):
   1. Recurrent unexpected panic attacks
   2. At least one of the attacks has been followed by 1 month (or more) of one (or more) of the following:
      a. Persistent concern about having additional attacks
      b. Worry about the implications of the attack or its consequences (e.g., losing control, having a heart attack, "going crazy")
      c. A significant change in behavior related to the attacks

B. Absence/presence of agoraphobia

C. The panic attacks are not due to the direct physiologic effects of a substance (e.g., a drug of abuse, a medication) or a general medical condition (e.g., hyperthyroidism).

D. The panic attacks are not better accounted for by another mental disorder.

Adapted from Diagnostic and Statistical Manual of Mental Disorders. 4th ed. Washington, DC. American Psychiatric Association, 1994.

Table 16.7.   Diagnostic Criteria for Generalized Anxiety Disorder

A. Excessive anxiety and worry (apprehensive expectation), occurring more days than not for at least 6 months, about a number of events or activities (such as work or school performance).

B. The person finds it difficult to control the worry.

C. The anxiety and worry are associated with three (or more) of the following six symptoms (with at least some symptoms present for more days than not for the past 6 months).
   1. Restlessness or feeling keyed up or on edge
   2. Being easily fatigued
   3. Difficulty concentrating or mind going blank
   4. Irritability
   5. Muscle tension
   6. Sleep Disturbance (difficulty falling or staying asleep, or restless unsatisfying sleep)

D. The focus of the anxiety and worry is not confined to features of an axis I disorder, e.g., the anxiety or worry is not about having a panic attack (as in panic disorder).

E. The anxiety, worry, or physical symptoms cause clinically significant distress or impairment in social, occupational, or other important areas of functioning.

F. The disturbance is not due to the direct physiologic effects of a substance (e.g., a drug of abuse, a medication) or a general medical condition (e.g., hyperthyroidism) and does not occur exclusively during a mood disorder, or a psychotic disorder.

Adapted from the Diagnostic and Statistical Manual of Mental Disorders, 4th ed. Washington, DC. American Psychiatric Association, 1994.

Prevalence of Anxiety Disorders in Cardiac Patients

Anxiety symptoms and anxiety disorders are common in cardiac settings. Panic disorder has been identified in 5% to 23% of patients with angiographic evidence of CAD (55) and in 30% to 61% of patients with chest pain and normal angiography (54, 55). Increasing attention is being given to sorting out when unexplained chest pain may be attributed to PD (54, 67) because unrecognized PD has significant psychosocial and health economics consequences (54). Goldberg et al. (68) reviewed patients with documented cardiac disease being followed up in an outpatient cardiology practice and found that 6.3% met criteria for PD (approximately 10 times the rate in the general population). They described two groups of patients—those with longstanding PD and those with PD of a shorter duration that seemed to develop secondary to the cardiac disease. This shorter-duration group differed in terms of being more likely to have had current or recent affective disorder, and to exhibit less phobic avoidance. Morris et al. (69) found a PD prevalence of 12.5% in a cardiology outpatient clinic, and 62.5% of the PD patients had significant heart disease. These findings contrast with community epidemiologic studies that have documented a 1-month prevalence rate of 0.3% in men and 0.5% in women (70). Generalized anxiety disorder is the most common anxiety disorder in community settings, accounting for up to one-half of all anxiety disorder diagnoses, and has a 1-month to 1-year prevalence of 2.5% to 6.4% (66, 70). About half of patients with GAD complain of chest pain (71). Studies of GAD in cardiac patients are just beginning.

Clinical Significance of Anxiety Disorders in Cardiac Patients

There have been a number of studies examining the negative impact of anxiety on recovery from MI (72–89) and cardiac surgery (90–97) and adjustment to implanted defibrillators (98, 99). Recent studies suggest that PD (100, 101) and phobic anxiety (102) are associated with increased risk of cardiovascular mortality. A prospective study of 33,999 male U.S. health professionals documented an age-adjusted relative risk of fatal coronary heart disease among men with the highest levels of phobic anxiety of 3.01 (95% CI 1.31–6.90) compared to men with the lowest levels of phobic anxiety (103). This risk was associated with sudden rather than nonsudden cardiac death (103). Similar findings were reported in a sample of 2,280 men taking part in the Normative Aging Study (104). To date, research has focused on men, although studies of these issues in women are now underway.

In addition to increased mortality, anxiety disorders may interfere with cardiac rehabilitation patients in terms of their ability to comply with the program. As well, patients with anxiety disorders may be unduly bodily preoccupied and may place unnecessary restrictions on their activity, thus impeding their progress in returning to full occupational and social functioning.

Pathophysiologic Relationships Between Anxiety Disorders and Cardiac Disorders

There is a developing literature on the relationship between the central nervous system and the cardiovascular system and an increasing awareness of the relationship between stress, the autonomic nervous system, and the neural regulation of the cardiovascular system (105, 106). There is an association between emotion and changes in heart rate and blood pressure and thus myocardial oxygen requirements (107, 108). The studies of mental stress induced in CAD patients in experimental settings have documented reduction in left ventricular function, regional wall motion abnormalities, and coronary artery spasm (109). Postulated mechanisms for the impact of anxiety on the heart include induction of coronary artery spasm secondary to hyperventilation during an anxiety attack (110, 111), triggering of fatal ventricular arrhythmias (112, 113), and diminished heart rate variability, which increases the risk for ventricular arrhythmia (114–116). Associations have been reported between PD and microvascular angina (117, 118), idiopathic cardiomyopathy (119), and hypertension (107, 120). Byrne (121) has reviewed the evidence that anxiety disorders and stress may also act by "exacerbating the levels of established risk factors for coronary heart disease" and concluded that there is some support for the short-term influence of stress on smoking behavior and hypertension, but that long-term influences are debatable.

Issues in the Diagnosis of Anxiety Disorders in Cardiac Rehabilitation Patients

Patients presenting with anxiety symptoms must be evaluated for a medical cause for the anxiety (Table 16.8) before reviewing the psychiatric differential diagnosis. Cardiac rehabilitation patients should be evaluated for PD if they are 1) describing cardiovascular or respiratory symptoms that cannot be accounted for on a physiologic basis; 2) showing excessive preoccupation with their body and reporting a variety of nonspecific symptoms; or 3) demonstrating avoidance behavior such as difficulties in being in public places or driving a car.

Treatment of Anxiety Disorders

As previously discussed with regard to major depression, the patient with an anxiety disorder typically requires an integrated biopsychosocial approach. A variety of forms of talking therapy are helpful to patients with anxiety disorders, and the parameters for therapy are similar to those in pa-

Table 16.8.   Medical Differential Diagnosis of Anxiety

Neurologic	Drugs
Seizure disorder	Amphetamine
Vertigo	Aminophylline
Encephalopathy	Anticholinergics
Postconcussion syndrome	Antihypertensives
Restless legs syndrome	Reserpine, hydralazine
Syncope	Antituberculous agents
Endocrine	Isoniazid, cycloserine
Thyroid dysfunction	Caffeine
Hypocalcemia	Cocaine
Hyperadrenalism	Digitalis toxicity
Rheumatoid/Collagen Vascular	Dopamine
Systemic lupus erythematosus	Ephedrine
Temporal arteritis	Epinephrine
Metabolic Conditions	Hallucinogens
Anemia	Levodopa
Hypoglycemia	Lidocaine
Hyponatremia	Methylphenidate
Hyperkalemia	Monusodium glutamate
Porphyria	Nonsteroidal anti-inflammatory drugs
Respiratory Conditions	Phenylephrine
Asthma	Phenylpropanolamine
Chronic obstructive pulmonary disease	Procarbazine
Pneumonia	Pseudoephedrine
Pneumothorax	Salicylates
Pulmonary edema	Steroids
Pulmonary embolus	Theophylline
Respiratory dependence	Thyroid preparations
Circulatory	Withdrawal—alcohol and
Myocardial ischemia (angina	sedative/hypnotics
pectoris, myocardial infarction)	
Hypovolemia	
Congestive heart failure	
Arrhythmia	
Valvular disease	
Infections	
Mononucleosis	
Viral hepatitis	
Tuberculosis	
Secreting Tumors	
Carcinoid	
Insulinoma	
Pheochromocytoma	

tients with depression. However, there is often a stronger focus on cognitive and behavioral techniques in patients with PD to help them to confront and overcome those situations that they have begun to avoid. All forms of behavior therapy attempt to expose the patient to the avoided situation and to help them in tolerating the ensuing anxiety until it has abated. Relaxation techniques can be used to help diminish any anxiety that is experienced. The literature on cognitive and behavioral management in cardiac patients has been reviewed (67, 122). Other forms of individual psychotherapy or marital or family therapy may be required in those patients who have become highly dysfunctional with their symptoms and do not show progress with a combination of pharmacotherapy and cognitive or behavior therapy.

Pharmacologic Therapy of Anxiety in Patients with Cardiovascular Disease

There are a number of effective pharmacologic treatments for PD and GAD. Pharmacologic treatment is warranted if patients report frequent or severe symptoms; show significant occupational or social dysfunction because of symptoms; experience demoralization or suicidal ideation because of distress related to the symptoms; or develop a comorbid condition such as a major depressive episode or substance abuse (123). General principles of pharmacotherapy in the medically ill include appropriate diagnosis, delineation of target symptoms against which the success of the pharmacotherapy can be assessed (e.g., zero panic attacks), education of the patient and family about the appropriate use of medication, and dealing with misunderstandings about the role of medication and fears of addiction and stigmatization. Although the principle of "start low, go slow" is often helpful, it is important to remember that many patients will require a full therapeutic dose of the medication for an appropriate duration of treatment to obtain full benefit.

Panic Disorder

The primary goal of pharmacotherapy is to completely block panic attacks from occurring (123). A second important goal is to reverse any avoidance behavior that the patient has developed and to restore the patient to normal functioning—achieving this may require cognitive or behavior therapy or other forms of psychother-apy, although many patients show a complete resolution in symptomatology when effective pharmacologic blockade of panic has occurred.

Deciding which medication is best for which patient is influenced by several factors, including 1) how quickly panic blockade must be achieved (antipanic benzodiazepines work quickly whereas there is a delayed onset of action of up to 8 weeks with SSRIs, TCAs, and MAOIs); 2) concerns about both general and cardiovascular-specific side effects of medication; and 3) concerns about physical dependence and withdrawal symptoms on discontinuation of treatment (123). Benzodiazepines should be avoided in patients with a past or current history of alcohol or drug abuse, and there is some evidence to suggest that they should not be used as a first-line treatment in patients with personality disorders or chronic pain conditions (57).

In treating patients with PD, the basic choice is between 1) a benzodiazepine with antipanic efficacy—alprazolam has been documented to have antipanic efficacy equivalent to imipramine or phenelzine, and clonazepam, lorazepam, and high-dose diazepam also appear to have antipanic efficacy (124); or 2) an antidepressant—SSRIs such as paroxetine, sertraline, and fluoxetine are now first-line treatments rather than TCAs in both cardiac and noncardiac patients. Imipramine is the most thoroughly and rigorously studied of the TCAs but there is also evidence for the antipanic efficacy of clomipramine, desipramine, nortriptyline, amitriptyline, and doxepin (125). Phenelzine is the best studied of the MAOIs (123).

Benzodiazepines offer the advantage of rapid onset of antipanic activity, in contrast to antidepressants, which have a 2- to 8-week delay in onset of action (124). However, benzodiazepines also hold the potential for withdrawal problems when it is time for treatment to be discontinued (123, 126), and this must be discussed with the patient before initiating medication.

Dosage

Selective serotonin-reuptake inhibitors are used in doses similar to those used in treating major depression with the exception of paroxetine, which typically requires 40 to 60 mg to achieve full benefit. Tricyclic antidepressants and MAOIs must be used in doses similar to those used in treating major depression (Table 16.3). The dosage requirement for benzodiazepines varies considerably between patients and must be titrated to the point at which there is complete blockade of panic attacks. This may require doses of 3 to 6 mg alprazolam or 1.5 to 3 mg of clonazepam, but some patients may require as much as 10 mg of alprazolam equivalents per day to obtain complete blockade of attacks (124). Table 16.9 shows the equivalency doses of the antipanic benzodiazepines. Antipanic benzodiazepines should be started at the equivalent of alprazolam 0.5 mg three times a day and increased by 0.5 mg every 2 to 3 days until there are no further panic attacks. Some patients using alprazolam or lorazepam may require a four-times-a-day dosing schedule, and there are a minority who will experience "clock-watching" in whom there is a breakthrough of symptoms before the time for the next dose. Patients with breakthrough symptoms may require a change to a longer-acting benzodiazepine (i.e. clonazepam or diazepam) that can be used on a twice or thrice daily dosing schedule. Patients should also be monitored for "breakthrough depression," which has been reported during treatment with clonazepam, lorazepam, and alprazolam (57).

SIDE EFFECTS

The general and cardiovascular side effects of the SSRIs, TCAs, and MAOIs have been discussed earlier. Benzodiazepines tend to be well tolerated, with the most prominent side effects being sedation and psychomotor impairment; however, these tend to diminish during the first few weeks for the majority of patients. Nonetheless, it is important to caution patients about the potential harmful effects of sedation in terms of safety issues such as driving a car, operating heavy equipment, or taking part in activities in which a high degree of alertness is required. Other side effects include fatigue, ataxia, slurred speech, amnesia, and difficulty in learning new material (124). Benzodiazepines may decrease the metabolism and elimination of digoxin (109).

It should be noted that some patients will experience an exacerbation of panic in the first week that they are on an antidepressant and should be cautioned about this. It is often helpful to provide alprazolam or another benzodiazepine to use as needed during this time (e.g., alprazolam 0.5 mg three times a day).

DURATION OF THERAPY

There is some debate as to the optimal duration of therapy. Most clinicians would recommend 6 to 12 months of treatment once a remission in symptomatology has been achieved. The medication

Table 16.9. Use of Benzodiazepines in the Treatment of Panic Disorder and Generalized Anxiety Disorder

Drug	Comparable Oral Dose (mg)	Time to Peak Plasma Level (hr)	Half-life (hr)	Active Metabolites Present	Comments
Benzodiazepines with antipanic efficacy					
Alprazolam (Xanax)	0.5	1–2	6–20	Yes	Typically TID or QID dosing; extra caution on withdrawal
Clonazepam (Klonopin, Rivotril)	0.25	1–4	19–60	No	BID or TID dosing
Diazepam (Valium)	5.0	1–2	14–100	Yes	BID or daily dosing
Lorazepam (Ativan)	1.0	2 (p.o.) 1 (s.l.)	8–24	No	BID or TID
Other benzodiazepines					
Oxazepam (Serax)	15	2–3	3–25	No	Slow onset of action; BID dosing; kinetics relatively unaffected by age or liver disease
Prazepam (Centrax)	10	2.5–6	30–100	Yes	Low sedative potential

should be tapered slowly, thus allowing identification of continuing PD that may become manifest during the tapering phase. A gradual reduction is particularly important with benzodiazepines; if symptoms recur after a dosage reduction, they may be the result of withdrawal, symptom rebound (the same symptoms as the patient had before treatment but much more intense and resolving with time off of the medication), or symptom recurrence (the same symptoms with original intensity, which will not resolve without further treatment) (124, 126). A gradual reduction of no more than 10% of the total dose per week will minimize withdrawal problems—in the patient who is having a difficult time withdrawing from medication, the rate of reduction may be slowed. It is easiest to reduce the first 50% of the total benzodiazepine dose whereas the reduction of the final 50% must be done more slowly (126). There are a variety of more sophisticated strategies for medication tapering that can be used for those patients who are having difficulty (128).

The timing of the attempt at discontinuing drug therapy deserves attention (128). Ideally, discontinuation should not be attempted until the patient is stable and there is a complete resolution of any avoidance behavior and a return to full social and occupational functioning. Before starting to taper the medication, the possibility of symptom reemergence should be discussed with the patient. The patient's medical status must be reevaluated in light of the potential for adverse results should the PD return. It is also important to time the discontinuation to avoid periods of high life stress.

Some patients may require long-term therapy with an antipanic medication. Panic disorder and GAD tend to have chronic, relapsing courses necessitating repeated treatment. There is general agreement that continued maintenance treatment is justified in those individuals with 1) a history of longstanding and severe PD; 2) ongoing panic attacks or avoidance behavior while on medication; and 3) continued presence of secondary depression or substance abuse (123). Medication should also be continued if the patient's cardiac status is precarious and there would be risk associated with the return of panic attacks.

GENERALIZED ANXIETY DISORDER

Benzodiazepines, SSRIs, TCAs, and buspirone are used to treat GAD. Doses are similar to those used in PD, with the goal of alleviating anxiety. All benzodiazepines seem to be equally effective. Buspirone is a novel anxiolytic agent. It is an azaspirone that is free of problems of psychomotor impairment, withdrawal syndromes, abuse potential, and interaction with alcohol (127). It is suitable for use in patients with past histories of substance abuse and stimulates respiration; thus, it can be used in patients with lung disease when a benzodiazepine might be contraindicated. Side effects associated with its use include dizziness, nausea, headaches, nervousness, lightheadedness, and excitement. There is a delayed onset of action—most patients require a minimum of 1 to 2 weeks of therapy before noticing improvement; however, as much as 6 weeks may be required. The average daily dosage range is 20 to 30 mg with a starting dose of 5 mg three times a day and an increase in 5-mg increments every 2 to 3 days.

References

1. Wells KB, Golding JM, Burnam MA. Psychiatric disorder in a sample of the general population with and without chronic medical conditions. Am J Psychiatry 1988;145:976–981.
2. Kaplan HI, Sadock BJ, eds. Comprehensive textbook of psychiatry. 5th ed. Baltimore: Williams & Wilkins, 1989.
3. Groves JE. Taking care of the hateful patient. N Engl J Med 1978;298:883–887.
4. Littman AB. Prevention of disability due to cardiovascular diseases. Heart Dis Stroke 1993;2:274–277.
5. Wells KB, Stewart A, Hays RD, et al. The functioning and well-being of depressed patients. Results from the Medical Outcomes Study. JAMA 1989;262:914–919.
6. Katon W, Sullivan MD. Depression and chronic medical illness. Clin Psychiatry 1990;51(Suppl 6):3–11.
7. Robins LN, Helzer JE, Weissman M, et al. Lifetime prevalence of specific psychiatric disorders in three sites. Arch Gen Psychiatry 1984;41:949–958.
8. American Psychiatric Association. Diagnostic and statistical manual of mental disorders. 4th ed. Washington, DC: American Psychiatric Association, 1994.
9. Popkin MK, Callies AL, Mackenzie TB. The outcome of antidepressant use in the medically ill. Arch Gen Psychiatry 1985;42:1160–1163.
10. Sherbourne CD, Wells KB, Hays RD, et al. Subthreshold depression and depressive disorder: clinical characteristics of general medical and mental health specialty outpatients. Am J Psychiatry 1994;151:1777–1784.
11. Anderson D, Deshaies G, Jobin J. Social support, social networks and coronary artery disease rehabilitation: a review. Can J Cardiol 1996;12:739–744.
12. Berkman LF, Leo-Summers L, Horwitz RI. Emotional support and survival after myocardial infarction. Ann Intern Med 1992;117:1003–1009.
13. Jones DA, West RR. Psychological rehabilitation after

myocardial infarction: multicentre randomised controlled trial. BMJ 1996;313:1517–1521.

14. Frasure-Smith N, Lespérance F, Prince RH, et al. Randomised trial of home-based psychosocial nursing intervention for patients recovering from myocardial infarction. Lancet 1997;350:473–479.

15. Oldridge N, Streiner D, Hoffmann R, et al. Profile of mood states and cardiac rehabilitation after acute myocardial infarction. Med Sci Sports Exerc 1995;27: 900–905.

16. Finnegan DL, Suler JR. Psychological factors associated with maintenance of improved health behaviors in postcoronary patients. J Psychol 1985;119:87–94.

17. Blumenthal JA, Williams RS, Wallace AG, et al. Physiological and psychological variables predict compliance to prescribed exercise therapy in patients recovering from myocardial infarction. Psychosom Med 1982;44:519–527.

18. Hill DR, Kelleher K, Shumaker SA. Psychosocial interventions in adult patients with coronary heart disease and cancer. A literature review. Gen Hosp Psychiatry 1992;14S:28S–42S.

19. Elkin I, Shea MT, Watkins JT, et al. National Institute of Mental Health treatment of depression collaborative research program: general effectiveness of treatments. Arch Gen Psychiatry 1989;46:971–982.

20. Kahn D. The dichotomy of drugs and psychotherapy. Psychiatr Clin North Am 1990;13:197–208.

21. Shapiro PA. Nortriptyline treatment of depressed cardiac transplant recipients. Am J Psychiatry 1991;148: 371–373.

22. Glassman, AH, Bigger JT Jr. Cardiovascular effects of therapeutic doses of tricyclic antidepressants: a review. Arch Gen Psychiatry 1981;38:815–820.

23. Glassman AH, Roose SP, Biggar JT Jr. The safety of tricyclic antidepressants in cardiac patients: risk/benefit reconsidered. JAMA 1993;269:2673–2675.

24. Preskorn SH. Clinical pharmacology of selective serotonin reuptake inhibitors. 1st ed. Caddo, OK: Professional Communications, 1996.

25. Askinazi C. SSRI treatment of depression with comorbid cardiac disease. Am J Psychiatry 1996;153:135–136.

26. Ellison JM, Milofsky JE, Ely E. Fluoxetine-induced bradycardia and syncope in two patients. J Clin Psychiatry 1990;51:385–386.

27. Feder R. Bradycardia and syncope induced by fluoxetine [letter]. J Clin Psychiatry 1991;52:139.

28. Buff DD, Brenner R, Kirtane SS, et al. Dysrhythmia associated with fluoxetine treatment in an elderly patient with cardiac disease. J Clin Psychiatry 1991;52:174–176.

29. Schulman RW. The serotonin syndrome: a tabular guide. Can J Pharmacol 1995;2:139–144.

30. Sternbach HS. The serotonin syndrome. Am J Psychiatry 1991;148:705–713.

31. Burgraff GW. Are psychotropic drugs at therapeutic levels a concern for cardiologists? Can J Cardiol 1997;13:75–80.

32. Ereshefsky L. Treating depression: potential drug interactions. Psychiatr Ann 1997;244–258.

33. Richelson E. Pharmacokinetic drug interactions of new antidepressants: a review of the effects on the metabolism of other drugs. Mayo Clin Proc 1997;72: 835–847.

34. Roose SP, Glassman AH, Giardina EGV, et al. Tricyclic antidepressants in depressed patients with cardiac conduction disease. Arch Gen Psychiatry 1987;44:273–275.

35. Roose SP, Glassman AH, Siris SG, et al. Comparison of imipramine- and nortriptyline-induced orthostatic hypotension. A meaningful difference. J Clin Psychopharmacol 1981;1:316–319.

36. Boehnert MT, Lovejoy FH Jr. Value of the QRS duration vs the serum drug level in predicting seizures and ventricular arrhythmias after an acute overdose of tricyclic antidepressants. N Engl J Med 1985;313:474–479.

37. Foulke GE, Albertson TE. QRS interval in tricyclic antidepressant overdose: inaccuracy as a toxicity indicator in emergency settings. Ann Emerg Med 1987;16: 160–163.

38. Roose SP, Glassman AH, Giardina EGV, et al. Nortriptyline in depressed patients with left ventricular impairment. JAMA 1986;256:3253–3257.

39. Glassman AH, Johnson LL, Giardina EGV, et al. The use of imipramine in depressed patients with congestive heart failure. JAMA 1983;250:1997–2001.

40. Dalack GW, Roose SP, Glassman AH. Tricyclics and heart failure [letter]. Am J Psychiatry 1991;148:1601.

41. Ereshefsky L. Drug–drug interactions involving antidepressants: focus on venlafaxine. J Clin Psychopharmacol 1996;16(Suppl 2):37S–53S.

42. Preskorn SH. Comparison of the tolerability of bupropion, fluoxetine, imipramine, nefazodone, paroxetine, sertraline, and venlafaxine. J Clin Psychiatry 1995;56 (Suppl 6):12–21.

43. Janowsky D, Curtis G, Zisook S, et al. Ventricular arrhythmias possibly aggravated by trazodone. Am J Psychiatry 1983;140:796–797.

44. Roose SP, Glassman AH, Giardina EGV, et al. Cardiovascular effects of imipramine and bupropion in depressed patients with congestive heart failure. J Clin Psychopharmacol 1987;7:247–251.

45. Roose SP, Dalack GW, Glassman AH, et al. Cardiovascular effects of bupropion in depressed patients with heart disease. Am J Psychiatry 1991;148: 512–516.

46. Gelenberg AJ, Schooneover SC. Depression. In: Gelenberg AJ, Bassuk EL, Schoonover SC, eds. The practitioner's guide to psychoactive drugs. 3rd ed. New York: Plenum, 1991:23–89.

47. Davidson J. Seizures and bupropion: a review. J Clin Psychiatry 1989;50:256–261.

48. Babb SV, Dunlop SR, Hoffman MA. Protracted ventricular arrhythmias occurring after abrupt tricyclic antidepressant withdrawal. Psychosomatics 1990;31: 452–456.

49. Regan WM, Margolin RA, Mathew RJ. Cardiac arrhythmia following rapid imipramine withdrawal. Biol Psychiatry 1989;25:482–484.

50. Zielinski RJ, Roose SP, Devanand DP, et al. Cardiovascular complications of ECT in depressed patients with cardiac disease. Am J Psychiatry 1993;150:904–909.

51. Green SA. Mind and body: the psychology of physical illness. Washington, DC: American Psychiatric Press, 1985.

52. Skerritt PW. Anxiety and the heart—a historical review. Psychol Med 1983;13:17–25.

53. Byrne DG, Rosenman RH, eds. Anxiety and the heart. New York: Hemisphere Publishing, 1990.

54. Fleet PR, Dupuis G, Marchand A, et al. Panic disorder, chest pain and coronary artery disease: literature review. Can J Cardiol 1994;10:827–834.

55. Zaubler TS, Katon W. Panic disorder and medical comorbidity: a review of the medical and psychiatric literature. Bull Menninger Clin 1996;60(2, Suppl A): A12–A38.

56. Rosenbaum JF. Current concepts in psychiatry: the drug treatment of anxiety. N Engl J Med 1982;306: 401–404.

57. Katon W. Panic disorder in the medical setting. Washington, DC: American Psychiatric Press, 1991.

58. Wise MG, Taylor SE. Anxiety and mood disorders in medically ill patients. J Clin Psychiatry 1990;51 (Suppl):27–32.

59. Shalev AY, Schreiber S, Galai T. Post-traumatic stress disorder following medical events. Br J Clin Psychol 1993;32:247–253.

60. Doerfler LA, Pbert L, DeCosimo D. Symptoms of post-traumatic stress disorder following myocardial infarction and coronary artery bypass surgery. Gen Hosp Psychiatry 1994;16:193–199.

61. Lydiard RB. Coexisting depression and anxiety: special diagnostic and treatment issues. J Clin Psychiatry 1991;52(Suppl):48–54.

62. Weissman MM, Klerman GL, Markowitz JS, et al. Suicidal ideation and suicide attempts in panic disorder and attacks. N Engl J Med 1989;321:1209–1214.

63. Weissman MM. The hidden patient: unrecognized panic disorder. J Clin Psychiatry 1990;51(Suppl):5–8.

64. Rosenbaum JF. Limited-symptom panic attacks: missed and masked diagnosis. Psychosomatics 1987; 28:407–412.

65. Brown TA, Barlow DH, Liebowitz MR. The empirical basis of generalized anxiety disorder. Am J Psychiatry 1994;151:1272–1280.

66. Brawman-Mintzer O, Lydiard RB. Biological basis of generalized anxiety disorder. J Clin Psychiatry 1997;58(Suppl 3):16–25.

67. Fleet RP, Beitman BD. Unexplained chest pain: when is it panic disorder? Clin Cardiol 1997;20:187–194.

68. Goldberg R, Morris P, Christian F, et al. Panic disorder in cardiac outpatients. Psychosomatics 1990;31:168–173.

69. Morris A, Baker B, Devins GM, et al. Prevalence of panic disorder in cardiac outpatients. Can J Psychiatry 1997;42:185–190.

70. Regier DA, Narrow WE, Rae DS. The epidemiology of anxiety disorders: the epidemiologic catchment area (ECA) experience. J Psychiatr Res 1990;24(Suppl 2): 3–14.

71. Carter CS, Servan-Schreiber D, Perlstein WM. Anxiety disorders and the syndrome of chest pain with normal coronary arteries: prevalence and pathophysiology. J Clin Psychiatry 1997;58(Suppl 3):70–73.

72. Hackett TP, Cassem NH. Psychological hazards of convalescence following myocardial infarction. JAMA 1971;215:1292–1296.

73. Rahe RH, Ward WH, Hayes V. Brief group therapy in myocardial infarction rehabilitation. Three to four year follow-up of a controlled trial. Psychosom Med 1978;41:229–241.

74. Ibrahim MA, Feldman JG, Sultz HA, et al. Management after myocardial infarction: a controlled trial of the effect of group psychotherapy. Int J Psychiatr Med 1974;5:253–268.

75. Bilodeau CB, Hackett TP. Issues raised in a group setting by patients recovering from myocardial infarction. Am J Psychiatry 1971;128:105–110.

76. Cay EL, Vetter NJ, Philip AE, et al. Return to work after a heart attack. J Psychosom Res 1973;17:231–243.

77. Garrity TF, Klein RF. Emotional response and clinical severity as early determinants of six-month mortality after myocardial infarction. Heart Lung 1975;4:730–737.

78. Dellipiani AW, Cay EL, Philip AE, et al. Anxiety after heart attack. Br Heart J 1976;38:752–757.

79. Doerhman ST. Psychosocial aspects of recovery from coronary heart disease: a review. Soc Sci Med 1977;11:199–218.

80. Mayou R. The course and determinants of reactions to myocardial infarction. Br J Psychiatry 1979;134: 588–594.

81. Byrne DG. Anxiety as state and trait following survived myocardial infarction. Br J Soc Clin Psychology 1979;18:417–423.

82. Byrne DG, Whyte HM, Butler KL. Illness behaviour and outcome following survived myocardial infarction: a prospective study. J Psychosom Res 1981;25:97–107.

83. Degre-Coustry C, Grevisse M. Psychological problems in rehabilitation after myocardial infarction. Adv Cardiol 1982;29:126–131.

84. Lloyd GG, Cawley RH. Psychiatric morbidity after myocardial infarction. Q J Med 1982;51:33–42.

85. Stern MJ, Gorman PA, Kaslow L. The group counselling vs exercise therapy study: a controlled intervention with subjects following myocardial infarction. Arch Intern Med 1983;143:1719–1725.

86. Oldenburg B, Perkins RJ, Andrews G. Controlled trial of psychological intervention in myocardial infarction. J Consult Clin Psychol 1985;53:852–859.

87. Faller H. Coping with myocardial infarction: a cognitive-emotional perspective. Psychother Psychosom 1990;54:8–17.

88. Thompson DR, Webster RA, Cordle CJ, et al. Specific sources and patterns of anxiety in male patients with first myocardial infarction. Br J Med Psychol 1987;60: 343–348.

89. Frasure-Smith N, Lesperance F, Talajic M. The impact of negative emotions on prognosis following myocardial infarction: is it more than depression. Health Psychol 1995;14:388–398.

90. Kornfeld DS, Zimberg S, Malm JR. Psychiatric complications of open-heart surgery. N Engl J Med 1965; 273:287–292.

91. Frank KA, Heller SS, Kornfeld DS. A survey of adjustment to cardiac surgery. Arch Intern Med 1972;130: 735–738.

92. Heller SS, Frank KA, Kornfeld DS, et al. Psychological outcome following open-heart surgery. Arch Intern Med 1974;134:908–914.

93. Gundle M, Reeves BR, Tate S, et al. Psychosocial outcome after coronary artery surgery. Am J Psychiatry 1980;137:1591–1544.

94. Jenkins CD, Stanton BA, Savageau JA, et al. Physical, psychologic, social and economic outcomes after cardiac valve surgery. Arch Intern Med 1983;143:2107–2113.

95. Jenkins CD, Stanton BA, Savageau JA, et al. Coronary artery bypass surgery: physical, psychological, social and economic outcomes six months later. JAMA 1983;250:782–788.

96. Magni G, Unger HP, Valfre C, et al. Psychosocial outcome one year after heart surgery: a prospective study. Arch Intern Med 1987;147:473–477.

97. Sokol RS, Folks DG, Herrick RW, et al. Psychiatric outcome in men and women after coronary bypass surgery. Psychosomatics 1987;28:11–16.

98. Fricchione GL, Vlay SC. Psychiatric aspects of patients with malignant ventricular arrhythmias. Am J Psychiatry 1986;143:1518–1525.

99. Morris PL, Badger J, Chmielewski C, et al. Psychiatric morbidity following implantation of the automatic implantable cardioverter defibrillator. Psychosomatics 1991:32:58–64.

100. Coryell W, Noyes R, Clancy J. Excess mortality in panic disorder: a comparison with primary unipolar depression. Arch Gen Psychiatry 1982;39:701–703.

101. Coryell W, Noyes R, House DJ. Mortality among outpatients with anxiety disorders. Am J Psychiatry 1986;143:508–510.

102. Haines AP, Imeson JD, Meade TW. Phobic anxiety and ischaemic heart disease. Br Med J 1987;295:297–299.

103. Kawachi I, Colditz GA, Ascherio A, et al. Prospective study of phobic anxiety and risk of coronary heart disease in men. Circulation 1994;89:1992–1997.

104. Kawachi I, Sparrow D, Vokonas PS, et al. Symptoms of anxiety and risk of coronary heart disease: the normative aging study. Circulation 1994;90:2225–2229.

105. Hjemdahl P. Physiology of the autonomic nervous system as related to cardiovascular function: implications for stress research. In: Byrne DG, Rosenman RH, eds. Anxiety and the heart. New York: Hemisphere Publishing, 1990:95–158.

106. Esler M. Neural regulation of the cardiovascular system. In: Byrne DG, Rosenman RH, eds. Anxiety and the heart. New York: Hemisphere Publishing, 1990:159–186.

107. Balon R, Ortiz A, Pohl R, et al. Heart rate and blood pressure during placebo-associated panic attacks. Psychosom Med 1988;50:434–438.

108. Volicer BJ, Volicer L. Cardiovascular changes associated with stress during hospitalization. J Psychosom Res 1978;22:159–168.

109. Shapiro PA. Psychiatric aspects of cardiovascular disease. Psychiatr Clin North Am 1996;19:613–629.

110. Freeman LJ, Nixon PG. Are coronary artery spasm and progressive damage to the heart associated with the hyperventilation syndrome? Br Med J 1985;291:851–852.

111. Myerburg RJ, Kessler KM, Mallon SM, et al. Life-threatening ventricular arrhythmias in patients with silent myocardial ischemia due to coronary artery spasm. N Engl J Med 1992;326:1451–1455.

112. Lown B. Mental stress, arrhythmias, and sudden death. Am J Med 1982;72:177–180.

113. Katz C, Martin RD, Landa B, et al. Relationship of psychological factors to frequent symptomatic ventricular arrhythmia. Am J Med 1985;78:589–594.

114. Yeragaani VK, Pohl R, Berger R, et al. Decreased heart rate variability in panic disorder patients: a study of power-spectral analysis of heart rate. Psychiatr Res 1993;46:89–103.

115. Kawachi I, Sparrow D, Vokonas PS, et al. Decreased heart rate variability in men with phobic anxiety (data from the normative aging study). Am J Cardiol 1995;75:882–885.

116. Yeragani VK, Berger R, Songer DA, et al. Power spectrum of the QRS complex in patients with panic disorder and normal controls. Psychiatr Res 1997;66:167–174.

117. Wielgosz AT. Connecting the ceruleus and the coronaries. Am J Cardiol 1988;62:308–309.

118. Roy-Byrne PP, Schmidt P, Cannon RO, et al. Microvascular angina and panic disorder. Int J Psychiatr Med 1989;19:315–325.

119. Kahn JP, Gorman JM, King DL, et al. Cardiac left ventricular hypertrophy and chamber dilatation in panic disorder patients: implications for idiopathic dilated cardiomyopathy. Psychiatr Res 1990;32:55–61.

120. White WB, Baker CH. Episodic hypertension secondary to panic disorder. Arch Intern Med 1986;146:1129–1130.

121. Byrne DG. Anxiety and the heart: a psychological perspective. In: Byrne DG, Rosenman RH, eds. Anxiety and the heart. New York: Hemisphere Publishing, 1990:483–491.

122. Byrne DG. The behavioral management of the cardiac patient. Norwood, NJ: Ablex Publishing, 1987.

123. Rosenbaum JF, Pollack RA, Jordan SK, et al. The pharmacotherapy of panic disorder. Bull Menninger Clin 1996;60(2, Suppl A):A54–A75.

124. Davidson JRT. Use of benzodiazepines in panic disorder. J Clin Psychiatry 1997;58(Suppl 2):26–28.

125. Jefferson JW. Antidepressants in panic disorder. J Clin Psychiatry 1997;58(Suppl 2):20–24.

126. Roy-Byrne PP, Hommer D. Benzodiazepine withdrawal: overview and implications for the treatment of anxiety. Am J Med 1988;84:1041–1052.

127. Bezchlibnyk-Butler KZ, Jeffries JJ. Clinical handbook of psychotropic drugs. 7th ed. Toronto: Hogrefe & Huber Publishers, 1997.

128. Dupont RL. Thinking about stopping treatment for panic disorder. J Clin Psychiatry 1990;51(Suppl A):38–45.

Vocational Issues: Maximizing the Patient's Potential for Returning to Work

William A. Dafoe, Barry A. Franklin, and Laura Cupper

Rehabilitation of the cardiac patient involves restoring and maintaining optimal physical, psychological, occupational, social, and recreational status. To facilitate these objectives, contemporary cardiac rehabilitation services may include exercise training, risk factor modification, medical surveillance, and psychosocial or vocational counseling. For many cardiac patients, returning to work is an important objective. Work is considered psychologically therapeutic for the recovering cardiac patient. Moreover, the economic survival of many patients and their families depends on gainful employment.

Cardiac rehabilitation has achieved dramatic improvements in patients' functional capacity, coronary risk factors, psychological well-being, and survival (1–3), but there is contradictory evidence regarding whether rehabilitation programs can influence the resumption of gainful employment (4–8). The Clinical Practice Guidelines on Cardiac Rehabilitation (9) state that "return to work as a measure of outcome of exercise-based cardiac rehabilitation may not be appropriate unless formal vocational rehabilitation services are provided to patients as part of the rehabilitative process." Although the patient's return to work is generally viewed as one measure of a successful rehabilitation outcome, whether it be after a myocardial infarction (MI) or coronary artery bypass graft (CABG) surgery, some symptomatic or high-risk patients may be unable to return to jobs that are physically demanding. The process of evaluating the patient for returning to work often occurs during the early outpatient rehabilitation program. "Rehabilitation constitutes a path from total temporary inability to work, connected with

the gravity of the illness, to a substantially normal return to the habits of before. This is a crucial phase in the treatment of the patient, both from the physical and psychological points of view" (10). It is important, therefore, that the physician address vocational issues in concert with rehabilitation services.

THE PROBLEM: CARDIAC COSTS AND DISABILITY

Patients who fail to return to work within 6 months after an MI or CABG surgery are unlikely to do so (11). This highlights the need for early counseling to encourage resumption of work. Indeed, many patients fail to return to work because they lack the medical assurance that they can resume vocational activities safely. Perhaps even more disturbing are studies that show no differences in return-to-work rates for CABG patients than for MI or angioplasty patients (12, 13). After both MI and bypass surgery, the rate of returning to work for women is also lower than that for men. An older age at the time of the cardiac event, a longer period of convalescence, and more severe disease seem to negatively affect the return-to-work rate for women (14, 15).

In the United States, approximately 30% of the total cost of disability payments can be attributed to cardiovascular disease. In 1992 approximately 7.9 million persons aged 15 and older were listed as disabled because of cardiovascular disease; these cases were about five times as costly as the average claim (16). Unfortunately, uniform standards for determining the degree of residual cardiac impairment are not available. Persons who have similar symptoms may be treated differently with regard to disability status, compensation, or both.

The goals of vocational rehabilitation are to evaluate whether returning to work is safe and realistic and to expedite the resumption of gainful employment, while assisting individuals to remain at work. During the last three decades, work classification clinics and research studies have done much to dispel the myth that cardiac patients are unemployable. It is estimated that up to 80% of patients with uncomplicated MI will return to work (5, 12). Moreover, the time for returning to work and resuming full activities for these patients has decreased from 4 months after an event in 1970 to approximately 60 to 70 days in 1990 (17, 18). Froelicher et al. (5) reported that 21% of post-MI patients returned to work by week 3, 62% returned between weeks 4 and 12, 11% returned between weeks 12 and 24, and 6% did not return. Nevertheless, the socioeconomic consequences of failure to return to work for such a prevalent disease are significant (16). For example, Fitzgerald et al. (19) prospectively studied patients employed in the 6-month period before percutaneous transluminal coronary angioplasty (PTCA) was conducted to assess the total cost associated with their absence from work. The total direct and indirect costs for this sample (n = 53) were $273,480 and $150,944, respectively. When these costs are generalized to all patients in the United States undergoing uncomplicated PTCA, the costs are more than $1.2 billion. Facilitating an earlier return to work, particularly among low-risk patients, could result in a significant savings in disability compensation (20, 21).

ROLE OF THE PHYSICIAN

The patient's physician plays a major role in assessing the return to work. There is an expectation that the physician is the patient's advocate and, in this regard, takes into account the job requirements (physical and mental) and the patient's capacity to meet these demands. The physician also is influenced by societal norms (a patient is expected to return to work), agency pressures (governmental agencies and insurance companies with more stringent disability requirements), and demographic factors (there may be limited employment in a certain area for cardiac patients). If the financial integrity of the family is threatened by the patient's failure to return to work (e.g., pension plans may be discontinued), the physician may feel an obligation to protect these funds. Thus, conflict over the return-to-work issue can affect the ongoing physician-patient-family relationship. Some physicians may feel that certain patients require an extended convalescence because of the perceived stressful nature of their job or its physical demands. Unfortunately, this may reduce the likelihood of a successful return to work. Physician attitude and encouragement with regard to returning to work plays a vital role in its actualization (22).

The focus of occupational work evaluation is to determine whether the cardiovascular demands produced by physical, psychological, and environmental stressors exceed the threshold for a safe working capacity (22, 23). Because the return-to-work decision is complex, it is important for physicians to have as much information as possible about these factors. The patient and family are expecting an uneventful course; most employers want assurance that their employees are safe on the job, despite their cardiac status; and the physician has a legal responsibility to ensure, as much as possible, that the patient does not endanger himself or the lives of others. Employability, therefore, should consider three factors: 1) the capability of the person to perform the job; 2) the risk involved in performing the job; and 3) the risk to society if the person performs the job (24).

In the first week of hospitalization, the opposite ends of the spectrum with regard to returning to work can be identified. For example, the low-risk patient with an uncomplicated MI can be assured that a return to work after hospitalization and rehabilitation in all likelihood poses no problems. Conversely, patients who are class IV, according to the New York Heart Association (NYHA) Functional and Therapeutic Scheme (Table 17.1) (25), that is, symptomatic at rest, are unlikely to return to work unless their medical status can be improved. Patients at intermediate risk may require additional diagnostic studies (coronary angiograms, exercise radionuclide testing) and therapeutic interventions (including adjustment of medications, PTCA, or revascularization surgery) before returning to work (18, 22).

Table 17.1. New York Heart Association Functional and Therapeutic Classification

Class	Restrictions[a]	Peak Exercise Tolerance METs	Cardiac Impairment %
I	None	≥7.0	0–15
II	Slight	5.0–6.0	20–40
III	Marked	3.0–4.0	50–70
IV	Severe	≤2.0	80–95

[a]Class I patients can perform ordinary physical activity without undue fatigue or symptoms. Class II and III patients may experience fatigue or symptoms (e.g., dyspnea, anginal pain) with ordinary or lighter than ordinary activity. Class IV patients have symptoms at rest and cannot perform any physical activity without discomfort.

At times, differing views exist between the various treating physicians about whether a patient can go back to work. Health insurers may place more emphasis on the specialist's opinion. It is important for all treating physicians to communicate effectively their recommendations regarding the patient's capability for returning to work or to delineate who will make this decision.

PHILOSOPHY OF WORK AND CAREER STAGES

The importance of employment has been clearly documented as central to well-being. Long-term unemployment often results in depression, self-imposed restrictions, lowered self-esteem, and declining health status. Early plans for the resumption of work may induce an optimistic attitude toward life, signifying the transition from a "sick role" to an active, productive social position. In contrast, the cessation of work can represent the turning point between contributing to self, family, and society or becoming a "drain on others" (26, 27).

Because cardiac events generally occur between the ages of 35 and 65, the patient's concerns are often aligned with those of workers of similar age—career advancement, maintenance and stabilization, or retirement (28). The career advancement phase, when workers often consider their careers a top priority, usually extends to age 45 or 50. Cardiac difficulties during these years and the need for lifestyle modification (e.g., smoking cessation, low-fat diet, regular exercise) may appear to conflict with a concentrated focus on work. Employers and coworkers may believe that their colleague who has cardiovascular dis-

ease should no longer compete or be promoted. During career maintenance, there can be more stability; however, there may be considerable responsibility with regard to administration, management issues, budget and finance, and staff supervision. Accordingly, absence from work can profoundly affect the worker and employer. Finally, patients approaching their late 50s or early 60s may elect not to return to work if they can retire without undue economic hardship (28).

INFLUENTIAL AND PREDICTIVE FACTORS

National and cultural customs, as well as national and local economic conditions, seem to influence return-to-work percentages (24). Table 17.2 shows that complex factors govern failure to return to work, including numerous nonmedical variables, employer stereotypes, and coworkers' attitudes (4, 12). To counteract these deterrents, vocational counseling should be implemented to facilitate the resumption of gainful employment.

Prognostic Variables

DEMOGRAPHICS

Age is negatively correlated with return to work. Although educational levels have not been consistently associated with resumption of work, there is a higher rate of return for white-collar workers, many of whom have graduate or postgraduate training (12, 15, 29). This may also reflect that many white-collar workers work for intrinsic as well as extrinsic reasons.

CLINICAL STATUS

Numerous medical factors play a predictive role in returning to work. Patients who have clinically evident severe pump failure or left ventricular (LV) dysfunction, with or without angina pectoris, have a poorer prognosis and are less likely to return to work. The number of previous cardiac events also has been related to subsequent work status (12, 15, 29). Patients who fail to return to work are more likely to have had an MI or bypass surgery before the current event and less relief of angina postoperatively than those who resume occupational activities. Physician attitude and the patient's perception of the physician's expectations also are predictive of the return to work (29).

Mark and associates (12) found that those patients at high risk for departure from the work

Table 17.2. Factors Influencing Work Return

Factor	More Likely to Return to Work	Less Likely to Return to Work
Individual		
Age	≤ 55 years old	> 55 years old
Education	Postgraduate degree	Less education
Clinical status		
LV impairment	None or mild	Significant
No. of cardiac events	One	Numerous
Self-perception of work return	Strong self-efficacy	Poor self-efficacy
Self-perception of illness	Transient and less serious	Permanent and serious
Perception of physician's view	Favors return to work	Does not approve
Societal Issues		
Family attitudes	Supportive	Not supportive
	Involved in rehabilitation	May sabotage efforts regarding work return
Labor market	Previous job or other jobs available	Job market poor
Employment aspects		
Career stage	Advancement/maintenance	Retirement stage
Job satisfaction	High	Low
Work stress	Manageable	High
		"Stress caused heart problems"
Type of work	"White collar," self employed	"Blue collar"
Time off work	Working at time of event	Off work before event
		Has not worked for 6 months
Financial	Needs work for income	Sufficent funds from other sources
Employer	Job modification possible	No job modification possible
	Contact maintained with employee	No contact while off work
Coworkers' attitudes	Help reduce work stressors	Minimal assistance
	Supportive and encouraging	Resentful

force can be prospectively identified at angiography (i.e., a time when it may be possible to intervene to help preserve employment). Functional status as measured by the Duke Activity Survey Index (an indicator of functional capacity) was the single most important predictor of 1-year employment status, followed by older age, black race, presence of congestive heart failure, lower education level, presence of extracardiac vascular disease, poorer psychological status, and lower job classification. Standard clinical variables, functional measures, and demographic and socioeconomic characteristics provided 20%, 27%, and 45%, respectively, of the total predictive information about follow-up work outcomes. Although PTCA patients who went back to work returned substantially earlier than their CABG or medical counterparts, the investigators found no evidence that coronary revascularization with either PTCA or CABG provided any long-term employment benefit over initial medical therapy.

GENDER

As mentioned earlier, women are generally older than men at the time of their acute cardiac event and have a longer period of convalescence and more severe disease, factors that can negatively affect their return-to-work rate. Women often undertake more household responsibilities so that the combined workload between home and work is greater than that of their male counterparts. It has also been suggested that less vocational and general counseling is provided for women after an acute MI (30). Accordingly, more research is needed concerning women with heart disease and work.

SELF-EFFICACY

Self-efficacy is defined as an evaluation of the ability to execute a specific action with confidence (31) and, from a vocational perspective, refers to the patient's perception of the ability to resume work successfully. The patient's in-hospital expectations of future vocational status have been shown to be an important predictor for returning to work. Patients who anticipated few future work problems had a higher work return rate compared to those who had negative expectations (15, 32, 33). Petrie et al. (34) studied the relationship between the post-MI patients' perception of their illness and their subsequent rate of returning to work. The men who perceived their illness as transient and less serious returned to work earlier. Thus, to promote a more favorable work return, dysfunctional perceptions, beliefs, and behavioral intentions need to be identified at an early stage and modified.

TIME OFF WORK

Work status at the time of the cardiovascular event is considered predictive of returning to work. Persons who are working productively at the time of their cardiac event are more likely to return to work sooner and to remain at work (15). If a patient has not returned to work within 6 months after an MI, then employment prospects are further diminished. Early intervention by health care professionals may help anticipate, identify, and modify barriers to returning to work and alleviate, at least in part, the anxiety often found in such patients (35).

FAMILY ATTITUDES

Concern for the patient's well-being or lack of encouragement by the family can represent negative influences that affect the return to work (36). Often, overprotection results, and work (stress) is postponed as long as possible (24, 37). The optimal situation is for the family, particularly the spouse, to have appropriate information, to lend support, and to participate in the rehabilitation and decision-making process. Thus, the rehabilitation process and the patient's confidence are enhanced. It appears that too much support is better than not enough (38).

FINANCIAL DISINCENTIVES

Returning to work after a cardiac event also depends on financial and logistic considerations, including the availability of adequate compensation during sick leave (e.g., disability insurance) and for retirement (e.g., pension plans). Often individuals are unaware of the provisions of their disability insurance. Long-term disability plans vary; however, generally the individual is eligible

for payments for the first 24 months provided that the former occupation can no longer be performed. Thereafter, the individual must be totally disabled "for all occupations" for disability payments to continue. In addition, labor market factors, such as the level of unemployment and related job opportunities, influence the rate of work resumption after a major illness (39).

During challenging economic times, some employers offer an early retirement package to encourage those who would not otherwise qualify for retirement, thereby decreasing the employer's work force and costs. Although financial compensation ensures economic survival and may allow for retraining in work more appropriate for the patient, it also may act as a deterrent (40). Use of trial periods for reentering the work force while maintaining partial benefits may be helpful in this regard.

JOB SATISFACTION

The degree of job satisfaction before the cardiac event is positively correlated with the rapidity of work return. For example, if a person feels like a significant contributor to the success of a business or profession, then that person is motivated by the job, and fears and anxieties about returning to work are attenuated (37). In contrast, considerable work stress correlates with a lower rate of returning to work (39). It is a widely held perception that work stress is a contributing factor to a cardiac event. Abbot and Berry (41) reported that individuals who returned to work early were more likely to have attributed their MI to occupational stressors. This result appears paradoxical; however, the authors concluded that these subjects found their work challenging and interesting despite the heavy workload.

THE EMPLOYER'S ROLE

Employer stereotypes of employees who have disabilities (e.g., cardiovascular disease) as being unable to compete in the labor market may act as barriers to returning to work (42). Stolz and Erdelyi (43) suggest that an employer's willingness to modify jobs and reduce work-related stress may have some effect on the patient's morbidity and early mortality. Failure to contact the employee is demoralizing and, in some cases, devastating to self-esteem (44, 45). It is important to provide reassurance to the employer or company physician that persons with cardiovascular disease can resume work without adverse sequelae. Appropriate factual information serves to decrease concerns regarding potential liability issues, increased health care costs, and insurance premiums (40). For example, most employers are unaware that at least 60% of cardiac patients can be expected to work effectively to retirement age (37). Although some studies have shown that employees with cardiac problems lose more work days than their contemporaries without heart disease, participants in rehabilitation programs fare well vis-à-vis attendance and productivity (46). An individual may be able to assume modified duties for a certain time, provided that there will eventually be a resumption of all job responsibilities and demands. In some cases union or company policy may not allow for job modification in terms of hours, work responsibilities, or a gradual resumption of activities. Moreover, employers who do not want to take back an employee because of previous work-related problems (e.g., interpersonal difficulties) may use the cardiac condition as a reason for terminating employment.

Attitude of Coworkers

Coworkers' attitudes toward a returning employee can range from hostility to supportive encouragement. For example, if coworkers must work harder to compensate for their colleague who is perceived to be sick, resentment may ensue. One study of 350 patients with MI or CABG surgery conducted 12 months after hospital discharge showed that one of the factors that made it easier to return to work was the support of coworkers (47). If coworkers harbor negative feelings for the workplace, they may perceive their nonworking colleague with cardiovascular disease as fortunate for having acquired such a reprieve.

Capacity for Job Modification

Job modifications can allow a person to return to a work environment that represents a safe and familiar way of life (37). Furthermore, modifying job tasks is often cheaper than recruiting and training new employees. The employer should be assured that workers generally perform job requirements well below their maximal physical work capacity. Even if the employee's functional capacity is reduced, most jobs can still be performed in a safe and efficient way, with considerable cardiorespiratory reserve (46).

JOB EVALUATION

Job titles generally provide little insight into the requirements of a particular position. It is important for the physician to acquire accurate information about the specific work-related tasks, the corresponding energy expenditure, and the degree of isometric and upper body exertion. This evaluation is essential for decisions on work capabilities and should include information about the physical requirements, psychological stress, superimposed environmental factors, and safety of work resumption.

Physical Requirements

The underlying assumption for a safe return to work is that a patient should work below metabolic loads that evoke abnormal clinical signs or symptoms, including ischemic ST-segment depression (± 0.1 mV), angina pectoris, serious arrhythmias, or wall-motion abnormalities. Moreover, the associated energy expenditure should be considerably less than the patient's peak or symptom-limited functional capacity. Accordingly, the physical demands of the job should be determined for the peak and average aerobic requirements and myocardial demands.

AEROBIC REQUIREMENTS: THE MET CONCEPT

A critical measure of metabolism and energy expenditure is oxygen (O_2) consumption ($\dot{V}O_2$), expressed in terms of a rearrangement of the Fick equation:

$$\dot{V}O_2 = HR \times SV \times (CaO_2 - C\bar{v}O_2)$$

where $\dot{V}O_2$ = oxygen consumption (mL/min); HR = heart rate (beats per minute); SV = stroke volume (mL/beat); and $CaO_2 - C\bar{v}O_2$ = arteriovenous oxygen difference (mL of O_2/dL blood). It is apparent that both central and peripheral regulatory mechanisms affect the magnitude of body oxygen consumption.

Typical circulatory data at rest and during maximal exercise in a healthy, sedentary 30-year-old man are shown in Table 17.3. By dividing the absolute resting oxygen consumption (250 mL/min) by the man's body weight in kilograms

17.3.   Circulatory Data at Rest and During Maximal Exercise for a Healthy Sedentary Man (70 kg)

	$\dot{V}O_2$				HR		SV		$(CaO_2-C\bar{v}O_2$
Condition	(mL/kg/min)	(L/min)	METs	=	(beats/min)	×	(mL/beat)	×	(mL/dL blood)
Rest	3.5[a]	0.25	1.0[a]		70		70		5.1
Maximal exercise	42.0	3.0	12.0		190		100		15.8

[a]3.5 mL/kg/min= 1 MET (metabolic equivalent); average resting metabolic rate for all persons regardless of body weight.

(70 kg), one derives the energy requirement for basal homeostasis, termed one MET (metabolic equivalent), approximating 3.5 mL O_2/kg per minute. This relative expression of oxygen consumption is extremely important in exercise physiology, being independent of body weight and, thus, relatively constant for all persons (48). Furthermore, multiples of this value often are used to quantify respective levels of energy expenditure. For example, if stair climbing requires three times the resting energy expenditure, then the requirement is 3 METs or 10.5 mL O_2/kg per minute.

The typical 12-fold increase in oxygen transport and utilization achieved at maximal exercise is brought about by respective increases in the hemodynamic correlates of $\dot{V}O_2$ (e.g., a fourfold increase in cardiac output and a threefold increase in arteriovenous oxygen difference [$4 \times 3 = 12$ METs]). Table 17.4 provides representative maximal MET values for healthy adults, cardiac patients, and endurance athletes. In contrast to the healthy adult, the reduced functional capacity (in METs) in the cardiac patient appears to be caused primarily by decreased maximal cardiac output, secondary to reduced SV or HR, rather than impairment in the peripheral extraction of oxygen (49). Because the maximal arteriovenous oxygen difference appears to be little affected by exercise training or heart disease, the maximal MET capacity is a good indication of maximal pump function (50). It is an important value in the functional evaluation of the severity of heart disease.

The metabolic costs of many occupational activities have been defined in terms of kilocalorie expenditure (kcal/min) or oxygen uptake (appendix A) (51). Physicians may find such tables helpful in matching a patient's aerobic capacity to a task, assuming that patients can sustain work output throughout an 8-hour day at a level in the range of 25% to 40% of the $\dot{V}O_2$max (52). If the patient achieved a peak workload of 10 METs during exercise testing, then a safe and manageable work rate would be in the range of 2.5 to 4.0 METs. There are, however, several inherent limitations to using the MET concept as a guide to vocational planning (53).

One limitation in using MET tables of selected vocational activities lies in the fact that these represent average energy expenditures that may vary considerably from person to person, depending on the pace at which the activity is performed, the participant's size, previous job training, and work efficiency.

Another problem with this method is that the energy (MET) requirements were obtained during sustained or "steady-state" work, whereas most occupational activities are intermittent in nature. Accordingly, a patient with a 5-MET capacity might be discouraged from returning to the occupation of lawn maintenance (a requirement of 5 to 6 METs), because presumably it represents maximal or supermaximal effort; however, if the activity is performed intermittently, for example, 2 minutes of work, followed by 1 minute of rest, then the task can be accomplished easily at oxygen consumption and HR levels well below those estimated for it (Fig. 17.1). By using the MET concept in its strictest sense, a patient's capacity for certain activities may be underestimated considerably.

Perhaps the greatest limitation of the MET concept in activity prescription lies in the assumption that work oxygen consumption equal to that obtained during leg exercise testing produces similar HR and blood pressure (BP) demands, and vice versa. Factors such as psychological stress, climate (temperature and humidity), and the acti-

Table 17.4.   Maximal Aerobic Capacity (METs) for Different Populations

Group	METs
Healthy adults	10–12
Cardiac patients	6–8
Endurance athletes	15–20

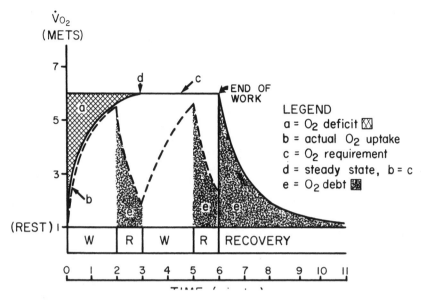

Figure 17.1. Oxygen requirements during work. An activity that requires 6 METs when performed continuously (*curved line reaching peak at d*) requires less than 6 METs when performed intermittently (*broken lines*), because rest periods permit partial repayment of oxygen debt. W, work; R, rest. (Adapted from Franklin BA, Hellerstein HK. Realistic stress testing for activity prescription. J Cardiovasc Med 1982;7:570–576.)

vation of muscles not used during the exercise test (i.e., upper extremities) may alter the linear relationship between myocardial and total body oxygen demands during exercise testing, creating disproportionate cardiac demands at relatively low levels of energy expenditure. For example, although desk work requires only 1.5 to 2 METs, if psychologically stressful, it may provoke HR and systolic BP responses comparable to those attained at higher metabolic rates (e.g., 3 to 4 METs) during exercise testing. Consideration of only the oxygen consumption or MET level during work may not provide an accurate index of the cardiac demands.

MYOCARDIAL DEMANDS

Isometric or static effort (sustained muscle contraction with little or no movement) occurs when straining to lift, push, or pull heavy loads. The excessive myocardial demands may be dangerously camouflaged by relatively low metabolic requirements, so that the usual warning signs of overexertion (tachycardia, sweating, and dyspnea) are absent.

The cardiovascular response to static exertion apparently is mediated by a neurogenic mechanism (54). Heart rate increases in relation to the tension exerted; in contrast, SV remains essen-

tially unchanged except at higher levels of tension (greater than 50%), at which it may decrease. The result is a moderate increase in cardiac output, which is nevertheless disproportionately high for the increase in metabolism. Despite the increased cardiac output, blood flow to the noncontracting muscle does not increase significantly, probably because of reflex vasoconstriction. The combination of vasoconstriction and increased cardiac output causes a disproportionate rise in systolic and diastolic BP, as well as in myocardial oxygen requirements.

The magnitude of the pressor response during isometric work depends on the total muscle mass involved (55), the types of muscles used (i.e., fast versus slow twitch), the duration of the muscle contraction, and the tension exerted relative to the greatest possible tension in the muscle group (percent of maximal voluntary contraction) (54). A relatively mild isometric contraction by weakened arm muscles, therefore, may evoke an excessive pressor response.

Although isometric or combined static-dynamic efforts traditionally have been contraindicated for patients with coronary artery disease (CAD), it appears that static exercise may be less hazardous than was once presumed, particularly in patients with reasonable cardiorespiratory fitness (more than 7 METs) and good LV function (56). Isometric exertion, regardless of the percentage of maximal voluntary contraction used, generally fails to elicit angina, ischemic ST-segment depression, or significant ventricular arrhythmias among selected cardiac patients (57, 58). The rate-pressure product and myocardial oxygen demands are less during maximal isometric than during maximal dynamic exercise, primarily because of a lower peak HR response in the former (57). Increased subendocardial perfusion, secondary to elevated diastolic BP, may also contribute to the lower incidence of ischemic responses reported during isometric or combined isometric-dynamic effort. Furthermore, the myocardial oxygen supply–demand relationship appears to be altered favorably by superimposing static on dynamic effort, so that the rate-pressure product at ischemia is actually increased (58). Although LV function deteriorates during progressive work loads in patients with myocardial ischemia, mild ischemia may be tolerated during steady-state exercise without a deterioration of LV function (59). These findings are changing the cautious attitude toward isometric exertion for coronary patients. Rather than arbitrarily proscribing occupational activities with isometric requirements (carrying luggage or other weights, operating a jackhammer, performing construction or carpentry work), the physician should evaluate the person's response to such predominantly static activities and give advice about how to minimize adverse responses; for example, a yoke or shoulder strap for carrying weights can be used to avoid the Valsalva maneuver.

If a job requires sustained upper extremity work, it is important to consider that, although maximal physiologic responses are generally greater during leg exercise than arm exercise, the HR, BP, minute ventilation, perceived exertion, and oxygen consumption for arm exercise are greater for any given work rate (60). The disparity in cardiorespiratory and hemodynamic responses to arm exercise versus leg exercise at identical work rates may be attributed to reduced mechanical efficiency during arm exercise, the involvement of smaller muscle groups, the static effort required with arm work, increased sympathetic tone during arm exertion, concomitant isometric contraction, vasoconstriction in the nonexercising leg muscles, or all these factors. Aerobic capacity

($\dot{V}O_2max$) during arm work generally approximates 70% $\pm$ 15% of the $\dot{V}O_2max$ during leg work (60). The significantly greater $\dot{V}O_2max$ with the legs may be attributed to their greater muscle mass, or perhaps leg musculature contains more tissue capable of high oxygen extraction than does arm musculature.

Psychological Stress

Stress has been described as excessive environmental demands combined with inadequate coping resources yielding the presence of emotional distress or characteristic patterns of maladaptive behaviors, or both (61). Many patients cite mental stressors as important contributors to their cardiac disease (12). Stress is a difficult construct to measure quantitatively; however, it is strongly associated with heavy workloads, meeting deadlines, changes in technology and the work environment, poor interpersonal work relationships, and even boredom (37).

Psychological stress can elicit myocardial ischemia, manifested by significant ST-segment depression, the provocation of angina pectoris, or both. The rate-pressure product at the onset of ischemia may be lower than for exercise stress. Postulated mechanisms for this discrepancy include peripheral vasoconstriction, increased norepinephrine secretion, and changes in platelet aggregability (62). Frimerman et al. (63) studied changes in hemostatic function in 30 accountants (26 men and 4 women, aged 34.5 $\pm$ 9 years) at the end of the fiscal year, a period associated with the longest working hours and peak stress, as compared with a calm work period. Under both conditions, the subjects were asked to complete a questionnaire that graded their subjective feelings of stress caused by work overload on a scale from 1 to 10, and blood samples were obtained. During the stressful period, 83% of the accountants graded their occupational stress as more than 5. In contrast, during the control period (i.e., after a vacation or lightened workload) all graded their occupational stress as less than 5. Results showed a significant elevation in coagulation factors VII and VIII, fibrinogen, thrombocyte count, and thrombin- and ADP-induced platelet aggregation during the period of mental stress (caused by increased workload) as compared with a calm work period. These findings suggest that occupational stress can precipitate a hypercoagulable state that can favor focal thrombosis and, as a consequence, the development and progression of CAD. Chronic stress can have adverse effects on cardiovascular risk factors, either directly or indirectly (64).

There is no clear consensus in the literature with regards to the relationship between work stress and the development of heart disease or its subsequent prognosis. Theorell et al. (65) reviewed seven studies that showed an association between stressful environments and an increased risk of MI. In 1991, these authors studied 127 men in the Stockholm area who returned to work after an MI, and they reported an increased death rate in those subjects who returned to high stress jobs as defined by "demanding jobs with limited possibilities of influencing decisions and developing skills." Karasek and colleagues (66, 67) developed the concept of "job strain," which purports to measure the interaction between the worker and the job environment. Job strain was correlated with cardiac death in Swedish men (66) and with the prevalence of MIs in the National Health and Nutrition Examination (68). Because circadian rhythms and seasonal variability influence the rates of MI, it would be interesting to compare any differences between workers and retirees. Spielberg et al. (69) found that both groups had similar early morning peak times for MIs; however, the workers had a second daily peak in the afternoon around 4 pm. The authors concluded that the biphasic circadian incidence of MIs suggests a possible relation to professional activity.

Conversely, a number of studies show no relationship between job stress and cardiovascular end points. The Honolulu Heart Study, a prospective cohort study, showed no relationship between job strain and incidence of CAD (70). Hlatky et al. (71) used the same job strain index and found no relationship to the degree of atherosclerosis as determined on angiography. Indeed, job strain was more common in those with normal coronary arteries. As seen with other studies, the traditional risk factors did correlate with the extent of disease. Further evaluation by Hlatky and associates found no relationship between job strain and subsequent cardiac end points (cardiac death or nonfatal infarction). Rost and Smith (26) studied the relationship between early return to work after an initial MI and the patient's subsequent emotional well-being as assessed by a series of psychosocial inventories. Ninety of 143 patients (63%) who had been employed at the time of initial MI returned to work by 4 months and remained employed at 12 months. Those patients who returned to work displayed significantly lower levels of emotional distress than patients who did not return to work independent of multiple indicators of initial physical and psychological adjustment (Fig. 17.2). These findings suggest that the trajectory of emotional adaptation after an acute cardiac event differs for individuals who do and do not return to work. Thus, there is insufficient evidence to implicate job stress as a distinct cardiac risk at this time. Nevertheless changes in work demands may be required for individuals who report high levels of job stress or demonstrate signs and symptoms of myocardial ischemia while at work.

Because adults spend up to 50% of their time in work-related activities, any stressors in this domain must be addressed. Providing a stress management program that is oriented to occupational issues has proved to be beneficial in modifying deleterious behavior patterns and in reinforcing confidence in the patient's ability to return to work (20). In some cases, a brief sabbatical from work may be required to provide intensive counseling for job-related stressors.

Environmental Factors

SHIFT WORK

Shift work can increase the energy requirements of any given job. Moreover, the ability to cope with shift work decreases with age, dropping significantly after age 40, with the duration of sleep also declining with age (72, 73). Night shift workers average 25% to 33% less sleep than day or swing shift workers (74). When a person attempts to return to work after an acute cardiac event, it is beneficial to return to the day shift. Working day shifts allows for a reintegration to the workplace at reduced energy demands. In addition, the person is better able to access the social support system. After an acclimation period, resumption of shift duties may be feasible.

FUMES

Workplace fumes must be considered when evaluating the patient's vocational setting. Exposure to carbon monoxide can result in the formation of carboxyhemoglobin, decreasing the oxygen carrying capacity of blood. Carbon monoxide can be generated by oxyacetylene

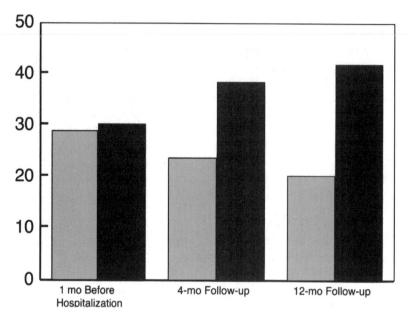

Figure 17.2.   Levels of emotional distress (0–50 scale) for patients who did (*shaded bars;* n = 90) and did not (*black bars:* n = 42) return to work by 4 months after myocardial infarction and at 12-month follow-up.

welding in a poorly ventilated area and exposure to automobile exhaust fumes (75).

TEMPERATURE

A cold environment can lower significantly the work rate at which the ischemic or anginal threshold occurs (76). Excessive cooling may trigger reflexes that cause constriction of coronary blood vessels and decrease myocardial oxygen supply. For those who suffer from angina when inhaling cold air (77), discomfort can be reduced or alleviated by wearing a face mask or scarf to warm the inspired air. The weight of additional outdoor clothing increases the metabolic demands for any tasks and decreases the mean exercise time (78, 79). Although the peak and sign- or symptom-limited workloads are diminished by cold, the incidence of arrhythmias appears similar to that with dynamic exercise (20).

The occurrence of cardiovascular complications is relatively high among men who have heart disease and who perform hard work that involves an isometric component in a cold environment. The increase in myocardial oxygen consumption related to the increased HR, coupled with the substantial rise in BP prompted by isometric work, makes activities such as snow shoveling a concern (80, 81).

Working in hot, humid weather may consti-

tute an even greater hazard for the heart disease patient. First, body temperature rises rapidly in response to physical exertion. This leads to a shunting of blood from the core to the periphery (skin) and causes excessive sweating. These mechanisms cause a reduction in effective circulating blood volume and a subsequent drop in BP (82). Heart rate and myocardial oxygen consumption increase disproportionately to keep up with increasing metabolic demands. Individuals who are not acclimated to heat and who are exposed to temperatures greater than 24°C experience added HR increases of 1 beat per minute for each degree Celsius when exercising (Fig. 17.3) and 2 to 4 beats per minute for each degree Celsius with concomitant increased humidity (83). Finally, loss of sweat causes changes in serum and cellular electrolytes (sodium and potassium) that can precipitate arrhythmias. These alterations, singly and collectively, may be deleterious to the compromised myocardium (84).

Safety of Work Resumption

On-the-job studies in the 1950s revealed that the energy cost of most jobs was lower than anticipated. The physical stresses of factory and steel mill jobs generally were low and of brief duration, rarely sustained at high levels for more than 2 or 3 minutes. Furthermore, the pattern of

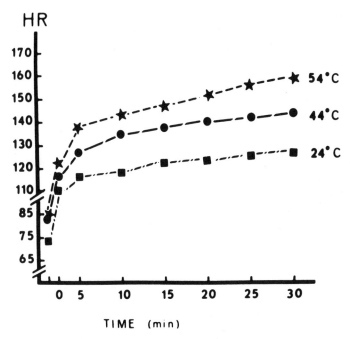

Figure 17.3.   Influence of environmental temperature on heart rate (HR) responses at a constant exercise workload. Heart rate increases approximately 1 beat per minute for each degree Celsius increment in ambient temperature above 24°C. (Adapted from Pandolf KB, Cafarelli E, Noble BJ, et al. Hyperthermia: effect on exercise prescription. Arch Phys Med Rehabil 1975;56:524–526.)

energy expenditure was intermittent, not continuous, with 30% to 45% of the working shift spent sitting or standing quietly (85). Many tasks involved greater demands on the upper than on the lower extremities.

Automation has decreased the energy demands of all occupational work even more during the past 40 years. For example, only 5% of patients now perform "heavy" occupational work, as compared with 65% in the 1950s (86). Today, heavy work in entry-level jobs usually is performed by younger workers. There is also considerable evidence that work-related isometric exertion is not as hazardous as once believed, especially in low-risk patients (56–58, 87).

Although the workplace traditionally is presumed to be more stressful than the home environment, cardiovascular complications occur no more frequently on the job than at home (86). It appears that the physical demands of most jobs can be performed safely by patients classified as low-risk. Moreover, some patients classified as high-risk on the basis of impaired LV function demonstrate a relatively well-preserved physical work capacity and, thus, are capable of gainful employment (88); however, those who have

strenuous occupations may require job modifications or reassignment.

The proposed job should be assessed in terms of safety to the patient and to the public in the event of incapacitation from exertional signs or symptoms. Certain vocations have high physical demands combined with emotional stress. For example, firefighters are required to wear heavy equipment while performing strenuous work in hot, dangerous conditions. If the firefighter were to become incapacitated by severe angina or syncope, his safety, as well as the safety of others, would be compromised. Similar problems for airline pilots who have peak psychological stress during takeoffs and landings could have disastrous consequences.

The probability of angina or syncope relates to the variables that determine prognosis after MI. Because of the vagaries of the atherosclerotic process, however, the accuracy in predicting which patient will develop such clinical manifestations remains imperfect. A summary tool for prognosis was developed by Pryor et al. (89) using weighted pathophysiologic constructs that include descriptors of myocardial function, myocardial jeopardy, and myocardial ischemia

(Table 17.5). An added difficulty is the realization that the disease may progress suddenly from accelerated atherosclerosis, plaque rupture, or both. The clinician who evaluates the patient for returning to work or ongoing employment needs to consider all these factors. Accordingly, regular cardiologic assessment may be required for high-risk vocations.

How Early Is Safe?

Dennis et al. (17) conducted a randomized trial to assess the efficacy of symptom-limited exercise testing about 3 weeks after uncomplicated MI in facilitating an earlier return to work. Participants were previously employed men and women who were younger than 60 years. Screening yielded 201 subjects (mean age, 50 years); of these, 99 and 102 were randomized to the intervention and usual-care groups, respectively. Patients in the intervention group who did not exhibit marked ischemic ST-segment depression (more than 2 mm) during exercise testing (n = 91) were advised to return to work about 35 to 42 days after their MI. Patients in the usual-care group returned to work when they believed it was appropriate. On average, patients in the intervention group went back to work 3 weeks earlier than those who received usual care (51 compared to 75 days) without adverse effects. If these figures are extrapolated to acute MI patients in general, it appears that facilitating an earlier return to work can yield $500 million each year in medical cost savings and additional earnings alone.

ASSESSMENT OF THE PATIENT

Several noninvasive procedures can be used in formulating a prescription for work resumption. These may involve a clinical assessment of the patient and a job evaluation, including an analysis of the type of work, energy requirements, environmental conditions and psychological stresses, simulated work testing (i.e., weight carrying, repetitive weight lifting, arm wrench work, machine operation), and ambulatory electrocardiographic (ECG) monitoring (76). Conventional exercise testing, however, is still the most widely used technique to evaluate quantitatively the following variables: chronotropic capacity, aerobic capacity of the body, myocardial aerobic capacity, and associated changes in electrical functions of the heart (90).

Exercise Testing

A World Health Organization (WHO) expert committee on rehabilitation stated that "the primary purpose of an exercise test is to determine the responses of the individual to efforts at given levels and from this information to estimate probable performance in specific life and occupational situations" (53). Standard lower extremity exercise tests, using either the treadmill or cycle ergometer, as discussed in chapter 4, have the advantage of reproducibility and quantification of physiologic responses to known external workloads. Protocols are progressive in intensity and may include increases in speed or

Table 17.5. Prognostic Characteristics Classified by Pathophysiologic Constructs and Weighted According to Power in Predicting Prognosis for Patients with Manifest Coronary Artery Disease

Characteristics	Relative Importance
Myocardial Function	
Congestive heart failure	4
Function class	3
Diuretic use	2
Digitalis use	2
Cardiomegaly	3
S_3 gallop	3
Prior myocardial infarction	2
Exercise systolic pressure	3
Exercise capacity	4
Ventricular arrhythmias	2
Ejection fraction	4
Wall motion score	4
Left ventricular end-diastolic pressure	2
Myocardial Jeopardy	
Angina frequency	1
Duration of angina	1
Level of exercise inducing angina	3
Degree of exercise-induced ST depression	3
Exercise systolic pressure	3
Reversible thallium perfusion defects	3
Number and distribution of obstructed coronary vessels	3
Myocardial Ischemia	
Rest or nocturnal angina	3
Progressive angina	2
Unstable angina	3
Failure to respond to nitroglycerin	2
ST-segment depression (resting ECG)	3

Adapted from Prior DB, Bruce RA, Chaitman BR, et al. Task force I. Determination of prognosis in patients with ischemic heart disease. J Am Coll Cardiol 1989; 14:1016–1025.

grade, or both, in treadmill testing, and increases in external load (watts) or pedaling speed in cycle ergometer testing. A treadmill protocol that includes large work increments between stages (e.g., Bruce test) is more likely to unmask ischemic ECG changes (91), but is less accurate in estimating functional capacity (92).

The functional information derived from exercise testing is based on the oxygen requirement of the peak external workload attained. Typically, this is evaluated by direct measurement or by estimation of the peak or maximal rate of oxygen consumption ($\dot{V}O_2max$), expressed as mL/kg per minute, or as METs. It should be emphasized, however, that the cardiac patient's $\dot{V}O_2max$ may be markedly overestimated when it is predicted from exercise time or workload. Several explanations have been offered to account for this phenomenon (93). Moreover, because leg and arm $\dot{V}O_2max$ generally provides a marginal estimate at best of reciprocal arm and leg aerobic capacity, arm exercise testing appears to be the evaluation of choice for persons whose occupational activity is dominated by dynamic upper extremity efforts (94).

The time course of the patient in relation to the acute cardiac event also should be considered. If a patient undergoes exercise testing soon after hospital discharge (e.g., 3 weeks), his physical work capacity may be spuriously low because of deconditioning, fatigue, or fear of physical exertion. A significant increase in aerobic capacity, corresponding to 2 to 3 METs, generally occurs between 3 and 11 weeks after clinically uncomplicated MI, even in patients who undergo no formal exercise training (95, 96). Greater improvements occur, however, in patients who simultaneously undergo home or gymnasium exercise training programs, approximating 3 and 4.4 METs, respectively (95). The magnitude of cardiovascular improvement subsequent to physical conditioning depends on several factors, including the subject's initial fitness, clinical cardiac status, LV dysfunction, total amount of exercise accomplished or calories expended, and patient compliance. If work return is deemed unfeasible with the patient's current fitness level, then another exercise test should be scheduled after a 3-month exercise training regimen.

PREDICTIVE VALUE

Exercise testing has proved useful in predicting who will return to work after an MI or CABG surgery. The peak HR and workload achieved are correlated directly with return-to-work rates. In one study performed soon after MI, those patients who had 2 mm or more of exercise-induced ST-segment depression had a return-to-work percentage only half of that for those with lesser degrees of ischemic ECG change (97). Another study showed that MI patients who had a physical work capacity less than 100 W were less likely to return to work (98). Early cycle ergometer testing after CABG surgery also has been shown to be helpful in discriminating between those who would return to work and those who would not. Patients who attained peak workloads of 60 W or less returned to work less than half as often as those who achieved 120 W or more (99).

Work Simulation

Work simulation may be appropriate for patients with reduced exercise tolerance (less than 7 METs) or those with LV dysfunction who have jobs that require a significant isometric component. Standard lower extremity exercise tests for work prescription may not necessarily reflect the requirements for lifting and carrying (76). Work simulation testing attempts to mimic, as closely as possible, the physical demands that will be encountered. The usual tasks used for simulated testing include repetitive lifting, carrying, stacking, or shoveling. Because some investigators have reported an increased incidence of ventricular arrhythmias during static compared to dynamic exertion (100, 101), there should be continuous ECG and BP monitoring before, during, and after the testing. Blood pressure should be taken in the nonexercising arm immediately before the weight is lifted and just before the weight is released (Table 17.6).

Mental Stress Testing

Emotional stressors have been shown to induce myocardial ischemia, wall-motion abnormalities, and serious ventricular arrhythmias. Although mental stress has been evaluated in the laboratory with BP and ECG monitoring, radionuclide scanning, and echocardiography, such testing is not routinely performed. The most practical method to assess ECG responses is to have the patient evaluated with a Holter monitor (76), use a diary to record daily activities, and attempt to correlate ischemic ST-segment changes and arrhythmias with concomitant emotional stress.

Table 17.6.　Designing a Weight-Lifting and Carrying Test

Information that needs to be obtained from the individual or observed at the work-site includes the following:

1. The type of weight lifting performed in the workplace
    - object is lifted and stacked
    - object is lifted and carried
    - object is lifted and held
2. The differing amounts of weight that are lifted
3. How the object is lifted and carried
    - carried with one arm
    - lifted and carried on the shoulder
    - held against the body
4. The amount of time per lifting episode and rest period between lifting episodes
5. The position of the object before lifting and after being put down
    - floor level
    - waist height
    - above the shoulders

Weight-lifting and carrying tests can be designed using this information.

Blood pressure should be taken in the nonexercising arm immediately before lifting and just before releasing each weight.

Continuous ECG monitoring should be performed.

Individual should lift weights with no warm-up and at a rate that would be followed in the workplace (i.e., self-determined).

EXERCISE TRAINING TO IMPROVE FUNCTIONAL CAPACITY

A major objective of an exercise training program after MI or CABG surgery is to help patients return to work successfully by improving functional capacity. Decreased HR and BP responses to submaximal exercise also are beneficial, signifying a reduction in myocardial oxygen consumption at a given level of work. The physical conditioning program should restore patients' work tolerances gradually so that they will be able to return to work soon after hospital discharge. Exercise training studies in patients with CAD generally have demonstrated an 11% to 56% increase (mean 20%) in preconditioning values of $\dot{V}o_2max$ (102). For those patients whose jobs require upper extremity efforts, static-dynamic work, or both, the program should include exercises such as upper extremity strengthening using weights, arm cranking (Fig. 17.4), or rowing, as well as more traditional aerobic activities such as walking or jogging and stationary cycle ergometry.

VOCATIONAL COUNSELING SERVICES

Each state is legislated to provide vocational rehabilitation, and these services have been available since the 1920s. The general eligibility for services is that a person must have a diag-

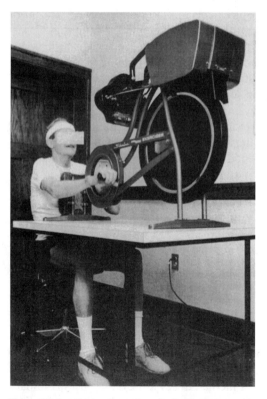

Figure 17.4.　Cycle ergometer adapted for arm exercise training. Bicycle handgrips fit over the pedals, clamps secure the ergometer to a sturdy metal table, and a padded breastplate helps standardize arm position.

nosed disabling condition that is a job handicap and a reasonable expectation of successful return to work. Provision of these services varies, with some agencies having a vocational rehabilitation counselor in a liaison capacity with the local cardiac rehabilitation program.

Persons who anticipate difficulties with work return can apply for vocational rehabilitation services or be referred by their physicians. Vocational rehabilitation counselors then can provide counseling that may include work hardening, job analysis, job simulation, job stabilization, establishment of a new vocational direction, and training for job placement. Occasionally, if it is near the end of the fiscal year, resources may be exhausted and the person may have to await further funding.

Preparation for Return to Work

Once it has been determined that an individual can safely and feasibly return to work, preparation will facilitate the work return process. Planning to phase in by working part-time hours can smooth the transition. Discussion with a vocational counselor as well as with other cardiac patients who have returned successfully to work can help identify the difficulties or pitfalls and the rewards of returning to work. Returning to the job at a nonpeak time is beneficial; for example, a produce clerk might return after the busy Christmas period. Individuals need to decide how they will continue to implement their lifestyle changes and work in a more healthy fashion.

Work Hardening

If a person needs to increase physical tolerance or self-confidence to return to a former occupation, a work hardening program can be developed. This service can be performed in the rehabilitation program or within a competitive work environment. It generally entails work with the participant and the employer to negotiate a mutually agreeable arrangement to facilitate the "hardening" process. The procedure can include increasing the work hours or adding job tasks by increments until optimal levels are achieved.

Job Stabilization

Job stabilization involves monitoring a participant's work return for at least 3 months and providing supportive counseling. Individual stress management techniques, time management, and assertiveness training may be required.

Establishing a New Vocational Direction

For clients who require a new occupation, vocational counseling begins with an exploration of past work history, interests, and aptitudes. Transferable skills analysis may suggest other jobs that an individual could undertake with minimal or no retraining. Testing by a psychologist can be included to further explore potential job interests and aptitudes. In addition, a comprehensive work assessment that uses a vocational evaluation unit may be required. This evaluation can assist clients in exploring new vocational directions and provide a detailed job assessment in terms of skills and interests. A 4- to 8-week employer placement in a given job helps assess the client's physical tolerance and aptitude for a specific occupation. During this time, the participant can acquire an understanding of the tasks or responsibilities required for a job while building self-confidence and reestablishing a work routine.

Assessments usually are unpaid work experiences within a competitive work environment. Employers are requested to participate in these experiences and generally are accommodating. Although the assessment is individualized for the participant, that person is expected to meet the employment standards of the position and to work under the same conditions as other employees. The goals of the assessment are clearly defined, with specific tasks agreed to by the client, vocational counselor, and the employer. Regular meetings with all parties assist in facilitating an optimal learning experience for the client and serve to ensure that the needs of the employer are met. After exploration of new career directions and possible employer assessments to test feasibility, a vocational goal is determined. The participant then can be assisted with job search activities, such as writing a résumé and appropriate cover letters, assistance regarding job interviews, obtaining job leads, and networking in a given field. Supportive counseling is offered during the job search.

CONCLUSIONS

Unfortunately, vocational counseling often is underemphasized in contemporary cardiac rehabilitation programs. Certainly, there is room for improvement in return-to-work rates, especially in the CABG surgery patient. We must conclude, as Brinkley (103) so elegantly summarized, that " . . . work is an essential ingredient for quality of living. We have seen too many people who quit too soon, sitting on porches, watching cars go by. I have also been impressed by the numbers who die within a year or two after retirement. I have wondered if the stimulus of work did not, in fact, give life itself."

A comprehensive cardiac rehabilitation program must include three complementary components—medical, psychological, and social—if it is going to favorably influence the return-to-work rate. Moreover, program personnel should be aware of the services provided through their state vocational rehabilitation agencies, and they should establish contact with the appropriate counselors to facilitate referrals.

The physician, in conjunction with these programs and services, should help to ensure that the cardiac patient is returned to an optimal vocational status and, if employable, is provided an opportunity to work.

References

1. Leon A, Certo C, Comoss P, et al. Scientific evidence of the value of cardiac rehabilitation services with emphasis on patients following myocardial infarction: Section 1. Exercise conditioning component. Position paper of the American Association of Cardiovascular and Pulmonary Rehabilitation. J Cardpulm Rehabil 1990;10:79–87.
2. Oldridge N, Guyatt G, Jones N, et al. Effects on quality of life with comprehensive rehabilitation after acute myocardial infarction. Am J Cardiol 1991;67:1084–1089.
3. O'Connor G, Buring G, Yusuf S, et al. An overview of randomized trials of rehabilitation with exercise after myocardial infarction. Circulation 1989;80:234–244.
4. Franklin B. Getting patients back to work after myocardial infarction or coronary bypass surgery. Physician Sportsmed 1986;14:183–194.
5. Froelicher ES, Kee LL, Newton KM, et al. Return to work, sexual activity, and other activities after acute myocardial infarction. Heart Lung 1994;23:423–435.
6. Hamalainen H, Kallio V, Knuts L, et al. Community approach in rehabilitation and secondary prevention after acute myocardial infarction: results of a randomized clinical trial. J Cardpulm Rehabil 1991;11:221–226.
7. Worcester M, Hare D, Oliver R, et al. Early programmes of high and low intensity exercise and quality of life after acute myocardial infarction. BMJ 1993;307:1244–1247.
8. Hedback B, Perk J, Wodlin P. Long-term reduction of cardiac mortality after myocardial infarction: 10-year results of a comprehensive rehabilitation programme. Eur Heart J 1993;14:831–835.
9. Wenger N, Froelicher E, Smith L, et al. Cardiac rehabilitation. Clinical practice guideline no. 17. Rockville, MD: US Department of Health and Human Services, Public Health Service, Agency for Health Care Policy and Research and the National Heart, Lung, and Blood Institute, 1995.
10. Renzulli A, Gobbato F, Maisano G. The interaction between man-work environment and the return to work of coronary patients. The philosophical aspects. Eur Heart J 1988;9(Suppl L):5–7.
11. Wenger N. Rehabilitation of the patient with coronary heart disease: new information for improved care. Postgrad Med 1989;85:369–380.
12. Mark DB, Lam LC, Lee KL, et al. Identification of patients with coronary disease at high risk for loss of employment. A prospective validation study. Circulation 1992;86:1485–1494.
13. Allen JK. Physical and psychosocial outcomes after coronary artery bypass graft surgery: review of the literature. Heart Lung 1990;19:49–55.
14. Shanfield SB. Return to work after an acute myocardial infarction: a review. Heart Lung 1990;19:109–117.
15. Gutmann MC, Sheldahl LM, Tristani FE, et al. Returning the patient to work. In: Pollock ML, Schmidt DH, eds. Heart disease and rehabilitation. 3rd ed. Champaign, IL: Human Kinetics, 1995:405–421.
16. American Heart Association. Heart and stroke statistical update. Dallas, TX: American Heart Association, 1997.
17. Dennis C, Houston-Miller N, Schwartz RG, et al. Early return to work after uncomplicated myocardial infarction: results of a randomized trial. JAMA 1988;260:214–220.
18. DeBusk R. The Stanford University cardiac rehabilitation program. J Myocard Ischem 1990;1:28–45.
19. Fitzgerald S, Merrill A, Aversano T, et al. Direct and indirect cost of percutaneous transluminal coronary angioplasty. Cardiology 1994;85:298–302.
20. DeBusk R, Dennis C. Occupational work evaluation of patients with cardiac disease: a guide for physicians. West J Med 1982;137:515–520.
21. Nair C, Colburn H, McLean D, et al. Cardiovascular disease in Canada. In: Bray D, ed. Health reports. Ottawa: Statistics Canada—Canadian Centre for Health Information, 1989;1:1–22.
22. Dennis C. Vocational capacity with cardiac impairment. In: Scheer SJ, ed. Medical perspectives in vocational assessment of impaired workers. Gaithersburg, MD: Aspen, 1991:301–334.
23. Scheer S. The physician's responsibility in assessing vocational capacity. In: Scheer SJ, ed. Medical perspectives in vocational assessment of impaired workers. Gaithersburg, MD: Aspen, 1991:1–18.
24. Davidson D. Return to work after cardiac events. A review. J Cardiac Rehabil 1983;3:60–69.
25. Criteria Committee of the New York Heart Association. Diseases of the heart and blood vessels: nomenclature and criteria for diagnosis. 6th ed. Boston: Little, Brown and Company, 1953:112–113.
26. Rost K, Smith GR. Return to work after an initial myocardial infarction and subsequent emotional distress. Arch Intern Med 1992;152:381–385.

27. Flynn RJ. Effect of unemployment on depressive affect. In: Cappeliez P, Flynn R, eds. Depression and the social environment: research and intervention with neglected populations. Montreal, Quebec: McGill-Queens University Press, 1993:185–217.

28. Super D. A life span, life space perspective in convergence. In: Lent SA, ed. Convergence in career development theories: implications for science and practice. Palo Alto, CA: CPP Books, 1994:184–196.

29. Lundbom J, Myhre HO, Ystgaard B, et al. Factors influencing return to work after aortocoronary bypass surgery. Scand J Thorac Cardiovasc Surg 1992;26:187–192.

30. Franklin B, Bonzheim K, Berg T. Gender differences in rehabilitation. In: Julian D, Wenger N, eds. Women and heart disease. London: Martin Dunitz, 1997:151–172.

31. Bandura A, Cervone D. Differential engagement of self-reactive influences in cognitive motivation. Organ Behav Hum Decis Processes 1986;38:92–113.

32. Maeland J, Havik O. Psychological predictors for return to work after a myocardial infarction. J Psychosom Res 1987;31:471–481.

33. Dennis C. Rehabilitation of patients with cardiac disease. In: Braunwald E, ed. Heart disease: a textbook of cardiovascular medicine. Philadelphia: WB Saunders, 1991:1388–1393.

34. Petrie KJ, Weinman J, Sharpe N, et al. Role of patients' view of their illness in predicting return to work and functioning after myocardial infarction: longitudinal study. BMJ 1996;312:1191–1194.

35. Mitchell DK. Principles of vocational rehabilitation: a contemporary view. In: Long C, ed. Prevention and rehabilitation in ischemic heart disease. Baltimore: Williams & Wilkins, 1981:314–344.

36. Mulcahy R, Kennedy C, Conroy R. The long term work record of post-infarction patients subjected to a rehabilitation and secondary prevention program. Eur Heart J 1988;9(Suppl L):84–88.

37. Cay E, Walker D. Psychological factors and return to work. Eur Heart J 1988;9(Suppl L):74–81.

38. Riegel BJ. Contributors to cardiac invalidism after acute myocardial infarction. Coron Artery Dis 1993;4:215–220.

39. Maeland J, Havik O. Return to work after a myocardial infarction: the influence of background factors, work characteristics, and illness severity. Scand J Soc Med 1986;14:183–195.

40. Sagall EL. Legal aspects of rehabilitation after myocardial infarction and coronary artery bypass surgery. In: Wenger NK, Hellerstein HK, eds. Rehabilitation of the coronary patient. 2nd ed. New York: John Wiley & Sons, 1984:493–511.

41. Abbott J, Berry N. Return to work during the year following first myocardial infarction. Br J Clin Psychol 1991;30:268–270.

42. Bowe F. Coming back: directions for rehabilitation and disabled workers. Hot Springs, AK: Arkansas Research Training Center in Vocational Rehabilitation, 1986.

43. Stolz I, Erdelyi A. Practical aspects of identifying and correcting worksite stress in post-infarction patients returning to work. Eur Heart J 1988;9(Suppl L):82–83.

44. Hester E. Disability and disincentives: prospective models for change. In: Scheer S, ed. Multidisciplinary perspectives in vocational assessment of impaired workers. Rockville, MD: Aspen, 1990:205–218.

45. Mital A, Shrey DE. Cardiac rehabilitation: potential for ergonomic interventions with special reference to return to work and the Americans with Disabilities Act. Disabil Rehabil 1996;18:149–158.

46. National Institute on Disability and Rehabilitation Research. Rehab brief—cardiac rehabilitation. Washington, DC: US Department of Education, 1980:111.

47. Flynn R, Cupper L, Cavner G, et al. Early identification of return to work difficulties among cardiac patients. Canadian Congress of Rehabilitation, 1989.

48. Balke B. Experimental studies on the functional capacities of middle-aged and aging persons. J Okla Med Assoc 1961;54:120–123.

49. Franklin BA, Rubenfire M. Exercise training in coronary heart disease: mechanisms of improvement. Pract Cardiol 1980;6:84–99.

50. Bruce RA. Principles of exercise testing. In: Naughton JP, Hellerstein HK, eds. Exercise testing and exercise training in coronary heart disease. New York: Academic Press, 1973:45–61.

51. Fox SM, Naughton JP, Haskell WL. Physical activity and the prevention of coronary heart disease. Ann Clin Res 1971;3:404–432.

52. Astrand PO, Rodahl K. Textbook of work physiology. New York: McGraw-Hill, 1970.

53. Hellerstein HK, Franklin BA. Exercise testing and prescription. In: Wenger NK, Hellerstein HK, eds. Rehabilitation of the coronary patient. 2nd ed. New York: John Wiley & Sons, 1984:197–284.

54. Lind A, McNichol G. Muscular factors which determine the cardiovascular responses to sustained and rhythmic exercise. Can Med Assoc J 1967;96:706–715.

55. Mitchell J, Payne P, Saltin B. The role of muscle mass in the cardiovascular response to static contractions. J Physiol (Lond) 1980;309:45–54.

56. Fardy P. Isometric exercise and the cardiovascular system. Physician Sportsmed 1981;9:43–56.

57. Ferguson R, Cote P, Bourassa M. Coronary blood flow during isometric and dynamic exercise in angina pectoris patients. J Cardiac Rehabil 1981;1:21–27.

58. DeBusk R, Pitts W, Haskell W. Comparison of cardiovascular responses to static-dynamic and dynamic effort alone in patients with ischemic heart disease. Circulation 1979;59:977–984.

59. Foster C, Gal RA, Murphy P, et al. Left ventricular function during exercise testing and training. Med Sci Sports Exerc 1996;29:297–305.

60. Franklin B. Exercise testing, training and arm ergometry. Sports Med 1985;2:100–119.

61. Blumenthal J, Bradley W, Dimsdale J, et al. Task force III: assessment of psychological status in patients with ischemic heart disease. J Am Coll Cardiol 1989;14:1034–1041.

62. Williams R, Lane T, Kuhn C, et al. Physiological and neuroendocrine response patterns during different behavioral challenges: differential hyper-responsivity of type A men. Science 1982;218:483–485.

63. Frimerman A, Miller HI, Laniado S, et al. Changes in hemostatic function at times of cyclic variation in occupational stress. Am J Cardiol 1997;79:72–75.

64. Hillbrand M, Spitz RT, eds. Lipids, health, and behavior. Washington, DC: American Psychological Association, 1997:16–46.

65. Theorell T, Perski A, Orth GK, et al. The effects of the strain of returning to work on the risk of cardiac death after a first myocardial infarction before the age of 45. Int J Cardiol 1991;30:61–67.

66. Karasek R, Baker D, Marxer F, et al. Job decision latitude, job demands, and cardiovascular disease: a prospective study of Swedish men. Am J Public Health 1981;71:694–705.

67. Schwartz JE, Pieper CF, Karasek RA. A procedure for linking psychosocial job characteristics to health surveys. Am J Public Health 1988;78:904–909.

68. Karasek RA, Theorell T, Schwartz JE, et al. Job characteristics in relation to the prevalence of myocardial infarction in the US Health Examination Survey (HES) and the Health and Nutrition Examination Study (HANES). Am J Public Health 1988;78:910–918.

69. Spielberg C, Falkenhahn D, Willich SN, et al. Circadian, day-of-week, and seasonal variability in myocardial infarction: comparison between working and retired patients. Am Heart J 1996;132:579–585.

70. Reed DM, LaCroix AZ, Karasek RA, et al. Occupational strain and the incidence of coronary artery disease. Am J Epidemiol 1989;129:459–502.

71. Hlatky MA, Lam LC, Lee KL, et al. Job strain and the prevalence and outcome of coronary artery disease. Circulation 1995;92:327–333.

72. Shearer J. Report of a workshop for the Hamilton Academy of Medicine's section of emergency medicine. Can Med Assoc J 1989;141:243–244.

73. Tepas DI, Duchon JC, Gersten AH. Shiftwork and the older worker. Exp Aging Res 1993;19:295–320.

74. Akerstedt T. Shift-work, shift-dependent well-being and individual differences. Ergonomics 1981;24:265–273.

75. Petronio L. Chemical and physical agents of work-related cardiovascular diseases. Eur Heart J 1988;9(Suppl L):26–34.

76. Sheldahl LW, Wilke NA, Tristani FE. Exercise prescription for return to work. J Cardpulm Rehabil 1985;5:567–575.

77. Hattenhauer M, Neill WA. The effect of cold air inhalation on angina pectoris and myocardial oxygen supply—effect of antianginal medications. Circulation 1975;51:1053–1058.

78. Juneau M, Johnstone M, Dempsey E, et al. Exercise-induced myocardial ischemia in a cold environment—effect of antianginal medications. Circulation 1989;79:1015–1020.

79. Lassvik C, Areskog HH. Angina pectoris during inhalation of cold air. Br Heart J 1980;43:661–667.

80. Franklin B, Bonzheim K, Gordon S, et al. Snow shoveling: a trigger for acute myocardial infarction and sudden coronary death. Am J Cardiol 1996;77:855–858.

81. Willich SN, Lewis M, Lowel H, et al. Physical exertion as a trigger of acute myocardial infarction. Triggers and Mechanisms of Myocardial Infarction Study Group. N Engl J Med 1993;329:1684–1690.

82. Rowell LB, Marz JH, Bruce RA, et al. Reductions in cardiac output, central blood volume, and stroke volume with thermal stress in normal men during exercise. J Clin Invest 1966;45:1801–1816.

83. Pandolf KB, Cafarelli E, Noble BJ, et al. Hyperthermia: effect on exercise prescription. Arch Phys Med Rehabil 1975;56:524–526.

84. Haskell WL, Brachfeld N, Bruce RA, et al. Task Force II: determination of occupational working capacity in patients with ischemic heart disease. J Am Coll Cardiol 1989;14:1025–1034.

85. Hellerstein HK. Prescription of vocational and leisure activities. Adv Cardiol 1978;24:105–115.

86. DeBusk RF, Blomqvist CG, Kouchoukos NT, et al. Identification and treatment of low-risk patients after acute myocardial infarction and coronary-artery bypass surgery. N Engl J Med 1986;314:161–166.

87. DeBusk R, Valdez R, Houston N. Cardiovascular responses to dynamic and static effort soon after myocardial infarction: application to occupational work assessment. Circulation 1978;58:368–375.

88. Litchfield RL, Kerber RE, Benge W, et al. Normal exercise capacity in patients with severe left ventricular dysfunction: compensatory mechanisms. Circulation 1982;66:129–134.

89. Pryor DB, Bruce RA, Chaitman BR, et al. Task Force I. Determination of prognosis in patients with ischemic heart disease. J Am Coll Cardiol 1989;14:1016–1025.

90. Franklin BA, DeBusk RF, Gordon NF, et al. Exercise testing update: with or without CAD—when is activity safe? Physician Sportsmed 1991;19:111–120.

91. Starling MR, Crawford MH, O'Rourke RA. Superiority of selected treadmill exercise protocols predischarge and six weeks postinfarction for detecting ischemic abnormalities. Am Heart J 1982;104:1054–1060.

92. Haskell WL, Savin W, Oldridge N, et al. Factors influencing estimated oxygen uptake during exercise testing soon after myocardial infarction. Am J Cardiol 1982;50:299–307.

93. Franklin BA. Pitfalls in estimating aerobic capacity from exercise time or workload. Appl Cardiol 1986;14:25–26.

94. Franklin BA, Vander L, Wrisley D, et al. Aerobic requirements of arm ergometry: implications for exercise testing and training. Physician Sportsmed 1983;11:81–90.

95. DeBusk RF, Houston N, Haskell W, et al. Exercise training soon after myocardial infarction. Am J Cardiol 1979;44:1223–1229.

96. Savin WM, Haskell WL, Houston-Miller N, et al. Improvement in aerobic capacity soon after myocardial infarction. J Cardiac Rehabil 1981;1:337–342.

97. Weintraub M, Jacoby J, Wigler J, et al. The prognostic value of ECG stress test in postmyocardial infarction patients [abstract]. World Congress on Cardiac Rehabilitation, Jerusalem 1981:82.

98. Velasco JA, Tormo V, Ridocci F, et al. From Spain: return to work after a comprehensive cardiac rehabilitation program. J Cardiac Rehabil 1983;3:735–738.

99. Roskamm H, Gohlke H, Samek L. Long-term effect of aortocoronary bypass surgery on exercise tolerance and vocational rehabilitation [abstract]. World Congress on Cardiac Rehabilitation, Jerusalem 1981:10.

100. Atkins JM, Matthews OA, Blomqvist CG, et al. Incidence of arrhythmias induced by isometric and dynamic exercise. Br Heart J 1976;38:456–471.

101. Blomqvist CG. Upper extremity exercise testing and training. Cardiovasc Clin 1981;15:175–183.

102. Thompson PD. The benefits and risks of exercise training in patients with chronic coronary artery disease. JAMA 1988;259:1537–1540.

103. Brinkley SB. The use of exercise test results in vocational rehabilitation of cardiac clients. In: Naughton JP, Hellerstein HK, eds. Exercise testing and exercise training in coronary heart disease. New York: Academic Press, 1973:307–309.

SECTION V.

Selected Issues
in Secondary Prevention

Sophisticated Lipid Diagnosis and Management: The Potential for Plaque Stabilization and Regression in the Cardiac Rehabilitation Setting

H. Robert Superko and Pat Dunn

ADVANCES IN LIPIDOLOGY AND ATHEROSCLEROSIS

Several issues in the field of lipidology and metabolism recently have become clinically important and can be applied to clinical care. Without knowledge of these advances, many patients will receive treatment that is of little benefit to their disease, despite improved cholesterol values, and some can have significant progression of their disease despite low-density lipoprotein cholesterol (LDL-C) less than 80 mg/dL (1, 2). Advances in the field of metabolic atherosclerosis manipulation now permit physicians to apply these research findings to patient care. To treat coronary artery disease (CAD) appropriately, it is necessary to understand the implications of these findings and how to approach them therapeutically. They include the importance of genetics, lipoprotein heterogeneity associated with insulin resistance, apoprotein E (apo E) polymorphisms, lipoprotein(a) (Lp(a)), postprandial lipemia, low-density lipoprotein (LDL) modification, hypoalphalipoproteinemia, familial defective apoprotein B (apo B), homocysteinemia, cost-effectiveness, and application in the cardiac rehabilitation setting. These topics are important because they are often associated with CAD risk as great or greater than hypercholesterolemia, and are often more common than hypercholesterolemia (Fig. 18.1) (3).

Although elevated blood cholesterol is well established as a cardiovascular (CV) risk factor, it is important to note that approximately 80% of patients who go on to develop CAD have the same blood cholesterol values as those who do not develop CAD (Fig. 18.2) (4). Although the reduction of elevated blood cholesterol can result in a significant reduction in CV events, a large percentage of the groups assigned to receive cholesterol-lowering drugs and able to achieve a reduced blood cholesterol continue to have CV events (Fig. 18.3) (1). This chapter will address many of the important, and common, metabolic issues associated with CAD and how they can be addressed in the cardiac rehabilitation setting.

The laboratory capability to diagnose and treat all the disorders discussed in this chapter is now available to every clinician through a blood mail-in program from laboratories such as those at the Lawrence Orlando Berkeley National Laboratory at the University of California–Berkeley and the Berkeley HeartLab (5). In 80% of CAD patients, an inherited lipoprotein disorder can be identified that is linked to CAD risk. Most of these disorders are inherited in a dominant fashion. This suggests that 50% of first-degree relatives may be at increased risk for CAD.

Lipoprotein Heterogeneity

Most lipoproteins, such as the LDL and high-density lipoprotein (HDL) classes, are not composed of homogeneous lipoproteins but, rather, a spectrum of particles that are quite heterogeneous. Lipoprotein research has led to the delineation of two major forms of HDL, HDL_2 and HDL_3, and to the definition of individual subpopulations within

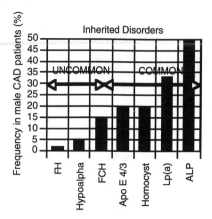

Figure 18.1. Frequency of inherited disorders in the CAD population. The uncommon disorders of familial heterozygous hypercholesterolemia (*FH*), hypoalphalipoproteinemia (*hypoalpha*), and familial combined hyperlipidemia (*FCH*) can be detected by routine lipid panels but are relatively uncommon. The four most common disorders, apo E 4/3, homocysteinemia (*homocyst*), elevated Lp(a), and the Atherogenic Lipoprotein Profile or LDL subclass pattern B (*ALP*) are present in 20% to 50% of CAD patients and are not detected by routine laboratory tests.

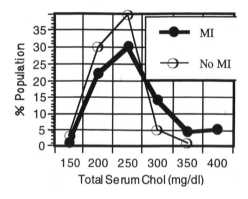

Figure 18.2. Total serum cholesterol (*chol*) values in the Framingham Study and the percent of the population having a myocardial infarction (*MI*) or not (*No MI*). Approximately 80% of MI patients have the same TC values as those who do not have an MI.

these two categories termed HDL_{2b}, HDL_{2a}, HDL_{3a}, HDL_{3b}, and HDL_{3c} (6, 7). Cross-sectional studies reveal that a deficit of HDL_2 is associated with CAD (8). Abnormalities in HDL subclass distribution can exist in the setting of normal high-density lipoprotein cholesterol (HDL-C) values.

Similarly, LDL is not a homogeneous category of lipoproteins but consists of a set of discrete subspecies with distinct molecular properties, including size and density (9, 10). In normal subjects, at least four major LDL sub-

species can be identified (10): LDL-I is the largest and least dense, and, the smallest, LDL-IV, is the most dense (9, 10). Analysis of LDL subspecies is made possible by numerous techniques, including gradient gel electrophoresis, which separates LDL particles into seven regions on the basis of their differing size, and analytic ultracentrifugation, which separates the particles into 12 regions on the basis of their differing density (6, 8, 9). In most healthy people, the major subspecies is large or buoyant, whereas the smaller, denser LDL subspecies are generally present in small amounts.

After a treatment, clinically important LDL subclass distribution changes can occur that are not evident on measures of LDL-C. For example, significant differences in LDL subclass distribution exist despite almost identical LDL-C in persons treated with various combinations of alpha or beta blockers (11, 12). This may be of importance because the Milan regression trial has shown significant arteriographic progression in CAD patients randomized to receive propranolol compared to nitroglycerine (13). Similar significant changes in LDL subclass distribution, despite no change in LDL-C, have been reported with weight loss and gemfibrozil (14, 15).

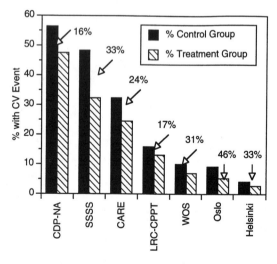

Figure 18.3. The percent of the control and treatment groups who experienced a CV event in seven large clinical trials involving blood lipid and cholesterol reduction. *CDP-NA*, Coronary Drug Project, nicotinic acid arm; *SSSS*, Scandinavian Symvastatin Survival Study; *CARE*, Coronary Artery Recurrent Event; *LRC-CPPT*, Lipid Research Clinic–Coronary Primary Prevention Trial; *WOS*, West of Scotland; *Oslo*, Oslo Heart Study; *Helsinki*, Helsinki Heart Study.

The clinical importance of this issue involves the identification of a highly atherogenic milieu by the presence of specific LDL subclasses. The dense LDL subclass pattern, also referred to as the Atherogenic Lipoprotein Profile (ALP) or LDL pattern B, is a heritable trait determined by a single major dominant gene (the *alp* locus) (16, 17). The gene for this trait has been localized to chromosome 19, near the LDL receptor loci, and to three other loci (18, 19). Thirty percent to 35% of people are heterozygous for *alp,* and another 5% are homozygous. The full expression of this trait occurs after puberty in men and after menopause in women. Hypertriglyceridemia is often associated with LDL pattern B, and epidemiologic analysis has now identified elevated triglycerides (TGs) as an independent CAD risk factor, but it is the presence of ALP that is associated with moderately elevated TGs that create the atherogenic conditions (20, 21). In addition to increased risk for CAD, pattern B trait is also associated with in-

sulin resistance, low HDL$_{2b}$, elevated intermediate-density lipoprotein (IDL), enhanced postprandial lipemia, low vitamin E lipoprotein particle content, and increased susceptibility to oxidation (22–24).

Low-density lipoprotein subclass distribution is best determined by analytic ultracentrifugation (ANUC) (6), but a less expensive method, gradient gel electrophoresis (GGE), has been successfully used in parallel with ANUC in several clinical trials at the Lawrence Berkeley National Laboratory and Berkeley HeartLab (25).

The LDL pattern B trait is associated with a tendency toward elevated levels of TG, very low-density lipoprotein (VLDL), and IDL, as well as reduced levels of HDL. The LDL pattern B can persist, however, even when levels of TG and HDL are normal (Fig. 18.4). In general, the higher the TG values, the greater the likelihood the LDL particles will be small and dense. It is important to note the significant overlap between LDL pattern

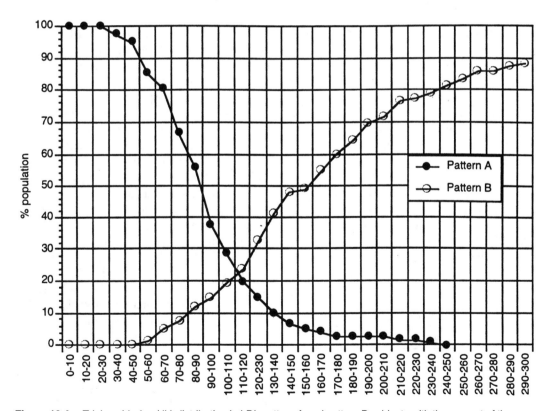

Figure 18.4.   Triglyceride (mg/dL) distribution in LDL pattern A and pattern B subjects with the percent of the population who are LDL pattern A or B for a given fasting TG represented. Individuals with fasting TGs in excess of 250 mg/dL are most likely LDL pattern B whereas individuals with fasting TGs less than 70 mg/dL are most likely LDL pattern A. Individuals with TGs between 70 and 250 mg/dL can be either LDL pattern A or pattern B and a GGE analysis is required to properly classify them as LDL pattern A or pattern B.

A and LDL pattern B for the TG range of 70 to 250 mg/dL. Within this range, Tgs are an unreliable predictor of LDL subclass pattern (26).

Studies have found that LDL size is a powerful predictor of CAD risk, independent of TGs, HDL-C, LDL-C, and body mass index. An early study, the Boston Area Health Study, reported that in myocardial infarction (MI) patients versus control subjects only HDL-C was significantly lower and TGs significantly higher while LDL-C was not different between the groups (Table 18.1). Analysis of this early study indicated that LDL subclass pattern B carried a threefold greater risk of CAD, despite no difference in LDL-C (17).

In 1996 and 1997, three prospective trials that investigated the predictive nature of LDL size were reported. The Physicians Health Study investigated the importance of LDL subclass pattern on CAD risk in 14,916 men (27). After 7 years of follow-up in 266 patients and 308 control subjects, statistical modeling revealed that LDL diameter was related to CAD risk and was statistically significant before including nonfasting TG values.

The Stanford Five City Project prospectively investigated the relationship of LDL size to the incidence of CAD in 124 matched pairs of CAD patients and control subjects between 1979 and 1992 (28). Low-density lipoprotein size was significantly smaller ($P < 0.001$) among CAD patients compared with control subjects. The association was graded across quintiles of LDL size. This difference was statistically independent of HDL-C, non-HDL-C, TG, smoking, blood pressure, and body mass index. It was not statistically independent of the total cholesterol (TC) to HDL-C ratio. Among all the physiologic risk factors, LDL size was the best differentiator of CAD status in conditional logistic regression, whereas

TC/HDL-C was a stronger independent predictor of CAD status.

The Quebec Cardiovascular study was a prospective investigation of CAD risk factors in 2103 asymptomatic men in seven counties of the Quebec metropolitan area (29). After 5 years of follow-up, LDL diameter proved to be an independent predictor of CAD risk. The power of LDL size as a risk predictor was independent of age, body mass index, alcohol consumption, smoking, fasting TGs, apo B, and LDL-C and HDL-C. The combined presence of small LDL and elevated apo B produced an even greater (sixfold) increase in CAD risk.

Because each LDL particle carries only one apo B-100, measuring apo B may be a more precise determination of the number of LDL particles than measuring LDL-C (30). Unfortunately, few studies that involve TGs and CAD report apo B values. This is important because of the high incidence of hyperapobetalipoproteinemia (81%) in the post-MI population that exhibits relatively "normal" LDL-C and moderately elevated plasma TGs (30). Persons with this condition have an overabundance of small, dense LDL particles similar to those noted in patients who have ALP or familial combined hyperlipidemia and in patients who have more progression of CAD demonstrated on arteriography (31–33). This interaction of a dense LDL pattern and elevations in plasma TGs eventually may help clarify the association of TGs and CAD. Unfortunately, a ratio of LDL-C to apo B is not an effective predictor of LDL subclass pattern (34).

Coronary arteriographic evidence indicates that subjects who exhibited arrest of angiographically determined CAD progression, or regression, had significantly greater reductions in IDL ($S_f12–20$) and "dense" LDL ($S_f0–7$), compared with subjects who exhibited CAD progression (31, 33, 35–37). In some of these investigations, change in lipoprotein subclass distribution was a better predictor of arteriographic outcome than was change in LDL-C (35, 38).

The clinical implications of LDL heterogeneity are profound. Although elevated LDL-C increases CAD risk, it appears that an LDL subclass distribution abnormality is a more common and powerful predictor of risk. It is present in 50% of men with CAD and identifies a group of people who can respond particularly well to appropriate

Table 18.1. Analysis of Cholesterol and Triglycerides in Patients with Myocardial Infarction and in Normal Volunteers (17)

	MI Cases	Controls	P
Total cholesterol (mg/dL)	226	215	NS
LDL-C (mg/dL)	144	138	NS
HDL-C (mg/dL)	33	40	<0.01
Triglycerides (mg/dL)	214	157	<0.01

MI = myocardial infarction; LDL-C = low-density lipoprotein cholesterol; HDL-C = high-density lipoprotein cholesterol.

treatment and are good arteriographic responders to treatment. Total cholesterol and LDL-C are frequently within normal limits in these individuals, and thus their high risk status is not identified on routine blood lipid tests.

Apoprotein E Polymorphism

Another common inherited trait that affects LDL-C levels is differences in apo E isoforms. There are three major isoforms: E2, E3, and E4 (39–41). The E protein is attached to TG-rich lipoproteins, but not LDL. One of its roles is to regulate lipoprotein particle uptake by the hepatic B-E receptor. The hepatic B-E receptor recognizes both apo B and apo E. The most common allele, E3, has a frequency of approximately 0.78, whereas E4 has a frequency of 0.15, and E2, a frequency of 0.07 (42). Several studies have established that the E4 allele is associated with higher and E2 with lower levels of LDL-C and apo B (compared with the E3 allele). Hepatic LDL receptor activity is relatively higher in persons who have the apo E2 genotype (41–43). Postprandial lipid metabolism differences exist between E3/E4 subjects and normal E3/E3 subjects (44–46). Persons with the E4 allele have enhanced postprandial lipemia, which may contribute to CAD (45). This difference is not apparent in the fasting state.

The disease type III hyperlipoproteinemia is an example of an interaction of the apo E2 homozygous state with another genetic or environmental factor, leading to marked accumulation of TG-rich lipoprotein remnants and accelerated atherosclerosis (46, 47). More than 90% of persons who have type III hyperlipoproteinemia are apo E2 homozygotes; however, the disease is caused by interaction of the apo E2/E2 state with another genetic or environmental factor because most persons with E2/E2 do not exhibit the abnormal lipid profile characteristic of Type III.

The clinical relevance of apo E genotypes relates to the association of abnormal lipoprotein metabolism, differential effects on therapy, and possible association with CAD. Because the apo E isoform is a genetically fixed characteristic, it need only be determined once for each patient. It is useful in analyzing potential differences in response to a therapeutic intervention because a subgroup may respond more favorably to the treatment, but the response in the entire group may be diluted because of the inclusion of a non-responsive E isoform group in the analysis (48). Apoprotein E4 can now be considered a CV risk factor, and apo E4 has been shown to be related to CAD in young men, independent of plasma cholesterol concentrations (49). This suggests that apo E genotypic effects on arterial lesions may not be mediated entirely by differences in plasma cholesterol concentrations.

Apoprotein E isoforms explain part of the individual differences in LDL-C response to a reduced fat diet (50). Men with the apo E 3/4 pattern respond to a reduced fat diet with significantly greater LDL-C reduction compared to men with the apo E 3/3 pattern (48). Postprandial lipid responses to a fat meal exist between E 3/4 subjects and normal E 3/3 subjects (44, 45). Individuals with the E4 allele have enhanced postprandial lipemia, which may contribute to CAD, and this difference is not apparent in the fasting state (51). This differential response to diet has implications for clinical decision on who may benefit most from nutrition counseling in the era of limited health care dollars.

An association between the apo E4 allele and Alzheimer's disease has recently been elucidated. In families with a history of Alzheimer's disease, the presence of one E4 allele increases the risk of developing Alzheimer's to approximately 49% and in those family members with two E4 alleles, to approximately 91% (52). This relationship certainly involves both other genetic and environmental interactions (53). At the present time it is recommended that the E4 allele not be used to predict Alzheimer's risk in the general population (Table 18.2) (54).

Table 18.2.   Clinical Implications of Apoprotein E Isoform Patterns

E3/3	E2/2	E4/3(4/4)
"Normal" pattern	Potential to express type III HLP Good fibrate responders	Increased CAD risk 1.3-fold Good LDL-C responders to low-fat diet Good LDL-C responders to probucol Enhanced postprandial lipemia Alzheimer's link?

CAD = coronary artery disease; HLP = ; LDL-C = low-density lipoprotein cholesterol.

Lipoprotein(a)

Lipoprotein(a) is an LDL particle with a second protein, called [a], attached by a disulfide bridge to apo B. This protein [a] is homologous to plasminogen and appears to be composed of 35 to 45 repeating units, similar to plasminogen kringle number 4 (55). Lipoprotein(a) is an independent risk factor for MI in young men and is independently associated with arteriographically defined coronary disease (56, 57). The Framingham trial has revealed that values in excess of 35 mg/dL are associated with a twofold increased CAD risk and the level of risk is similar to TC greater than 240 mg/dL or HDL-C less than 35 mg/dL (58). The CAD risk associated with elevated Lp(a) is greatly enhanced by the presence of other risk factors, such as elevated LDL-C and ALP (59).

Although no prospective human trials designed to lower Lp(a) and monitor CAD events have been reported, it is interesting to note that in the Familial Atherosclerosis Treatment Study (FATS), the mean Lp(a) in subjects who experienced a clinical event was 51 mg/dL, whereas in the group free of clinical events, it was 25 mg/dL (60). Medications have little effect on Lp(a) levels, although recent evidence suggests that nicotinic acid, and perhaps estrogen and testosterone, may have some effect (61–63). Plasmapheresis has also been used to effectively lower Lp(a) and was associated with a significant reduction in restenosis following angioplasty (64).

Despite the importance of Lp(a) in determining CAD risk, there is no international standard for Lp(a) determination, and commercial sources of Lp(a) measurements do not appear to have the same quality control standards as research laboratories, which have internal standards. This means that results published in the medical literature may not be applicable to values obtained in commercial laboratories. A survey conducted at Berkeley HeartLab of repeat measurements revealed a small range of error (-1 mg/dL to $+5$ mg/dL) in blinded specimens analyzed internally versus a large range of error (-145 mg/dL to $+25$ mg/dL) among the same specimens submitted to commercial labs (1).

Postprandial Lipemia

After a meal, plasma TGs and lipoproteins undergo dynamic change, which is a period called postprandial lipemia. The atherogenic process probably occurs during the entire 24 hours of a typical day, and blood lipid measurements obtained at 8 am, after an overnight fast, often do not reflect nonfasting lipid status (65). Indeed, it has been hypothesized that atherosclerosis is a postprandial phenomenon (66).

The association of abnormalities in postprandial lipemia (PPL) and CAD is not a new concept. In 1963, Harlan and Beischer (67) described a greater PPL period in patients who had CAD, compared to "normals" (68). Although the association of postprandial lipoprotein abnormalities and CAD has yet to be fully clarified, postprandial abnormalities are present in patients who have LDL pattern B, hyperapobetalipoproteinemia, and abnormalities in apo E isoforms (11, 69, 70). Abnormal postprendial lipemia has also been identified as a CAD risk factor (71). Genetic differences in Lp(a) response to fat meals are suggested by the finding that the greatest increase in TG-rich lipoprotein-associated [a] occurs in subjects who show the lowest fasting Lp(a) levels (69). The apo[a] from postprandial with d less than 1.006 lipoproteins was larger than two other apo[a] subspecies obtained at d = 1.05 − 1.09 (69). Gender differences appear to affect postprandial lipemia, and significantly greater increases in HDL_2 ($P < 0.05$) occur 4.5 hours after a meal in women compared to men (72). This may reflect the efficiency of reverse cholesterol transport.

Therapeutic maneuvers that can alter PPL often are not reflected on fasting blood tests. Treatment of hypertension with β-blocking medication significantly ($P < 0.008$) increases PPL despite no significant difference in fasting TG concentrations, whereas α-blocking medication shows a decrease in PPL. Physical activity can be associated with significant reductions in PPL and may be one mechanism of the beneficial CV effect of chronic physical activity (73). Chronic alcohol consumption is known to have a significant effect on fasting plasma TGs, HDL-C, and HDL_3-C. Alcohol also enhances the postprandial response twofold when taken with a meal, compared to consuming alcohol with no food (74).

Lipid-lowering medications, such as nicotinic acid and gemfibrozil, that have an effect on fasting TGs can lower PPL significantly (15, 75). Other medications, such as the hydroxymethylglutaryl-CoA (HMG-CoA) reductase inhibitor fluvastatin—

described as having only a mild effect on fasting TGs—actually have significant effects on PPL not reflected in changes in fasting measurements (76). Bile acid binding resins can increase PPL, particularly in subjects who have elevated TGs (77).

Low-density Lipoprotein Modification (Oxidation)

Modification, or oxidation, of apoproteins may contribute to atherosclerosis in humans. Oxidation of apo B has been shown to result in a modified LDL particle that is taken up rapidly by a scavenger receptor on tissue macrophages, resulting in atherogenic foam cell formation, inhibition of macrophage egress from the artery wall, and damage to the endothelial border that contributes to atherosclerosis in animal models (78).

This in vitro modification can occur in the presence of endothelial cells. Incubation of LDL with cultured endothelial cells results in a modified LDL (m-LDL) that is taken up by macrophages 3 to 10 times more rapidly than native LDL, resulting in atherogenic foam cell formation (79–81). This m-LDL undergoes many structural changes, most of which depend on peroxidation of polyunsaturated fatty acids in the LDL lipids that can be inhibited by vitamin E (82, 83).

The human pathologic effects of m-LDL are believed to occur in the arterial wall because addition of plasma to the in vitro system results in inhibition of cell-induced oxidation, in part caused by naturally circulating plasma antioxidants (84). Once the LDL contains fatty acid lipid peroxides, a propagation follows that amplifies the number of free radicals and leads to extensive fragmentation of the fatty acid chains (85, 86). High-density lipoprotein and the associated apoproteins, A-I and A-II, may play a protective role in inhibiting oxidation of apo B on the LDL particle. Apoproteins A-I and A-I/A-II, and HDL itself, have a protective effect on Cu^{2+}-catalyzed oxidation of human LDL (87). A portion of lipoprotein oxidative susceptibility involves lipoprotein vitamin E content.

Evidence in humans that vitamin E supplementation may be of benefit can be found in two investigations. Analysis of CLAS data has revealed that patients who self-selected to consume vitamin E had significantly better arteriographic outcome compared to those who did not (88). The Cambridge Heart Attack and Antioxidant Study (CHAOS) randomly assigned 2000 male CAD patients to receive either 800 IU vitamin E per day or placebo (89). After 17 months, the vitamin E group was found to have significantly fewer nonfatal MIs.

Familial Defective Apoprotein B

Familial defective apo B (FDB) is a genetic disorder that results from a single nucleotide mutation (90). It occurs in approximately 1 in 500 people in the general population and is associated with LDL-C between 270 and 370 mg/dL (91). The LDL receptor function is normal; however, because of the abnormal apo B, only 32% of receptor-binding activity is found. This relatively uncommon cause for hypercholesterolemia exhibits LDL-C values in the same range as that of patients who have familial heterozygous hypercholesterolemia (FH). One major difference is that only one genetic defect has been found for FDB, whereas approximately 30 mutations have been found for the LDL receptor. Whether FDB patients frequently exhibit the clinical manifestations of FH, tendon xanthoma are uncommon.

Hypoalphalipoproteinemia

Low HDL-C has been determined to be a CAD risk factor in numerous epidemiologic and clinical trials. Low HDL (less than 25 mg/dL) is generally felt to have a genetic cause, which is transmitted in an autosomal dominant fashion, strongly linked to premature CAD and has been called hypoalphalipoproteinemia (92). One genetic cause is a polymorphism in the region between the apolipoprotein A-I and apolipoprotein C-III genes, which results in abnormally low HDL values (93). In these patients, elevated TGs or elevated LDL-C are not necessarily common, and isolated low HDL is the main contributor to premature CAD.

Homocysteinemia

In the 1800s, medical experts debated whether atherosclerosis was caused by diets rich in dairy fat or rich in protein (94). The supporters of the fat hypothesis won the day, in part because laboratory methods existed to measure cholesterol, but laboratory methods to measure amino acids had not been developed. Recent evidence suggests that homocysteine, a thiol-containing amino acid derived from methionine, is linked to coronary heart disease. The rare genetic disorder, homocystinuria, substantially increases the risk of thromboembolic disorders, and MI is not uncommon as the fatal event in young individuals who have homocystinuria (95).

The enzyme cystathionine β-synthase controls an early reaction in the transfersulfuration of homocysteine to cysteine and plays a pivotal role in the remethylation of homocysteine to methionine. Numerous investigations have now indicated that homocysteine blood levels are elevated in approximately 20% of CAD patients and 30% of peripheral vascular disease patients (96, 97). It has been suggested that persons heterozygous for cystathionine β-synthase may be at increased risk for CAD (98). Elevated plasma homocysteine levels are a strong predictor of mortality in CAD patients (99).

The disorder can be diagnosed by fasting homocyst(e)ine values or by a postmethionine load value. Abnormal range for fasting values has been suggested to be more than 14 μmol/L (100, 101). Fasting values in excess of 14 μmol/L and post postmethionine load values greater than 38 mmol/L at 6 hours have been suggested as levels at which treatment may be beneficial (101, 102). It is important to note that even in the setting of very low CAD risk, because of an HDL-C greater than 90 mg/dL, CAD and PVD (peripheral vascular disease) can still occur in hyperhomocystinemic patients (103). The commonly used lipid-altering medication nicotinic acid may impair folate absorption and result in elevated homocystine values (104). Therapy is low risk and involves high doses of pyridoxine or folate (1 to 5 mg/day) (105).

Importance of Genetics

Findings suggest that much of CAD is genetically linked, and this has important diagnostic, family counseling, and therapeutic implications. The more precise the diagnosis of a specific cause, the more individualized can be the therapy. In this early era of metabolic manipulation of CAD, this is extremely important. Family counseling is important in cases in which a genetic abnormality can be identified. Often, CAD victims have offspring in their 20s to 30s, which is the prime time for an aggressive primary prevention effort if these children are found to have inherited the trait or traits that are present in their CAD-afflicted parent. Although the genetic

abnormality itself cannot be altered, expression of the trait can be suppressed and it is established that aggressive manipulation of other CAD risk factors can reduce the risk in the victim and in the offspring.

The previous sections in this chapter have demonstrated several atherogenic conditions that are genetically linked. In several, the chromosomal location for the abnormality is known. For example, the LDL receptor is located on the short arm of chromosome 19, and the Lp(a) gene is located in close proximity to the plasminogen gene located at chromosome 6q27 (18, 106, 107). Presently, more than 20 genetically linked lipoprotein abnormalities that contribute to CAD have been identified (108). Many of these inherited traits are transmitted in a Mendelian dominant fashion. Clinical identification of these abnormalities is important to diagnose accurately the cause of atherosclerosis, to help determine proper therapy, and to conduct appropriate family counseling. The last issue may be the most important because it can result in identification, risk stratification, and therapy in appropriate persons at an early age. Construction of a family pedigree can be of great help in identifying family members who may have inherited the same trait or combination of traits that are present in the family member with established CAD. Figure 18.5 represents one such family examined at the Cholesterol, Genetics, and Heart Disease Institute.

The future is bright with regard to potential gene therapy. Studies with transgenic mice suggest that genetic manipulation may offer substantial therapeutic options (109). Human genetic therapy is not in the far distant future. In mice, a transgenic line has been created that expresses high levels of human apo A-I and results in an HDL particle distribution similar in size to human HDL_2 and HDL_3 (109). In the next decade, transgenic human experiments may offer an alternative lipoprotein manipulation therapy to classic pharmacology.

CLINICAL TRIALS EVIDENCE

Epidemiologic Studies

Atherosclerosis is a fatal disease and only relatively recently have arteriographic studies documented that regression of this disease is a possibility. It is established that plasma cholesterol

Family Pedigree

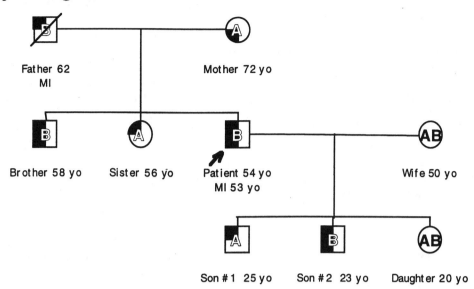

Figure 18.5. Pedigree example. A, AB, or B represents the presence of LDL pattern A, AB, or B. The father died of heart disease at the age of 62, and he had elevated Lp(a) and LDL pattern B. One of his sons (54 years old, *arrow*) had a heart attack at the age of 53, and his blood test results were identical to his father's except he additionally had homocystinemia that he inherited from his mother. Among the patient's siblings, the 58-year-old brother is the one to worry about the most because his test results are the same as the 54-year-old brother who already has had a heart attack. The sister has only elevated Lp(a) but does not have LDL pattern B or homocystinemia. This reflects a lower heart disease risk. Among the patient's children, the 23-year-old son is the one most at risk because his blood test results look like his father's in regard to the presence of the high-risk heart disease risk factors. By using such an analysis, families can identify those members at highest risk and implement preventive measures early to reduce their heart disease risk and, as in the case of the 58-year-old brother, consider noninvasive CV testing to determine whether heart disease is present but not yet apparent. This can be lifesaving.

and the family of plasma lipoproteins are major factors in the pathogenesis of coronary atherosclerosis (110). Evidence that these lipoproteins play a major causal role in the etiology of atherosclerosis is abundant and convincing (111–115). Observation and intervention trials have demonstrated that elevated plasma cholesterol increases CAD risk, and that reduction in elevated plasma cholesterol results in fewer CV events. However, as mentioned at the beginning of this chapter, 80% of CAD patients have the same TC as those who do not develop CAD. This means that if clinicians focus only on reducing LDL-C, it will be a disservice for the majority of their patients. A brief review of these investigations will contribute to clarifying this issue.

The Framingham Heart Study is an ongoing surveillance study conducted in more than 5000 men and women and has been in progress for more than 35 years (4). A stepwise increase in serum cholesterol and the associated increase in 24-year incidence of CAD were particularly powerful factors in young men but were much less apparent in women. The contribution of LDL to CAD risk in young men was apparent in the Framingham study (116). In an older population of men and women (aged 50 to 80 years), LDL-C was associated significantly ($P < 0.05$) with CAD after 7 years of follow-up (4).

The Multiple Risk Factor Intervention Trial (MRFIT) investigated the effect of hypertension control, diet advice, and smoking cessation on the development of CAD (117). In this study, 361,662 men were screened, and a 6-year mortality rate was calculated in relation to serum cholesterol (118). Three important clinical lessons resulted from this analysis. First, for men who have serum cholesterol higher than 181 mg/dL, the risk of CAD death increased progressively, which suggests that defining a "safe" cholesterol level may lull many persons into a false sense of security. Second, for men who had serum cholesterol levels in excess of 253 mg/dL, the relative risk was 3.8 times greater than for men with levels lower than 181 mg/dL. Finally, although serum cholesterol higher than the 90th percentile is often used to define "hypercholesterolemia," 54% of the CAD occurred in men whose levels fell between the 20th (181 mg/dL) and 85th (253 mg/dL) percentiles, and the other 46% occurred in men above the 85th percentile. This last lesson may be the most important and indicates that targeting only persons who have "hypercholesterolemia" for treatment misses the majority of high-risk persons. It also indicates that total serum cholesterol may not be an adequate laboratory measurement to define lipoprotein-mediated CAD risk.

The independent relationship between plasma TGs and CAD has now been established (21). The Dresden hyperlipoproteinemia study (119) supports the need to lower elevated plasma lipids and, in particular, TGs. Using a nonblinded protocol, this study investigated the efficacy of TG and cholesterol reduction on CV complications and mortality in 260 patients who had hyperlipoproteinemia for a mean of 67 months (119). The appearance of angina seemed to cluster in the "moderate" reduction group. Myocardial infarction was significantly lower, however, in the "effective" control group, compared with the "insufficient" lipid reduction group. The Stockholm Prospective Study (120) contributed powerful information that treatment of elevated TGs results in clinical benefit. The Stockholm Study investigated the relation of plasma TGs to CAD in 3486 subjects. During a 14-year period 176 MIs occurred. Although cholesterol and TGs were independent risk factors for CAD, TGs were the more important of the two. The MI rate for the bottom quintile of TGs and cholesterol was 16/1000 and 27/1000, respectively, and for the top quintile of TGs and cholesterol, it was 65/1000 and 47/1000, respectively. Additional investigative work in Stockholm revealed that treatment with clofibrate and nicotinic acid resulted in a significant reduction in fatal CV events (120). The benefit of treatment in this investigation was particularly beneficial in patients who had a fasting TG of more than 200 mg/dL at baseline, and in those in whom greater than 30% reduction in TGs was

achieved. This finding assumes added clinical importance with the recent knowledge that mild to moderate elevations in TGs often indicate the presence of LDL pattern B.

High-density lipoprotein cholesterol and HDL subclass distributions commonly demonstrate an inverse relationship to CAD. The observation that low HDL-C was associated with CAD was verified by the Lipid Research Clinics (LRC) Study, which revealed HDL-C to have the strongest standard lipoprotein relation (inverse) to CAD (121). In men who have HDL-C lower than 25 mg/dL, the CAD incidence during 4 years was 180/1000 compared to 25/1000 in men who had HDL-C in excess of 64 mg/dL. Furthermore, this relationship persisted above the age of 60 years. The Livermore Study monitored 1961 men for 10 years and reported significant associations between HDL subclasses and CAD (122). Both HDL_2 and HDL_3 were correlated inversely to CAD events, and in men who developed CAD events, the antecedent reduction in HDL_2 concentration was disproportionately large. The clinical relevance of this observation is that reductions in HDL_2 may be a harbinger of CV events and reflects impaired "reverse cholesterol transport."

This investigation, conducted at the Lawrence Berkeley National Laboratory, is important because it is one of the few large trials that used ultracentrifugation to determine the lipoprotein profile as a continuous spectrum of particles. This allowed for the fine discrimination and definition of lipoprotein classes. Most other investigations have used the standard precipitation techniques to separate lipoprotein classes into heterogeneous groups that may obscure clinically important changes in lipoprotein subclasses. When precipitation methods are used to determine HDL-C and estimate LDL-C, IDL is included in the LDL-C measurement. Thus, an important question for studies that reveal an association between LDL-C change and outcome is how much of the benefit is caused by changes in IDL that are obscured by the laboratory methodology. In the setting of relatively "normal" LDL-C, IDL is a more powerful predictor of CAD severity than is LDL (123). Elevated IDL is found in LDL subclass pattern B.

In the Tromso Heart Study, 6595 relatively young men (20 to 49 years) were observed for 2 years (124). Seventeen had MIs, and each case was matched with two control subjects for age, residence, ethnic origin, and physical activity. The HDL-C made a threefold greater contribution to the prediction of CAD events than LDL-C in the "young" population (d < 1.063). Total cholesterol and TGs were not different between the groups. Mean LDL-C was 222 mg/dL and 190 mg/dL in the MI patients and control subjects (*P* < 0.005), respectively, and HDL-C was 25.6 mg/dL and 39.4 mg/dL (*P* < 0.005), respectively.

A gender difference exists in the relationship of HDL-C to CAD: 7569 men and women free of CAD were followed in the LRC prevalence study for 8.4 years (121). It was concluded that HDL-C was inversely related to CAD in both men and women. In women HDL-C was more closely related to CV disease than LDL-C. The HDL-C increments of 10 mg/dL were similar to a CV disease mortality rate ratio of LDL-C increments of 30 mg/dL. In the 7-year Framingham Study follow-up, HDL-C has the strongest correlation with CAD events of all the lipoprotein measurements (*P* < 0.001) (116). From the Framingham data, an HDL-C risk multiplier table has been developed. These data demonstrate the gender difference in HDL-C and CAD risk and are illustrated in Table 18.3.

A combined analysis of the relationship between HDL-C and CAD in four large investigations confirms the inverse relationship of HDL-C to heart disease, as well as its independent role in CAD risk prediction (122). The Framingham Heart Study (FHS), Lipid Research Clinics Prevalence Mortality Follow-Up Study (LRCF), the LRC-Coronary Primary Prevention Trial Placebo Group, and the Multiple Risk Factor Intervention

Trial (MRFIT) control groups were used for the analysis. In general, a 1-mg/dL increase in HDL-C was associated with a significant reduction in CAD risk of 2% in men and 3% in women. In the LRCF, in which only fatal end points were documented, a 1-mg/dL increase in HDL-C was associated with a significant reduction of fatal end points of 3.7% in men and 4.7% in women. The HDL-C level was unrelated to non-CV disease mortality.

As discussed above, LDL subclass determination is actually more informative in determining CAD risk than is total, LDL-C, HDL-C, or TGs. The Boston Area Health Study, the Physicians Health Survey, the Stanford Five City Project, and the Quebec Cardiovascular Study all confirmed the high risk of LDL pattern B (17, 27–29). Low-density lipoprotein pattern B is associated with low HDL_2 and low HDL_{2b}. This is clinically important because this common, genetically determined CAD risk factor is not reflected by measurement of LDL-C. Furthermore, the Quebec Study revealed that if the LDL particle is small, it increases CV risk three- to fivefold independent of all other risk factors and lipid measurements. It helps explain the high incidence of CAD in the majority of patients who do not have classic hypercholesterolemia.

Clinical Trials

Many large, randomized clinical trials have confirmed the cholesterol hypothesis—that is, that actively lowering elevated blood cholesterol results in reduced CAD events. The World Health Organization (WHO) Cooperative Trial was a double-blind trial using the medication clofibrate to reduce blood cholesterol (125). In this 5-year trial, 15,745 men were enrolled, half of whom had serum cholesterol in the upper third of the normal distribution. The subjects were randomly assigned into three groups: one was treated with clofibrate, the second was a control group with cholesterol in the upper third distribution, and the third was a control group with cholesterol in the lower third distribution. Serum cholesterol was reduced approximately 9% by the medication and resulted in a significant reduction in nonfatal MIs (*P* < 0.05). This reduction in nonfatal MIs was seen to the greatest extent in those men who smoked cigarettes and in those who had elevated blood pressure.

Table 18.3. Relative Risk for Coronary Disease Based on HDL-C Value (mg/dl)

HDL-C	Men	Women
30	1.8	NA
35	1.5	NA
40	1.2	1.9
45	1.0	1.6
50	0.8	1.3
55	0.7	1.0
60	0.6	0.8
65	0.5	0.6
70	NA	0.5

HDL-C = high-density lipoprotein cholesterol; NA = not available.

Unfortunately, 25% more deaths from all causes ($P < 0.01$) and a greater number of cholecystectomies were reported in the clofibrate-treated group ($P < 0.001$).

The Coronary Drug Project (CDP) was a double-blind, randomized, placebo-controlled clinical trial designed to use several medications to reduce elevated blood cholesterol in patients who previously had survived an MI (126). Five medications initially were used, but three of them, two estrogen doses (5.0 mg/day, 2.5 mg/day) and dextrothyroxine, were discontinued prematurely because of excessive drug-related morbidity and mortality. Estrogen was discontinued because of an excessive number of nonfatal CV events, excessive thromboembolism, and increased cancer mortality compared with the placebo group. One of the two remaining medications, clofibrate, resulted in approximately a 6% reduction in serum cholesterol but was associated with an increased incidence of complications.

The remaining medication, nicotinic acid, resulted in approximately a 10% reduction in serum cholesterol. When compared to the placebo group, almost identical death rates caused by CAD were evident, but the incidence of nonfatal MI was 27% lower in the nicotinic acid group than in the placebo group (nicotinic acid = 8.9%, placebo = 12.2%; $P < 0.01$). The incidence of saphenous vein bypass surgery was lower in patients treated with nicotinic acid, and cerebral vascular accidents were 24% lower in the nicotinic acid group, which approached statistical significance. A 15-year follow-up analysis was conducted 9 years after completion of the trial and nicotinic acid therapy. Surprisingly, this follow-up study found that mortality from all causes in each group was similar, except for the group treated with nicotinic acid. In the nicotinic acid group, mortality was 11% lower ($P < 0.002$) than in the placebo group (127). This cholesterol-lowering study revealed a significant reduction in all-cause mortality in the nicotinic acid group (128).

The Coronary Primary Prevention Trial (CPPT) was a 10-year clinical investigation of the effect of LDL-C reduction in 3806 asymptomatic men who had TC in excess of 265 mg/dL (129). The cholestyramine-treatment group revealed 8.5% and 12.6% greater reductions in TC and LDL-C, respectively, compared to the placebo group. This resulted in a 24% reduction in definite CAD death and a 19% reduction in nonfatal MI. The difference between the cholestyramine and placebo groups was statistically significant, using a one-tailed Student's t test. From this data, the proportional hazards statistical model predicts that a 25% reduction in TC will result in a 49% reduction in CAD risk. This is the origin of the generalization that for every 1% reduction in total plasma cholesterol, a 2% reduction in CAD risk can be expected in men with elevated LDL-C.

The HDL-C increase in the cholestyramine group was associated with fewer CV end points. For each 1-mg/dL increase in HDL-C, there was a 5.5% reduction in risk of definite CAD death or MI. Similar associations were seen in the placebo group. The higher the HDL-C, the more risk reduction was achieved for a given amount of LDL-C reduction. In the group with the lowest HDL-C at the start of the trial, reduction in LDL-C did not result in a significant reduction in CV events. This suggests that the low HDL-C group may remain a high-risk group for reasons other than LDL-C levels. Because this group was identified by low HDL-C, it was probably enriched in LDL pattern B subjects, and resins are not the drug of choice for this disorder.

The Helsinki Trial was a 5-year, double-blind, randomized trial on the effects of gemfibrozil on CAD events in 4081 healthy, middle-aged men, 63% of whom were classified as Fredrickson type IIa, 28% as type IIb, and 9% as type IV (130). The drop-out rate was 29.9%. After a mean follow-up of 60 months, the total number of CAD events was significantly lower ($P < 0.02$, two-tailed Student's t test) in the gemfibrozil group than in the placebo group. The greatest reduction was in nonfatal MIs (37%; $P < 0.05$), which is consistent with the CDP results. A second analysis of the Helsinki results indicated that in a group with fasting TGs greater than 200 mg/dL, and an elevated TC/HDL-C ratio, a 74% reduction in clinical events was observed (131). This cohort comprised approximately 10% of the study population and supports the concept that the treatment should match the disorder. If treatment is not individualized, many patients will expend time and money on a therapy that is of no benefit to them.

Most recently several additional investigations strengthen the evidence. The Scandinavian Simvastatin Survival Study (SSSS) was a 5-year inves-

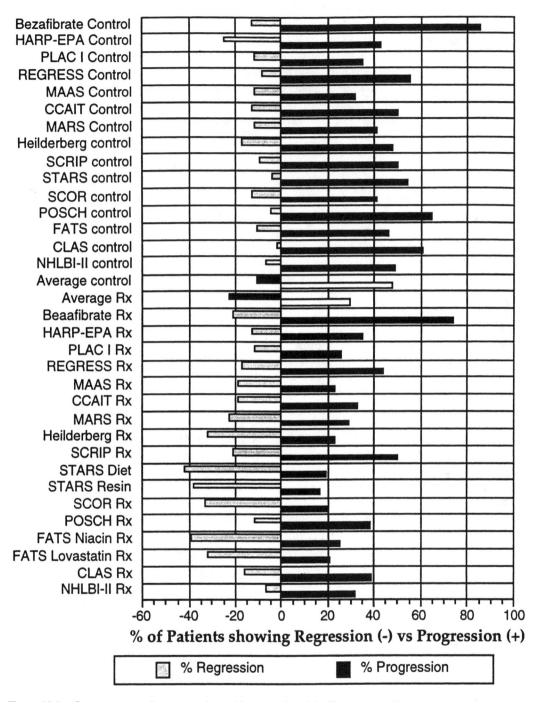

Figure 18.6.   Coronary artery disease arteriographic regression trials. The percent of the control population reported to show arteriographic progression is represented in the upper half of the figure by the bars to the right, and the percent reported to show regression is represented by the bars to the left. The treatment groups are represented in the lower half of the figure. Despite aggressive treatment, 20% to 40% of treated patients continue to have arteriographic progression of CAD. See text for full names of trials and other details.

tigation in 4444 subjects with CAD and a mean LDL-C of 188 mg/dL. Treatment resulted in a 35% reduction in LDL-C and a 31% reduction ($P <$ 0.0001) in major coronary events (132). The West of Scotland (WOS) study was a 5-year investigation in 6595 subjects believed to be clinically free of CAD. Treatment resulted in a 26% reduction in LDL-C, and significant (30%) reduction in definite coronary events (133). The Cholesterol and Recurrent Events (CARE) study recently reported results in 4159 post-MI patients who were randomized to receive placebo (n = 2078) or 40 mg pravastatin (n = 2081) for 5 years (134). The mean LDL-C at baseline was 139 mg/dL and represents a nonhypercholesterolemic CAD population typically found in cardiology practices. Low-density lipoprotein cholesterol was reduced approximately 32% in the pravastatin group. Although a significant reduction in total MI and the need for coronary artery bypass graft (CABG) surgery and percutaneous transluminal coronary angioplasty were demonstrated for the entire group, the study reported that the significant reduction in CV events appeared to cluster in subjects with a baseline LDL-C greater than 125 mg/dL and no significant reduction in events attributable to prevastatin was seen in subjects with a baseline LDL-C less than 125 mg/dL.

We analyzed the Stanford Coronary Risk Intervention Project arteriographic data in regard to potential benefit in CAD patients with an entry LDL-C less than 125 mg/dL, not on lipid-lowering medications (135). In patients treated with multiple risk factor intervention, including lipid-lowering medications, such as niacin and gemfibrozil, significant arteriographic benefit was seen in LDL pattern B subjects, but not in patients with pattern A who had a baseline LDL-C less than 125 mg/dL. Thus, there is a group of "low" LDL-C CAD patients who will benefit from treatment. The CARE study did not observe this, perhaps because their analysis did not include determination of LDL subclass pattern A or B.

These large clinical trials indicate that a mild to moderate reduction in blood cholesterol can be achieved with drugs, and this reduction is associated with a statistically significant reduction in CV events. The amount of cholesterol reduction achieved in the earlier trials can be considered moderate and averaged around 10%. The SSSS, WOS, and CARE trials achieved greater

LDL-C reduction and appropriately greater reduction in CV events. However, as Figure 18.6 illustrates, even a 25% to 30% reduction in events, although laudable, is not sufficient to claim optimal metabolic control of atherosclerosis since many patients taking the drug have lowered LDL-C yet continue to have cardiovascular events. The WHO and CDP (clofibrate, estrogen, thyroxine) trials raise the question of safety of long-term drug treatment of elevated cholesterol with some medications, but the experience of the CPPT, CDP (nicotinic acid), SSSS, WOS, and CARE trials suggests that drug-related risk may be drug-specific, because few significant adverse medical effects were detected with long-term use of bile acid binding resins, nicotinic acid, or HMG-CoA reductase inhibitors.

Coronary Arteriographic Trial Evidence That Coronary Artery Disease Progression Can Be Delayed, Prevented, or Regressed

Coronary arteriography can be used to determine the extent of CAD, and repeat arteriograms can indicate whether progression, regression, or no change has occurred. Reports that use arteriography for the definition of CAD change date back to 1967. These earlier studies did not include control groups, and they did not adhere to strict clinical trial design; thus, interpretation of their results is unclear (136). Arteriographic results are clinically important because change in arteriographic appearance has a significant relationship to clinical events (137, 138). Despite the blood cholesterol benefit of treatment, 20% to 40% of treated patients showed progression (Fig. 18.6).

Three investigations that used relatively unconventional methods have been reported. The Program on the Surgical Control of the Hyperlipidemias (POSCH) trial used partial ileal bypass to lower blood cholesterol in 421 hypercholesterolemic subjects (139). A significant reduction in LDL-C was achieved with the surgery, and this was correlated with CAD regression in some but not all patients. This investigation raises the interesting issue of the risks and side effects of partial ileal bypass versus the risks and side effects of long-term drug therapy. There are pros and cons to both approaches, but the results of POSCH at least offer an additional therapeutic approach, especially for patients unresponsive to more conventional approaches.

The Heidelberg Study investigated the arteriographic effect of a low-fat diet and exercise therapy on men with CAD randomly assigned to a low-fat diet and exercise group or a control group (140). The treatment group had significantly better arteriographic outcome than the control group. The amount of exercise performed by the patients who ended up in the "regression" group was the equivalent of approximately 22 miles of walking or jogging per week (141).

The Lifestyle Heart Trial used a vegetarian diet, moderate exercise, stress management, smoking cessation, and group support to induce CAD regression in some but not all patients (142). After entry examination and arteriography, 53 subjects were assigned randomly to the intervention group, but only 53% subsequently agreed to take part. Forty-three patients were assigned to the control group, and only 42% agreed to participate. The findings of this investigation are difficult to interpret, in part because of the unusual nature of the selection procedure, the high dropout after randomization, the difference in baseline group characteristics, and the group bias potential. After 1 year, the investigators reported that the average diameter of stenosis decreased from 40.0% to 37.8% in the intervention group and increased from 42.7% to 46.1% in the control group ($P = 0.001$).

Coronary arteries respond to the atherosclerotic process initially by enlarging their diameters, and functionally important lumen stenosis may be delayed until the lesion occupies 40% or more of the internal elastic lamina area (143). Measurements of coronary artery lumen maximum diameter reduction obtained with quantitative coronary arteriography in the Coronary Artery Surgery Study (CASS) indicate that a natural mean reduction in maximum diameter of approximately 1% to 6% per year can be expected (144); however, the change was highly variable. Coronary artery disease progression has been related significantly to the number of diseased vessels, age, smoking status, and blood cholesterol (145). Patients who showed progression had a mean TC of 250 ± 42 mg/dL, compared to patients who showed no progression and who had a mean TC of 216 ± 48 mg/dL. With multivariate logistic regression, the number of segments ($P = 0.001$),

smoking status ($P < 0.05$), and cholesterol level ($P < 0.05$) were significant predictors of progression. This may be even more important in the CABG population, in which CAD progression is three to six times greater in grafted versus ungrafted arteries, and 45% of all grafts have significant occlusive disease 5 years after surgery (146).

In CAD patients without elevated LDL-C, lipoprotein subclasses are more important than LDL-C. The Montreal Heart Study attempted to identify factors that contribute to CAD progression (36). In the population of CAD patients studied, the mean LDL-C was 147 mg/dl and IDL and inversely HDL-C significantly predicted both clinical events and arteriographic progression, whereas LDL-C did not predict either clinical events or arteriographic progression. In this investigation of the "natural" arteriographic progression of CAD, progression was reported to be related to characteristics found in LDL pattern B subjects, namely elevated IDL-C ($P = 0.06$) and low HDL-C ($P = 0.002$), and these characteristics were also associated with clinical events (IDL, $P = 0.01$; HDL, $P = 0.02$). With IDL-C and HDL-C taken into account, there was no independent association between either LDL-C or VLDL-C and arteriographic measures of progression. In young post-MI patients, dense LDL particles are related to arteriographically determined CAD severity (147). The relationship of small LDL to IDL and HDL-C suggests a role for the small, dense LDL pattern B trait in these investigations that is not apparent from measures of TC or LDL-C.

The National Heart, Lung, and Blood Institute (NHLBI) type II study involved 116 subjects, all of whom were classified as type II hyperlipidemia patients, who were treated with diet therapy and either placebo or cholestyramine for 5 years (150, 151). The study revealed that among the lesions that caused 50% or greater stenosis at baseline, 33% of placebo-treated and 12% of cholestyramine-treated patients revealed lesion progression ($P < 0.05$). When the patients' arteriograms were examined independent of treatment group, a significant ($P < 0.05$) association was seen with LDL-C reduction, HDL-C increase, and the extent of coronary atherosclerosis progression. In the group who had the smaller change in HDL-C, 47% demonstrated progression; in the group who had the greater HDL-C change, 15% demonstrated progression. Unfortunately, this investigation met with some difficulty because of adherence problems, but it did demonstrate that lack of disease progression correlated significantly with changes in LDL-C and HDL-C values and, in particular, in the HDL-C subspecies HDL_{2a} and HDL_{2b}.

The St. Thomas' Arteriographic Regression Study (STARS) was conducted at the St. Thomas Hospital in London, England (152). After coronary arteriography, 90 men whose TCs were between 232 and 386 mg/dL were assigned randomly to a control group, a group treated with a low-fat, high-fiber (3.6 g/1000 kcal pectin) diet, or a group treated with the low-fat, high-fiber diet plus cholestyramine (16 g/day).

No substantial differences were reported among the groups for HDL-C. Arteriographically defined progression was reported to have occurred in 54% of the control group, compared with 19% of the diet group and 17% of the diet plus cholestyramine group. Regression occurred in 4% of the control group, compared with 42% of the diet group and 38% of the diet plus cholestyramine group. Dense LDL reduction was reported to be the best predictor of arteriographic change (35).

The Cholesterol Lowering Atherosclerosis Study (CLAS) involved 162 post-CABG patients randomly assigned to receive either placebo or treatment with colestipol and nicotinic acid (153). After 2 years of treatment, the average number of lesions that progressed was significantly lower ($P < 0.03$) in the drug-treatment group. The number of subjects who showed new atheroma formation in native coronary arteries ($P < 0.03$) and changes in bypass grafts ($P < 0.04$) was also significantly lower. Atherosclerosis regression was reported to have occurred in 16.2% of the drug-treated patients ($P < 0.002$). Drug treatment resulted in a 43% reduction in LDL-C, 22% reduction in TGs, and a 37% increase in HDL-C. The mean LDL-C values in the treatment and control groups were 97 mg/dL and 160 mg/dL, respectively. A post hoc analysis of the CLAS data, performed at the Lawrence Berkeley National Laboratory, revealed that benefit of intervention with diet, nicotinic acid, and colestipol was confined to subjects in the top third of the TG distribution (more than 190 mg/dL), a group that is enriched in LDL subclass

pattern B subjects (154, 155). Subjects with lower TGs received no significant arteriographic benefit compared with the control group despite substantial blood lipid changes.

Additional information regarding the effect of lipid treatment in CABS patients has been presented from the POSCH study and Coronary Artery Bypass Study (139, 156, 157). The POSCH study is an investigation of the effect of blood cholesterol reduction by means of abdominal surgery that involves an ileal loop resection (139). The need for CABG surgery and the redoing of CABG surgeries is dramatically less in the treatment compared to control groups (156).

The Coronary Artery Bypass Study investigated the effect of aggressive LDL-C reduction (goal of LDL-C, 60 to 85 mg/dL) versus moderate LDL-C reduction (goal LDL-C, 130 to 140 mg/dL) for 4 years in 1351 subjects who had a previous CABG surgery. The main finding was that aggressive treatment resulted in significantly better arteriographic outcome than did moderate treatment (158). Thirty-five percent of the moderate treatment group had substantial progression of their grafts compared with 24% in the aggressive treatment group ($P < 0.001$). Although this indicates benefit from aggressive treatment, it also indicates that 24% of CABG patients who achieved LDL-C values less then 100 mg/dL continued to show arteriographic progression.

The Familial Atherosclerosis Treatment Study (FATS) was a randomized, blinded 2.5-year trial of drug therapy in patients who had CAD documented with quantitative coronary arteriography (60). It is the first arteriographic investigation to use quantitative coronary arteriography, which allows for greatly enhanced precision of arterial lumen measurements (149, 159). One-hundred forty-six subjects were recruited on the basis of apo B greater than 125 mg/dL (TC more than 270 mg/dL). All subjects received diet instruction and were assigned randomly into three groups: placebo with and without colestipol (n = 46), lovastatin (40 mg/day) plus colestipol (n = 38), and nicotinic acid (4 g/day) plus colestipol (n = 36). The goal of therapy was to achieve an LDL-C less than 120 mg/dL. Change in apo B and HDL-C concentration revealed a significant relation to coronary artery lesion change. Additional reports from this investigation have revealed that most clinical and arteriographic benefit occurred in the subjects with moderate, not severely elevated, LDL-C (160).

Two important clinical event lessons were gleaned from a retrospective analysis of the FATS data. First, no asymptomatic patient had an event (161). Second, the greatest benefit occurred in symptomatic patients and those with LDL-C less than 160 mg/dL at baseline. The difference between events in the control versus treatment groups for subjects with initial LDL-C more than 160 mg/dL was four versus three, whereas in subjects with LDL-C less than 160 mg/dL , the difference was six versus two. Thus, patients with CAD symptoms and those with LDL-C less than 160 mg/dL received the most benefit from treatment (161, 162).

The results of the University of California–San Francisco Specialized Center for Atherosclerosis Research (SCOR) trial provides insight into familial heterozygous hypercholesterolemia patients treated with triple-drug therapy (163). Seventy-two patients who had familial hypercholesterolemia were randomly assigned either to a control group (n = 32) or to a treatment group (n = 40). The control group was treated with colestipol, and the treatment group received a combination of colestipol, nicotinic acid, and lovastatin. Quantitative coronary arteriography was performed and evaluated in a way similar to that of the FATS trial. This study is unique in that it included relatively equal numbers of men and women, and the patients did not have obvious CAD. Treatment with a combination of colestipol, nicotinic acid, and lovastatin resulted in 32.5% of the treatment group revealing "regression" compared with 12.5% in the control group. More important clinically, 41% of the control group exhibited arteriographic progression compared to 20% in the treatment group. Women had slightly greater reduction in TGs than men (25% versus 11%, $P = 0.10$), and the change in percent area coronary stenosis was significant in women ($P = 0.05$) but not in men.

Recently reported investigations using single statin therapy have consistently reported significant reductions in LDL-C and the rate of progression of arteriographically determined CAD. The Multicentre Anti-Atheroma Study (MAAS) treated 167 placebo and 178 simvastatin (20 mg/day) patients for 4 years with arteriograms at baseline, 2 years, and 4 years (165). Forty-two percent were on β-blockers, which may tend to complicate interpretation because of the effect of β-blockers on plasma lipoproteins and, in particular, small LDL (12). A 32% reduction in LDL-C with simvastatin was associated with significantly less progression and more regression. Although clinical events were less in the simvastatin group, this finding was not statistically significant.

The Regression Growth Evaluation Statin Study (REGRESS) treated 885 hypercholesterolemic men with either pravastatin or a placebo for 2 years (166). The mean segment diameter worsened by 0.10 mm in the placebo group and 0.06 mm in the pravastatin group, which represents a significant ($P = 0.02$) reduction in the rate of progression.

The Pravastatin Limitation of Atherosclerosis in the Coronary Arteries (PLAC-I) study treated 408 CAD patients with either pravastatin or placebo for 3 years (167). There was a trend for overall decreased progression ($P = 0.07$) and a significant reduction in progression for lesions less than 50% at baseline ($P < 0.04$).

The Canadian Coronary Artery Intervention Trial (CCAIT) used lovastatin in 331 CAD patients to reduce LDL-C and affect CAD progression (168). Progression with no regression occurred in 48 of 146 (32.9%) lovastatin-treated patients and in 76 of 153 (49.7%) placebo-treated patients. Lovastatin significantly slowed the progression of CAD in patients with a mean baseline LDL-C of 173 mg/dL, but there was no significant effect on regression (168).

The Monitored Atheroma Regression Study (MARS) was similar to CCAIT in the treatment of CAD patients with lovastatin or placebo (169). After 2 years of treatment, the lovastatin group had a 38% reduction in LDL-C and a trend for reduced arteriographic progression (2.2% increase with placebo, 1.6% with lovastatin; $P < .20$) but was significantly reduced for lesions obstructed more than 50%. In MARS, only those patients with mid-density LDL particles exhibited significant regression while, despite a similar 70 mg/dL, those with dense, or buoyant, LDL particles revealed no arteriographic benefit from lovastatin treatment (170).

The Stanford Coronary Risk Intervention Project (SCRIP) used quantitative coronary arteriography to assess the effect of 4 years of multifactorial risk intervention in a group of 300 subjects with documented CAD who were assigned randomly to a usual-care group or a special intervention group (172). The special intervention group received diet, exercise, weight reduction, and smoking cessation advice. Bile acid binding resins, nicotinic acid, gemfibrozil, and lovastatin were used to achieve an LDL-C goal of 110 mg/dL. Baseline plasma lipids were representative of a typical CAD population. The LDL-C was reduced approximately 18% more, and HDL-C increased approximately 7% more, in the special intervention group than the usual-care group. A significantly greater ($P < 0.01$) annualized rate of minimum diameter change for diseased vessels appeared in the usual-care group (0.046 mm/year), compared with that of the special intervention group (0.022 mm/year). Coronary artery disease regression was reported to be significantly greater ($P < 0.025$) in the special intervention group (21%) than in the usual-care group (10%). For the final 3 years of the study, significantly ($P < 0.006$) fewer deaths and nonfatal MIs occurred in the special intervention group (n = 2) than in the usual-care group (n = 13).

In the only arteriographic investigation to prospectively test the hypothesis that LDL pattern A and B have an impact on arteriographic outcome, SCRIP found that in the control group, the annual rate of arteriographic progression was twice as fast in LDL pattern B compared with LDL pattern A patients (33). In 1996, SCRIP reported that heart disease patients who were classified as LDL pattern B at the beginning of the study received significant benefit in regard to their arteriographic obstruction in response to 4 years of multiple risk intervention. The patients received low-fat diet, exercise, weight loss, smoking cessation, and lipid-lowering medications. The LDL pattern A patients revealed no significant arteriographic benefit despite the same treatment and almost identical LDL-C reduction.

Despite the well-deserved optimism that surrounds the results of these investigations, it is important to appreciate that like the clinical end point trials, a large number of patients in the treatment groups were found to exhibit arteriographic progression despite what was believed to be adequate lipid-lowering therapy. For the studies listed in Figure 18.6, on average, 48% of the control groups demonstrated "progression," but 30% of patients in the treatment groups also demonstrated "progression." On average 23% of the treated groups demonstrated "regression" whereas 11% of the control groups also demonstrated "regression." It is clear, from a detailed analysis of all the trials, that although the rate of progression can be reduced, lipid reduction delays progression but does not "cure" the disease. This is an important concept because research must continue vigorously to provide physicians and patients improved odds of "regression."

Although clinical events were not primary end points in the arteriographic investigations, most trials did demonstrate a reduction in clinical events (173). Although the event difference was generally statistically significant, as with arteriographic change, events continued to occur in the treatment groups despite aggressive therapy. This illustrates the reduction, but not elimination, of events with lipid treatment. For example, in SCRIP, after 4 years of treatment there were 34 events in the control group versus 20 in the treatment group ($P = 0.07$) (172). Although this is a big step in the right direction, the therapeutic approaches are clearly not adequate to treat this disease with a degree of success and consistency that is acceptable to patients and physicians alike.

Use of a single therapy may blunt the event reduction power of these investigations because of the presence of subgroups who do, and do not, respond favorably to the single therapy. Thompson and colleagues presented data in support of this concept by analyzing the CAD regression trials and showing that CV event reduction was more common in trials that used multifactorial intervention compared with those using a single intervention (174). This makes physiologic sense as multiple metabolic abnormalities cannot be treated successfully with a single therapy (175).

An important additional lesson from these trials is the finding that LDL pattern B and TG-rich lipoproteins are perhaps more important than LDL-C in predicting clinical events and arteriographic progression. Optimal metabolic assessment goes beyond determination of only TGs, total TC, LDL-C, and HDL-C. Although TG, HDL-C, and apo B values have a statistical relationship to LDL subclass pattern, they are not completely accurate. Measurement of LDL subclass distribution and peak LDL particle diameter, with classification as LDL pattern A or B, is highly desirable (176).

TREATMENT—EXERCISE AND WEIGHT LOSS

Studies that use physical activity as the main intervention often involve changes in diet composition and body fat content that may or may not be intentional. It is important to interpret plasma lipoprotein changes in view of the effect that these confounding variables may have on plasma lipoprotein values. The effect of physical activity on lipoprotein metabolism differs between normolipidemic and hyperlipidemic persons.

Effect of Physical Training on Plasma Lipids in Normolipemic Subjects

Articles have been published that review the effect of exercise on lipid metabolism in normolipemic and hyperlipidemic subjects (177–180). Interpretation of investigations can be confused because of the many factors that affect blood lipid values. For example, variables such as diet composition, caloric content, coffee and alcohol consumption, medications, and body weight change often were not reported in earlier studies. These variables confound the accurate interpretation of clinical investigations significantly. Physical training studies often involve dietary and weight change. A meta-analysis of 95 exercise studies suggests that reduction in TC and LDL-C is greatest when exercise training is associated with body weight loss (181). By this statistical approach, decreases in TC, LDL-C, TGs, and TC/HDL-C values were found to be significantly associated with decreases in body weight ($P < 0.05$). For example, young men who exercised for 4 days on either a high-fat or high-carbohydrate diet demonstrated a significant increase in HDL-C ($P < 0.001$) and particularly HDL_{2b} ($P < 0.01$) on a high-fat diet compared to the high-carbohydrate diet (182).

TRIGLYCERIDES

Investigations consistently have demonstrated lower plasma TG values in association with reported greater physical activity. This is clearly apparent in athletes such as long-distance runners and cross-country skiers, compared with sedentary subjects (183, 184). This difference becomes less apparent when comparing levels of reported physical activity in the general population. Studies of exercise training in normolipidemic subjects frequently indicate a re- duction in plasma TG after training (185). This change is less apparent in persons who have relatively low initial TG values (186, 187).

CHOLESTEROL

Plasma TC is no different in physically active persons than in sedentary ones, and undertaking a physical training program does not alter plasma TC values significantly, although a trend to lowered TC with greater activity has been reported (188, 189). Overwhelmingly, prospective studies support this observational data. Completing a period of exercise training and obtaining greater fitness does not appear to result in significant changes in TC. Even when weight loss is associated with increased physical activity, no significant change in plasma TC occurs (185).

Low-density lipoprotein cholesterol responds in a similar way to TC. It may be lower in highly active persons, but diet and body fat differences may account for this. The lack of change in LDL-C concentration after exercise or diet-induced weight reduction, however, masks significant changes in LDL subclass distribution, specifically significant reductions in small LDL (S_f0–7) and significant increases in large LDL (S_f7–12) (14, 185). These significant changes disappeared when adjusted for body mass change. This latter finding suggests that lipoprotein change attributed to exercise may in large part be related to the associated change in body fat content.

Reflecting this change in LDL subclass distribution, a significant change also is seen in HDL mass and HDL-C with increased physical activity. Both cross-sectional and longitudinal studies indicate that HDL values increase in association with a physical training program (190, 191). The amount and frequency of physical training are important aspects of a therapeutic exercise prescription, and evidence suggests that a threshold of more than the equivalent of 10 miles per week of jogging (for a period of several months) may be required before achieving HDL effects independent of the often associated effects of weight loss and dietary change (185). The major component of HDL increased by physical activity is the HDL_2 subclass and specifically HDL_{2b} (17). Approximately 50% of HDL-C is contained in the HDL_2 fraction in runners, compared to approximately 30% in sedentary controls (192).

Apoproteins

Apolipoprotein B concentrations have been reported in several studies, and physical training appears to have little effect on plasma concentration (193). Cross-sectional studies suggest that runners have higher apo A-I values than sedentary controls (180). Prospective exercise studies, however, both have and have not revealed significant increases in apo A-I and A-II after exercise training (187, 194). Exercise training that induces weight loss appears to increase apo A-I to a greater extent than a similar amount of weight loss produced by caloric restriction (185). The mechanism of increased apo A-I levels in physically active subjects may be related to increased biologic half-life, reduced fractional catabolic rate, and some increased synthetic rate.

Enzymes

Change in enzyme activity can play a significant role in altering plasma lipid values. Lecithin cholesterol acyltransferase (LCAT), lipoprotein lipase (LPL), and hepatic lipase (HL) are the major enzymes in lipid metabolism thought to be affected by exercise in healthy persons. Lecithin cholesterol acyltransferase is reported to be higher in endurance athletes and to increase after a training program (195). Substantial evidence exists to support an increase in LPL activity after physical training programs in healthy persons (196–198). Conversely, HL activity has been shown to decrease after a physical training program (197, 199).

Cholesterol esterification rate (CER), which is an indirect measure of LCAT activity, increases in both hypercholesterolemic (not significant) and normolipemic men ($P < 0.05$) after physical training (200). This may be caused by increased LCAT activity or increased availability of substrate, cofactors, or decreased inhibitors of the LCAT-mediated reaction. The significant decrease in red blood cell cholesterol in both groups suggests that the lower CER in the hypercholesterolemic group may contribute to an abnormal plasma lipid response to exercise therapy.

Lipoprotein lipase plays a major role in the mechanism of exercise effect on blood lipids. Hydrolysis of the lipid components of VLDL by LPL results in lipoprotein components that are transferred to small HDL particles, which creates an increased HDL mass (201). Evidence for increased adipose and muscle tissue LPL activity in chronic exercisers, as well as for increased LPL activity after an intravenous heparin infusion, is present in cross-sectional studies of endurance-trained athletes (compared with sedentary controls) (199, 202, 203). A local muscle lipase effect probably plays a significant role in exercise-induced lipoprotein change. Using a one-leg training technique, a significant change in arterial-venous degradation of VLDL-TG ($r = 0.91$) and production of HDL-C have been associated with muscle LPL ($r = 0.90$) (194).

Whether the training stimulus is a power or endurance activity appears to be important. Lipoprotein values and LPL activity do not differ significantly between control subjects and male sprinters, whereas long-distance runners of both sexes have higher HDL-C values and LPL activity than control subjects ($P < 0.05$) (202). A strong correlation exists between HDL-C and adipose tissue LPL ($r = 0.94$). Prolonged heavy exercise is associated with higher LPL activity, and adipose tissue LPL is highly correlated with HDL-C ($r = 0.94$) (196, 197).

Hepatic lipase responds to exercise in a way that is inverse to that of LPL (199). Cross-sectional studies indicate that runners have higher HDL-C values and lower HL activity than sedentary subjects (195). This observation is supported by the finding that exercise training in middle-aged men results in a decrease in HL activity (197). This inverse relationship between exercise training and HL is important because HL is correlated negatively with HDL_2 and positively with HDL_3 (204). Thus, HL appears to play a role in the conversion of HDL_2 to HDL_3, and decreased HL activity because of physical training may be a major factor in increasing the HDL_2/HDL_3 ratio observed after physical activity (205, 206).

Effect of Physical Training on Plasma Lipids in Hyperlipidemic Patients

The effect of exercise therapy on patients who have genetic defects or errors of metabolism that result in abnormal lipid profiles may be substantially different from those of persons who are free of these difficulties. Patients who demonstrate clear metabolic defects can be well defined, and their responses to exercise therapy can be predicted based on the known mechanism. Many hypercholesterolemic and hypertriglyceridemic patients, however, have a mixed or unclear cause for their lipid abnormality. In these subjects, physical training may be beneficial in improving their lipid abnormalities through a direct mechanism or through an indirect mechanism (reduction of excess body fat and diet modification). There are randomized, controlled studies of the effects of exercise on patients with specific hyperlipidemias.

HYPERTRIGLYCERIDEMIA

Percent ideal body fat in Class IIb patients has a strong positive correlation with TG ($r = 0.54$; $P < 0.001$) and a negative correlation with HDL-C ($r = -0.42$; $P < 0.01$) (207). Prospective trials in hypertriglyceridemic subjects indicate that physical training can result in TG reductions of 15% to 40%. This high-risk lipoprotein profile (elevated TG and reduced HDL-C) is associated with a high waist-to-hip girth ratio, as is commonly seen in men, and may help explain gender differences in CAD (208). Often, body fat and diet composition are altered simultaneously, and these confounders confuse the interpretation of any isolated effects of physical activity.

Although the role of exercise is important in altering TG values, the inverse relationships among TG, small LDL, and HDL levels appear to have important pathologic consequences and should be viewed as potential therapeutic results of exercise therapy in patients who have hypertriglyceridemia, even when LDL and HDL subclass distributions cannot be measured. In men who have mild TG elevation and who are slightly overweight, physical activity associated with fat weight loss results in significant reductions in "small" LDL despite no change in LDL-C (14).

Enhanced postprandial lipemia is associated with hypertriglyceridemia and atherogenic conditions such as combined hyperlipidemia, hyperapobetalipoproteinemia, LDL pattern B, and the presence of apo E isoform 3/4 (23, 46, 49). Physical activity can substantially reduce the postprandial elevation in TG-rich lipoproteins in normotriglyceridemic patients, and it is reasonable to expect a similar effect in hypertriglyceridemic patients (209).

In hypertriglyceridemic persons, exercise therapy in adequate doses results in reduced TG and increased HDL-C. Thus, exercise may be beneficial to patients who have lipoprotein abnormalities associated with an excess of TG-rich particles. This includes hypertriglyceridemia, combined hyperlipidemia, hyperapobetalipoproteinemia, and LDL subclass pattern B.

HYPERCHOLESTEROLEMIA

Many large epidemiologic investigations have failed to demonstrate consistently a correlation between reported physical activity and lipid values in populations not specifically selected for hyperlipidemia (210, 211). A paucity of cross-sectional studies have investigated physical activity and hypercholesterolemia. In the Coronary Primary Prevention Trial-Lipid Research Clinics (CPPT-LRC) analysis done in 7106 type II hyperlipidemic men, results of analysis of variance and regression models indicated that TC and LDL-C were not related to self-reported physical activity (212).

Large, controlled prospective studies of the effects of exercise on patients who have hypercholesterolemia are few. The studies that are available indicate no significant change in TC with physical training (200, 213–215). Some studies have reported a reduction in TC or LDL-C after exercise training in type IIa or IIb patients, but changes in diet and body mass complicate the interpretation (216).

The largest controlled exercise study of plasma lipoprotein change in a population with known CAD is the National Exercise and Heart Disease Project (NEHDP) (217). In this investigation, 223 post-MI men were assigned randomly to participate in moderate exercise or no exercise (control group). Mean TC and LDL-C values before training were 223 mg/dL and 150 mg/dL, respectively. This places the subjects in approximately the 65th percentile of age-matched normal persons (218). After 1 year of exercise training, no change was detected in TC, LDL-C, or HDL-C. A significant, but slight, reduction ($P = 0.04$) in TGs was noted. A physical training effect was confirmed by a significant ($P < 0.001$) increase in work capacity and a significant ($P < 0.05$) reduction in body fat.

The NEHDP study also raises the issue of a possible threshold dose of activity required to achieve exercise-induced lipoprotein change. Subjects in the NEHDP were encouraged to attend exercise sessions three times per week and to achieve 30 to 40 minutes of endurance activity at 70% to 85% of peak heart rate. This is the equivalent of approximately 600 kcal expended per week. In healthy persons, an energy expenditure of more than 1000 kcal/week may be required to achieve an increase in HDL-C that can be attributed to an exercise stimulus and not to associated weight loss (219). The lack of a significant HDL-C change may be related to an insufficient dose of exercise. Low HDL-C (hypoalphalipoproteinemia) in the absence of elevated TGs or excess body fat does not respond well to a physical training stimulus (220).

INSULIN

Despite a lack of profound changes in fasting lipoproteins after low- to moderate-intensity exercise programs, physiologic benefit may occur in carbohydrate metabolism. Insulin availability and activity have major effects on lipid metabolism and are abnormal in some persons who have dyslipidemias associated with hypertriglyceridemia. Acutely, insulin has been shown to decrease TG levels in subjects who have hypertriglyceridemia (221). Physiologically, however, insulin appears to have an effect on both VLDL secretion and TG removal. In animal models, physical training results in reduced insulin concentrations, decreased hepatic VLDL-TG secretion, and no change in adipose LPL activity, all of which suggest an increased insulin sensitivity that attenuates dietary carbohydrate-induced hypertriglyceridemia (222).

In states of chronic hyperinsulinemia, such as obesity in humans, a positive correlation between TGs and insulin values has been observed (223). Hepatic VLDL production also is increased by insulin (224). Contrary to this VLDL production and enhanced TG role is a TG catabolism produced through LPL. Adipose tissue LPL is stimulated by insulin, whereas the effect on muscle tissue LPL is less clear (223).

The effects of exercise on the insulin–lipid interaction in persons who have pathologic conditions can be complex. A glucose tolerance test (GTT) obtained 1 day after exercise in obese subjects revealed a stable basal insulin level but decreased insulin levels after the glucose load, compared to a nonexercising state, which suggests enhanced peripheral insulin sensitivity in response to the exercise stimulus (225). This is supported by studies in hypertriglyceridemic subjects (226–228). At least five training investigations measured plasma insulin. Investigations

that reported change in fasting insulin values after a physical training program have found both decreases and increases (214, 226, 229). In view of the association between hyperinsulinemia and low HDL-C with CAD, even moderate exercise may be metabolically beneficial and not reflected in routine measures of TC and TG (121). The question is whether it is the exercise, weight loss, or associated metabolic alterations that cause the change in insulin action (230).

GENDER

Most investigations of the interaction between exercise and lipoproteins have involved men. A meta-analysis of longitudinal studies that involved women (n = 27) indicates that TC and TG are significantly reduced ($P < 0.02$) in women after an exercise program. No significant change in HDL-C or LDL-C was observed, however, and there was a trend for women who had the highest levels to respond the most (231). Lipid differences in premenopausal women (compared with men or postmenopausal women) are linked to estradiol, 98% of which is protein bound (232). This may have a significant impact on any gender-difference response to exercise when considering the responses in premenopausal and postmenopausal women.

AGE

The effect of physical activity on lipoprotein metabolism in the elderly has not been investigated in any large prospective trial. Cross-sectional analysis in men aged 46 to 77 years indicates a significant inverse correlation ($r = -0.35; P < 0.01$) between functional capacity (maximal oxygen uptake) and the waist-to-hip ratio, and a strong correlation between percent fat and fasting glucose, insulin, and TGs and an inverse relationship with HDL-C (233). Japanese "old runners" and young runners have higher HDL-C and apo A-I and II levels and lower levels of VLDL-C and LDL-C than sedentary controls, regardless of age (234).

POSTPRANDIAL LIPEMIA

In cross-sectional investigations it has been demonstrated that athletes have significantly lower peak PPL and shorter PPL duration (209). As little as 15 miles per week resulted in a significant increase in LPL activity and a decrease in fasting TGs, as well as in postprandial TGs and TG-rich lipoprotein particles (73). After a train-

Table 18.4.   Pharmacologic Agents for Lipid Treatment

Drug Group	Indication	Effect	Primary Side Effects	Full-Dose Cost

BABR
  cholestyramine (Questran),
  colestipol (Cholestid, LoCholest)
	High LDLC	−28% LDL-C
		+4% HDL-C
			Constipation, GI distress	$1500

Fibric Acid Derivatives
  gemfibrozil (Lopid), clofibrate
  (Atromid-S) fenofibrate
	High TGs
	Low HDL-C
		−35% TGs
		+10% HDL-C
			GI distress	$750

HMGRI
  lovastatin (Mevacor), simvastatin
  (Zocor), fluvastatin (Lescol),
  prevastatin (Prevachol), atorvas-
  tatin (Lipitor), cerivastatin (Baycol)
	High LDL-C	−30% LDL-C	Elevated LFTs	$750–2,000

Nicotinic acid niacin (Niacor, Niaspan)	High LDL-C High TGs Low HDL-C	−20% LDL-C −30% TGs +25% HDL-C	Elevated LFTs Flushing, itching	$500

BABR = bile acid binding resin; LDL-C = low-density lipoprotein cholesterol; HDL-C = high-density lipoprotein cholesterol; GI = gastrointestinal; TG = triglyceride; HMGRI = hydroxymethylglutaryl-CoA reductase inhibitor; LFT = liver function tests; HDL = high-density lipoprotein.

ing program, postprandial increases in free fatty acids (FFAs) and TG values occur earlier, and the amplitude of the postprandial rise in FFA and TG is lower (235). This is interesting because it has been demonstrated that peak PPL is delayed in patients who have CAD (compared to controls without CAD), and two conditions associated with CAD, LDL subclass pattern B and hyperapo-betalipoproteinemia, have abnormally elevated and prolonged PPL (23, 68, 236). This suggests that not only do fasting lipid values reflect a CAD risk, but the total time that the arterial wall is exposed to atherogenic fat particles after a meal reflects a relative risk as well.

Low-density lipoprotein subclass pattern B is associated with enhanced postprandial lipemia (23). Four hours after a standard fat meal, LDL pattern A subjects will have TG values of approximately 200 mg/dL, whereas LDL pattern B individuals will have TG values of approximately 350 mg/dL.

Because of a paucity of studies, it is difficult to conclude anything about the effects of exercise therapy on dyslipidemias that result from rare dyslipidemias such as abetalipoproteinemia (237), hypoalphalipoproteinemia (233), Tangier disease, or other apo A-I abnormalities (238, 239). From current theories of lipoprotein metabolism, it appears unlikely that exercise has a significant effect on lipid metabolism in patients who have familial homozygous or heterozygous LDL receptor deficiency.

The use of therapeutic exercise to treat hyperlipidemia is a valid approach. Patients who have

hyperlipidemias and do not show a well-defined protein or enzymatic defect will respond to exercise therapy in a way similar to that of nor-molipemic subjects. The potential mechanism of this benefit probably involves classic systemic lipoprotein metabolism and also may involve changes in fecal steroid excretion through the gut, which has been shown to increase with aerobic training (240).

Many drug groups are available to treat lipid disorders. Table 18.4 lists the drugs used most often, along with their indications, effects, primary side effects, and dosages.

Bile Acid Binding Resins

MECHANISM

Bile acid binding resins have been used for more than 25 years (77). Intestinal binding of bile salts by the resin decreases bile salt reabsorption through the enterohepatic recirculation route. Hepatic cholesterol, HMG-CoA reductase activity, and hepatic cholesterol synthesis are increased. Inhibition of normal bile salt reabsorption also has been hypothesized as the cause of increased plasma TG concentrations by enhanced activity of phosphatidic acid phosphatase (77). In type II hyperlipidemia patients, resin therapy can result in LDL-C reductions of approximately 72 mg/dL, or 27%, and an HDL-C increase of 2 to 3 mg/dL, or 4% (241). There appears to be little effect on Lp(a).

INDICATION

Because of their long history for safety and efficacy, and because of their nonsystemic nature, bile acid binding resins are first-line drugs of choice for reduction of plasma LDL-C (242).

Resins are useful for patients with a mild elevation in plasma LDL-C who do not fall within the classic hyperlipidemia definition (greater than 90th percentile) and in whom reduction is warranted because of high CAD risk from other factors (243). In this group, it is important to note that low-dose resin therapy can have a significant effect on LDL-C reduction. One-half the recommended full dose of six packets per day can achieve approximately 75% of the full-dose LDL-C reduction (244–249). A colestipol dose of 5 g/day (16% full dose) can achieve 50% of the LDL-C reduction as that of a 50% full dose (250). Approximately 50% of moderately hypercholesterolemic subjects can achieve the U. S. National Cholesterol Education Program goal of an LDL-C less than 130 mg/dL with less than 50% full-dose resin. It is no longer necessary to dose patients two of three times per day. Once-a-day dosing achieves nearly the same effect as twice-a-day dosing (251). Colestipol is now available in a tablet form (252). Colestipol is effective in reducing small LDL particles in LDL pattern B patients, but not pattern A (253).

ADHERENCE ENHANCEMENT

Common patient complaints include difficulty in ingesting the resins, gastrointestinal distress, and constipation. Several tricks are available to enhance compliance. First, for all diet, exercise, weight reduction, and drug therapies, compliance can be enhanced greatly by effective use of a dedicated nurse (254). Second, the resins can be mixed in various liquid media, including juices and semisolid foods such as applesauce. Third, combining either mineral oil or supplemental fiber can reduce constipation complaints, and some fibers can further reduce LDL-C by approximately 10% (255). Bowel gas can be reduced by using simethicone.

Fibric Acid Derivatives

MECHANISM

Fibric acid derivatives enhance LPL activity and hepatic bile secretion and reduce hepatic TG production (256). Triglyceride and LDL-C responses to these agents depend on the lipoprotein abnormality and specific fibric acid derivative used (257). Triglyceride reductions between 8% and 72%, LDL-C reductions between 0% and 35%, and HDL-C increases between 0% and 25% have been reported. Generally, the greatest benefit is seen in patients who have elevations in plasma TG, although fenofibrate has been reported to produce significant LDL-C reduction (approximately 1.2 mmol/L) in type IIa patients (258). In hypertriglyceridemic patients who initially have low or normal LDL-C, gemfibrozil treatment may result in an increase in LDL-C, perhaps because of an increase in LDL production or a decrease in fractional LDL clearance rates (259). This response suggests a second lipoprotein abnormality that often requires two-drug therapy.

INDICATIONS

These agents are useful in the treatment of hypertriglyceridemia and in selected patients who have elevated LDL-C in combination with elevated TGs. The HDL-C level often is reported to increase significantly when initial HDL-C is low or when it is associated with reduction of TGs. These agents are the drugs of choice in type III hyperlipidemia. In the Helsinki Heart Study, gemfibrozil (600 mg two times a day) resulted in an overall 42% reduction in TGs, 10% reduction in LDL-C, and 10% increase in HDL-C (260). Although there was a 34% reduction in clinical events in the overall study, in a subgroup with elevated TGs (greater than 200 mg/dL) and a poor TC/HDL-C ratio, there was a 71% reduction in events (261). Virtually all the event reduction could be accounted for by this subgroup, which made up approximately 10% of the cohort. Cardiac end points were reduced most significantly in subjects who had high TGs or low HDL-C. The reduction in TGs achieved with gemfibrozil has been shown to be related to a reduction in small, dense LDL, and the combination of gemfibrozil and nicotinic acid is a particularly effective therapy for familial combined hyperlipidemia (15, 262).

ADHERENCE ENHANCEMENT

These drugs generally are well tolerated. Occasionally mild gastrointestinal distress (nausea) is experienced in the first week. To reduce this potential side effect, it can be useful to start therapy with one-half the normal dose for several days before increasing to full dose.

HMG-CoA Reductase Inhibitors

MECHANISM

Hydroxymethylglutaryl-CoA reductase inhibitors (HMGRI) competitively inhibit the rate-limiting enzyme in hepatic cholesterol synthesis, 3-hydroxy-3-methylglutaryl-coenzyme HMG-CoA reductase. This results in a compensatory increase in hepatic LDL receptor activity and appears to have some effect on LDL production rates (263). The Food and Drug Administration (FDA) has approved lovastatin (Merck & Co.), pravastatin (Bristol-Myers Squibb), simvastatin (Merck & Co.), fluvastatin (Sandoz Pharmaceuticals), atorvastatin (Parke-Davis), and in 1998, Cerivastatin (Bayer) for use in the United States (264–267).

INDICATIONS

In patients who have hypercholesterolemia, these compounds can achieve reductions of 30% to 50%, and when combined with a resin, reductions of 50% to 60% (268). They have a small effect on reducing fasting plasma TG concentrations, but this masks a significant reduction in postprandial triglyceridemia (76). Like the resins, these agents are useful in treating patients who have elevations in LDL-C but are not the agents of choice for treating hypertriglyceridemia or LDL subclass pattern B. They appear to have little effect on Lp(a) (269). Recommendations vary on what time of day to take the medication and whether it should be taken in conjunction with meals.

ADHERENCE ENHANCEMENT

These drugs generally are well tolerated and compliance issues usually center on remembering to take the medication.

Nicotinic Acid

MECHANISM

Nicotinic acid is a B vitamin that affects the lipoprotein system mediated through nicotinamide adenine dinucleotide (NAD), or NADP, by the inhibition of adenylate cyclase. Only nicotinic acid or its glycine conjugate (nicotinuric acid) has an antilipolytic effect (270). Nicotinamide is inactive with regard to lipoprotein change. Nicotinic acid inhibits endogenous cholesterol synthesis, increases catabolism, and reduces the plasma concentrations of nonesterified fatty acids by its action at the level of the adipocyte. Rapid release of prostaglandins from platelets is thought to be responsible, in part, for the vasodilation and flush response. Like other medications, nicotinic acid has pharmacologic effects that may benefit atherosclerosis and that are not reflected in plasma lipoprotein measure-

ments. These effects include prostaglandin and thromboxane perturbations, inhibition of platelet aggregation, and fibrinolysis (270). A long-acting, once-a-day nicotinic acid that is dosed at bedtime was recently approved by the FDA (271). This nicotinic acid has a significant effect in reducing small, dense LDL and, in LDL pattern B subjects, achieves a mean 40% reduction in LDL-C (75).

INDICATIONS

Nicotinic acid is useful in patients who have elevated TGs, TG-rich lipoproteins, and LDL-C, reductions in HDL-C, and the LDL subclass pattern B. Effects on lipids are commonly seen after the renal threshold is exceeded, which generally is approximately 1500 mg/day. The response of plasma lipoproteins is dose-dependent within the range of approximately 1500 to 6000 mg/day. Unmodified or time-release nicotinic acid can result in 10% to 25% LDL-C reductions in daily doses of 1500 to 3000 mg (272). Nicotinic acid is one of the few lipid medications that appears to have some effect on Lp(a). Nicotinic acid can suppress expression of LDL subclass pattern B when TGs are reduced below approximately 140 mg/dL (75, 273).

ADHERENCE ENHANCEMENT

Nicotinic acid is the lipid-altering drug with the most potential for side effects and, consequently, adherence problems. Because of its great potential benefit, it is worth expending extra effort on achieving compliance. Individual variability exists in the side effects to such an extent that it often can be attributed to differences in formulation. For this reason, obtaining several brands and testing each for individual tolerance can be helpful. Slowly titrating the dose from 100 mg three times a day to 500 mg three times a day over a 1-month period can ease the patient into a therapeutic dose range. The prostaglandin-mediated flush can be ameliorated in part by ingesting 2.5 grains of aspirin15 minutes before the nicotinic acid dose. Avoiding alcohol, monosodium glutamate, hot beverages, and spicy foods also can help ameliorate the flush. Gastrointestinal distress can be reduced by ingesting nicotinic acid with food. The most important tool to enhance adherence is a dedicated lipid nurse. The once-a-day timed-release nicotinic acid recently approved by the FDA appears to be well tolerated (271). Disorders and potential treatments are outlined in Table 18.5.

Table 18.5. Inherited Disorders Contributing to Coronary Artery Disease[a]

Disorder	Approximate Prevalence in CAD Patients	Treatment
ALP (LDL pattern B)	50%	Nicotinic acid–fibrates–low-fat diet
Lp(a)	33%	Nicotinic acid–estrogen
Homocysteinemia	20–30%	Folate–pyridoxine (B6)
High LDL-C	20–30%	Resin–statin–nicotinic acid
Apo E4	20%	Low-fat diet–probucol
High triglycerides	15%	Weight loss–exercise–nicotinic acid–fibrates
Hypoalpha	5%	Nicotinic acid–fibrates
Apo E2/2(type III)	2%	Fibrates–nicotinic acid

[a]Inherited disorders leading to CAD and the approximate prevalence in heart disease patients along with treatments for each of the disorders is shown. The most common disorders are treated by the least expensive therapies.
CAD = coronary artery disease; ALP = atherogenic lipoprotein profile; LDL = low-density lipoprotein; Lp(a) = lipoprotein(a); LDL-C = low-density lipoprotein cholesterol; hypoalpha = hypoalphalipoproteinemia; Apo = apoprotein.

Combination Drug Therapy

Lipidologists frequently use combinations of the drugs already mentioned. These combinations are tailored to the underlying lipoprotein abnormality and the patient's drug tolerance. One advantage is that substantial changes in lipid values can be achieved with relatively low doses of several drugs. This can be advantageous with regard to side effects, cost, and compliance. Triple-drug therapy is not uncommon in aggressive lipid clinics and was used in the SCOR and SCRIP arteriographic trials (163, 172).

To lower LDL-C, combinations of a resin with nicotinic acid, or an HMGRI, can be powerful and result in LDL-C reductions of 50% or more. In patients who have elevated LDL-C and TGs, the combination of resin or an HMGRI with nicotinic acid or gemfibrozil is useful. Without nicotinic acid or gemfibrozil, resins alone often can increase plasma TGs in these moderately hypertriglyceridemic patients.

In FH patients the combination of an HMGRI and nicotinic acid can be particularly successful in obtaining the desired lipid control. For patients who have elevated Lp(a), nicotinic acid is the only drug that appears to reduce Lp(a) levels, although this is not a consistent response.

Although there is a higher incidence of myositis in patients treated with the combination of HMGRI and a fibrate, it is a combination used by lipidologists. With this combination it is important to clearly discuss the potential risks and benefits with the patient (274).

The use of lipid-lowering agents in patients at risk for CAD and in those with diagnosed CAD is justified based on recent clinical and arteriographic trials. The primary lesson of these trials is that LDL-C should be reduced as low as possible without causing harm, and more importantly, small LDL and IDL should be aggressively treated. Conversion of LDL pattern B to pattern A and reduction of the dense LDLIIIa+b region to less than 15% is the appropriate strategy if CAD stability or regression is the clinical goal. Bile acid binding resins are safe and economical agents and can be considered as the initial drugs of choice for LDL-C reduction. When used in combination with other medications, LDL-C reduction can be particularly impressive. In the CAD population, an LDL-C goal of approximately 80 mg/dL is appropriate if cessation of disease progression or regression is the objective. Additional factors that will guide drug selection include Lp(a) levels and apo E isoforms, HDL subclass distribution, oxidation status, and homocysteine and fibrinogen values (32, 55, 78, 275, 276). Finally, it is important to remember that these medications have effects on the atherosclerotic phenomenon (other than lipoprotein changes) that include prostaglandins, thromboxanes, interleukin-1, and platelet aggregation (277). The analysis of cost-effectiveness based on LDL-C reduction is only a guide, and it is the clinician's duty to select a therapy that is most consistent with inhibiting the atherogenic process.

Some Final Thoughts Regarding Treatment of LDL Subclass Pattern B

Knowledge of LDL subclass pattern is useful because patterns A and B respond differently to many lipid-altering treatments. Pattern B subjects have a greater LDL-C and apo B reduction in response to dietary fat reduction than pattern A subjects (277a). After a low-fat diet, apo B decreased 10-fold more in the pattern B subjects compared to pattern A subjects. An additional investigation revealed that dietary fat reduction from 20% to 10% of total calories from fat resulted in conversion of pattern A subjects to pattern B, with significant increases in small LDL and IDL and reductions in HDL$_2$ (277b).

Lipid-lowering medications have variable effects on lipoprotein subclass distribution and a differential effect in LDL pattern A compared with pattern B subjects. Treatment with gemfibrozil alters the composition and distribution of LDL subspecies, with a shift from small LDL to larger LDL particles in most, but not all, hypertriglyceridemic patients. In relatively normolipemic pattern A and B subjects, gemfibrozil has a significantly greater effect on reduction in small LDL in pattern B compared with pattern A subjects (15). Nicotinic acid has a significantly greater effect on TG reduction, HDL-C increase, and increase in LDL particle diameter in LDL pattern B subjects compared with pattern A (75). Colestipol reduces small LDLs more in pattern B subjects compared with pattern A (253). Hydroxymethylglutaryl-CoA reductase inhibition effectively lowers LDL-C in patients with familial combined hyperlipidemia, but does not appear to improve the abnormal LDL composition or subclass distribution (278). Thus, part of the differential arteriographic response between pattern A versus pattern B subjects may be related to a differential response to many of the treatments used in the regression trials. Individuals with the LDL pattern B, or an abundance of TG-rich lipoproteins, appear to benefit most from therapies that reduce TGs, small LDL, and TG-rich lipoproteins (Table 18.6).

LDL patterns A and B are best determined by 2–16% polyacrylamide gradient gel electrophoresis with determination of the diameters of single or multiple LDL peaks, and percent distribution in seven LDL regions (26). This method has been used in multiple NIH-funded research investigations and at the Lawrence Berkeley National Laboratory (LBNL), University of California, Berkeley, correlated with the gold standard or lipoprotein subfraction determination, analytic ultracentrifugation, and clinical outcome. As part of the LBNL, office of technology transfer, and Berkeley HeartLab, such tests are now routinely available to clinicians worldwide and information discussed in this chapter is no longer esoteric but can be applied to clinical practice.

The clinical usefulness of the GGE information has been developed from numerous large clinical investigations dating back to the Lawrence Livermore Study in 1966 (180). More recently, case control and prospective studies have indicated that in a "healthy" population, the presence of the pattern B trait increases CAD risk 3-fold to 5-fold. These investigations include the Boston Area Health Study, the Physician's Health Survey, the Stanford Five City Project, and the Quebec study (17, 27–29). The risk attributed to the presence of the B trait was found to be independent of total, LDL, and HDL cholesterol, Apo B, triglycerides, TC/HDLC, and BMI. Thus, the presence of the LDL pattern B trait is an independent marker of significantly increased CAD risk. These investigations firmly establish the small LDL pattern B trait (ALP) as a major CAD risk factor independent of routine lipoprotein cholesterol measurements.

It is important to appreciate that many clinical and arteriographic investigations have reported that knowledge regarding LDL subclass pattern, or LDL particle size provides useful clinical information that guides treatment, and predicts outcome independent of routine lipid measurements (181). These investigations are outlined in Table 18.7.

Table 18.6. Summary of LDL Subclass Patterns and Their Clinical Implications.

Pattern A	Pattern B
Moderate diet responders	Increased CAD risk 3- to 5-fold
	Inherited (Mendelian dominant)
	Elevated IDL and insulin resistance
	High postprandial lipemia
	Susceptible to oxidation and low vitamin E content
	Low HDL_{2b} (reverse cholesterol transport)
	Great diet responders
	Possible enhanced expression with low-fat diet
	Good response to exercise and fat weight loss
	Good arteriographic responders
	Great nicotinic acid and gemfibrozil responders
	Good responders to colestipol

CAD = coronary artery disease; IDL = intermediate-density lipoprotein; HDL_{2b} = high-density lipoprotein of the 2b subclass.

PRACTICAL LIPID MANAGEMENT IN THE CARDIAC REHABILITATION SETTING

Advanced Lipoprotein Testing and Treatment in a Cardiac Rehabilitation Program

Cardiac rehabilitation has been validated as an effective model for secondary prevention of CAD. The Agency for Health Care Policy and Research published "Cardiac Rehabilitation: Clinical Practice Guidelines" in October 1995 (279). Thirty-seven reports in the scientific literature describe improvement in lipid profiles resulting from multifactorial cardiac rehabilitation. The rehabil-

Table 18.7.   Investigations Contributing Information to Clinical Decision Making on Lipoprotein Subclasses and CAD

Study	Type	Lipoprotein Subclass Finding
Livermore (182) risk	Prospective	Triglyceride rich Sf(20–100) lipoproteins associated with CAD. Lower HDL2 and HDL3 mass found in DeNova CAD subjects.
Framingham (182) risk	Prospective	Triglyceride rich Sf(20–400) lipoproteins associated with CAD.
Boston Heart (17)	Case Control	LDL pattern B associated with 3-fold increased CAD risk.
Physicians Health (27)	Prospective	LDL pattern B associated with 3.4-fold increased CAD risk independent of total and HDL cholesterol, and Apo B. Not statistically independent of TC/HDLC ratio.
Stanford FCP (28)	Prospective	LDL size is best predictor of CAD risk by conditional logistic regression. Not statistically independent of nonfasting triglycerides.
Quebec CV (29)	Prospective	LDL size independent predictor of CAD risk.
Montreal (153)	Arteriographic	IDL and HDL related to CAD progression but not LDLC.
NHLBI-II (157)	Arteriographic	Reduction in LDL, IDL, and small LDL mass related to atherosclerosis stability.
CLAS (161)	Arteriographic	Subjects with lower triglycerides benefited the least from niacin and resin treatment.
MARS (176)	Arteriographic	In treated subjects with LDLC < 85 mg/dl, triglyceride rich lipoproteins were correlated with disease progression.
SCRIP (33)	Arteriographic	Despite indentical LDLC reduction, subjects with a predominance of small LDL (pattern B) had significantly slower CAD progression compared to control subjects while those with a predominance of large LDL (pattern A) revealed no arteriographic effect of treatment compared to control subjects.
STARS (159)	Arteriographic	Change in dense LDL was the best predictor of arteriographic outcome.
FATS (168)	Arteriographic	Change in LDL buoyancy (inverse of density) was the best predictor of arteriographic outcome.
BECAIT (170)	Arteriographic	Triglyceride reduction but not LDL-C reduction is associated with arteriographic benefit equal to or greater than that seen in MAAS and REGRESS.

itation studies that reported the most favorable impact on lipid levels were multifactorial, that is, providing exercise training, dietary education, and counseling, and in some cases pharmacologic treatment, psychological support, and behavioral training. The report, however, does not recommend cardiac rehabilitation as a sole intervention in the treatment of lipid disorders (279).

Meta-analyses by O'Connor et al. (280) and Oldridge et al. (281) of randomized clinical trials of aerobic exercise training in post-MI patients have documented a powerful (20% to 30%) reduction in coronary deaths, but no reduction in CV morbidity. In comparison, numerous scientific investigations have shown that LDL-C reduction, by a variety of methods, can reduce heart disease events by 15% to 30% (282). In the largest secondary prevention study to date, the 4-S study (Scandinavian Simvastatin Survival Study) reported that treatment with simvastatin resulted in a significant 34% reduction in cardiac events (132). However, this 34% reduction represents the difference between 207 events in the placebo, and 136 events in the treatment groups. The reduction in events is remarkable progress, but a large number of patients are still experiencing events (Fig. 18.6).

Cardiac rehabilitation programs predominantly focus on nonpharmacologic approaches to reducing CV risk. It is becoming more apparent that a combination of therapies individualized to the underlying disorder is more effective than a single therapy. The combination of comprehensive cardiac rehabilitation involving medical evaluation, prescribed exercise, cardiac risk factor modification, and education and nutrition counseling with a sophisticated approach to lipoprotein management can improve CV health and reduce health care costs. Cardiac rehabilitation programs are ideally positioned to assume a pivotal role in delivering many components of comprehensive CV risk factor reduction in a secondary prevention setting.

One model for CV risk factor management is the Stanford Coronary Risk Intervention Project, which combined comprehensive risk factor management and sophisticated treatment of lipoprotein disorders (172). In this study, a 43% reduction in cardiac events was demonstrated. A comparison of the annual mean minimal diameter change in the coronary arteries showed that it was the LDL pattern B patients in the treatment group who experienced the most improvement, whereas pattern A patients in the treatment group were no different from the control group (33) (Table 18.8).

Sophisticated Lipoprotein Treatment in a Cardiac Rehabilitation Program

When advanced lipoprotein testing and the use of sophisticated treatment guidelines are combined with cardiac rehabilitation, the result is improved metabolic profiles, higher health status scores, better participation rates, lower readmission rates, and decreased health care costs (279).

Although only 20% of the patients in the cardiac rehabilitation program at one such program we are familiar with (Trinity Mother Frances

Table 18.8. Evolution of Cardiac Rehabilitation Toward Comprehensive Risk Factor Reduction Programs

Study	Major Findings
AHCPR Clinical Practice Guidelines Meta-analyses	Cardiac rehabilitation can be effective in improviding lipid profiles
	Not recommended as sole intervention
	Reduction in cardiovascular mortality
	No reduction in nonfatal cardiovascular events
	Significant reduction in cardiovascular events
	Large number of treatment group subjects still had events
SCRIP	Small arteriographic changes, significant reduction in events
	Patter B showed excellent arteriographic response to treatment
	Pattern A showed no benefit from treatment
Future	Cardiac rehabilitation programs will become comprehensive cardiovascular risk factor reduction programs including sophisticated treatment of risk factors, such as small, dense LDL, Lp(a), and homocysteine

AHCPR = Agency for Health Care Policy and Research; 4S = Scandinavian Simvastatin Survival Study; SCRIP = Stanford Coronary Risk Intervention Project; LDL = low-density lipoprotein; Lp(a) = lipoprotein(a).

Health System in Texas) had an abnormal lipid profile, the incidence of the pattern B (small, dense LDL) phenotype was 52% and Lp(a) was 41% (283). Diagnosis and treatment protocols in the lipid clinic were based on previous algorithms developed for Kaiser Hospital and Trinity Mother Frances Health System by members of Berkeley HeartLab, and improved by the use of sophisticated lipoprotein tests that guide drug use.

Perceived health status of patients is becoming increasingly important in our health care system. Lipid clinics that are becoming more sophisticated in the treatment of lipid disorders must also collect data showing their value as a preventive cardiology program. Fifty-six patients who had undergone CABG surgery and enrolled in the Trinity Mother Frances Cardiac Rehabilitation/Lipid Clinic were compared with 126 control CAD patients who had CABG surgery but did not enroll in the lipid clinic; patients were matched for age, gender, and CV status (283). General health perception was assessed by the SF36 health status questionnaire and there was a significant (p < 0.01) improvement after 1 year in the lipid clinic group (284).

Utilization of the health care system was also reduced in the CAD patients participating in the Cardiac Rehabilitation/Lipid Clinic program. End points were actual 1-year readmission rates and charges derived from hospital and clinic billing records that include clinic visits, inpatient readmissions, emergency room visits, outpatient cath lab procedures, and CV surgeries. Clinic visits were more frequent in the cardiac rehabilitation/lipid clinic group compared to the control (94 versus 24), hospitalizations were fewer in the rehabilitation/lipid clinic group (7 versus 22), as were ER visits (7 versus 22), but CV surgery and outpatient catheter lab procedures were similar (2 versus 5 and 4 versus 0) (283). Despite a greater number of clinic visits, a preventive cardiology program, guided by sophisticated lab tests and treatment protocols, is cost-effective in the real world and may save approximately $4120 per patient in the first year (Table 18.9).

One of the major limiting factors in the success of a cardiac rehabilitation program is the relatively low participation rates of patients in phase II cardiac rehabilitation programs. The participation rates for cardiac rehabilitation at Trinity Mother Frances dramatically improved with the commencement of sophisticated heart

Table 18.9. Heath Care System Utilization in 56 CAD Patients in a Cardiac Rehabilitation/Lipid Clinic Program Compared to 56 CAD Patients in a Usual Care Group

	Rehab/ Lipid	Control	Difference	P Value
n	56	56		
Clinic visits	94	24	70	.05
Hospitalizations	7	22	−15	.017
ER visits	7	22	−15	.023
CV surgery	2	5	3	NS
Outpatient cath	4	0	4	NS

CAD = coronary artery disease; Rehab/Lipid = cardiac rehabilitation/lipid clinic program; ER = emergency room; CV = cardiovascular; cath = catheterization; NS = not significant.

disease risk testing in a combined cardiac rehabilitation, lipid clinic, cardiopulmonary exercise testing and educational program format. Before the combined program, participation rates in 1994, 1995, and 1996 were 11%, 17%, and 24%. After the implementation of the combined program, participation rates rose to 52%.

The concept of "metabolic fitness" includes low-intensity exercise-induced improvement in lipid and carbohydrate metabolism that may not be linked to CV fitness. Patients who have small, dense LDL, high apo B, elevated TGs, low HDL, or obesity or who are diabetic are given a "metabolic" exercise prescription. Because exercise and weight loss can be effective in the treatment of TGs, low-intensity, longer duration exercise gives these patients a better chance of correcting their underlying disorder. Patients with elevated LDL-C are given a CV fitness exercise prescription because exercise alone is unlikely to be effective in reducing LDL-C. These patients can still benefit, however, from increasing their overall CV fitness. Recently, new insight into the details of the metabolic lipid response to exercise has been gained. The response to exercise can be affected by the underlying lipoprotein status, body fat composition, gender, age, carbohydrate tolerance, and, undoubtedly, factors yet to be identified.

CONCLUSIONS

The treatment of atherosclerosis and CAD has entered a new era with the advent of metabolic diagnosis and treatment of this common disorder. Significant advances have been made in the last decade that allow clinicians to use sophisticated laboratory tools to diagnosis the underlying metabolic disorder and customize treatment for the individual patient that provides the best environment for retarding the rate of CAD progression and perhaps achieving some degree of regression. Treatment is specific to the disorder, and no one drug or diet is optimal treatment for all patients. The small, dense LDL pattern B trait is the most common disorder found in CAD patients. It is more common than elevated LDL-C, and with appropriate treatment, patients can have a beneficial arteriographic outcome. Not only is a metabolic approach to CAD the proper scientific and medical approach, but it has also been shown to significantly reduce the financial impact of this disease by guiding specific therapies to the individual disorders. Thus, the most common underlying disorders contributing to CAD are treated by the least expensive of therapies (Table 18.5).

References

1. Superko HR. Beyond LDL-C reduction. Circulation 1996;94:2351–2354.
2. Hodis HN, Mack WJ, Azen SP, et al. Triglyceride- and cholesterol-rich lipoproteins have a differential effect on mild/moderate and severe lesion progression as assessed by quantitative coronary angiography in a controlled trial of lovastatin. Circulation 1994;90:42–49.
3. Superko HR. New aspects of cardiovascular risk factors including small, dense LDL, homocysteinemia, and Lp(a). Curr Opin Cardiol 1995;10:347–354.
4. Dawber TR. The Framingham study. Cambridge, MA: Harvard University Press, 1980.
5. Swift RL. Berkeley HeartLab. Start-Up 1996;1:15.
6. Lindgren FT, Jensen LC, Hatach FT. The isolation and quantitative analysis of serum lipoproteins. In: Nelson GJ, ed. Blood lipids and lipoproteins: quantitation, composition and metabolism. New York: Wiley-Interscience, 1972:181–274.
7. Blanche PJ, Gong EL, Forte TM, et al. Characterization of human high-density lipoproteins by gradient gel electrophoresis. Biochim Biophys Acta 1981;665:408–419.
8. Miller NE, Hammett G, Saltissi S, et al. Relation of angiographically defined coronary artery disease to plasma lipoprotein subfractions and apolipoproteins. Br Med J 1981;282:1741–1744.
9. Shen MMS, Krauss RM, Lindgren FT, et al. Heterogeneity of serum low density lipoproteins in normal human subjects. J Lipid Res 1981;22:236–244.
10. Krauss RM, Burke DJ. Identification of multiple subclasses of plasma low density lipoproteins in normal humans. J Lipid Res 1982;23:97–104.
11. Superko HR, Krauss RM. LDL and HDL particle subclass differences in CHD patients treated with selective and nonselective beta blocking medications. Thirteenth International Symposium on Atherosclerosis, Oct 9, 1988, Rome, Italy.
12. Superko HR, Wood PD, Krauss RM. Effect of alpha- and selective beta-blockade for hypertension control

on plasma lipoproteins, apoproteins, lipoprotein sub-classes, and postprandial lipemia. Am J Med 1989; 86(Suppl 1B):26–31.

13. Loaldi A, Montorsi P, Polese A, et al. Angiographic evolution of coronary atherosclerosis in patients receiving propranolol. Chest 1991;99:1238–1242.

14. Williams PT, Krauss RM, Vranizan KM, et al. Changes in lipoprotein subfractions during diet-induced and exercise-induced weight loss in moderately overweight men. Circulation 1990;81:1293–1304.

15. Superko HR, Krauss RM. Reduction of small, dense LDL by gemfibrozil in LDL subclass pattern B. Circulation 1995;92:I-250.

16. Austin MA, King MC, Vranizan KM, et al. Atherogenic lipoprotein phenotype. A proposed genetic marker for coronary heart disease risk. Circulation 1990;82: 495–506.

17. Austin MA, Breslow JL, Hennekens CH, et al. Low density lipoprotein subclass patterns and risk of myocardial infarction. JAMA 1988;260:1917–1921.

18. Nishina PM, Johnson JP, Naggert JK, et al. Linkage of atherogenic lipoprotein phenotype to the low-density lipoprotein receptor locus on the short arm of chromosome 19. Proc Natl Acad Sci USA 1992;89:708–712.

19. Rotter JI, Bu X, Cantor R, et al. Multilocus genetic determination of LDL particle size in coronary artery disease families [abstract]. Clin Res 1994;42:16A.

20. Hulley SB, Rosenman RH, Bawol RD, et al. Epidemiology as a guide to clinical decisions: the association between triglyceride and coronary heart disease. N Engl J Med 1980;302:1383–1389.

21. Austin MA. Review: plasma triglyceride and coronary heart disease. Arterioscler Thromb 1991;11:2–14.

22. Krauss RM. Heterogeneity of plasma low-density lipoproteins and atherosclerosis risk. Curr Opin Lipidol 1994;5:339–349.

23. Superko HR, Wood PD, Laughton C, et al. Low density lipoprotein (LDL) subclass patterns and postprandial lipemia. Arteriosclerosis 1990;10:826a.

24. Tribble DL, Holl LG, Wood PD, et al. Variations in oxidative susceptibility among six low density lipoprotein subfractions of differing density and particle size. Atherosclerosis 1992;93:189–199.

25. Krauss RM, Blanche PJ. Detection and quantitation of LDL subfractions. Curr Opin Lipidol 1992;3:377–383.

26. Superko HR, Krauss RM, Miller B. Prediction of LDL subclass pattern from Trig, HDLC, LDLC.apoB. Cardiovascular Health, Feb 19, 1998. San Francisco, California. Abstract.

27. Stampfer MJ, Krauss RM, Blanche PJ, et al. A prospective study of triglyceride level, low density lipoprotein particle diameter, and risk of myocardial infarction. JAMA 1996;276:882–888.

28. Gardner CD, Fortmann SP, Krauss RM. Small low-density lipoprotein particles are associated with the incidence of coronary artery disease in men and women. JAMA 1996;276:875–881.

29. Lamarche B, Tchernof A, Moorjani S, et al. Small, dense low-density lipoprotein particles as a predictor of the risk of ischemic heart disease in men. Prospective results from the Quebec cardiovascular study. Circulation 1997;95:69–75.

30. Sniderman AD, Wolfson C, Teng B, et al. Association of hyperapobetalipoproteinemia with endogenous hypertriglyceridemia and atherosclerosis. Ann Intern Med 1982;97:833–839.

31. Krauss RM, Lindgren FT, Williams PT, et al. Intermediate-density lipoproteins and progression of coronary artery disease in hypercholesterolaemic men. Lancet 1987;2:62–66.

32. Krauss RM. Relationship of intermediate and low-density lipoprotein subspecies to risk of coronary artery disease. Am Heart J 1987;113:578–582.

33. Miller BD, Alderman EL, Haskell WL, et al. Predominance of dense low-density lipoprotein particles predicts angiographic benefit or therapy in the Stanford Coronary Risk Intervention project. Circulation 1996;94:2146–2153.

34. Superko HR. Statistics don't tell the whole story. The Heart of the Matter? December 1996: 2.

35. Watts GF, Mandalia S, Brunt JN, et al. Independent associations between plasma lipoprotein subfraction levels and the course of coronary artery disease in the St Thomas' Atherosclerosis Regression Study (STARS). Metabolism 1993;42:1461–1467.

36. Phillips NR, Waters D, Havel RJ. Plasma lipoproteins and progression of coronary artery disease evaluated by angiography and clinical events. Circulation 1993;88:2762–2770.

37. Superko HR. Out with the old and in with the new thinking on lipids and heart disease. Curr Opin Cardiol 1997;12:180–187.

38. Superko HR. What can we learn about dense LDL and lipoprotein particles from clinical trials? Curr Opin Lipidol 1996;7:363–368.

39. Mahley RW. Apolipoprotein E: cholesterol transport protein with expanding role in cell biology. Science 1988;240:622–630.

40. Lusus AJ. Genetic factors affecting blood lipoproteins: the candidate gene approach. J Lipid Res 1988;29:397–429.

41. Gabelli C, Greff RE, Zech LA, et al. Abnormal low density lipoprotein metabolism in apolipoprotein E deficiency. J Lipid Res 1986;27:326–333.

42. Utermann G. Apolipoprotein E polymorphism in health and disease. Am Heart J 1987;113:433–440.

43. Brown MS, Goldstein JL. Lipoprotein receptors in the liver. J Clin Invest 1983;72:743–747.

44. Weintraub MS, Eisenberg S, Breslow JL. Different patterns of postprandial lipoprotein metabolism in normal, type IIa, type III, and type IV hyperlipoproteinemic individuals. J Clin Invest 1987;79:1110–1119.

45. Superko HR. The effect of apolipoprotein E isoform difference on postprandial lipoprotein composition in patients matched for triglycerides, LDL-cholesterol and HDL-cholesterol. Artery 1991:18:315–325.

46. Brown AJ, Roberts DCK. The effect of fasting triacylglyceride concentration and apolipoprotein E polymorphism on postprandial lipemia. Arterioscler Thromb 1991;11:1737–1744.

47. Mahley RW. Atherogenic hyperlipoproteinemia. The cellular and molecular biology of plasma lipoproteins altered by dietary fat and cholesterol. Med Clin North Am 1982;66:375–400.

48. Lopez-Miranda J, Ordovas JM, Mata P, et al. Effect of apolipoprotein E phenotype on diet-induced lowering

of plasma low density lipoprotein cholesterol. J Lipid Res 1994;35:1965–1975.

49. Superko HR. The effect of apolipoprotein E isoform difference on postprandial lipoprotein composition in patients matched for triglycerides, LDL-cholesterol and HDL-cholesterol. Artery 1991:18:315–325.

50. Dreon DM, Fernstrom HA, Miller B, et al. Apolipoprotein E isoform phenotype and LDL subclass response to a reduced-fat diet. Arterioscler Thromb Vasc Biol 1995;15:105–111.

51. Hixson JE, PDAY Research Group. Apolipoprotein E polymorphisms affect atherosclerosis in young males. Arterioscler Thromb 1991;11:1237–1244.

52. Corder EH, Saunders AM, Strittmatter WJ, et al. Gene dose of apolipoprotein E type 4 allele and the risk of Alzheimer's disease in late onset families. Science 1993;261:921–923.

53. St George-Hyslop P, McLachlan DC, Tuda T, et al. Alzheimer's disease and possible gene interaction. Science 1994;263:537.

54. American College of Medical Genetics/American Society of Human Genetics Working Group on ApoE and Alzheimer Disease. Statement on use of apolipoprotein E testing for Alzheimer disease. JAMA 1995;274:1627–1629.

55. Scanu AM, Gless GM. Lipoprotein(a). Heterogeneity and biological relevance. J Clin Invest 1990;85:1709–1715.

56. Sandkamp M, Funke H, Schelte H, et al. Lipoprotein(a) is an independent risk factor for myocardial infarction at a young age. Clin Chem 1990;36:20–23.

57. Dahlen GH, Guyton JR, Attar M, et al. Association of levels of lipoprotein Lp(a), plasma lipids, and other lipoproteins with coronary artery disease documented by angiography. Circulation 1986;74:758–765.

58. Bostrom AG, Cupples LA, Jenner JL, et al. Elevated plasma lipoprotein(a) and coronary heart disease in men aged 55 years and younger. JAMA 1996;276:544–548.

59. Schaefer EJ, Lamon-Fava S, Jenner JL, et al. Lipoprotein(a) levels and risk of coronary heart disease in men. JAMA 1994;271:999–1003.

60. Brown G, Albers JJ, Fisher LD, et al. Regression of coronary artery disease as a result of intensive lipid-lowering therapy in men with high levels of apolipoprotein B. N Engl J Med 1990;323:1289–1298.

61. Carlson LA, Hamsten A, Asplund A. Pronounced lowering of serum levels of lipoprotein Lp(a) in hyperlipidaemic subjects treated with nicotinic acid. J Intern Med 1989;226:271–276.

62. Soma M, Fumagalli R, Paoletti R, et al. Plasma Lp(a) concentration after oestrogen and progestogen in postmenopausal women [letter]. Lancet 1991;337:612.

63. Marcovina SM, Lippi G, Bagatell CJ, Bremmer WJ. Testosterone-induced suppression of lipoprotein(a) in normal men: relation to basal lipoprotein(a) level. Atherosclerosis 1996;122:89–95.

64. Daida H, Lee, YJ, Yokoi H, et al. Prevention of restenosis after percutaneous transluminal coronary angioplasty by reducing lipoprotein(a) levels with low-density lipoprotein apheresis. Am J Cardiol 1994;73:1037–1040.

65. Moreton JR. Chylomicronemia, fat tolerance, and atherosclerosis. J Lab Clin Med 1950;35:373–384.

66. Zilversmit DB. Atherogenesis: a post prandial phenomenon. Circulation 1979;60:473–485.

67. Harlan WR, Beischer DE. Changes in serum lipoproteins after a large fat meal in normal individuals and in patients with ischemic heart disease. Am Heart J 1963:61–67.

68. Genest J, Sniderman A, Cianflone K, et al. Hyperapobetalipoproteinemia. Arteriosclerosis 1986;6:297–304.

69. Bersot TP, Innerarity TL, Pitas RE, et al. Fat feeding in humans induces lipoproteins of density less than 1.006 that are enriched in apolipoprotein (a) and that cause lipid accumulation in macrophages. J Clin Invest 1986;77:622–630.

70. Bersot TP, Innerarity TL, Pitas RE, et al. Fat feeding in humans induces lipoproteins of density less than 1.006 that are enriched in apolipoprotein (a) and that cause lipid accumulation in macrophages. J Clin Invest 1986;77:622–630.

71. Patsch JR, Misesenbock G, Hopferwieser T, et al. Relation of triglyceride metabolism and coronary artery disease. Studies in the postprandial state. Arteriosclerosis and Thrombosis 1992;12:1336–1345.

72. Fellin R, Baggio G, Baiocchi R, et al. HDL2 and HDL3 variations during the postprandial phase in humans. In: Nosdea G, Lewis B, Paoletti R, eds. Diet and drugs in atherosclerosis. New York: Raven Press, 1980:85–91.

73. Weintraub MS, Rosen Y, Otto R, et al. Physical exercise conditioning in the absence of weight loss reduces fasting and postprandial triglyceride-rich lipoprotein levels. Circulation 1989;79:1007–1014.

74. Superko HR. Effects of acute and chronic alcohol consumption on postprandial lipemia in healthy normotriglyceridemic men. Am J Cardiol 1992;69:701–704.

75. Superko HR, KOS Investigators. Effect of nicotinic acid on LDL subclass patterns. Circulation 1994;90:I-504.

76. Superko HR, Haskell WL, DiRicco CD. HMGCoA reductase inhibitor (Fluvastatin) on LDL peak particle diameter. Am J Cardiol 1997;80:78–81.

77. Packard CJ, Shepherd J. The hepatobiliary axis and lipoprotein metabolism: effects of bile acid sequestrants and ileal bypass surgery. J Lipid Res 1982;23:1081–1098.

78. Steinberg D, Parthasarathy S, Carew TE, et al. Beyond cholesterol. Modifications of low-density lipoprotein that increase its atherogenicity. N Engl J Med 1989;320:915–924.

79. Henriksen T, Mahoney EM, Steinberg D. Enhanced macrophage degradation of low density lipoprotein previously incubated with cultured endothelial cells: recognition by receptor for acetylated low density lipoproteins. Proc Natl Acad Sci USA 1981;78:6499–6503.

80. Henriksen T, Mahoney EM, Steinberg D. Enhanced macrophage degradation of biologically modified low density lipoprotein. Arteriosclerosis 1983;3:149–159.

81. Sparrow CP, Parthasarathy S, Steinberg D. A macrophage receptor that recognizes oxidized low density lipoprotein but not acetylated low density lipoprotein. J Biol Chem 1989;264:2599–2604.

82. Goldstein BD, Lodi C, Collinson C, et al. Ozone and lipid peroxidation. Arch Environ Health 1969;18:631–635.

83. Steinbrecher UP, Parthasarathy S, Leake DS, et al. Modification of low density lipoprotein by endothelial

cells involves lipid peroxidation and degradation of low density lipoprotein phospholipids. Proc Natl Acad Sci USA 1984;83:3883–3887.

84. Fogelman AM, Shechter I, Saeger J, et al. Malondialdehyde alteration of low density lipoproteins leads to cholesterol ester accumulation in human monocyte macrophage. Proc Natl Acad Sci USA 1980;77:2214–2218.

85. Jurgens G, Lang J, Esterbauer H. Modification of human low-density lipoprotein by the lipid peroxidation product 4-hydroxynonenal. Biochim Biophys Acta 1986;875:103–114.

86. Esterbauer H, Jurgens G, Quehenberger O, et al. Autooxidation of human low density lipoprotein: loss of polyunsaturated fatty acids and vitamin E and generation of aldehydes. J Lipid Res 1987;28:495–509.

87. Ohta T, Takata K, Horiuchi S, et al. Protective effect of lipoproteins containing apoprotein A-I on Cu^{2+} catalyzed oxidation of human low density lipoprotein. FEBS Lett 1989;257:435–438.

88. Hodis HN, Mack WJ, LaBree L, et al. Serial coronary angiographic evidence that antioxidant vitamin intake reduces progression of coronary artery atherosclerosis. JAMA 1995;273:1849–1854.

89. Stephens NG, Parsons A, Schofield PM, et al. Randomised controlled trial of vitamin E in patients with coronary disease: Cambridge Heart Antioxidant Study (CHAOS). Lancet 1996;347:781–786.

90. Soria LF, Ludwig EH, Clarke HRG, et al. Association between a specific apolipoprotein B mutation and familial defective apolipoprotein B-100. Proc Natl Acad Sci USA 1989;86:587–591.

91. Innerarity TL. Familial hypobetalipoproteinemia and familial defective apolipoprotein B100: genetic disorders associated with apolipoprotein B. Curr Opin Lipidol 1990;1:104–109.

92. Vergani C, Beattale G. Familial hypo-alpha-lipoproteinemia. Clin Chim Acta 1981;114:45–52.

93. Ordovas JM, Schaefer EJ, Salem D, et al. Apolipoprotein A-I gene polymorphism associated with premature coronary artery disease and familial hypoalphalipoproteinemia. N Engl J Med 1986;314:671–677.

94. Virchow R. von Gesammelte Abhandlungen Zur Wissenschaftlichen. Berlin: Medicia, Müller, 1856:485.

95. Mudd SH, Levy HL. Disorders of transsulfuration. In: Stanbury JB, Wingarden JB, Fredrickson DS, et al., eds. The metabolic basis of inherited disease. New York: McGraw-Hill, 1983:522–559.

96. Robinson K. Hyperhomocysteinemia and low pyridoxal phosphate: common and independent reversible risk factors for coronary artery disease. Circulation 1995;92(10):2825–2830.

97. Selhub J, Jacques PF, Bostom AG, et al. Association between plasma homocysteine concentrations and extracranial carotid artery stenosis. NEJM 1995;332:286–291.

98. Malinow MR. Hyperhomocysteinemia. A common and easily reversible risk factor for occlusive atherosclerosis. Circulation 1990;81:2004–2006.

99. Nygard O, Nordrehaug E, Refsum H, et al. Plasma homocysteine levels and mortality in patients with coronary artery disease. N Engl J Med 1997;337:230–236.

100. Malinow MR, Kang SS, Taylor LM, et al. Prevalence of hyperhomocyst(e)inemia in patients with peripheral arterial occlusive disease. Circulation 1989;79:1180–1188.

101. Graham IM, Daly LE, Refsum HM, et al. Plasma homocysteine as a risk factor for vascular disease. The European concerted action project. JAMA 1997;277:1775–1781.

102. Robinson K, Mayer E, Jacobsen DW. Homocysteine and coronary artery disease. Cleveland Clinic J of Med 1994;61:438–449.

103. Superko HR. High HDLC, not protective in the presence of homocysteinemia. Am J Cardiol 1997;79:705–706.

104. Blankenhorn DH, Malinow MR, Mack WJ. Colestipol plus niacin therapy elevates plasma homocyst(e)ine levels. Coron Artery Dis 1991;2:357–360.

105. Brattstrom LE, Israelsson B, Jeppsson J-O, et al. Folic acid—an innocuous means to reduce plasma homocysteine. Scand J Clin Lab Invest 1988;48:215–221.

106. Lusis AJ, Heinzmann C, Sparkes RS, et al. Regional mapping of human chromosome 19: organization of genes for plasma lipid transport (APOCI, -C2, and -E and LDLR) and the genes C3, PEPD and GPI. Proc Natl Acad Sci USA 1986;83:3929–3933.

107. Frank SL, Klisak I, Sparkes RS, et al. Apolipoprotein (a) gene resides on human chromosome 6Q26–27, in close proximity to the homologous gene for plasminogen. Hum Genet 1988;79:352–356.

108. Lusis AJ, Sparkes RS. Chromosomal organization of genes involved in plasma lipoprotein metabolism: human and mouse 'fat maps.' In: Lusus AJ, Sparkes SR, eds. Genetic factors in atherosclerosis: approaches and model systems. Monographs in human genetics. Basel: Karger, 1989:79–94.

109. Rubin EM, Ishida BY, Clift SM, et al. Expression of human apolipoprotein A-I in transgenic mice results in reduced plasma levels of murine apolipoprotein A-I and the appearance of two new high density lipoprotein size subclasses. Proc Natl Acad Sci USA 1991;88:434–438.

110. Steinberg D. The cholesterol controversy is over. Why did it take so long? Circulation 1989;80:1070–1078.

111. Henriksen T, Mahoney EM, Steinberg D. Interactions of plasma lipoproteins with endothelial cells. Ann NY Acad Sci 1982;401:102–116.

112. Hjermann I, Holm I, Gelve BK, et al. Effect of diet and smoking intervention on the incidence of coronary heart disease. Lancet 1981;2:1303–1310.

113. Carlson LA, Bottiger LE. Risk factors for ischaemic heart disease in men and women. Results of the 19-year follow-up of the Stockholm Prospective Study. Acta Med Scand 1985;218:207–211.

114. Thelle DS, Forde OH, Try K, et al. The Tromso Heart Study. Acta Med Scand 1976;200:107–118.

115. Kornitzer M, De Backer G, Dramaix M, et al. The Belgian Heart Disease Prevention Project. Circulation 1980;61:18–25.

116. Kannel WB, Castelli WP, Gordon T. Cholesterol in the prediction of atherosclerotic disease. Ann Intern Med 1979;90:85–91.

117. Multiple Risk Factor Intervention Trial Group. Risk factor changes and mortality results. Multiple Risk Factor Intervention Trial Research Group. JAMA 1982;248:1465–1477.

118. Martin MJ, Hulley SB, Browner WS, et al. Serum cho-

lesterol, blood pressure, and mortality: implications from a cohort of 361,662 men. Lancet 1986;2:933–936.

119. Hanefeld M, Hora C, Schulze J, et al. Reduced incidence of cardiovascular complications and mortality in hyperlipoproteinemia (HLP) with effective lipid correction. The Dresden HLP study. Atherosclerosis 1984;53:47–58.

120. Carlson LA, Rosenhamer G. Reduction of mortality in the Stockholm ischaemic heart disease secondary prevention study by combined treatment with clofibrate and nicotinic acid. Acta Med Scand 1988;223:405–418.

121. Jacobs DR, Mebane IL, Bangdiwala SI, et al. High density lipoprotein cholesterol as a predictor of cardiovascular disease mortality in men and women: the follow-up study of the lipid research clinics prevalence study. Am J Epidemiol 1990;131:32–47.

122. Gordon DJ, Probstfield JL, Garrison RJ, et al. High-density lipoprotein cholesterol and cardiovascular disease. Four prospective American studies. Circulation 1989;79:8–15.

123. Phillips NR, Waters D, Havel RJ. Plasma lipoproteins and progression of coronary artery disease evaluated by angiography and clinical events. Circulation 1993;88:2762–2770.

124. Miller NE, Forde OH, Thelle DS, et al. The Tromso Heart Study. Lancet 1977;1:965–968.

125. Oliver MF, Heady JA, Morris JN, et al. A cooperative trial in the primary prevention of ischemic heart disease using clofibrate. Report from the Committee of Principal Investigators. Br Heart J 1978;40:1069–1118.

126. Coronary Drug Project Research Group. Natural history of myocardial infarction in the coronary drug project: long-term prognostic importance of serum lipid levels. Am J Cardiol 1978;42:489–498.

127. Canner PL, Berge KG, Wenger NK, et al. Fifteen year mortality in coronary drug project patients: long-term benefit with niacin. J Am Coll Cardiol 1986;8:1245–1255.

128. Canner PL, Berge KG, Wenger NK, et al. Fifteen year mortality in coronary drug project patients: long-term benefit with niacin. J Am Coll Cardiol 1986;8:1245–1255.

129. Lipid Research Clinics Program. The lipid research clinics coronary primary prevention trial results. I. Reduction in incidence of coronary heart disease. II. The relationship of reduction in incidence of coronary heart disease to cholesterol lowering. JAMA 1984;251:351–374.

130. Frick MH, Elo O, Haapa K, et al. Helsinki Heart Study: primary-prevention trial with gemfibrozil in middle-aged men with dyslipidemia. N Engl J Med 1987;317:1237–1245.

131. Manninen V, Tenkanen L, Koskinen P, et al. Joint effects of serum triglyceride and LDL cholesterol and HDL cholesterol concentrations on coronary heart disease risk in the Helsinki Heart Study. Circulation 1992;85:37–45.

132. Scandinavian Simvastatin Survival Study Group. Randomised trial of cholesterol lowering in 4,444 patients with coronary heart disease: the Scandinavian Simvastatin Survival Study (4S). Lancet 1994;349:1383–1389.

133. Shepherd J, Cobbe SM, Isles CG, et al. Prevention of coronary heart disease with pravastatin in men with hypercholesterolemia. N Engl J Med 1995;333:1301–1307.

134. Sacks FM, Pfeffer MA, Moye LA, et al. The effect of pravastatin on coronary events after myocardial infarction in patients with average cholesterol levels. N Engl J Med 1996;335:1001–1009.

135. Superko HR, Krauss RM, SCRIP investigators. Arteriographic benefit of multifactorial risk reduction in patients with LDLC < 125 mg/dL is seen in LDL pattern B but not pattern A. Fourth International Symposium on Multiple Risk Factors in Cardiovascular Disease. Washington, DC, April 1997, abstract book, p. 32.

136. Superko HR, Wood PD, Haskell WL. Coronary heart disease and risk factor modification. Is there a threshold? Am J Med 1985;78:826–838.

137. Brown GB, Zhao XQ, Sacco DE, et al. Lipid lowering and plaque regression. Circulation 1993;87:1781–1791.

138. Waters D, Craven TE, Lesperance J. Prognostic significance of progression of coronary atherosclerosis. Circulation 1993;87:1067–1075.

139. Buchwald H, Varco RL, Matts JP, et al. Effect of partial ileal bypass surgery on mortality and morbidity from coronary heart disease in patients with hypercholesterolemia. N Engl J Med 1990;323:946–955.

140. Schuler G, Hambrecht R, Schlierf G, et al. Regular physical exercise and low-fat diet. Effects on progression of coronary artery disease. Circulation 1992;86:1–11.

141. Hambrecht R, Niebauer J, Marburger C, et al. Various intensities of leisure time physical activity in patients with coronary artery disease. J Am Coll Cardiol 1993;22:468–477.

142. Ornish D, Brown SE, Scherwitz LW, et al. Can lifestyle changes reverse coronary heart disease? Lancet 1990;336:129–133.

143. Glagov S, Weisenberg E, Zarins CK, et al. Compensatory enlargement of human atherosclerotic coronary arteries. N Engl J Med 1987;316:1371–1375.

144. Ellis S, Sanders W, Goulet C, et al. Optimal detection of the progression of coronary artery disease: comparison of methods suitable for risk factor intervention trials. Circulation 1986;74:1235–1242.

145. Moise A, Theroux P, Taeymans Y, et al. Factors associated with progression of coronary artery disease in patients with normal or minimally narrowed coronary arteries. Am J Cardiol 1985;56:30–34.

146. Kroncke GM, Kosolcharoen P, Clayman JA, et al. Five-year changes in coronary arteries of medical and surgical patients of the Veterans Administration randomized study of bypass surgery. Circulation 1988;78 (Suppl 1):I-144–I-150.

147. Hamsten A, Walldius G, Szamosi A, et al. Relationship of angiographically defined coronary artery disease to serum lipoproteins and apolipoproteins in young survivors of myocardial infarction. Circulation 1986;73:1097–1110.

148. Deleted in proof.

149. Brown BG, Bolson EL, Dodge HT. Arteriographic assessment of coronary atherosclerosis. Review of current methods, their limitations, and clinical applications. Arteriosclerosis 1982;2:2–15.

150. Levy RI, Brensike JF, Epstein SE, et al. The influence

of changes in lipid values induced by cholestyramine and diet on progression of coronary artery disease: results of the NHLBI type II coronary intervention study. Circulation 1984;69:325–337.

151. Brensike JF, Levy RI, Kelsey, et al. Effects of therapy with cholestyramine on progression of coronary atherosclerosis: results of the NHLBI type II coronary intervention study. Circulation 1984;69:313–324.

152. Watts GF, Lewis B, Brunt JNH, et al. Effects on coronary artery disease of lipid-lowering diet, or diet plus cholestyramine, in the St Thomas' Atherosclerosis Regression Study (STARS). Lancet 1992;339: 563–569.

153. Blankenhorn DH, Nessim SA, Johnson RD, et al. Beneficial effects of combined colestipol-niacin therapy on coronary atherosclerosis and coronary venous by-pass grafts. JAMA 1987;257:3233–3240.

154. Miller BD, Krauss RM, Cashin-Hemphill L, et al. Baseline triglyceride levels predict angiographic benefit of colestipol plus niacin therapy in the cholesterol-lowering atherosclerosis study (CLAS) [abstract]. Circulation 1993;88:I-363.

155. Cashin Hemphill L, Mack WJ, Pogoda JM, et al. Beneficial effects of colestipol-niacin on coronary atherosclerosis. JAMA 1990;264:3013–3017.

156. Buchwald H, Campos CT, Boen JR, et al. Disease-free intervals after partial ileal bypass in patients with coronary heart disease and hypercholesterolemia. J Am Coll Cardiol 1995;26:351–357.

157. Campeau L, Enjalbert M, Lesperance J, et al. The relation of risk factors to the development of atherosclerosis in saphenous-vein bypass grafts and the progression of disease on the native circulation. N Engl J Med 1984;311:1329–1332.

158. Campeau L, Knatterud GL, Domanski M, et al. The effect of aggressive lowering of low-density lipoprotein cholesterol levels and low-dose anticoagulation on obstructive changes in saphenous-vein coronary-artery bypass grafts. N Engl J Med 1997;336:153–162.

159. Alderman EL, Hamilton KK, Silverman J, et al. Anatomically flexible computer-assisted reporting system for coronary angiography. Am J Cardiol 1982;49: 1208–1218.

160. Zhao ZQ, Brown BG, Hillger L, et al. Effects of intensive lipid lowering therapy on the coronary arteries of asymptomatic subjects with elevated apolipoprotein B. Circulation 1993;88:2744–2753.

161. Stewart BR, Brown BG, Shao XQ, et al. Benefits of lipid-lowering therapy in men with elevated apolipoprotein B are not confined to those with very high low density lipoprotein cholesterol. J Am Coll Cardiol 1994;23:899–906.

162. Zambon A, Brown BG, Hokansen JE, et al. Hepatic lipase changes predicts coronary artery disease regression/progression in the Familial Atherosclerosis Treatment Study. Circulation 1996;94;I-539.

163. Kane JP, Malloy MJ, Ports TA, et al. Regression of coronary atherosclerosis during treatment of familial hypercholesterolemia with combined drug regimens. JAMA 1990;264:3007–3012.

164. Deleted in proof.

165. MAAS Investigators. Effect of simvastatin on coronary atheroma: the Multicentre anti-atheroma study (MAAS). Lancet 1994;344:633–638.

166. Jukema JW, Bruschke VG, van Boven AJ, et al. Effects of lipid lowering by pravastatin on progression and regression of coronary artery disease in symptomatic men with normal to moderately elevated serum cholesterol levels (REGRESS). Circulation 1995;91:2528–2540.

167. Pitt B, Mancini GBJ, Ellis SG, et al. Pravastatin limitation of atherosclerosis in the coronary arteries (PLAC I). J Am Coll Cardiol 1995;26:1133–1139.

168. Waters D, Higginson L, Gladstone P, et al. Effects of monotherapy with an HMG-CoA reductase inhibitor on the progression of coronary atherosclerosis as assessed by serial quantitative arteriography (CCAIT). Circulation 1994;89:959–968.

169. Blankenhorn DH, Azen SP, Kramsch DM, et al. Coronary angiographic changes with lovastatin therapy. Ann Intern Med 1993;119:969–976.

170. Miller BD, Cashin-Hemphill L, Mack WJ, et al. Predominance of mid-density/low density lipoproteins predicts angiographic benefit of lovastatin in the Monitored Atherosclerosis Regression Study. Circulation 1994;90:I-460.

171. Deleted in proof.

172. Alderman EL, Haskell WL, Fair JM, et al. Beneficial angiographic and clinical response to multifactor modification in the Stanford Coronary Risk Intervention Project (SCRIP). Circulation 1994;89:975–990.

173. Campos CT, Nguyen P, Buchwald, et al. Effect of cholesterol lowering on PTCA, CABG, and heart transplantation rates: POSCH long-term follow-up study. Circulation 1993;88:I-386.

174. Thompson GR, Hollyer J, Waters DD. Percentage change rather than plasma level of LDL-cholesterol determines therapeutic response in coronary heart disease. Curr Opin Lipidol 1995;6:386–388.

175. Gofman JW, Young W, Tandy R. Ischemic heart disease, atherosclerosis and longevity. Circulation 1966; 34:679–697.

176. Superko HR. The atherogenic lipoprotein profile. Sci Med 1997;4:36–45.

177. Dufaux B, Assmann G, Hollmann W. Plasma lipoproteins and physical activity: a review. Int J Sports Med 1982;3:123–136.

178. Superko HR. Exercise training, serum lipids and lipoprotein particles: is there a change threshold? Exerc Sports Sci Med 1991;23:677–685.

179. Superko HR, Haskell WL, Wood PD. Modification of plasma cholesterol through exercise. Postgrad Med 1985;78:64–75.

180. Wood PD, Williams PT, Haskell WL. Physical activity and high-density lipoproteins. In: Mill NE, Miller GJ, eds. Clinical and metabolic aspects of high-density lipoproteins. Elsevier Science, 1984.

181. Tran ZU, Weltman A. Differential effects of exercise on serum lipid and lipoprotein levels seen with changes in body weight. A meta-analysis. JAMA 1985;254:919–924.

182. Griffin BA, Skinner RE, Maughan RJ. The acute effect of prolonged walking and dietary changes on plasma lipoprotein concentrations and high-density lipoprotein subfractions. Metabolism 1989;37:535–541.

183. Lehtonen A, Viikari J. Serum triglycerides and cholesterol and serum high density lipoprotein cholesterol in highly physical active men. Acta Med Scand 1978;204:111–114.

184. Martin RP, Haskell WP, Wood PD. Blood chemistry and lipid profiles of elite distance runners. Ann NY Acad Sci 1977;301:346–360.

185. Wood PD, Stefanick ML, Dreon DM, et al. Changes in plasma lipids and lipoproteins during weight loss by dieting versus exercise in overweight men. N Engl J Med 1988;319:1173–1179.

186. Williams SR, Logur E, Lewis JL, et al. Physical conditioning augments the fibrinolytic response to venous occlusion in healthy adults. N Engl J Med 1980;302: 987–991.

187. Wood PD, Haskell WL, Blair SN, et al. Increased exercise level and plasma lipoprotein concentrations: a one-year randomized controlled study in sedentary middle-aged men. Metabolism 1983;32:31–39.

188. Hickey NR, Mulcahy GJ, Bourke I, et al. Study of coronary risk factors related to physical activity in 15,171 men. Br Med J 1975;3:507–509.

189. Hoffman AA, Nelson W, Goss FA. Effects of an exercise program on plasma lipids of senior Air Force officers. Am J Cardiol 1967;20:516–524.

190. Wood PD, Haskell WL, Klein H, et al. The distribution of plasma lipoproteins in middle-aged male runners. Metabolism 1976;25:1249–1257.

191. Wood PD, Haskell WL. The effect of exercise on plasma high density lipoproteins. Lipids 1979;14:417–427.

192. Herbert PN, Bernier DN, Cullinane EM, et al. High-density lipoprotein metabolism in runners and sedentary men. JAMA 1984;252:1034–1037.

193. Iltis PW, Thomas TR, Adeniran SB, et al. Different running programs: plasma lipids, apoproteins, and lecithin:cholesterol acyltransferase in middle-aged men. Ann Sports Med 1984;2:16–21.

194. Keins B, Jorgenson I, Lewis S, et al. Increased plasma HDL-cholesterol and apo A-I in sedentary middle-aged men after physical conditioning. Eur J Clin Invest 1980;10:203–209.

195. Marniemi J, Dahlstrom S, Kvist M, et al. Dependence of serum lipid and lecithin:cholesterol acyltransferase levels on physical training of young men. Eur J Appl Physiol 1982;49:25–35.

196. Lithell H, Orlander J, Shele R. Changes in lipoprotein lipase activity and lipid stores in human skeletal muscle with prolonged heavy exercise. Acta Physiol Scand 1979;107:257–261.

197. Peltonen P, Marniemi J, Hietanen E, et al. Changes in serum lipids, lipoproteins and heparin releasable lipolytic enzymes during moderate physical training in man: a longitudinal study. Metabolism 1981;30: 518–526.

198. Kantor MA, Cullinane EM, Herbert PW, et al. Acute increase in lipoprotein lipase following prolonged exercise. Metabolism 1984;33:454–457.

199. Krauss RM, Wood PD, Giotas C, et al. Heparin-released plasma lipase activities and lipoprotein levels in distance runners [abstract]. Circulation 1979;50:II-73.

200. Sutherland WHF, Nye ER, Woodhouse SP. Red blood cell cholesterol levels, plasma cholesterol esterifica-

tion rate and serum lipids and lipoproteins in men with hypercholesterolaemia and normal men during 16 weeks physical training. Atherosclerosis 1983;47: 145–157.

201. Krauss RM. Regulation of high density lipoprotein levels. Med Clin North Am 1982;66:403–430.

202. Nikkila EA, Taskinen MR, Rehunen S, et al. Lipoprotein lipase activity in adipose tissue and skeletal muscle of runners: relation to serum lipoproteins. Metabolism 1978;27:1661–1671.

203. Nikkila EA, Kuusi T, Taskinen MR. Role of lipoprotein lipase and hepatic endothelial lipase in the metabolism of high-density lipoproteins: a novel concept on cholesterol transport in HDL cycle. In: Carlson LA, Pernow B, eds. Metabolic risk factors in ischemic cardiovascular disease. New York: Raven Press, 205–215.

204. Nikkila EA, Kuusi T, Taskinen MJ, et al. Regulation of lipoprotein metabolism by endothelial lipolytic enzymes. In: Carlson LA, Olsson AG, eds. Treatment of hyperlipoproteinemia. New York: Raven Press, 1984: 77–84.

205. Goldberg IJ, Mazlen RG, Rubenstein A, et al. Plasma lipoprotein abnormalities associated with acquired hepatic triglyceride lipase deficiency. Metabolism 1985; 34:832–835.

206. Kuusi T, Nikkila EA, Saarinen P, et al. Plasma high density lipoproteins HDL_2, HDL_3 and postheparin plasma lipases in relation to parameters of physical fitness. Atherosclerosis 1982;41:209–219.

207. Moorjani S, Gagne C, Lupien PJ, et al. Plasma triglycerides related decrease in high-density lipoprotein cholesterol and its association with myocardial infarction in heterozygous familial hypercholesterolemia. Metabolism 1986;35:311–316.

208. Freedman SD, Jacobsen SJ, Barboriak JJ, et al. Body fat distribution and male/female differences in lipids and lipoproteins. Circulation 1990;81:1498–1506.

209. Merrill JR, Holly RG, Anderson RL, et al. Hyperlipemic response of young trained and untrained men after a high fat meal. Arteriosclerosis 1989;9:217–223.

210. Garcia-Palmieri MR, Costas R, Cruz-Vidal M, et al. Increased physical activity: a protective factor against heart attacks in Puerto Rico. Am J Cardiol 1982;50: 749–755.

211. Keys A. Seven Countries. Cambridge, MA: Harvard University Press, 1980:199.

212. Gordon DJ, Witztum JL, Hunninghake D, et al. Habitual physical activity and high-density lipoprotein cholesterol in men with primary hypercholesterolemia. Circulation 1983;67:512–520.

213. Holloszy JO, Skinner JS, Toro G, et al. Effects of a six month program of endurance exercise on the serum lipids of middle-aged men. Am J Cardiol 1964;14: 753–760.

214. Erklens WD, Albers JJ, Hazzard WR, et al. High-density lipoprotein-cholesterol in survivors of myocardial infarction. JAMA 1979;242:2185–2189.

215. Phillipson BE. Effects of walking upon plasma lipids in hyperlipidemic patients. Ala Med 1983;53:15–18.

216. Lederer J. Place de l'exercise physique dans le traitement des hyperlipoproteinemies chez l'homme. Sem Hop Paris 1982;58:1285–1290.

217. LaRosa JC, Cleary P, Muesing RA, et al. Effect of long-term moderate physical exercise on plasma lipoproteins. The national exercise and heart disease project. Arch Intern Med 1982;142:2269–2274.

218. US Department of Health and Human Services. Lipid Research Clinics Population Studies Data Book, Volume 1. The Prevalence Study. NIH Publication No. 80–1527, July 1980.

219. Williams PT, Wood PD, Krauss RM, et al. Does weight loss cause the exercise-induced increase in plasma high density lipoproteins? Atherosclerosis 1983;47:173–185.

220. Raz I, Rosenblit H, Kark JD. Effect of moderate exercise on serum lipids in young men with low high density lipoprotein cholesterol. Arteriosclerosis 1988;8:245–251.

221. Jones DP, Arky RA. Effects of insulin on triglyceride and free fatty acid metabolism in man. Metabolism 1965;14:1287–1293.

222. Zavaroni I, Ida Chen Y, Mondon CE, et al. Ability of exercise to inhibit carbohydrate-induced hypertriglyceridemia in rats. Metabolism 1981;30:476–480.

223. Barse RJ, Schnatz JD, Frohmann LA. Evidence for a role of insulin secretion in production of endogenous hypertriglyceridemia. J Clin Invest 1968;47:6–14.

224. Topping DL, Mayers PA. Immediate effects of insulin and fructose on metabolism of perfused liver—changes in lipoprotein secretion, fatty-acid oxidation and esterification, lipogenesis and carbohydrate metabolism. Biochem J 1972;126:295–311.

225. Fahlen M, Stenberg J, Bjorntorp P. Insulin secretion in obesity after exercise. Diabetologia 1972;8:141–144.

226. Lampman RM, Santinga JT, Savage PJ, et al. Effect of exercise training on glucose tolerance, in vivo insulin sensitivity, lipid and lipoprotein concentrations in middle-aged men with mild hypertriglyceridemia. Metabolism 1985;34:205–211.

227. Lampman RM, Santinga JT, Hodge MF, et al. Comparative effects of physical training and diet in normalizing serum lipids in men with type IV hyperlipoproteinemia. Circulation 1977;55:652–659.

228. Wirth A, Diehm C, Hanel W, et al. Training-induced changes in serum lipids, fat tolerance, and adipose tissue metabolism in patients with hypertriglyceridemia. Atherosclerosis 1985;54:263–271.

229. Streja D, Mymin D. Moderate exercise and high-density lipoprotein-cholesterol. JAMA 1979;242;2190–2192.

230. Olefsky JM, Farquhar JW, Reaven GM. Reappraisal of the role of insulin in hypertriglyceridemia. Am J Med 1974;57:551–560.

231. Lokey EA, Tran ZV. Effects of exercise training on serum lipid and lipoprotein concentrations in women: a meta-analysis. Int J Sports Med 1989;10:424–429.

232. Gorbach SL, Woods SM, Longcope C, et al. Plasma lipoprotein cholesterol and endogenous sex hormones in healthy young women. Metabolism 1989;38:1077–1081.

233. Coon PJ, Bleecker ER, Drinkwater DT, et al. Effects of body composition and exercise capacity on glucose tolerance, insulin and lipoprotein lipids in healthy older men: a cross-sectional and longitudinal intervention study. Metabolism 1989;38:1201–1209.

234. Tamai T, Nakai T, Takai H, et al. The effects of physical exercise on plasma lipoproteins and apolipoprotein metabolism in elderly men. J Gerontol 1988;43:M75–M79.

235. Altekruse EB, Wilmore JH. Changes in blood chemistries following a controlled exercise program. J Occup Med 1973;15:110–113.

236. Pomeranze J, Beinfield WH, Chessin M. Serum lipid and fat tolerance studies in normal, obese and atherosclerotic subjects. Circulation 1954;10:742–746.

237. Deckelbaum RJ, Eisenberg S, Oschry Y, et al. Abnormal high density lipoproteins of abetalipoproteinemia: relevance to normal HDL metabolism. J Lipid Res 1982;23:1274–1282.

238. Schaefer EJ, Kay LL, Zech LA, et al. Tangier disease: high density lipoprotein deficiency due to defective metabolism of an abnormal apolipoprotein A-I. J Clin Invest 1982;70:934–945.

239. Schaefer EJ. Clinical, biological, and genetic features in familial disorders of high density lipoprotein deficiency. Arteriosclerosis 1984;4:303–322.

240. Sutherland WH, Nye ER, Boulter CP, et al. Physical training plasma lipoproteins and fecal steroid excretion in sedentary men. Clin Physiol 1988;8:445–452.

241. Levy RI, Fredrickson DS, Stone NJ, et al. Cholestyramine in type II hyperlipoproteinemia. Ann Intern Med 1973;79:51–58.

242. The NCEP Expert Panel. Report of the National Cholesterol Education Program Expert Panel on detection, evaluation, and treatment of high blood cholesterol in adults. Arch Intern Med 1988;148:36–69.

243. Glueck CJ, Ford S, Scheel D, et al. Colestipol and cholestyramine resin. Comparative effects in familial type II hyperlipoproteinemia. JAMA 1972;222: 676–681.

244. Dorr AE, Gundersen K, Schneider JC, et al. Colestipol hydrochloride in hypercholesterolemic patients—effect on serum cholesterol and mortality. J Chronic Dis 1978;31:5–14.

245. Witztum JL, Schonfeld G, Weidman SW, et al. Bile sequestrant therapy alters the compositions of low-density and high-density lipoproteins. Metabolism 1979; 28:221–229.

246. Hunninghake DB, Probstfield JL, Crow LO, et al. Effect of colestipol and clofibrate on plasma lipid and lipoproteins in type IIa hyperlipoproteinemia. Metabolism 1981;30:605–609.

247. Vecchio TJ, Linden CV, O'Connell MJ, et al. Comparative efficacy of colestipol and clofibrate in type IIa hyperlipoproteinemia. Arch Intern Med 1982;142:721–723.

248. Angelin B, Einarsson K. Cholestyramine in type IIa hyperlipoproteinemia. Is low-dose treatment feasible? Atherosclerosis 1981;38:33–38.

249. Vessby B, Kostner G, Lithell H, et al. Diverging effects of cholestyramine on apolipoprotein B and lipoprotein Lp(a). Atherosclerosis 1982;44:61–71.

250. Superko HR, Greenland P, Manchester RA, et al. Effectiveness of low dose colestipol therapy in patients with moderate hypercholesterolemia. Am J Cardiol 1992;70:135–140.

251. Shawaryn GG, Corak DL, Goris GB. A study of the safety and efficacy of Colestid (10 g/d) at varying dose

intervals: a report on Protocol M-7000–0055. 1992. unpublished UPJOHN data.

252. Superko HR, Haskell WL, Cianciola C. LDLC reduction with colestipol granules versus new tablet. Arteriosclerosis 1989;9:766a.

253. Superko HR, Williams PT, Alderman EL, et al. Differential lipoprotein effects of bile acid binding resin in LDL subclass pattern A versus B. Circulation 1992;86:I-144.

254. Miller NH, Thomas RJ, Superko HR, et al. Lipid-lowering therapy in post-MI patients: efficacy of a nurse-managed intervention [abstract]. Circulation 1991.

255. Blankenhorn DH. Preventive treatment of atherosclerosis. Menlo Park, CA: Addison-Wesley Publishing, 1984.

256. Saku K, Gartside PS, Hynd BA, et al. Mechanism of action of gemfibrozil on lipoprotein metabolism. J Clin Invest 1985;75:1702–1712.

257. Superko HR. A review of combined hyperlipidaemia and its treatment with fenofibrate. J Int Med Res 1989;17:99–112.

258. Brown VW, Dujovne CA, Farquhar JW, et al. Effects of fenofibrate on plasma lipids. Arteriosclerosis 1986;6:670–678.

259. Vega GL, Grundy SM. Gemfibrozil therapy in primary hypertriglyceridemia associated with coronary heart disease. Effects on metabolism of low-density lipoproteins. JAMA 1985;253:2398–2403.

260. Manninen V, Elo O, Frick H, et al. Lipid alterations and decline in the incidence of coronary heart disease in the Helsinki Heart Study. JAMA 1988;260:641–651.

261. Manninen V, Elo O, Frick H, et al. Lipid alterations and decline in the incidence of coronary heart disease in the Helsinki Heart Study. JAMA 1988;260:641–651.

262. Superko HR, Krauss RM. LDL subclass distribution change in familial combined hyperlipidemia patients following gemfibrozil and niacin treatment. J Am Coll Cardiol 1997;29:46A.

263. Bilheimer DW, Grundy SM, Brown MS, et al. Mevinolin and colestipol stimulate receptor-mediated clearance of low density lipoprotein from plasma in familial hypercholesterolemia heterozygotes. Proc Natl Acad Sci USA 1983;80:4124–4128.

264. McTavish D, Sorkin EM. Pravastatin. A review of its pharmacological properties and therapeutic potential in hypercholesterolaemia. Drugs 1991;42:65–89.

265. Bard JM, Luc G, Douste-Blazy P, et al. Effect of simvastatin on plasma lipids, apolipoproteins and lipoprotein particles in patients with primary hypercholesterolaemia. Eur J Clin Pharmacol 1989;37: 545–550.

266. Herd JA, Ballantyne CM, Farmer JA, et al. Effects of fluvastatin on coronary atherosclerosis in patients with mild to moderate cholesterol elevations (LCAS). Am J Card 1997;80:278–286.

267. Bakker-Arkema RG, Davidson MH, Goldstein RJ, et al. Efficacy and safety of a new HMG-CoA reductase inhibitor, atorvastatin, in patients with hypertriglyceridemia. JAMA 1996;275:128–133.

268. Illingworth DR. Mevinolin plus colestipol in therapy for severe heterozygous familial hypercholesterolemia. Ann Intern Med 1984;101:598–604.

269. Kostner GM, Gavish D, Leopold B, et al. HMGCoA reductase inhibitors lower LDL cholesterol without reducing Lp(a) levels. Circulation 1989;80:1313–1319.

270. Hotz W. Nicotinic acid and its derivatives: a short survey. Adv Lipid Res 1983;20:195–217.

271. Knopp R, Superko HR, Davidson M, et al. Long-term blood cholesterol lowering effects of a dietary fiber supplement. Archives of Family Medicine (submitted).

272. Knopp RH, Ginsberg J, Albers JJ, et al. Contrasting effects of unmodified and time-release forms of niacin on lipoproteins in hyperlipidemic subjects: clues to mechanism of action of niacin. Metabolism 1985;34:642–650.

273. Superko HR, Krauss RM. Differential effects of nicotinic acid in subjects with different LDL subclass patterns. Atherosclerosis 1992;95:69–76.

274. Pierce LR, Wysowski DK, Gross TP. Myopathy and rhabdomyolysis associated with lovastatin-gemfibrozil combination therapy. JAMA 1990;264:71–75.

275. Malinow MR, Kang SS, Taylor LM, et al. Prevalence of hyperhomocyst(e)inemia in patients with peripheral arterial occlusive disease. Circulation 1989;79:1180–1188.

276. Kannel WB, Wolf PA, Castelli WP, D'Agostino RB. Fibrogen and risk of cardiovascular disease. JAMA 1987;258:1183–1186.

277a. Dreon DM, Fernstrom H, Miller B, Kraus RM. Low density lipoprotein subclass patterns and lipoprotein respose to a reduced-fat diet in men. FASEB J 1994;8:121–126.

277b. Dreon DM, Fernstrom H, Williams PT, Kraus RM. LDL subclass patterns and lipoprotein response to a low-fat, high-carbohydrate diet in women. Arterioscler Thromb Vasc Biol 1997;17:707–714.

278. Superko HR, Krauss RM, DiTicco C. Effect of HMGCoA reductase inhibitor (fluvastatin) on LDL peak particle diameter. Am J Cardiol 1997;80:78–81.

279. Wenger NK, Froelicher ES, Smith LK, et al. Cardiac rehabilitation. Clinical practice guidelines No 17. Rockville, MD: US Department of Health and Human Services, Public Health Service, Agency for Health Care Policy and Research and the National Heart, Lung and Blood Institute. AHCPR Publication No. 9600672. October, 1995.

280. O'Connor GT, Buring JE, Yusuf S, et al. An overview of randomized trials of rehabilitation with exercise after myocardial infarction. Circulation 1989;80:234–244.

281. Oldridge NB, Guyatt GH, Fischer ME, Rimm AA. Cardiac rehabilitation after myocardial infarction: combined experience of randomized clinical trials. JAMA 1988;260:945–950.

282. Superko HR, Krauss RM. Coronary artery disease regression: convincing evidence for the benefit of aggressive lipoprotein management. Circulation 1994;90:1056–1069.

283. Dunn P, Meese R, Superko R, Williams P. Cardiovascular risk reduction is cost-effective in the real world. Circulation 1997;96:I-67.

284. Lansky D, Butler JBV, Waller FT. Using health status measures in the hospital setting. Med Care 1992;30:MS57–MS73.

Smoking Cessation as a Critical Element of Cardiac Rehabilitation

Milagros C. Rosal, Ira S. Ockene, and Judith K. Ockene

Cigarette smoking is a major risk factor for the development of coronary heart disease (CHD) and for increased morbidity and mortality among people who have already developed CHD. Cessation rates of chronic cigarette smokers after a diagnosis of myocardial infarction (MI) or angina are reportedly between 20% and 60% (1), but a large proportion of patients continue to smoke or later relapse (2, 3). Given the high risk from continued smoking for CHD patients, there is a need to provide empirically based smoking cessation interventions to these patients during their rehabilitation period. These interventions must be tailored to patients' characteristics (usually older and less healthy individuals who may need to make multiple health-risk behavior changes) (4). It is also important to provide alternatives to group programs (which appeal only to a relatively small proportion of patients), and to provide programs that facilitate long-term abstinence given the high proportion of post-MI patients who stop smoking on their own but later relapse (5).

Cardiac rehabilitation providers are uniquely and powerfully situated in their routine practice to educate patients about the relationship between lifestyle and CHD, and to help patients develop the skills necessary to make behavioral changes, decrease morbidity and mortality, and improve quality of life. The continuity of care and extended contact between patients and the cardiac rehabilitation staff provides an excellent opportunity to provide smoking cessation interventions.

The purpose of this chapter is to 1) provide an overview of the health risks of smoking and benefits of cessation for CHD patients; 2) discuss the theoretical foundation of smoking cessation interventions; 3) review the multiple factors that affect smoking behaviors; and 4) present a model for intervention in the cardiac rehabilitation setting.

HEALTH RISKS OF SMOKING AND BENEFITS OF CESSATION

Cigarette smoking accounts for an estimated 30% of deaths caused by CHD (6–8). Cigarette smoke has many potentially toxic components, nicotine and carbon monoxide (CO) among them, that produce a variety of adverse cardiovascular effects. Nicotine causes the release of epinephrine and norepinephrine, resulting in increases in blood pressure, heart rate, cardiac output, coronary blood flow, and myocardial oxygen consumption. In patients with coronary artery narrowing, this can result in myocardial ischemia and cardiac arrhythmias (8). Carbon monoxide, a gas component, has a strong affinity for hemoglobin, displacing oxygen and causing the smoker to lose as much as 15% of his blood oxygen-carrying capacity, depending on the amount smoked and the depth of inhalation. Such a loss can exacerbate angina and provoke MI, arrhythmias, and sudden death. Other toxic gases present in cigarette smoke are responsible for additional physiologic processes that can potentially lead to chronic obstructive pulmonary disease and cancer among smokers as well as among those who do not smoke themselves but who are exposed to environmental tobacco smoke (8).

Most of the increased risk of suffering an initial MI largely abates within 2 to 3 years of quitting smoking (9). In addition, smoking cessation after the development of CHD has almost immediate health benefits and is associated with a reduction in risk of recurrent MI and sudden cardiac death of 50% or more (8, 10–14). Furthermore, increasing intervals of abstinence are associated with progressively lower CHD mortality rates with the risk of the ex-smoker approaching that of the never-smoker by 5 years (8, 15, 16). The benefits of smoking cessation for CHD patients go beyond the improvement in medical status. Cessation has clear psychosocial benefits, and those who quit are more likely to engage in additional health-promoting and disease-preventing behaviors than are those who continue to smoke (17).

THEORETICAL FOUNDATION OF SMOKING CESSATION INTERVENTIONS

Several theories and models provide a framework for understanding and intervening with smoking behavior. These include the consumer information processing theory, the social learning theory, the health belief model, the stages of change model, the patient-centered counseling model, and behavioral self-management.

The Consumer Information Processing Theory

According to the consumer information processing theory (CIP) (18), certain conditions are necessary for individuals to make use of information: information must be available; it must be wanted or believed to be useful by the consumer; and it must be able to be processed within the time, energy, and comprehension levels of the consumer (19). Thus, for information about smoking and health to influence action, the counselor must make the information available, present such information at "teachable moments" (times when the smoker may be more receptive, such as after an MI); and the information must be presented at a level that the patient can comprehend. The more the counselor is able to relate the patient's symptoms or problems to smoking and is confident that the patient understands and is able to use this information, the greater the likelihood that the smoker will be motivated to attempt cessation and maintain abstinence. Understanding the health impact of smoking is a critical factor in maintenance of cessation by cardiac patients (20).

The Health Belief Model

This model (21) asserts that cognitive factors influence motivation to and likelihood of changing a behavior. Thus, an individual will take action if he believes that he is vulnerable or at risk for worsening CHD or death; that there will be serious consequences if he does not quit smoking;

that he is capable of taking action to quit; that quitting will decrease the risk; and the potential costs (barriers) of taking action will be outweighed by the benefits. This model assumes that personal and environmental variables influence the individual's cognitions affecting change. For example, personalized information about the patient's atherosclerotic process and how smoking affects it must be available for the patient to develop a realistic appraisal of personal risk.

The Stages of Change Model

This model (22) describes smoking cessation as a process over time, defined by four stages: precontemplation (the smoker is neither considering quitting nor actively processing information on smoking and health); contemplation (the smoker is thinking about quitting and is processing information about the effects of smoking and ways to quit); action (the smoker is no longer smoking and has not done so for less than 6 months); maintenance (the individual has not smoked for more than 6 months, and may establish long-term abstinence or may relapse). When relapse occurs, the smoker recycles to any one of the previous stages. This model guides intervention and proposes that smokers at different stages benefit from different approaches.

Social Learning Theory

Social learning theory (SLT) (23, 24) states that behaviors are learned and therefore can be unlearned or altered; that behavior is determined by multiple influences; that the process of learning involves active participation of the individual; and that behavior is dynamic and is constantly interacting with and being influenced by multiple determinants (24, 25). According to this theory, two types of cognitions mediate the decision to change and the eventual behavior change: response-outcome expectancies and self-efficacy beliefs. The first type, response-outcome expectancy, is the degree to which an individual believes that a given course of action will lead to a particular outcome, e.g., how firmly the patient believes that quitting smoking will prevent his or her disease from progressing. These cognitions must be favorable for behavior change to occur. Self-efficacy expectations, on the other hand, refer to the patient's belief in his or her ability to make the desired change (i.e., to stop smoking). A positive belief that one has the necessary tools and resources to live comfortably and effectively without cigarettes leads to a greater commitment to change and to persistence of efforts. Research in this area strongly supports the idea that expectation of success is an important factor in quitting smoking and maintaining abstinence (26) independent of skill or knowledge (27, 28).

Patient-centered Counseling

The theoretical foundation of patient-centered counseling (PCC), social cognitive theory (23, 29) and the health belief model (21), emphasizes the importance of the patient's involvement, and confidence in his or her ability to change a specific behavior (self-efficacy) and maintain the change. In addition, similar to the principles articulated by Prochaska and DiClemente in their stages of change model (22), the patient-centered intervention model emphasizes to providers the need to meet the patient at the stage of change that he or she is at, and that whereas every patient may not completely succeed at altering a health-related behavior, most can be reached at some level through persistent effort. With a focus on all patients, no matter what stage of change they are at, the PCC approach facilitates the involvement of less motivated patients and helps the provider to develop more realistic expectations of what can be achieved in one encounter. The PCC model also uses principles articulated by Marlatt and colleagues (30) in their relapse prevention model, and teaches providers that continued reinforcement and planning to deal with high-risk situations is needed to help prevent relapse. The PCC model helps the patient to become actively involved in his or her own care, believe in his or her ability to make a change (no matter how small), and use past experiences on which to build.

Behavioral Self-Management

Using principles of behavior modification, behavioral self-management requires that an individual become aware of the triggers that cue a behavior and the consequences that reinforce it. The individual can then decide whether to avoid the trigger, alter it, or substitute an incompatible or CHD-preventive behavior when triggers to smoke occur. The acknowledgment of multiple influences as determinants of behavior renders this theory very valuable in integrating physiologic, psychological or personal, and environmental factors known to influence smoking behavior.

FACTORS THAT INFLUENCE SMOKING BEHAVIOR

Cigarette smoking is a complex behavior pattern affected by a variety of interacting variables including physiologic factors, personal characteristics, environmental influences, and even other behaviors of the individual (e.g., having a drink and smoking a cigarette).

Physiologic Factors

Cigarette smoking is often maintained to avoid nicotine withdrawal symptoms, which often accompany tobacco abstinence, and by a desire for the immediate peripheral and central effects of nicotine (e.g., anorectic impact, arousal from norepinephrine activity, increased concentration, and euphoric effects possibly mediated by β-endorphin release). The nicotine withdrawal syndrome is a psychiatric diagnosis described in the Diagnostic and Statistical Manual of Mental Disorders (DSM-IV) of the American Psychiatric Association (Fig. 19.1). Withdrawal symptoms elicited by acute deprivation from nicotine begin within 24 hours of cessation or significant reduction of tobacco use, increase for 3 to 4 days, and gradually decrease during 1 to 3 weeks (31). Changes in appetite and concentration problems tend to persist longer than do feelings of restlessness and irritability. Not all smokers are physiologically dependent. Although heavier smokers (those who take in more nicotine) usually have stronger withdrawal symptoms, there is great variability. Nicotine dependence interferes with immediate attempts to withdraw from cigarettes, and smokers with more intense withdrawal symptoms have more difficulties stopping smoking (32). Hospitalized patients often go through nicotine withdrawal during their hospitalization.

Conditioning mediates the role of physiologic factors in cessation and maintenance of cessation. Numerous internal or environmental stimuli, including activities, thoughts, feelings, and behaviors, become conditioned to or attached to the use of nicotine and evoke urges or cues to smoke. This conditioning ties smoking to the rituals of daily life and is an important contributor to the difficulty of breaking the addiction to nicotine. Thus, in addition to acute deprivation from nicotine, withdrawal symptoms may also be elicited by conditioned stim-

A. Daily use of nicotine for at least several weeks.

B. Abrupt cessation of nicotine use, or reduction in the amount of nicotine used, followed within 24 hours by four (or more) of the following signs:

    (1) dysphoric or depressed mood
    (2) insomnia
    (3) irritability, frustration, or anger
    (4) anxiety
    (5) difficulty concentrating
    (6) restlessness
    (7) decreased heart rate
    (8) increased appetite or weight gain

C. The symptoms in criterion B cause clinically significant distress or impairment in social, occupational, or other important areas of functioning.

D. The symptoms are not due to a general medical condition and are not better accounted for by another mental disorder.

Figure 19.1.   DSM-IV diagnostic criteria for nicotine withdrawal. (Based on information from the American Psychiatric Association. Diagnostic and Statistical Manual of Mental Disorders. 4th ed. Washington, DC: American Psychiatric Association, 1994. Copyright 1994 American Psychiatric Association.)

uli. Studies indicate that, even long after cessation, former smokers manifest physiologic reactivity to smoking cues (33, 34), which threatens abstinence. This conditioning influence is one of the reasons why individuals who are physiologically addicted to nicotine may require behavioral interventions in addition to pharmacologic treatment (i.e., nicotine replacement therapy or other medication).

Personal Characteristics

In addition to specific cognitive factors proposed by SLT, namely response-outcome expectancy and self-efficacy beliefs (described above), affective states also have been shown to influence smoking behavior. The temporary experience of negative affect, including depression, sadness, anxiety, and anger, is not an uncommon reaction to a cardiac event. Clinically significant negative affect, however, is associated with the experience of more severe withdrawal symptoms (35) and failure to quit smoking and maintain abstinence (36, 37). Nicotine is considered to reduce negative affect and stress, enhance positive affect, and provide stimulation during times of boredom or inac-

tivity (36). Several theories have been proposed to understand the association between smoking and affect (38–41), and laboratory studies have supported the conclusion that smoking significantly reduces fluctuations or changes in mood or affect during stress (39, 41).

Demographic factors also have been associated with smoking behavior. Older smokers, those better educated, and those with higher occupational level are more likely to quit smoking than the younger, less educated smoker in a lower occupational level (7, 42, 43). Another influential factor is the patient's medical condition. Patients diagnosed as having more severe CHD demonstrate a greater likelihood of cessation and long-term abstinence (26).

Weight gain, a possible undesirable outcome of smoking cessation, may also negatively influence an individual's motivation to quit smoking. Approximately 80% of all quitters will experience some weight gain, and the average weight gain after smoking cessation is 5 to 8 pounds (2.3 to 3.6 kg) (8, 44–46). Weight concerns may be greater for women in particular, as women often indicate weight gain to be related to their return to smoking (8, 47).

Environmental Influences

Successful cessation outcomes have been associated with greater social support for cessation and having fewer smokers in one's environment (43). Individuals who work in an environment with smokers are themselves more likely to smoke (48). In addition, different ethnic cultural groups provide different levels of support for smoking behavior. For example, cigarette smoking rates among Hispanics and African-Americans have been lower than among whites until recently, and are now on the increase while smoking rates for most other groups have decreased (7, 49).

INTERVENING WITH CHD PATIENTS WHO SMOKE

General Program Issues

IN-HOSPITAL VERSUS OUTPATIENT INTERVENTIONS

In-hospital interventions have been found to boost the cessation rate of cardiac patients (26, 50). Several factors make in-hospital interventions desirable, including 1) hospitalization is a period of enforced nonsmoking, 2) patients may be more receptive to the idea of quitting because of health concerns, and thus are more motivated to quit, and 3) patients can be more easily reached. Issues of concern for in-hospital interventions include the short time available for such intervention and the transient cognitive impairments (potentially interfering with the learning of new skills required to quit smoking) experienced by some patients after coronary artery bypass graft operations. In-hospital abstinence may be deceptively easy (i.e., hospitals' nonsmoking policy; smokers are removed from their usual triggers to smoke and are usually more motivated to quit because of the recent cardiac event) and maintained abstinence cannot be presumed. With a thorough assessment and knowing the difficulties with in-hospital abstinence, physicians can stratify patients before discharge by risk of relapse, and those at higher risk can be targeted for postdischarge outpatient intervention. In most cases, patients will benefit from outpatient follow-up, which can take place via telephone calls or face-to-face as part of the outpatient cardiac rehabilitation program.

PHYSICIAN INVOLVEMENT

The patient's physician plays an important role and must be included in the effort to help smoking patients quit. Physicians may participate in the smoking intervention effort by discussing with the patient the benefits of quitting and the risks of continued smoking, and encouraging and reinforcing quit and maintenance efforts. This brief intervention can be delivered in 2 to 3 minutes. Evidence from observational and clinical trials demonstrates that physicians who intervene with their smoking patients, no matter how briefly, have a significant impact on their cigarette smoking behavior (51).

Assessment and Intervention Strategies

Given that almost all hospitalized post-MI patients will be off cigarettes, and many at least temporarily very motivated, much attention needs to be paid at this point to maintenance of change and avoidance of relapse. A thorough assessment of the patient's recent (or current) smoking behavior pattern is necessary to tailor the smoking cessation intervention to the specific needs and circumstances of the patient. At least a minimum level of rapport must be established between provider and patient to enhance the patient's cooperation. In contrast with a provider-centered approach (which focuses on giving information and admonishing the patient to change, and assumes that the patient shares a common set of concerns or expectations with the provider), the patient-centered model (discussed above) encourages providers to tailor the intervention to the individual by 1) asking open-ended questions about relevant change variables (Fig. 19.2), and 2) providing positive reinforcement for attempted or planned behavioral changes. A smoking history questionnaire may be used when a face-to-face interview with the patient is not possible (Fig. 19.3). A 14-item self-efficacy questionnaire also is available to assess the patient's commitment to cessation and self-efficacy beliefs in achieving the goal of abstinence (52). This questionnaire has been shown to predict with a high degree of accuracy which patients will relapse within 6 months (28).

AFFECTIVE/MOOD STATE

The high rate of smokers with a history of depression suggests that screening for a history of negative affect is potentially clinically useful. Identification of patients with a history of depression allows the implementation of additional preventive strategies or the referral of the patient for psychological evaluation and treatment, or

A. Motivation to quit
   How do you feel about your smoking?
   Have you thought about trying to stop smoking?
   Why would you like to stop smoking?
   How confident are you in your ability to quit or stay off of cigarettes?

B. Past experience
   Have you ever stopped smoking in the past?
   For how long?
   What methods did you use?
   What problems did you encounter and how did you handle them?
   Why did you start smoking again?

C. Exploring triggers to smoking and coping strategies
   When are you more likely to smoke?
   Which cigarettes will be hardest to give up?
   What do you think you would do now to stop smoking?

D. Questions for follow-up
   How did you do with your plan?
   What helped you to not smoke?
   What problems did you have?

E. Questions after relapse
   What led to your first cigarette?
   How did you feel after that?
   What else could you have done to keep you from taking a cigarette?
   What would you like to do now?

Figure 19.2. A model for open-ended questioning. (Reproduced with permission of Karger S, Basel AG, Kristeller J, Merriam P, Ockene J, et al. Smoking intervention for cardiac patients: in search of more effective strategies. Cardiology 1993;82:317–324.)

both. A clinical interview conducted by a mental health professional, or by specially trained cardiac rehabilitation staff, and standardized assessment instruments provide an ideal means to diagnose clinically significant emotional distress. Some of the available instruments to screen for depression and mood state include the Beck Depression Inventory (53), the Profile of Mood States (54), and the Symptom Check-List-90-R (55) (results from these instruments must be interpreted by a psychologist).

For individuals with a history of dysphoric mood, treatment for depression (antidepressant medication or cognitive-behavior therapy or both) may result in increased self-esteem and self-efficacy to quit smoking, and facilitate the use of smoking cessation strategies (56, 57). Antidepressant medications may reduce cravings during withdrawal, secondary to effects on central neurotransmitter systems parallel to those of nicotine (58), and prevent weight gain (599); however, there is a paucity of data on how useful these medications are for smokers (60, 61), and only bupropion hydrochloride has been shown to have at least an initial benefit for smokers trying to quit (62). Cognitive-behavioral therapy, which focuses on the modification of negative affect and on increasing healthy behaviors in depressed patients, may also be beneficial (60). Teaching the smoking patient more effective methods to manage or regulate negative mood may decrease the risk of relapse. In addition, through its emphasis on increasing pleasant activities, cognitive-behavioral therapy may help replace the positive mood-engendering effect of nicotine and move the person toward environments that reinforce

Name:_____   Date: _____

1. What is your smoking status? (check one)
____ Ex-smoker   ___ Current smoker   ___ Never-smoker

2. If ex-smoker:
   a. When did you stop smoking? _____
   b. How did you stop? _____

3. If current smoker:
   a. How many cigarettes a day do you smoke? ___
   b. What brand of cigarettes do you usually smoke? _____
   c. How soon after you wake up do you smoke your first cigarette?
      ____within 15–30 minutes ___30 minutes to 1 hour ____ over 1 hour
   d. Do you find it difficult to refrain from smoking in places where it is forbidden, such as the theater, doctor's office?
      _____yes   _____no
   e. Do you smoke when you are so ill that you are in bed most of the day?
      _____yes   _____no
   f. How many times have you stopped smoking cigarettes for more than 1 day?
      _____never   _____once   _____2–3 times _____ 4 or more times
   g. When did you last stop? _____
   h. Why did you decide to stop smoking on your last attempt?_____
   i. If you have stopped smoking cigarettes in the past, which methods helped you? (check as many as apply)
      _____Individual or group counseling _____Hypnosis
      _____Self-help materials   _____Acupuncture
      _____Gradual reduction   _____Physician advice
      _____Special filters   _____Cold turkey
      _____Exercise   _____Nicotine replacement (gum, patch)
      _____Other (please specify):_____
   j. The last time you stopped smoking cigarettes, how difficult was it?
      _____Very difficult _____ Difficult _____Easy   _____Very easy
   k. Why did you start smoking again? _____
   l. How interested are you in stopping again?
      ____Not at all ____A little _____Some ____A lot _____Very much
   m. If you decided to stop smoking during the next two weeks, how confident are you that you would succeed?
      ____ Not at all ____ A little ____ Some ____A lot _____Very much

Figure 19.3.   Smoking history questionnaire. (Source: Ockene JK. Smoking intervention: a behavioral, educational, and pharmacological perspective. In: Ockene IS, Ockene JK, eds. Prevention of coronary heart disease. Reproduced with permission from Lippincott, Williams & Wilkins, Baltimore, MD.)

nonsmoking. Patients experiencing clinically significant negative affect should be seen more frequently, particularly immediately after cessation, to monitor withdrawal symptoms and exacerbation of negative mood and to enhance use of effective coping skills. With increased monitoring, signs of relapse may be quickly addressed.

INTERVENTION LEVEL

The level of intervention must be appropriate to the patient's stage of change, and the patient's beliefs, desire, and motivation to quit smoking are the first topics to be addressed. The goal of intervening with precontemplators is not to immediately get the patient to quit, but to simply motivate the patient and to move the patient along to the stage of contemplation. The precontemplator should be approached with a motivational approach based on personalized information on smoking and CHD, and correction of misperceptions. Response-outcome expectancies must be favorable if the decision to quit smoking is to occur; thus, information on how cigarette smoking affects the progression of CHD and other diseases should be provided, and the patient's understanding of this information should be assessed. Physiologic feedback also may be used to promote favorable response-outcome expectancies. For example, the use of a CO meter can demonstrate to the smoker the presence of elevated CO levels. The valuable feedback received from this test and information on the effects of CO on CHD can help to increase motivation for change if used in a nonconfrontational, information-sharing manner.

In addition to cardiac-related information, the provider should assess other possible reasons the patient might have for quitting smoking. The provider's concerns may differ from those of the patient. Most patients have thought about quitting at some time; thus, the provider may inquire about what reasons the patient had that elicited the thought of quitting, and then discuss these reasons. The provider should express concern about the patient's health and, in a nonconfrontational manner, ask the patient to consider stopping. Poorly motivated smokers may require interventions aimed at exploring alternative plans, including information on smoking and health, advice on cutting back or changing brands, encouragement for outpatient counseling, encouragement of assistance by significant others, and additional visits by the counselor depending on the length of the patient's hospital stay.

Different from the precontemplator, the contemplator needs support to attempt cessation and help to develop a realistic cessation strategy. For example, the patient may have concerns about withdrawal symptoms, and the provider may give information regarding strategies to reduce or to manage those symptoms. For some patients, their lack of motivation to quit may be related to a lack of confidence in their ability to quit smoking. An expectation of success (or high self-efficacy) is a critical factor in the degree of commitment and persistence that a patient will

make in his or her efforts to quit smoking and maintain abstinence. Low self-efficacy levels (little expectation of their ability to quit) may be related either to perceived or actual deficits in personal skills or environmental supports. For patients with low self-efficacy levels, treatment must begin with enhancing either mastery expectations or skills, depending on the case. Once treatment is initiated, self-efficacy expectations should continue to be assessed and enhanced. Several strategies may be used for this purpose, including the use of self-monitoring, successful performance accomplishments, cognitive restructuring, physiologic feedback, and mastery of physiologic and emotional arousal states.

For smokers approaching action, the provider should ask for a quit date. In cases when the smoker is unable to provide a quit date, the provider must state that he or she will ask again in a stated period of time. This approach emphasizes the importance and seriousness of the intervention process. For patients in the action stage, the emphasis of the intervention should be on preventing relapse by using the relapse prevention strategies described below.

ASSESSMENT AND MANAGEMENT OF NICOTINE DEPENDENCE

The provider must determine the level of the patient's nicotine dependence and estimate the extent to which the patient will require special assistance during the withdrawal phase. Withdrawal symptoms are more likely among patients who smoke within 30 minutes of waking, have difficulty refraining from smoking in public areas, have a history of intense withdrawal symptoms in the past, or have a pattern of relapsing within a few hours or days. The number of cigarettes smoked is not a reliable indicator given that not all heavy smokers (more than one pack per day) report intense withdrawal symptoms, whereas some relatively lighter smokers appear to experience intense withdrawal. A formal assessment of nicotine dependence can be made by administering the Fagerstrom Tolerance Questionnaire (FTQ) (Fig. 19.4) (63, 64) or the revised FTQ (65). Higher scores suggest the need to intervene to manage withdrawal symptoms.

Nicotine withdrawal symptoms are likely to occur during the hospital stay because most hospitals today enforce a nonsmoking policy. Although cardiac patients are as likely to be nicotine depen-

1. How many cigarettes a day do you smoke?

2. What is the nicotine yield per cigarette of your usual brand?
   0.3–0.8 g (Low to Medium)   0.9–1.5 g (Medium)   1.6–2.2 g (Medium to High)

3. Do you inhale?
   Never   Sometimes   Always

4. Do you smoke more during the morning than during the rest of the day?
   No   Yes

5. How soon after you wake up do you smoke your first cigarette?
   More than 30 minutes   Less than 30 minutes

6. Of all the cigarettes you smoke during the day, which would you most hate to give up?

7. Do you find it difficult to refrain from smoking in places where it is forbidden (e.g., in church, at the library, in a no-smoking cinema)?

8. Do you smoke even if you are so ill that you are in bed most of the day?
   No   Yes

Scoring: Add up the scores as follows:

1. 0–15, 0; 16–25, 1; 25+, 2
2. Low to medium, 0; Medium, 1; Medium to high, 2
3. Never, 0; Sometimes, 1; Always, 2
4. No, 0; Yes, 1
5. Less than 30 minutes, 1; more than 30 minutes, 0
6. Score one point if you answered: The first cigarette of the day; all others, 0
7. Yes, 1; No, 0
8. Yes, 1; No, 0

This questionnaire measures the degree of physical dependence on the nicotine in cigarettes: 0–3, light dependence; 4–7, medium dependence; 8–11, dependence.

Figure 19.4. Fagerstrom tolerance questionnaire. (Reproduced with permission from Carl O. Fagerstrom.)

dent as any other smoker, they may not always be good candidates for nicotine replacement therapy (NRT). Nicotine replacement therapies are contraindicated for patients during the immediate post-MI period, and for patients with life-threatening arrhythmias and those with severe or unstable angina. For patients who have relapsed after hospital discharge, the decision to use strategies to decrease withdrawal symptoms should be based on the assessment of physiologic dependency, the patient's stage of change, and his or her medical condition. For those patients who are ready to quit but are highly nicotine dependent, either nicotine fading or NRT can be effective strategies to minimize withdrawal symptoms.

Nicotine Fading

Nicotine fading (66) has two components: brand switching to a lower nicotine-level cigarette, and gradual reduction in the number of cigarettes (i.e., tapering). Both strategies reduce the likelihood or severity of withdrawal symptoms after cessation, and allow smokers to learn how to manage smoking urges and master skills helpful in quitting. Brand switching also helps to weaken pleasant associations attached to smoking.

Tapering is encouraged by reducing the number of cigarettes smoked by about 50% per week. When tapering, it is important to remind the smoker 1) not to inhale more deeply, 2) not to smoke more cigarettes than usual, and 3) not to cover the vents in the filter of lower-nicotine cigarettes, as this increases nicotine availability. Tapering should be combined with behavioral management such that lower-need cigarettes, as defined by the patient, are eliminated first. This approach tends to increase self-efficacy. Tapering to 10 to 15 cigarettes per day is a realistic goal before quitting completely. As the number of cigarettes smoked decreases, CO levels in expired air can be measured to provide the patient with feedback on dosage reduction. This feedback reinforces response-outcome expectation.

Nicotine Replacement Therapy

The rationale for use of NRT is that providing nicotine without the adverse health consequences of tars and gases present in cigarette smoking gives the smoker a mechanism for reducing withdrawal symptoms while managing the psychological and behavioral aspects of smoking cessation. Nicotine replacement therapy can be useful in the outpatient setting for patients whose cardiac condition has stabilized and for whom NRT is preferable to continued smoking. Nicotine replacement therapy is less likely to be beneficial to patients who have already been abstinent for 5 to 7 days (when the worst withdrawal symptoms occur). However, if withdrawal symptoms persist, or if the patient expresses marked concern about relapse after discharge, then NRT may reduce the likelihood of relapse. Several forms of NRT are available to nicotine-dependent patients, including nicotine-containing gum, the transdermal nicotine patch, and nicotine nasal spray. The former two are currently being sold over the counter. A comparison of currently available forms of NRT is provided in Figure 19.5.

When combined with behavioral treatment, nicotine-containing gum has been found effective in aiding cessation (67–69). However, the use and effectiveness of nicotine-containing gum has been limited by unpleasant side effects (i.e., unappealing taste and dislike for chewing, gastrointestinal problems) and compromised by inadequate instructions offered by providers and improper use by the patient. Frequent problems in the use of the gum include chewing too fast, us-

ing too few pieces (the recommended number being about half the number of cigarettes smoked), not "parking" it (i.e., letting it sit between the cheek and teeth for proper absorption), and using it for too short a period (the recommended time being 3 to 6 months with tapered use).

The transdermal nicotine patch has largely replaced nicotine gum (70, 71). The passive nature of this nicotine-delivery system enhances compliance with its use, allows for a more continuous administration of nicotine (thus avoiding peaks and valleys in its delivery), and avoids the side effects associated with the gum. The use of the transdermal nicotine patch in conjunction with a behavioral intervention has shown 6-month abstinence rates of 26% compared with 12% for placebo and a reduction in withdrawal symptoms, including craving.

Nicotine nasal spray (NNS) is the latest NRT approved by the Food and Drug Administration for use as an aid in smoking cessation. Nicotine nasal spray has been found significantly more effective than placebo in helping smokers quit (72). However, side effects include throat irritation, coughing, sneezing, runny eyes and nose, palpitations, and nausea.

Although NRTs may be safer than continued use of cigarettes for cardiac patients, there are contraindications for their use. Thus, whenever possible, cardiac patients should be encouraged to use fading techniques rather than NRT if a determination of nicotine dependence has been made.

ASSESSMENT AND MANAGEMENT OF BEHAVIORAL PATTERNS

Once the patient has made a decision to quit smoking and physiologic dependency issues have been addressed, emphasis should be placed on designing a plan to modify the patient's smoking behavior pattern. For this purpose, a detailed behavioral assessment (self-monitoring or interview, or both, depending on the setting) is essential. On hospital discharge, physical withdrawal symptoms represent less of a threat, as most patients have already experienced the nicotine withdrawal syndrome during their hospitalization. However, conditioned responses to environmental cues represent an important influence that may lead to relapse. Thus, the maintenance of abstinence depends on how prepared a patient is to manage internal and environmental stimuli conditioned to his or her smoking behavior. For this reason,

	Transdermal Patches (Patches)			Nicotine Polacrilex (Gum)	Nicotine Nasal Spray
	OTC* Patches		Rx Patch	OTC Gum	Rx Spray
Brand name	Nicotrol	Nicoderm	Pro-step	Nicorette	Nicotrol NS
Dosage Frequency	15 mg 1 patch/16 h	21, 14, 7 mg 1 patch/24 h 16 h	22, 11 mg 1 patch/24 h	2, 4 mg 1 piece/1 to 2 h	10 mg/mL 1–2 doses/h Max 5 doses/h
Duration	6 weeks	10 weeks	6–12 weeks	12 weeks	3 months
Cost**	$155	$265	$45.99/box of 10 $42.69/box of 7	$300 full duration	$37 per bottle

*OTC = over the counter.
**These are approximate costs in the Northeast as of March 1997.

Figure 19.5. Comparison of currently available forms of nicotine replacement therapy (NRT).

training in behavioral management is an essential component of a sound smoking cessation and relapse prevention intervention. Behavioral management also is crucial in helping relapsers quit. A thorough in-hospital behavioral assessment must inquire about recent or current smoking patterns as well as past experiences with cessation, resources that helped and factors that hindered maintained cessation in past quit attempts, experience with other behavioral changes, factors that may have led to relapse, highest- and lowest-"need" cigarettes, and anticipated "high-risk-for-relapse" situations.

Patients who relapse after hospital discharge should be introduced to behavioral self-monitoring, which requires recording the times when the patient smokes, the need or importance of each cigarette, the cues or antecedents that trigger the urge to smoke (place, mood, thoughts associated with each cigarette smoked), and the rewards or consequences that follow smoking. Compliance with self-monitoring is enhanced by asking the patient to wrap the self-monitoring form ("wrap sheet") around his or her cigarette pack, and fill it out at the time that each cigarette is smoked, emphasizing that delayed recall is very unreliable. After a single week, wrap sheets are helpful to the patient and the provider because they increase knowledge about what stimuli (i.e., behaviors, cognitions, and environmental factors) are related to smoking. The patient is first asked to identify

any patterns observed; the clinician then proceeds to examine patterns further with the patient. Self-monitoring is an effective way of gathering more information, engaging the patient immediately in the treatment process, and assessing the level of motivation. Self-monitoring can also assist patients in cutting back, particularly the cigarettes smoked automatically. Unfortunately, not all patients are receptive to self-monitoring. The rationale and benefits of self-monitoring should be discussed with such patients; however, patients should not be pressured to do so. If this is the case, an attempt at a 24-hour recall of cigarettes smoked can be a reasonable replacement, and attempts to identify smoking patterns should be made by using open-ended questions such as "In what situations did you tend to smoke today?" and "Which cigarettes tended to be 'automatic' for you today, that you really wouldn't miss?"

Because self-monitoring reveals specific areas that need attention (i.e., high-need and high-risk situations), strategies for managing such situations can then be discussed and planned. Appropriate and realistic planning of strategies to manage critical situations will enhance the patient's self-efficacy beliefs and increase the likelihood of total cessation. Open-ended questions such as "What might you be able to do to cope with this specific situation instead of smoking?" can help plan realistic strategies. The most commonly used strategies for the behavioral management of high-need and high-risk situations include 1) stimulus control (avoidance of, or modified response to, high-need and high-risk situations), and 2) reinforcement (use of rewards or incentives).

Stimulus Control

When a behavior is differentially controlled by antecedent stimuli (the behavior is more likely to occur after some situations but not others), the behavior is considered to be under stimulus control. Modification of such behavior takes place by 1) avoiding the antecedent stimuli, 2) engaging in behaviors incompatible with the usual behavior in the presence of such stimuli, or 3) developing alternative coping skills to use in the presence of such stimuli.

1. Avoiding antecedent stimuli: Self-monitoring records can be used to identify the antecedent stimuli indicative of high-need and high-risk situations, and the provider can aid the patient in deciding ways to avoid such trigger situations. For instance, a patient who usually smokes a cigarette whenever he or she drinks coffee may decide to temporarily not drink coffee or to drink it only in nonsmoking places to break its conditioning to smoking. Although avoidance of high-need or high-risk situations is a commonly recommended behavioral strategy at the beginning of a smoking cessation intervention, its use is less critical in later stages of intervention as the patient develops alternative coping skills to manage these situations.
2. Engaging in incompatible behaviors: Engagement in situations or activities incompatible with smoking when a high-need or high-risk situation is present is an effective strategy for the management of such situations. For example, a patient who is used to smoking after a meal may decide to leave the table as soon as he or she finishes the meal and go for a walk or take a shower.
3. Developing alternative coping skills: Commonly taught coping skills include relaxation methods, assertive communication skills, cognitive restructuring, and effective use of social support networks, depending on the patient's needs. Learning stress management skills may be helpful particularly to patients who report stress as the reason for their difficulties in quitting or for their relapse (73).

Relaxation techniques such as diaphragmatic breathing, brief meditation, visualization exercises, and self-hypnosis may serve functions previously served by smoking by providing a break from the stressful situation and having a physiologically active relaxation effect. These are also important techniques for weight management.

Assertive communication is important in refusing offers to smoke and in managing social situations that have served as antecedent stimuli for smoking behavior. The provider can ask "Are there situations where you feel that you might have difficulties refusing a cigarette offer?" or "How comfortable do you feel asking your friends to not smoke in your car or home?" The provider may then role-play similar and related social scenarios with the patient and coach the patient to develop assertive ways of verbalizing his or her needs to effectively manage the challenges of such scenarios.

Cognitive restructuring techniques are often used as part of smoking cessation interventions for the purpose of identification and modification of faulty thought patterns associated with smoking. The patient is taught how to challenge irrational thinking associated with high-need and high-risk situations, and is helped in developing alternative thought responses to stressful situations. Examples of such situations and self-statements are nostalgia ("I remember how great it felt smoking after lunch"), testing oneself ("I bet I could smoke just one and then put it down"), crisis ("I really need a cigarette now"), and self-doubts ("I don't have much will power").

Cognitive strategies that can be used to manage these thoughts include the following:

1. Challenging: This involves directly confronting the logic of the thoughts and rehearsing positive responses to them. For example, the patient may think, "Feeling stressed does not mean that I need a cigarette. I can breath deeply and use a brief meditation technique to confront this stressful situation more effectively."
2. Recall and visualization of benefits of nonsmoking: The patient can remind himself or herself about the personal benefits experienced as a result of quitting.
3. Recall and visualization of unpleasant smoking experiences: The patient can practice recalling unpleasant aspects of smoking such as

smell or physical discomfort experienced after heavy smoking.

4. Distraction: Rather than confronting the undermining thoughts, the patient can be assisted in recognizing them and diverting attention from smoking to another, preferably pleasant, subject (e.g., calling a friend).

Reinforcement

Planning of rewards and incentives throughout the process of smoking cessation and maintenance is an important intervention component. Rewards should be planned for successes in meeting predefined behavioral goals for a week, a month, and so on, and should not be associated with smoking. Rewards should be decided on by the patient. In addition to patient self-rewards, clinicians also can provide rewards for signs of effort and progress, and reinforce the belief in the patient's ability to change.

SOCIAL SUPPORT

Providers need to assess social influences that affect smoking behavior in their patients to tailor interventions to the patient's social and cultural context. Important social variables that should be assessed include the number of smokers among the patient's friends, family, and coworkers and whether or not there are any smokers in the patient's household. Quality of social support to quit smoking also should be assessed, as well as the patient's use of support sources. In addition, the patient should be asked how confident he or she feels in his or her ability to resist social pressures to smoke. These variables can be assessed either during the assessment interview or through a questionnaire. If social support is lacking, smoking patients should be encouraged to identify potential sources of support and to build up social support systems in their environment. Friends, family members, and coworkers can be part of such a support network, and significant others may be invited to attend intervention sessions if this seems appropriate. Clinicians must encourage patients to use such systems whenever they need help to ensure their maintained abstinence, and at times may need to help patients develop their ability to ask for help. This is a particularly critical issue when working with women. Women are often less inclined to ask for help from their family and friends because they tend to have difficulties

shifting their caretaking role to the role of being cared for. The clinician can ask questions such as "Has anyone in your family or any friend ever expressed concern about your smoking?" or "Who could you call when you are having a difficult time coping with an urge to smoke?" Patients who lack a supportive environment may need more frequent contacts. These patients also can be instructed to call a help line anytime they experience difficulties that threaten their abstinence.

Additional Intervention Tools

BEHAVIORAL CONTRACTS

Contracts can help the clinician and the patient in goal setting and clarifying the specific steps that the patient will take to accomplish the goal of quitting smoking. Behavioral contracts require a great degree of explicitness to serve their purpose, including 1) whether the patient will taper, use NRT, or stop smoking; 2) a quit date; 3) reasons for stopping; 4) steps to follow in response to high-need and high-risk situations; 5) alternative strategies in case the first choice of coping methods cannot be accomplished; and 6) a plan for follow-up. Behavioral contracts can also be used to set weekly goals for specific changes. Written contracts can help the patient keep the plan in mind and emphasize the seriousness of smoking cessation (Fig. 19.6).

SELF-HELP MATERIALS

Self-help materials must be appropriate to the needs of the cardiac population and meet the individual needs of patients in terms of readiness to quit smoking. Other important considerations include language, text size, readability, and graphic material. In addition to self-help booklets, patients may benefit from a relaxation tape, self-monitoring sheets, and printed relapse prevention strategies (Fig. 19.7).

WEIGHT MANAGEMENT

The potential weight gain associated with smoking cessation should be acknowledged and addressed as part of the intervention. Other components of outpatient cardiac rehabilitation, namely dietary and exercise components, along with behavior modification counseling, can be integrated to prevent or decrease the likelihood of weight gain and thus its negative influence on the smoker's efforts.

Quit Smoking Contract

After careful consideration, I have decided to quit smoking on _____.
                                                                (date)

I am responsible for this decision and understand that my own commitment to quit smoking is of primary importance.

My personal reasons for stopping are:
_____
_____

To prepare for the quit date, I plan to do the following:

Trigger situations: My personal strategies to deal with these situations:
_____   _____
_____   _____

Resources:

  Support team: _____

  Stress reducers: _____

  Rewards: _____

_____   _____   _____
Patient signature   Provider signature   Today's date

Figure 19.6.   Quit smoking contract sample.

Follow-up Contact

Follow-up serves as a reminder of the importance health care providers attach to smoking cessation. Maintenance of cessation is often difficult. In the general population, relapse rates after cessation range between 75% and 80% at 6 months or earlier (8), and individuals continue to relapse, although at lower rates, even after 6 years (2, 3). Follow-up contact is important to monitor progress toward the goal and to examine how helpful the smoking cessation plan is in helping the patient to manage high-need and high-risk situations. During the follow-up period patients are most vulnerable to relapse because of stressors associated with adjustment to illness and return to daily activities. Questions such as "What part of your plan was helpful?" and "What part of the plan did you have problems with?" can assist the clinician in revising the plan and determining future goals. Substantial health benefits of maintaining abstinence should be addressed. Telephone counseling can be helpful with patients who are unable to attend follow-up sessions.

Relapse Prevention

Relapse prevention techniques, initially introduced by Marlatt and Gordon (74) to deal with preventing relapse among alcohol abusers, have been extrapolated for use with smokers (75). The use of relapse prevention techniques aids patients in maintaining cessation longer, and helps them to smoke fewer cigarettes if they relapse (76). Four key elements can provide preparation for the maintenance of nonsmoking behavior:

1. Identifying high-risk situations: Continued awareness of situations in which a "slip" or lapse is likely to occur is essential to maintenance of cessation, even after nicotine withdrawal effects have ceased. The initial self-monitoring can help guide the identification or prediction of situations that may pose challenges to the former smoker in the future.

For Physicians:
_____

Clinical Practice Guideline: Smoking Cessation. Agency for Healthcare Policy and Research. To order: (202) 512–1800

How to Help Your Patients Stop Smoking: A National Cancer Institute Manual for Physicians. To order: (800) 4-CANCER

Clinical Opportunities for Smoking Intervention: A Guide for the Busy Physician. To order: (301) 251–1222

AAFP Stop Smoking Kit. American Academy of Family Physicians. To order: (800) 944–0000

For Patients:
_____

Clearing the Air. National Cancer Institute. To order: (800) 4-CANCER

Smart Move. American Cancer Society. To order: contact local ACS Chapter

Freedom from Smoking for You and Your Baby. American Lung Association. To order: contact local ALA Chapter

Quitting Times: A Magazine for Women Who Smoke. Fox Chase Cancer Center. To order: Contact Massachusetts Tobacco Clearinghouse (617) 482–9485

Figure 19.7.   Self-help materials for smoking cessation.

2. Coping rehearsal: The clinician can help the patient prepare to manage high-risk situations by asking the patient to vividly imagine each specific high-risk situation (details of the people, place, time, etc.), and then asking him or her to visualize what could be done to cope with the situation other than smoking.

3. Identifying and combating undermining self-statements: Certain thoughts or self-statements can be a setup for possible slips if they undermine the goal of remaining an ex-smoker. Understanding habitual rationalizations can help guard against relapse by returning the sense of control to the patient. The patient must learn to expect that such thoughts can occur and prepare to respond to them effectively (see cognitive restructuring above).

4. Avoiding the abstinence violation effect (AVE): The AVE is a common negative emotional response, involving depression, guilt, and lowered self-esteem, to a slip or lapse while the person is committed to abstinence. The individual then attributes the lapse to internal weakness and personal failure (i.e., lack of will power) rather than to external or situational factors, and a resulting decrease in motivation to exert control ("I might as well keep on smoking") and lowered self-efficacy ("I can't quit") follow. The following strategies may be helpful to prevent the AVE:

a. Awareness that the AVE reaction is common: Helping the patient anticipate the AVE as a predictable and common reaction to a slip can be very useful. It is important to point out that the challenge is to let the AVE reaction pass without smoking another cigarette to cope with the associated stress.

b. A slip or lapse is different from a relapse: A slip is no more than an error or mistake and everyone makes mistakes. Making one error does not imply personal weakness or lack of will power. A relapse, on the other hand, involves a complete resumption of smoking.

  c. You can learn from your slips: Slips can be conceptualized as learning experiences that allow patients to examine what works and what does not in helping them to avoid slips.

  d. Irrational interpretation of a slip: The clinician must emphasize that one slip does not make a smoker, unless the person chooses to make it so.

Helping Relapsers

If relapse occurs, the clinician must emphasize the positive aspects of having stopped even briefly, identify what triggered the relapse, and problem-solve for future cessation attempts. The patient should be reminded that relapse is a normal part of the cessation process and that most smokers have stopped several times before they quit for good. The patient's readiness to attempt another cessation trial should be reassessed. Once the patient decides to quit smoking again, training in behavioral management should be emphasized as part of a negotiated plan for quitting. This plan includes setting a quit date, reviewing strategies for quitting, providing self-help materials, and scheduling of follow-up contact with emphasis on relapse prevention.

References

1. Schwartz J. Review and evaluation of smoking cessation methods: the United States and Canada, 1978–1985. Bethesda, MD: National Cancer Institute, NIH Publication No. 87–2940, 1987.
2. Scott R, Mayer J, Denier C, et al. Long-term smoking status of cardiac patients following symptom-specific cessation advice. Addict Behav 1990;15:549–552.
3. Havik O, Maeland J. Changes in smoking behavior after a myocardial infarction. Health Psychol 1988;7:403–420.
4. Ockene J, Hosmer D, Rippe J, et al. Factors affecting cigarette smoking status in patients with ischemic heart disease. J Chronic Dis 1985;38:985–994.
5. Kristeller J, Merriam P, Ockene J, et al. Smoking intervention for cardiac patients: in search of more effective strategies. Cardiology 1993;82:317–324.
6. The health consequences of smoking: cardiovascular disease: a report of the Surgeon General. Rockville, MD: US Department of Health and Human Services, Office on Smoking and Health, Publication No. PHS 84–50204, 1983.
7. The Surgeon General's report. Reducing the health consequences of smoking: 25 years of progress. Washington, DC: US Department of Health and Human Services, Publication No. 89–8411, 1989.
8. The health benefits of smoking cessation: a report of the Surgeon General. Washington, DC: US Department of Health and Human Services, Publication No. CDC 90–8416, 1990.
9. Rosenberg L, Palmer J, Shapiro S. Decline in risk of myocardial infarction among women who stop smoking. N Engl J Med 1990;322:213–217.
10. Hammond E, Horn D. Smoking and death rates. Report on forty-four months of followup of 187,783 men. II. Death rates by cause. JAMA 1958;166:1294–1308.
11. Doll R, Peto R. Mortality in relation to smoking: twenty years' observations on male British doctors. Br Med J 1976;2:1525–1536.
12. Friedman G, Petitti D, Bawal R, et al. Mortality in cigarette smokers and quitters: effect of baseline differences. N Engl J Med 1981;304:1407–1410.
13. Gordon T, Kannel W, McGee D, et al. Death and coronary attacks in men giving up cigarette smoking: a report from the Framingham Study. Lancet 1983;2:1345–1348.
14. Ockene J, Kuller L, Svendsen K, et al. The relationship of smoking cessation to coronary heart disease and lung cancer in the Multiple Risk Factor Intervention Trial (MRFIT). Am J Public Health 1990;80:954–958.
15. Sparrow D, Dawber T, Colton T. The influence of cigarette smoking on prognosis after a first myocardial infarction. A report from the Framingham Study. J Chronic Dis 1978;31:425–432.
16. Salonen J. Stopping smoking and long-term mortality after acute myocardial infarction. Br Heart J 1980;43:463–469.
17. Gerace T, Hollis J, Ockene J, et al. Smoking cessation and change in diastolic blood pressure, body weight, and plasma lipids. Prev Med 1991;20:602–628.
18. Bettman J. An information processing theory of consumer choice. Reading, MA: Addison-Wesley, 1979.
19. Rudd J, Glanz K. How individuals use information for health action and consumer information processing. In: Glanz K, Lewis F, Rimer B, eds. Health behavior and health education: theory, research and practice. San Francisco: Jossey-Bass, 1990.
20. Strecher V, DeVellis B, Becker M, et al. The role of self-efficacy in achieving health behavior change. Health Educ Q 1986;13:73–92.
21. Rosenstock I. The health belief model: explaining health behavior through expectancies. In: Glanz K, Lewis F, Rimer R, eds. Health behavior and health education: theory, research, and practice. San Francisco: Jossey-Bass, 1990.
22. Prochaska J, DiClemente C. Stages and processes of self-change of smoking: toward an integrative model of change. J Consult Clin Psychol 1983;51:390–395.
23. Bandura A. Self-efficacy: toward a unifying theory of behavioral change. Psychol Rev 1977;84:191–215.
24. Bandura A. Self-efficacy: the exercise of control. New York: WH Freeman, 1997:604.
25. Bandura A. Social foundation of thought and action: a social cognitive theory. Englewood Cliffs, NJ: Prentice-Hall, 1986.
26. Ockene J, Kristeller J, Goldberg R, et al. Smoking cessation and severity of disease: The Coronary Artery Smoking Intervention Study. Health Psychol 1992;11:119–126.

27. DiClemente C. Self-efficacy and smoking cessation maintenance: a preliminary report. Cognit Ther Res 1981;5:175–187.

28. Condiotte M, Lichtenstein E. Self-efficacy and relapse in smoking cessation programs. J Consult Clin Psychol 1981;49:648–658.

29. Bandura A. Self-efficacy: the exercise of control. New York: WH Freeman, 1997.

30. Marlatt A, Gordon J, McClellan W. Current perspectives: patient education in medical practice. Patient Educ Counsel 1986;8:151–163.

31. Hughes J, Hatsukami D. The nicotine withdrawal syndrome: a brief review and update. Int J Smoking Cessation 1992;1:21–26.

32. West R, Hajek P, Belcher M. Severity of withdrawal symptoms as a predictor of outcome of an attempt to quit smoking. Psychol Med 1989;19:981–985.

33. Abrams D, Monti P, Carey K, et al. Reactivity to smoking cues and relapse: two studies of discriminant validity. Behav Res Ther 1988;26:224–233.

34. Abrams D, Wilson G. Clinical advances in treatment of smoking and alcohol addiction. Washington, DC: American Psychiatric Association Press, 1986:606–626.

35. Covey L, Glassman A, Stetner F. Depression and depressive symptoms in smoking cessation. Compr Psychiatry 1990;31:350–354.

36. The health consequences of smoking: nicotine addiction. A report of the Surgeon General. Rockville, MD: US Department of Health and Human Services, Public Health Service, Centers for Disease Control, Center for Health Promotion and Education, Office on Smoking and Health, Publication No. CDC 88–8406:5233, 1988.

37. Pomerleau O, Adkins D, Pertschuk M. Predictors of outcome and recidivism in smoking cessation treatment. Addict Behav 1978;3:65–70.

38. Tomkins S. Psychological model for smoking behavior. Am J Public Health 1966;56:17–20.

39. Pomerleau C, Pomerleau O. The effects of a psychosocial stressor on cigarette smoking and subsequent behavioral and physiological responses. Psychophysiology 1987;24:278–285.

40. Pomerleau O, Pomerleau C. Research on stress and smoking: progress and problems. Br J Addict 1991;86: 599–603.

41. Schachter S. Pharmacological and psychological determinants of smoking. Ann Intern Med 1978;88: 104–114.

42. Ockene J, Camic P. Public health approaches to cigarette smoking cessation. Ann Behav Med 1985;7: 14–18.

43. Ockene J, Benfari R, Hurwitz I, et al. Relationship of psychosocial factors to smoking behavior change in an intervention program. Prev Med 1982;11:13–28.

44. Williamson D, Madans J, Anda R, et al. Smoking cessation and severity of weight gain in a national cohort. N Engl J Med 1991;324:739–745.

45. Flegal K, Troiano R, Pamik E, et al. The influence of smoking cessation on the prevalence of overweight in the U.S. N Engl J Med 1995;333:1165–1170.

46. Hall S, Ginsberg D, Jones R. Smoking cessation and weight gain. J Consult Clin Psychol 1986;54:342–346.

47. Pomerleau C. Smoking and nicotine replacement

48. Sorensen G, Pechacek T, Pallonen U. Occupational and worksite norms and attitudes about smoking cessation. Am J Public Health 1986;76:544–549.

49. Novotny T, Warner K, Kendrick J, et al. Smoking by blacks and whites: socioeconomic and demographic differences. Am J Public Health 1988;78:1187–1189.

50. Taylor C, Houston-Miller N, Killen J, et al. Smoking cessation after acute myocardial infarction: effects of a nurse-managed intervention. Ann Intern Med 1990; 113:118–123.

51. Fiore M, Bailey W, Cohen S, et al. Smoking cessation: Clinical Practice Guideline No. 18. Rockville, MD: US Department of Public Health and Human Services, Public Health Service, Agency for Health Care Policy and Research, 1996.

52. Yates A, Thain J. Self-efficacy as a predictor or relapse following voluntary cessation of smoking. Addict Behav 1985;10:291–298.

53. Beck A. The Beck depression inventory. Philadelphia: Center for Cognitive Therapy, 1978.

54. McNair D, Lorr M, Droppleman L. Profile of mood states. San Diego: Educational and Industrial Testing Service, 1971.

55. Derogatis L. SCL-90-R: administration, scoring and procedures manual—II. Baltimore: Clinical Psychometric Research, 1983.

56. Glassman A, Helzer J, Covey L, et al. Smoking, smoking cessation, and major depression. JAMA 1990;264: 1546–1549.

57. Edwards N, Murphy J, Downs A, et al. Doxepin as an adjunct to smoking cessation. A double-blind pilot study. Am J Psychiatry 1989;146:373–376.

58. Labbate L. Nicotine cessation, mania, and depression. Am J Psychiatry 1992;149:708.

59. Lief H. Bupropion treatment of depression to assist smoking cessation [letter to the editor]. Am J Psychiatry 1996;153:3.

60. Hall S, Munoz R, Reus V, et al. Nicotine, negative affect, and depression. J Consult Clin Psychol 1993;61: 761–767.

61. Hughes J. Non-nicotine pharmacotherapies for smoking cessation. J Drug Dev 1994;6:197–203.

62. Ferry L, Robbins A, Scariati P, et al. Enhancement of smoking cessation using the antidepressant bupropion hydrochloride [abstract]. Circulation 1992;86: 671.

63. Fagerstrom K. Measuring degree of physical dependency to tobacco smoking with reference to individualization of treatment. Addict Behav 1978;3:235–241.

64. Fagerstrom K, Schneider N. Measuring nicotine dependence: a review of the Fagerstrom tolerance questionnaire. J Behav Med 1989;12:159–182.

65. Heatherton T, Kozlowski L, Frecker R, et al. The Fagerstrom test for nicotine dependence: a revision of the Fagerstrom tolerance questionnaire. Br J Addict 1991;86:1119–1127.

66. Foxx R, Brown R. Nicotine fading and self-monitoring for cigarette abstinence or controlled smoking. J Appl Behav Anal 1979;12:111–125.

67. Lam W, Sze P, Sacks H, et al. Meta-analysis of ran-

domized controlled trials of nicotine chewing gum. Lancet 1987;2:27–29.

68. Cepeda-Benito A. Meta-analytical review of the efficacy of nicotine chewing gum in smoking treatment programs. J Consult Clin Psychol 1993;61:822–830.

69. Rosal M, Ockene J, Hurley T, et al. Effectiveness of nicotine-containing gum in the physician-delivered smoking intervention study (PDSIP). Prev Med 1998;27:262–267.

70. Tonnesen P, Norregaard J, Simonsen K, et al. A double-blind trial of a 16-hour transdermal nicotine patch in smoking cessation. N Engl J Med 1991;325:311–315.

71. Transdermal Nicotine Study Group. Transdermal nicotine for smoking cessation. JAMA 1992;266: 3133–3138.

72. Schneider N, Olmstead R, Mody F, et al. Efficacy of a nicotine nasal spray in smoking cessation: a placebo-controlled, double-blind trial. Addiction 1995;90: 1671–1682.

73. Shiffman S. Relapse following smoking cessation: a situational analysis. J Consult Clin Psychol 1982;50: 71–86.

74. Marlatt G, Gordon J. Determinants of relapse: implications for the maintenance of behavior change. In: Davidson P, Davidson S, eds. Behavioral medicine: changing health lifestyles. New York: Brunner/Mazel, 1980:410–452.

75. Lichtenstein E, Brown A. Current trends in the modification of cigarette dependence. In: Bellack A, Hersen M, Kazdin A, eds. International handbook of behavior modification and therapy. New York: Plenum, 1985.

76. Davis J, Glaros A. Relapse prevention and smoking cessation. Addict Behav 1986;11:105–114.

77. American Psychiatric Association. Diagnostic and statistical manual of mental disorders. 4th ed. Washington, DC: American Psychiatric Association, 1994.

Gender-specific Issues Related to Coronary Risk Factors in Women

JoAnne Micale Foody and Fredric J. Pashkow

CORONARY DISEASE RISK FACTORS IN WOMEN

Introduction

Contrary to popular belief, cardiovascular disease (CVD)—not cancer—is the leading cause of death in women in the United States (1). The incidence of CVD—including fatal and nonfatal coronary heart disease (CHD), stroke, and hypertension—increases with age in women. In fact, CVD is almost twice as common in postmenopausal women as in their premenopausal counterparts, probably because of declining levels of endogenous estrogen. Numerous factors account for these age-related differences. For example, alterations in serum lipids and lipoproteins increase with age in women, placing older women at increased risk for CHD (2). Blood pressure also rises with age in women, placing older women at increased risk for stroke and other hypertensive complications. In addition, blood glucose levels increase with age in women, again placing older women at increased risk of CHD. These and other age-related physiologic changes—separately or in combination—greatly increase the risk of cardiovascular morbidity and mortality in postmenopausal women and pose a major individual and public health challenge.

Epidemiology

Coronary heart disease is the leading cause of morbidity and mortality for women in the United States: it claims the lives of more than a quarter of a million women each year. Deaths from CVD are almost twice those caused by cancer. Approximately one of every two women in the United States will die of some cardiovascular event—most likely, myocardial infarction (MI), hypertensive heart disease, or stroke. The impact of CVD is even greater for black women in whom the overall annual mortality rate caused by CVD is approximately 67% higher than that in white women (2.25 per 1000 versus 1.35 per 1000, respectively) (1).

Risk factors for CVD in women include 1) those that are innate and, hence, not modifiable (e.g., increasing age or gender), and 2) those that can be modified through behavioral interventions, dietary regulation, exercise, or pharmacologic means (e.g., high cholesterol or hypertension) (Table 20.1). These risk factors are the same in women as in men, although the impact of individual coronary risk factors and the results of their interventions differ dramatically by gender. Special emphasis must also be placed on those uniquely female attributes that modify coronary risk: specifically, oral contraceptives, pregnancy, menopausal status, and the use of postmenopausal hormone therapy.

Coronary risk factors are highly prevalent in women in the United States. In women aged 20 to 74, 33% have hypertension, more than one-quarter have hypercholesterolemia, more than one-quarter are cigarette smokers, more than a quarter are overweight, and more than a quarter report sedentary lifestyles. Although these risk factors are more prevalent in men than in women, as women age, their risk factor profile approaches and in some instances surpasses that of their male counterparts.

Cholesterol and Dyslipidemia

It is well established that the higher the level of serum cholesterol, the higher the risk of CHD (3). Multiple studies have borne out these results

Table 20.1.   Risk Factors for Cardiovascular Disease in Women

Modifiable Risk Factors	Unmodifiable Risk Factors
Dyslipidemias	Increasing age
Hypertension	Gender
Diabetes mellitus	Genetics
Cigarette smoking	Race
Obesity	Menopause(?)
Physical inactivity	

(Table 20.2). According to the Lipid Research Clinics Prevalence Study (4), lipid and lipoprotein concentrations vary according to a woman's ovarian function. Women who have undergone natural menopause or oophorectomy have significantly higher concentrations of total cholesterol (TC) when compared with menstruating women or those who have undergone hysterectomy with preservation of ovarian function (5–8). Similar findings have been observed for changes in low-density lipoprotein cholesterol (LDL-C) levels (9).

There is virtually no risk of CHD in women with a "desirable" level of TC (<205 mg/dL [5.30 mmol/L]) whereas even a slight elevation in cholesterol (up to a "borderline" high level of 220 to 250 mg/dL [5.69 to 6.47 mmol/L]) results in an approximate doubling of risk (3, 10). The incidence of CHD continues to rise steeply as cholesterol concentrations reach the "high" level (>280 mg/dL [>7.24 mmol/L]). The annual rate of CHD in women also rises sharply in relation to age, plateauing at the age of 65 to 74, and then begins to decline. Fewer than 10 per 1000 women younger than 55 years (presumed to be premenopausal or perimenopausal) have CHD, whereas the rate of CHD jumps to almost 25 per 1000 in women between the ages of 55 and 64 (presumed to be postmenopausal) and to more than 30 per 1000 in women between the ages of 65 and 74 (3, 10). Thus the risk of CHD is strongly correlated to both increasing age and serum TC level in women.

High-density Lipoprotein Cholesterol

Elevated high-density lipoprotein cholesterol (HDL-C) levels play a key role in protecting both men and women against the development of CHD (11–13). The Lipid Research Clinics follow-up study showed that HDL-C was the major lipid predictor of CHD mortality in women (4). Some more recent data suggest that HDL-C levels decline in association with natural menopause, thus placing postmenopausal women at greater risk for CHD than their male counterparts. A prospective study in 541 women who were premenopausal at the time of study enrollment revealed that the mean HDL-C level of 65 women who entered natural menopause declined significantly ($P < .01$) when compared with that of an age-matched group of 65 premenopausal women who served as control subjects (14). These differences between premenopausal and postmenopausal groups remained statistically significant, even after multivariate analysis adjusted for age, body mass index (BMI), and cigarette smoking.

Some investigators have suggested that the TC:HDL-C ratio is the best predictor of angiographically documented CHD in women (15). In women a desirable HDL-C level is between 50 and 60 mg/dL (1.29 and 1.55 mmol/L). Given that a desirable TC level has been established as less than 205 mg/dL (5.30 mmol/L), the TC:HDL-C ratio should be 4.0 or less. The Framingham Study illustrated that the ratio rises steadily with age in women. The ratio of TC:HDL-C in women between the ages of 15 and 34 (presumed to be premenopausal) was only 3.4 whereas that of women older than 55 years (presumed to be postmenopausal) was greater than 4.5 (16).

Low-density Lipoprotein Cholesterol

The Framingham study found LDL-C to be a significant positive predictor of coronary disease in women, although less powerful than HDL-C (17). In contrast, The Lipid Research Clinics study did not find LDL-C to be a significant independent predictor of CVD in women (4).

Low-density lipoprotein cholesterol level was a poor predictor of CVD mortality in female participants in The Lipid Research Clinics follow-up study after adjustment for other CVD factors. In fact, after stratification by HDL-C category, the highest CVD death rates were noted among women with low HDL-C and normal LDL-C levels (4). This finding is contrary to what is observed in men, in whom CVD risk increases with levels of either TC or LDL-C.

Very high LDL-C concentrations carry the same poor prognosis in both sexes. Men and women who are homozygous for familial hyper-

Table 20.2. Major Studies That Implicate Cholesterol as a Coronary Disease Risk for Women

Studies	Women(n)	Ages(years)	Results
Framingham Heart Study	2873	35–94	TC >265 mg/dl: twofold risk of CHD compared with women with TC <205 mg/dl
Dono-Tel Aviv	1325	25–69	TC >265 mg/dl: threefold increase compared with TC< 200mg/dl
Rancho -Bernardo	2048	59–79	TC >260: 2.5 fold increase in risk
Nurses' Health Study	120,343	30–55	Self-reported hypercholesterolemia increases risk of nonfatal MI 2 times and fatal CHD 3 times TC < 200 mg/dL

cholesterolemia have a similar increased risk for CHD (18). However, women who are heterozygous have a lower risk attributable to LDL-C compared with heterozygous men (18). This finding may be merely because of the higher HDL-C levels found in women.

Postmenopausal women with high levels of LDL-C are not protected by estrogen, nor by the generally higher levels of HDL-C. The higher levels of LDL-C are most likely associated with a greater percentage of small, dense LDL-C particles. Premenopausal women are relatively protected by estrogen and high levels of HDL-C (17), but for postmenopausal women, LDL-C level might be a stronger and perhaps more independent risk factor (16).

Triglycerides

The role of triglycerides (TGs) in the development of CHD is still the subject of some debate. For the most part, TGs have not been shown to be a statistically independent predictor of CHD risk when HDL-C and LDL-C are considered in a multivariate analysis. But studies have demonstrated TGs as a strong and independent risk factor for women (6, 19, 20) and some experts feel they should be conscientiously addressed.

Lapidus et al. (21) demonstrated the continued importance of TG levels as a risk factor for CVD even after adjustment for multiple risk factors, including TC levels in a longitudinal study involving more than 1,400 women. A large study involving 25,058 middle-aged men and 24,535 middle-aged women for 15 years of follow-up showed that a high level of TGs is an independent risk factor for mortality from CHD after adjustment for other risk factors in women but not in men (22, 23).

In the Lipid Research Clinics follow-up study (4), age-adjusted mortality relative risk in women was 1.6 for TG levels of 200 to 300 mg/dL (2.26 to 3.39 mmol/L), and 3.4 for levels more than 400 mg/dL (4.52 mmol/L) compared with levels less than 200 mg/dL (2.26 mmol/L). Cardiovascular disease death rates in women with high TG levels were more than 11 times the rates of women with normal TG levels. The risk was stronger if HDL-C level was low (<50 mg/dL [1.29 mmol/L]).

Elevated TG levels are likely to be prevalent in older postmenopausal women, in whom TGs may be markers for the presence of other atherogenic lipoproteins. We see that as women age and progress through menopause, the percentage of smaller, denser LDL-C rises; the occurrence of small, dense LDL-C has been associated with hypertriglyceridemia. We know that small, dense LDL-C may be more susceptible to oxidation and thus more atherogenic; therefore, its association with TGs may explain the predictive power of TGs in older postmenopausal women (24, 25).

Diabetes Mellitus

Diabetes mellitus (DM) is the single most powerful risk factor for CHD in women. Its impact is greater in women than in men. Women with diabetes have a fivefold increase in CVD than women without diabetes. Follow-up data from the Framingham study (11, 26) showed that the prevalence of DM among women rises sharply with age. The prevalence among women younger than 44 years (presumed to be premenopausal) is only 6.9 per 1000, but almost triples to 18.6 per 1000 in women between the ages of 45 and 54 (presumed to be approaching menopause or perimenopause) (Table 20.3).

High blood glucose levels are a strong predictor of CHD risk, independent of whether or not

Table 20.3.   Ratio of Total: HDL Cholesterol in Women by Age: The Framingham Study

Age (yr)	Mean ± SD
15–24	3.4 ± 0.9
25–34	3.4 ± 1.1
35–44	3.6 ± 1.2
45–54	4.0 ± 1.5
55–64	4.5 ± 1.5
65–74	4.6 ± 1.5
75–79	4.7 ± 1.4

HDL = high-density lipoprotein.

the individual has clinical diabetes. Based on the 16-year follow-up data from the Framingham study, the conclusion that the annual incidence of CHD increases with blood glucose levels and increasing age was drawn (27). There is, for example, little risk of CHD in women with blood glucose levels less than 60 mg/dL ("low"). Greater than about 130 mg/dL, however, the CHD risk escalates sharply—doubling and even tripling that associated with lower glucose levels.

Women with DM have been found to have twice the risk of MI as nondiabetic women of the same age; the risk of MI in diabetic women equals that of nondiabetic men of the same age (27). In diabetic women, the incidence of CHD is almost three times that of nondiabetic women as compared with a twofold increase in incidence in men. Diabetes cancels the female hormonal advantage over men. There is also some indication that DM predisposes women to more lethal coronary events, almost doubling the case fatality rates.

According to the 20-year follow-up data from the Framingham study, the presence of DM tends to attenuate any gender-related differences in cardiovascular morbidity and mortality. In fact, the risk of CHD in diabetic women is higher than that of both diabetic men and nondiabetic women, even after adjustment has been made for age and other CHD risk factors. The higher risk among diabetic women may be partially explained by the "clustering" of multiple risk factors in diabetic individuals, such as hypertension, smoking, and obesity (26). Diabetic women in the Framingham population had significantly higher levels of four CHD risk factors (other than diabetes or high blood glucose levels): 1) HDL-C, 2) TGs, 3) systolic blood pressure, and 4) relative body weight (Table 20.4). Only systolic blood pressure and relative body weight were signifi-

cantly higher in male diabetics compared with nondiabetic males (26).

Differences in lipoprotein profiles are largely explained by insulin activity (28). In both men and women, insulin promotes lipoprotein lipase-mediated TG removal. Thus, a deficiency of insulin results in hypertriglyceridemia. Diabetes increases endogenous hepatic very low-density lipoprotein cholesterol (VLDL-C) secretion. Activity of the LDL-C receptors is also insulin-dependent and is downregulated in the absence of insulin. Concentrations of HDL-C are increased by insulin administration in men and women with insulin-dependent diabetes (28).

Hypertension

The two other leading causes of cardiovascular mortality and morbidity in women are stroke and hypertension. Stroke is the second leading cause of cardiovascular mortality in women, accounting for 87,391 deaths among women in the United States in 1990 (1). This was substantially higher than the number of men who died of stroke in that year. The incidence of both fatal and nonfatal stroke rises steadily with age in both genders. Among women aged 30 to 44 years the estimated incidence of stroke is only 8,000 annually. This figure rises sharply to 50,000 in women between the ages of 45 and 65 and more than triples to 179,000 in women older than 65 years. Thus, postmenopausal women are at significantly higher risk of stroke than are premenopausal women. Although the incidence of stroke is higher for men of all ages compared with women of all ages, the mortality rate is higher in women. This is in large part because of an almost 80% higher death rate from stroke in black women than in white women (1).

Table 20.4.   Coronary Heart Disease Risk Factors in Diabetic Versus Nondiabetic Women: The Framingham Study

Risk Factor	Diabetic	Nondiabetic
Serum cholesterol (mg/dL)	259	250
HDL-C (mg/dL)	54	58
LDL-C (mg/dL)	157	155
Triglycerides (mg/dL)	141	133
Systolic BP (mm Hg)	150	139
Relative weight (% ideal)	129	121
Cigarettes/day	6	5

HDL-C = high-density lipoprotein cholesterol; LDL-C = low-density lipoprotein cholesterol; BP = blood pressure.

The 20-year follow-up data from the Framingham study indicate that the risk of hypertensive complications increases markedly after about the age of 45 to 55 (presumed to be approaching menopause or perimenopause) in women with both borderline and frank hypertension. However, the attributable risk percent (i.e., the proportion of cardiovascular end points attributable to hypertension) is higher for postmenopausal women than for men of comparable ages: 74.3% versus 64.5% for ages 55 to 64, and 75.8% versus 66.5% for ages 65 to 74. The prevalence of hypertension in white men and women is about equal, whereas the prevalence is greater in black women compared with black men (29).

The relationship between hypertension and atherosclerosis is complex. Hypertension in the presence of other risk factors, in particular hypercholesterolemia, clearly accelerates the progression of atherosclerosis. Among participants of the Normal Health and Nutrition Examination Survey II (NHANES II) 40% of persons with hypertension had blood cholesterol levels greater than 240 mg/dL (6.21 mmol/L) and 46% of those with blood cholesterol levels more than 240 mg/dL (6.21 mmol/L) had hypertension (30). Persons with hypertension and dyslipidemia often have glucose intolerance and upper body obesity. This constellation of risk factors, variously referred to as syndrome X, the deadly quartet, or familial dyslipidemic hypertension, confers a markedly increased risk of CHD.

Obesity

The Nurses' Health Study (31) showed that women with a BMI (defined as weight in kilograms per height in square meters) of 25 to 29 kg/m², compared with the leanest women, had an age-adjusted relative risk for CHD of 1.8, whereas morbidly obese women (BMI > 29 kg/m²) had a relative risk for CHD of 3.3. In 115,886 American women 30 to 55 years of age, who were participants in the Nurses' Health Study, 40% of coronary events were attributable to excess body weight. Twenty-five percent of American women 35 to 64 years of age have a BMI of 29 kg/m² or higher—the category of women having relative risks of nonfatal MI and fatal CHD of 3.2 and 3.5, respectively (31).

The cumulative effect obesity has on an individual's heart remains unclear partly as a result of

1) the use of different obesity measurements, and 2) the failure to account for confounding slimming effects of smoking and preexisting disease in several studies. The measurement of obesity has shifted from the BMI to the waist-to-hip ratio (WHR). Although both BMI and WHR have indicated a clear linear association between obesity and CHD, the WHR, which accounts for abdominal adiposity, is viewed as a more accurate predictor of CHD (32). The distribution of fat appears to be a more significant predictor than total fat, according to recent studies, because android fat patterns are more metabolically active (33) and highly associated with dyslipidemia (34). Despite this, the National Center for Health Statistics still uses BMI as the recognized measurement of obesity. The guidelines for obesity are defined as a BMI of 27.8 or more in men and 27.3 kg/m² or more in women, and morbid obesity has been defined as a BMI of 31.1 in men and 32.3 kg/m² in women (35).

Obesity has been shown to be an independent risk factor for the development of CHD in women. In a 26-year follow-up of participants in the Framingham Heart Study (10), relative weight in women was positively and independently associated with coronary disease and coronary and CVD death. The study further showed that weight gain after the young adult years conveyed an increased risk of CVD in both genders that could not be attributed either to the initial weight or the levels of the risk factors that may have resulted from weight gain. Evidence from other epidemiologic studies indicates that 30% of the CHD occurring in obese women can be attributed to the excess weight alone, and even being mildly to moderately overweight increases the risk of coronary disease in middle-aged women (10).

Truncal, android, or male-pattern obesity, manifest as an increase in the WHR, correlates with higher LDL-C and lower HDL-C levels. Truncal obesity is associated with both higher blood pressure and hyperinsulinemia, which lead to increases in atherogenic lipoproteins and decreases in HDL-C (36, 37). The mechanism for this is unclear, although it has been hypothesized that it may somehow be related to an increase in peripheral insulin resistance: the portal venous drainage of abdominal fat may induce hepatic insulin resistance, elevated circulating insulin, higher TG levels, and lower HDL-C levels.

Women tend to carry the majority of their

weight through their hips (gynoid pattern) This pattern is not associated with a high risk for CVD. Women with truncal obesity have the same risk conferred as men.

Smoking

Although diabetes is the most biologically gender-differentiated risk factor for coronary disease in women, cigarette smoking may be the most psychologically and sociologically distinguishing risk behavior for men and women. Cigarette smoking in women is an especially serious risk (38). Cigarette smoking carries an especially increased hazard for young women because it is often accompanied by oral contraceptive use, a combination that promotes thrombogenesis (38).

Smoking is deadly, claiming nearly 200,000 lives in the United States in 1994, or nearly one-fifth of all heart disease deaths (38). Among adult Americans, the prevalence of cigarette smoking declined markedly from its peak in 1965, when 40% smoked. Smoking prevalence has declined more rapidly among men than women, so that the gender gap in smoking prevalence has narrowed considerably. This difference is likely to continue to narrow, because adolescent girls are starting to smoke at the same rate as boys. This is likely to contribute to a substantially greater female burden of CVD.

For several decades it has been clear that smoking is associated with an elevated risk of CHD among men. For some time, it was believed that cigarette smoking was not associated with CHD among women. However, positive correlations have been observed in both case-control and prospective cohort studies of nonfatal MI and fatal coronary disease.

The Nurses' Health Study, a large, prospective cohort study of women, examined the incidence of CHD in relation to cigarette smoking in a cohort of 119,404 female nurses from the age of 30 to 55 (39). The number of cigarettes smoked per day was positively correlated with the risk of CHD (relative risk of 5.5 for more than 25 cigarettes per day), nonfatal MI (relative risk of 5.8), and angina pectoris (relative risk of 2.6). Overall, cigarette smoking accounted for approximately half these events. This attributable risk was highest among women who were already at increased risk because of older age, family history of MI, obesity, hypertension, hypercholesterolemia, or diabetes. These data emphasize the importance

of cigarette smoking as a determinant of CHD in women, as well as the markedly increased hazards associated with this habit in combination with other risk factors for this disease.

New evidence points to the significant role of passive smoking in the development of CHD (40). Women are seriously threatened by this new, emerging risk factor for CHD. Passive smoke reduces the ability of the blood to deliver oxygen to the myocardium and impairs the heart's ability to use oxygen. After only 2 cigarettes, a nonsmoker's platelet activity matches that of a habitual smoker. Second-hand smoke causes increased intimal wall damage, accelerates atherosclerotic lesions, and increases intimal wall damage after ischemia or MI. In a prospective trial published recently, men and women were found to have increased aortic thickening in both smokers and passive smokers (41).

Young women constitute the major group that is increasing smoking. The reasons for this are complex. More than a third of women perceive that they must smoke to maintain their weight, and more than two-thirds believe they will gain weight if they quit (42–45).

Smoking has been equated with physical attractiveness, social desirability, and even feminine self-assertion and independence. Cigarette advertising in magazines downplays the hazards of smoking, and this is particularly true of women's-interest publications (46). "Low-yield" cigarettes are specifically targeted at women, with the implication that the lower levels of tar and nicotine are safer, but these cigarettes have been shown not to lower the risk of a first nonfatal MI than higher-yield brands (47).

Physical Activity

Sedentary lifestyle is now recognized as a major risk for CHD. However, studies that specifically address the effects of increased physical activity on coronary disease risk factors beyond lipids are uncommon, and until recently the findings have been equivocal (48). Even moderately fit women demonstrate significantly better blood sugars, blood pressures, and anthropometric indices in addition to improvement in the lipid profile when compared with women in the lowest fitness category (49, 50).

Increasing evidence shows that inactivity and a sedentary lifestyle may be independent risk factors for the development of CHD in both men and women. Few studies have addressed the relationship between physical fitness or habitual activity level and CVD in women (51).

Cross-sectional studies comparing active and sedentary women report a positive association between exercise and HDL-C in both premenopausal and postmenopausal women (51–53). Significant differences between groups remained for HDL-C values when results were corrected for differences in percent body fat. Two studies compared plasma lipids with menopausal status in female runners (49, 54). They showed no differences in HDL-C between premenopausal and postmenopausal women who exercised, but when inactive and exercising women were compared, it appeared that younger premenopausal women responded with lipoprotein changes less strongly than older postmenopausal women. Hence, exercise appeared to attenuate the age-related increase in LDL-C and decrease in HDL-C. Otherwise, in these cross-sectional studies, women on hormone replacement therapy (HRT) who reported exercising had higher HDL-C than sedentary women not on HRT (55).

Psychosocial Aspects of Heart Disease in Women

During the past decade, a large body of evidence has accumulated regarding the relationship of socioeconomic status, employment, type A behavior, hostility, depression, and social support to CVD.

Socioeconomic factors, including educational attainment, are important contributors to coronary disease risk. There is a remarkable gradient of death rates from heart disease in women from 1971 to 1984, ranging from 14.0 per 1000 for women with 0 to 7 years of education to 7.5 per 1000 for women with 13 or more years of education completed (56).

Women with a low educational level had a significantly increased age-specific incidence of angina pectoris. There was no significant correlation between marital status or number of children and incidence of ischemic heart disease or overall mortality. Multivariate analyses showed that the association between low educational level and incidence of angina pectoris was independent of socioeconomic group itself, cigarette smoking, systolic blood pressure, indices of obesity, serum TGs, and serum cholesterol (57).

Matthews et al. (58) investigated the association between educational attainment and biologic and behavioral risk factors for CHD in a community sample of 2138 middle-aged, perimenopausal women. Among 541 eligible participants, the lower the education level the women reported, the more atherogenic was their risk factor profile, including higher systolic blood pressure, LDL-C, apolipoprotein B, TGs, fasting and 2-hour postprandial glucose values, BMI, and lower HDL-C and HDL-C:LDL-C ratio. The attainment of lower educational level also correlated with being a cigarette smoker, participating in little physical exercise, and consuming alcohol less than 1 day a week. These individuals more often reported on standardized psychological tests being type B, angry, pessimistic, depressed, and dissatisfied with their jobs, and having little social support and self-esteem. Similar associations were obtained between educational attainment and risk factors reported by the 1588 nonparticipants during the telephone screening interview. These results suggest many biologic and behavioral factors by which women with little education are at elevated risk for CHD, and thus, education may be a potentially important public health intervention for women.

As women have assumed different roles in the workplace, the impact of these roles on cardiovascular and women's health in general has been questioned. In a review of the literature, Haynes and colleagues (59) found, on the basis of nine published studies, that working women appear to be healthier than nonworking or unemployed women according to several health indicators.

The Unique Cardiovascular Role of Estrogen

The protective effect of estrogen appears to be strongest among women who are currently using this therapy. That is, former users have a higher risk of heart disease than current users, but lower than women who have never taken estrogen. Estrogen appears to be protective against many forms of CVD, including heart attack, stroke, and blockage of coronary blood vessels (60, 61).

These observations have led researchers to hypothesize that estrogen may directly or indirectly retard the development of plaques, favorably affect the vulnerability of existing plaques, or reduce the risk of coronary occlusion by preventing the formation of an occlusive thrombus, a consequence of plaque rupture. In addition, estrogen may alter endothelial function and attenuate vasomotor dysfunction, possible triggers of plaque rupture.

Estrogen may protect women through modification of the lipid profile. Postmenopausal women have reduced LDL-C and elevated HDL-C compared to men (62). After menopause, women take on a more atherogenic lipid profile as LDL-C rises, HDL-C falls, and lipoprotein(a) increases. Estrogen replacement reverses these adverse changes in lipoprotein profile and diminishes cardiovascular risk.

Recent observational epidemiologic studies have strongly suggested that estrogen replacement therapy (ERT) in women reduced cardiovascular death significantly (63). The marked reduction in cardiovascular mortality seen in women who have received ERT strongly suggests that the majority of older women, particularly those with atherosclerotic heart disease or who are at high risk for atherosclerotic heart disease, should be considered for ERT on this basis alone.

The Postmenopausal Estrogen/Progestin Intervention Trial (PEPI) (64) demonstrated that there is a significant lowering of LDL-C even with the addition of medroxyprogesterone acetate (MPA) or micronized progesterone. Of the four regimens studied, continuous conjugated estrogens (Premarin, 0.625 mg) without any progestin had the most favorable effect on HDL-C; however, the high rate of endometrial hyperplasia (10% per year) makes this an unacceptable regimen for women with a uterus. Premarin (0.625 mg) in combination with micronized progesterone had a more favorable HDL-C effect when compared to the same dose of Premarin in combination with daily MPA (2.5 mg) or with cycled MPA (10 mg). All four regimens lowered LDL-C and fibrinogen levels and did not elevate blood pressure or have detectable effects on insulin levels after a challenge.

The beneficial effects of ERT on CHD morbidity and mortality are now appreciated. Studies suggest that the risk of CHD is reduced by about 35% to 50% among healthy postmenopausal women who take estrogen. Among women with CHD, the degree of protection appears to be even more substantial—several studies reported up to an 80% reduction in the risk for subsequent CHD events (65). Although one of the earliest reports from the Framingham study noted that the relative risk of cardiovascular events was increased in estrogen users, a reanalysis of these data, which corrected for errors in reporting of estrogen use, found that an insignificant protective effect of estrogen (relative risk, 0.40) was noted in younger women and that there was an insignificant adverse effect (relative risk, 1.8) in women aged 50 to 59 years (66). In the Nurses' Health Study (67), the largest prospective study published to date, involving more than 48,000 postmenopausal women, a 46% reduction in MI or death was noted (relative risk, 0.56) among postmenopausal estrogen users (Table 20.5).

Primary Prevention

Primary prevention focuses on reducing risk factors in large populations of women who have no evidence of disease, but who have dyslipidemia or other cardiac risk factors. Primary prevention of CVD in women is problematic and faces obstacles to its implementation for several reasons. Women themselves have difficulty recognizing the benefits of the recommendations. The issue is often raised that there are insufficient data from clinical trials to justify cholesterol-lowering interventions in women because most studies have been performed in male subjects. The National Cholesterol Education Program (NCEP) recommendations (68, 69) may be less appropriate for women in that some who are screened may have TC levels in the desirable range but LDL-C or HDL-C levels that put them at risk.

The guidelines provide for the detection, evaluation, and treatment of hypercholesterolemia and related disorders (68, 69). In these recommendations, TC and HDL-C are the primary screening parameters. Patients are categorized by age, gender, hormonal status, number of risk factors, and fasting LDL-C level. Patients with two or more risk factors are considered to be at "high risk." Evaluation beyond TC and HDL-C measurement is recommended for those with screening TC levels more than 240 mg/dL (6.21 mmol/L), or TC levels of 200 to 239 mg/dL (5.17 to 6.20 mmol/L) associated with other risk factors or established CHD. An HDL-C level greater than 60 mg/dL (1.55 mmol/L) allows "credit" of one risk factor; on the other hand, individuals with low levels of HDL-C (<35 mg/dL [0.91 mmol/L]) are considered to have an additional risk factor, and lipoprotein analysis is recommended. Neither TC nor HDL-C are parameters actually targeted for intervention; only LDL-C is

Table 20.5. Risk of Cardiovascular Disease and Post Menopausal Hormone Use

Group	Person-Years	Major Coronary Disease		Fatal Cardiovascular Disease		Total Stroke	
		Cases (95%CI)	RR	Cases (95%CI)	RR	Cases (95%CI)	RR
Non-users	179,194	250		129	1.0	123	1.0
		250					
Current users	73,532	45	0.51(0.37–0.70)	21	0.48(0.31–0.74)	39	0.96(0.67–1.37)
Former users	85,128	110		55		62	
			0.91(0.73–1.14)		0.84(0.61–1.15)		1.00(0.74–1.36)

Modified from Stampfer MJ, Colditz GA, Willett WC, et al. Postmenopausal estrogen therapy and cardiovascular disease. Ten-year follow-up from the nurses' health study. N Engl J Med 1991;325:756–762.

specifically targeted. Little consideration for gender is present in the guidelines as originally published, and the normal values for lipoproteins are considered to be the same for men and women.

Dietary modification is recommended for low-risk patients (one risk factor) with LDL-C levels greater than 160 mg/dL (4.14 mmol/L) and high-risk patients (two or more risk factors) with LDL-C less than 160 mg/dL (4.14 mmol/L). Low-risk patients whose LDL-C levels reach 190 mg/dL (4.91 mmol/L) or high-risk patients whose LDL-C levels reach 160 mg/dL (4.14 mmol/L) are recommended to start drug therapy. Drug therapy is not recommended in men younger than 35 years and in premenopausal women unless LDL-C levels are more than 220 mg/dL (5.67 mmol/L). The guidelines set higher LDL-C thresholds for drug intervention in premenopausal women (LDL-C >220 mg/dL [>5.67 mmol/L]) than in postmenopausal women (LDL-C >190 mg/dL [>4.91 mmol/L]). Hormone replacement therapy is currently recommended by NCEP as an option for postmenopausal women with hypercholesterolemia (68, 69).

The NCEP guidelines prove problematic in women for the following reasons. First, treatment is based on LDL-C levels, which are probably less important in women than other lipoproteins. Second, a cutoff of 35 mg/dL (0.91 mmol/L) is given for HDL-C, instead of the more relevant level of 45 or 50 mg/dL (1.16 or 1.29 mmol/L) in women, considering that 50 mg/dL (1.29 mmol/L) is in fact an average HDL-C value for women (68, 69). Third, TG levels (and for that matter, diabetes) are not considered to be independent risk factors, although they have been demonstrated to be a risk in certain subsets of women. Nonpharmacologic therapy (weight reduction, alcohol restriction, and increased phys-

ical activity) is recommended for all patients with elevated TGs. Drugs are started to lower TGs only if other lipoprotein abnormalities are present, TGs are very high (>1000 mg/dL [>11.25 mmol/L]; necessary to prevent acute pancreatitis), or there is a personal family history of CHD or other manifestations of atherosclerosis (68, 69).

Secondary Prevention

Secondary prevention is aimed at individuals who already have CHD and are therefore at highest risk for having progressive disease. Women in this group generally accept treatment to reduce risk. Lipoprotein analysis is required in all patients, but again classification is based on LDL-C. For these patients, the optimal LDL-C is 100 mg/dL (2.59 mmol/L) or less. If it is more than this value, a cholesterol-lowering therapy must be initiated: a nonpharmacologic approach for LDL-C between 100 and 130 mg/dL (2.59 and 3.36 mmol/L), and drug therapy when LDL-C is 130 mg/dL (3.36 mmol/L) despite a trial of dietary therapy and physical activity (68, 69).

Lowering LDL-C to less than 100 mg/dL (2.59 mmol/L) has been shown to result in a significant decrease in recurrent MI and CHD mortality (45, 70). Drugs to lower TGs are recommended for all patients with elevated TGs (>200 mg/dL [>2.26 mmol/L]) in the context of secondary prevention. Lastly, HRT maintains its position between diet and lipid-lowering drugs. However, HRT has an even greater benefit in secondary prevention than in primary prevention of CHD. There is a 73% reduction in CHD mortality in users of postmenopausal estrogen who have CHD at baseline, compared with the 55% reduction seen in all women regardless of baseline CHD status (71).

Diet

The NCEP dietary intervention should occur in two steps. Step I involves an intake of saturated fat of 8% to 10% of total calories, 30% or less of the total calories should be derived from fat, and less than 300 mg of cholesterol per day. If this diet proves inadequate to achieve the goals, the patient should proceed to the step II diet. Step II calls for further reductions in saturated fat intake to less than 7% of calories and in cholesterol to less than 200 mg per day. The polyunsaturated:saturated fat ratio should thus be increased (68, 69).

All reduced-fat diets have a beneficial effect on LDL-C, but consistently also reduce HDL-C, which is disadvantageous for women (72). Furthermore, the literature observes specific gender differences for diet responsiveness (73).

Two studies in women who switched from a "typical American diet" to the NCEP step I diet showed that LDL-C levels fell by 32% and 29%, and HDL-C levels decreased by 16% and 20% (74, 75). Two similar studies in men showed decreases in LDL-C of 24% and 26% and either no change or an insignificant 12% fall in HDL-C (76, 77). These results suggest that LDL-C falls comparably in men and women with dietary modification, but that the decrease of HDL-C is more drastic in women (78). However, prospective studies that compare men and women after a comparable dietary protocol are necessary for a real gender analysis.

Furthermore, menopausal status may affect dietary responsiveness. In one small study, a similar response to diet was observed in both premenopausal and postmenopausal women (79). A large study of 2222 postmenopausal women compared with men of corresponding ages found greater declines in LDL-C and TG levels in men than in women and a greater decline in HDL-C levels in women than in men when all subjects followed a very low-fat diet (80).

From a woman's perspective, the most important problem with diet therapy appears to be the accompanying decrease of HDL-C. The decrease is more severe in women than in men, and even more extreme in postmenopausal women. Given that the inverse relationship of HDL-C to cardiac events may be more emphatic in women than the adverse risk imparted by LDL-C, the conclusion is that diet may have an effect opposite the desired one. As suggested, for women with a very high LDL-C and at risk for CHD, all available techniques must be used to lower LDL-C. For low-risk women, unless they have a weight problem, the benefits of a low-fat diet are far from clear.

Weight Loss

Efforts to prevent or treat obesity have had only limited success. Striking excesses in morbidity and mortality from CHD attributable to obesity in middle-aged women have stimulated greater efforts to understand and treat the problem of obesity in women.

Studies indicate that serum lipid responses to weight loss differ for women compared with men. A 10% reduction in body weight caused HDL-C to rise in men, but to fall slightly in women, and LDL-C levels declined in both men and women but to a greater extent in men (81).

LaRosa et al. (82) suggest that the presence of excess truncal fat in both men and women correlates with increases in LDL-C and decreases in HDL-C, accounting for the increased risk of CHD observed in central obesity. As stated previously, postmenopausal women have a tendency for truncal fat disposition. Adipose tissue in postmenopausal women can serve as a source of estrogen synthesis. Thus, the benefits of weight reduction in older women may be offset by the loss of estrogen-producing adipose tissue. As an additional consequence, the expected increases in HDL-C and decline in LDL-C with weight loss may be less evident than in men.

Among the recent developments that advanced the current understanding of obesity are the 1994 discovery of the obesity gene, *ob*, which produces the food-intake regulating enzyme, leptin (83, 84); the development of behavioral programs that modify unhealthy eating behavior; and the use of pharmacologic drugs such as nonadrenergic and serotonin-reuptake inhibitors (85). There are several medications currently available for the temporary treatment of obesity; these medications are categorized by their affects on energy intake, storage, and output. Drugs that affect the brain include serotonergic and noradrenergic medications (86). Noradrenergic drugs influence weight loss through stimulation of the hypothalamus. The use of dexfenfluramine and fenfluramine, serotonin reuptake inhibitors, has been discontinued because of an increase in valvular heart defects and pulmonary hypertension.

Although these pharmacologic agents temporarily aid in the patient's struggle against obesity, the National Task Force on Obesity cautions against the use of these agents for long-term maintenance in light of unknown side effects. In the most extreme cases, surgical therapy can be used for treatment. In morbidly obese patients (BMI >40 kg/m^2) and severely obese patients (BMI, 35 to 40 kg/m^2) with coexisting conditions, jejunoileal shunts and gastroplasty can aid in the maintenance of weight loss, as 80% of patients do maintain a weight 10% below their preoperative weight about 10 years after surgery (35).

In addition to caloric restriction, behavior modification, and pharmacologic therapy, exercise figures as one of the most popular and effective methods of weight loss for the obese patient. The greatest weight losses have been reported in a combined regimen of diet and exercise rather than diet or exercise alone (88–92).

Two issues important to weight-loss effectiveness are degree of loss and duration of loss. Even if weight is lost, studies indicate that in the vast majority of cases, weight-loss maintenance frequently fails because of the many physiologic and psychological factors that contribute to obesity. Approximately two-thirds of persons who lose weight will regain it within 1 year, and almost all persons who lose weight will regain it within 5 years. As evidenced by a substantial body of research, this short-term weight loss is ineffective in modifying coronary risk factors. Additional health risks that accompany "weight cycling" are increased cardiovascular morbidity and mortality, as well as increased abdominal fat, blood pressure, and insulin resistance (35).

Exercise

Exercise is generally accepted as a mechanism to increase HDL-C and reduce LDL-C levels in men. Although a number of studies have been carried out in women, they unfortunately fail to consider potential confounders such as hormonal status and body composition.

Exercise improves the lipid profile, but probably less strongly for women than for men. Again, hormonal status may influence the response. Postmenopausal women seem to exhibit a greater response to exercise, even if some train-ing studies are controversial. Exercise at least seems to attenuate the age-related modifications in the lipid profile (93).

The physiologic reasons for differences between men and women and their lipoprotein response to diet, weight loss, and exercise are not well defined. The role of circulating estrogen could be involved. LaRosa et al. (94) proposed that further investigations should include studies of different responses to these therapeutic modalities in postmenopausal women with and without exogenous hormone replacement.

In reviews on the effects of cardiac rehabilitation on morbidity and mortality, reductions in all-cause mortality of 20% to 24% and in CHD mortality of 23% to 25% among rehabilitation program participants were demonstrated (95, 96). Only 3 of the 22 studies that were reviewed included women, however, and in these 3 studies, women made up only 3% (143 of 4554 patients) of the entire sample. No separate analyses were performed related to the effect of participation in cardiac rehabilitation programs on clinical outcomes in women. Lavie and Milani (97) have reported that cardiac rehabilitation and exercise training produced improvements in exercise capacity and body fat comparable to men, but improvements in BMI and lipids were not statistically significant. Thus, inadequate data exist for determining whether women experience reductions in CVD similar to those in men who participate in formal cardiac rehabilitation.

Generally, intervention studies suggest that exercise training programs in the absence of other interventions attenuate the age-related increase in TC levels but do not cause HDL-C levels to rise appreciably in older women. In younger women, high levels of exercise (accompanied by decreased body fat) may increase HDL-C. Given the results in the cross-sectional studies, we note that two of the longitudinal investigations do not compare premenopausal and postmenopausal women but focus on postmenopausal women (98, 99).

In conclusion, exercise improves the lipid profile, but probably less strongly for women than for men. Again, hormonal status may influence the response. Postmenopausal women seem to exhibit a greater response to exercise, even if some training studies are controversial. Exercise at least seems to attenuate the age-related modifications in the lipid profile.

Cholesterol-altering Drugs

Few studies include women and very few analyze women in a separate group. However, recent studies suggest a significant decrease in coronary morbidity and mortality with the aggressive lowering of cholesterol levels in women (100–102).

PRIMARY PREVENTION

In a randomized study of 431 elderly patients (mean age, 71 years) with hypercholesterolemia, 71% of whom were women, two doses of lovastatin were compared with placebo. Total cholesterol fell 17% to 20%; LDL-C 24% to 28%; and TGs 4.4% to 9.9%. High-density lipoprotein cholesterol levels rose 7.0% to 9.0%. No changes were observed in the placebo group. Gender, race, and age did not significantly affect responses (103). However, in another study of 1815 patients, 43.1% of whom were women, a more favorable impact on lipid profile was observed in women taking fluvastatin compared with placebo than in men. Although a similar impact of therapy was observed for TGs, there was a stronger effect on LDL-C and HDL-C in women than in men: in women, the change from baseline was −26.7% for LDL-C and 5.3% for HDL-C (104).

The Air Force/Texas Coronary Atherosclerosis Prevention Study (AFCAPS/TexCAPS), a primary prevention trial using lovastatin again revealed that women with elevated LDL-C (130 to 190 mg/dL [3.36 to 4.91 mmol/L]) had a significantly higher reduction in first coronary events than their male counterparts (102). These new data further extend the utility of cholesterol-lowering to an even broader section of the population.

Thus, although the impact of drug therapy appears comparable or even more effective in altering lipid levels in women compared with men, the evidence is not completely certain, and further investigation will be required before it can be concluded that primary treatment reduces CHD morbidity or mortality similarly in men and women.

SECONDARY PREVENTION

A recent, large, randomized study of 4,444 patients (70), 18% of whom were women, was designed to evaluate the effect of cholesterol-lowering with simvastatin on mortality and morbidity in patients with CHD. During the 5.4-year median follow-up, simvastatin produced mean changes in TC, LDL-C, and HDL-C of −25%, −35%, and +8%, respectively. The probability that a woman avoided a major coronary event was 77.5% in the placebo group and 85.1% in the treatment group. Total mortality and risk for a major coronary event were similar for both genders. Other benefits of treatment included a 37% reduction ($P <$ .00001) in the risk of undergoing myocardial revascularization procedures.

Of particular importance is the Cholesterol and Recurrent Events (CARE) study (100). The CARE study was specifically designed to address the question of whether lowering LDL-C with pravastatin in patients with CHD and normal or only mildly elevated LDL-C concentrations provided clinical benefit. Mean baseline LDL-C in the CARE study was 139 mg/dL (3.59 mmol/L). A 24% reduction in the study's primary end point of CHD death or nonfatal MI was observed with treatment with pravastatin ($P <$ .002). Because a large portion of the population with CHD does not have severely elevated cholesterol, risk reduction in this group could have major public health implications.

Significantly, a greater reduction in CHD death and nonfatal MI was observed in the subset of women in this study compared to men. Formal subset analysis on women is pending. These data corroborate the findings from other trials that the benefits of lipid-lowering therapy appear relatively soon after the initiation of therapy. Women may have a greater benefit from cholesterol-reduction interventions.

Postmenopausal women with a history of CHD may need more aggressive treatment for elevated cholesterol, according to a recent study. The Heart and Estrogen/Progestin Replacement Study (HERS), involving 2763 women with a known history of CHD, found that although 47% of the HERS participants were currently receiving some form of cholesterol-lowering medication, 63% had LDL-C levels that exceeded the NCEP guidelines. Therefore, many of the women who were eligible to receive cholesterol-lowering drug therapy based on their elevated cholesterol levels either were not receiving drug treatment or were not treated aggressively enough. Fully 91% of the study's participants had LDL-C levels that exceeded the 1993 Adult Treatment Panel (ATP) goal of less than 100 mg/dL (2.59 mmol/L) (65).

Most of the women were white (88.7% white, 7.9% African American, 2% Hispanic) and, generally, most were inactive and overweight. Many were ex-smokers (49%) and more than 13% still smoked. More than half (59.5%) had high blood pressure and 23% had diabetes. The researchers found that women with one or more of the following characteristics were less likely to be on a cholesterol-lowering agent: African American, Hispanic, or other nonwhite ethnic identity; higher BMI; sedentary lifestyle; a consumer of alcohol or tobacco; or having a diagnosis of CHD that preceded 1985. Women with lower LDL-C levels tended to have postgraduate education, participate in an exercise program, and have never married (65).

Cholesterol should be treated in women as in men, and women may benefit more. The fact that premenopausal women are at lower risk of heart disease than men of the same age has been misinterpreted by many to mean that risk factors are not as important to treat in women as in men.

Antioxidant Therapy

Antioxidants may suppress the formation of oxidized LDL and thereby influence the formation of atherosclerotic plaque. Both epidemiologic and laboratory studies suggest that antioxidants can provide a protective effect on coronary arteries.

The Nurses' Health Study assessed the relative risk of a major CHD event in 87,245 female nurses studied for up to 8 years (105). Relative risk of major coronary disease of those in the lowest quintile of vitamin E intake was compared with risk in the highest quintile (relative risk, 0.66 after adjustment for age and smoking). Adjustment for a variety of other coronary risk factors and nutrients, including other antioxidants, had little effect on the results. As the authors point out: "Although these prospective data do not prove a cause-and-effect relation, they suggest that among middle-aged women the use of vitamin E supplements is associated with a reduced risk of coronary heart disease." No large randomized clinical trials of antioxidants have yet been reported, albeit two such trials, the Women's Health Initiative and an ancillary Trial of Antioxidant Therapy, are in progress.

Smoking Cessation

Significant gender differences exist in smoking cessation behavior. Some are ascribed to chemistry, others to a lack of confidence in the ability to quit, and still others are concerns regarding weight gain after cessation. In addition, nicotine may have different effects on women and men.

Cigarette smoking carries an especially increased hazard for young women because it is often accompanied by oral contraceptive use, a combination that promotes thrombogenesis (106). In general, women are less likely to contemplate smoking cessation than men and are likely to smoke to reduce tension and control weight. Although women quit smoking at the same rate as men, they are less able to maintain cessation over the long term. Recent data from the Lung Health Study (107) indicate that long-term relapse rates may be higher in women than in men. The study, sponsored by the National Heart, Lung, and Blood Institute (NHLBI), evaluated the efficacy of early smoking cessation intervention for patients with chronic obstructive pulmonary disease. Men had significantly higher cessation rates than women, but other factors were seen to be important predictors of successful quitting. Participants who were better educated, married, and older were more likely to stay away from tobacco. Those who had larger body mass were among the successful quitters as were those who had made cessation attempts in the past without the help of nicotine gum. Women tended to fit the categories of participants less likely to remain abstinent. This study offers evidence for gender differences in the subjective effects of nicotine withdrawal. Women reported a greater dependence on cigarettes and used more nicotine gum during the study. Biochemically, nicotine clearance is more rapid in men than in women, even after correction for body weight.

Finally, women's anxiety about weight gain after cessation is a major impediment to their even attempting to quit smoking. Smoking cessation has also been suggested as a possible contributing factor to the increase in prevalence of being overweight in the United States (108). Weight gain after cessation, an average of 10 pounds or more during a 10-year period, appears to be caused by both increased eating and the metabolic changes produced by nicotine withdrawal. Nicotine gum has been shown to partially reduce or delay weight gain.

The clinical implications are that smoking cessation programs for women may have to emphasize strategies to help them develop confidence to stop smoking, to make a commitment to quitting, and to develop strategies for maintaining cessation for extended periods of time (109). Smoking cessation programs for women should emphasize techniques for reducing tension and for weight control (110).

The Surgeon General's report (111, 112) states that former smokers live longer than continuing smokers and that a person 50 years or younger who quits smoking has a 50% reduction in mortality during the next 15 years as compared with a smoker. In the Nurses' Health Study (113) the CHD risk is decreased by 30% within only 2 years after cessation. These benefits extend to the population with diagnosed coronary artery disease. During 5 years, the CHD population in the Coronary Artery Surgery Study (CASS) (114) that quit smoking benefited from a 32% lower rate of mortality. Overall, the bulk of studies indicates a 30% to 50% reduction in CHD mortality in the first 2 years and a more gradual decline in the next 10 to 20 years before the smoker mirrors the CHD mortality risk of a never-smoker (115).

The 12-year follow-up data from the Nurses' Health Study examined the relationship of time since smoking with reduction in CHD incidence and mortality in middle-aged women (114). On stopping smoking, one-third of the excess risk of CHD was eliminated within 2 years of cessation. Thereafter the excess risk returned to the level of those who had never smoked during the interval 10 to 14 years after cessation.

Aspirin Therapy

Aspirin in doses of 325 mg or less per day appears to be beneficial in preventing the incidence of MI in men and women without clinically apparent CHD. This benefit is magnified in those patients older than 50 years and in those with risk factors for CHD. Its use does not appear to reduce overall mortality and may be associated with an increased risk of hemorrhagic stroke, particularly in larger doses (116).

Data also support the use of aspirin in survivors of MI to reduce the incidence of reinfarction and death. Aspirin may provide the best opportunity for secondary prevention after acute MI because of its effectiveness, low cost, safety profile, and lack of strong contraindications. More than 18,000 patients have been enrolled in randomized trials to assess the role of antiplatelet therapy for sec-

ondary prevention of MI. The guidelines for treatment of acute MI published by the American Heart Association and American College of Cardiology in 1990 strongly recommend the use of aspirin for all survivors of acute MI to prevent the late recurrence of MI and death (117).

Estrogen Therapy

Hormonal status must be carefully considered because of the important effects of estrogen not only on lipids, but also on endothelial function and other risk factors. After menopause, women often have an increase in weight, higher levels of LDL-C, and lower levels of HDL-C. Oral estrogen replacement is useful in improving the lipid profiles in women with decreases in LDL-C and increases in HDL-C. One study showed that oral therapy with 2 mg estradiol or 6.25 mg conjugated estrogens lowered LDL-C and raised HDL-C by 14% to 16% (118). The decrease in LDL particles results from accelerated catabolism, which increased 36%.

Although prospective cohort data are suggestive, there are no clinical trials that show that estrogen use in primary prevention is beneficial. The benefits for postmenopausal women with increased risk for CHD are considerable. The Postmenopausal Estrogen/Progestin Intervention (PEPI) study (53) was designed to show the benefits of combined estrogen/progestin therapy in a 3-year study involving 875 postmenopausal women who ranged from 45 to 64 years of age. Baseline TG values were less than 500 mg/dL (5.64 mmol/L). There were five treatment arms that compared estrogen alone versus estrogen and different regimens of associated progestin use. The various treatment regimens lowered LDL-C to levels about 15 mg/dL (0.39 mmol/L) less than those in the placebo group; they all raised TGs.

More definite recommendations await the results of two ongoing studies that are examining the effects of estrogen on cardiovascular endpoints. These include a secondary prevention trial known as the Heart and Estrogen Replacement Study (HERS) (65), along with a 15-year disease prevention study involving more than 160,000 women, known as the Women's Health Initiative (WHI).

In women starting postmenopausal hormone therapy, it seems reasonable to check cholesterol, TGs, LDL-C, and HDL-C. If TGs are more than 300 mg/dL (3.39 mmol/L), attention should be given toward nonpharmacologic interventions, such as regular exercise and a weight-reducing diet low in simple sugars. Also, a search for secondary causes and family screening for familial lipid disease would be reasonable. Although only a small group of women who take postmenopausal estrogen develop severe hypertriglyceridemia or pancreatitis, the number could be reduced if more women were screened for lipid abnormalities.

Conclusion

Cardiovascular disease is the leading cause of morbidity and mortality in women, with the vast majority of cardiovascular events occurring in the postmenopausal years. Most of our knowledge of CVD comes from studies in middle-aged men. Recent emphasis on women's health in general and in cardiovascular health in particular has led to increasing evidence that significant gender differences do exist in CHD incidence, risk factors, and modification of cardiovascular risk in women.

Health care providers must coordinate their efforts to effectively treat and prevent CVD in women in such a way as to take into account the unique biology, physiology, and epidemiology of CVD in women. There is increasing evidence of the roles of traditional and nontraditional risk factors in the development of CVD in women and in developing new strategies to incorporate this evidence into programs of prevention.

References

1. American Heart Association. Heart and stroke statistical update. Dallas, TX: American Heart Association, 1997.
2. Matthews KA, Meilahn E, Kuller LH, et al. Menopause and risk factors for coronary heart disease. N Engl J Med 1989;321:641–646.
3. Kannel WB, Castelli WD, Gordon T, et al. Serum cholesterol, lipoproteins and risk of coronary artery disease: The Framingham Study. Ann Intern Med 1971; 74:1–12.
4. Family Study Committee for the Lipid Research Clinics Program. The Collaborative Lipid Research Clinics Program Family Study. I. Study design and description of data. Am J Epidemiol 1984;119:931–943.
5. Rosenberg L, Palmer JR, Shapiro S. Decline in the risk of myocardial infarction among women who stop smoking. N Engl J Med 1990;322:213–217.
6. Gordon T, Kannel WB, Hjortland MC, et al. Menopause and coronary heart disease. The Framingham Study. Ann Intern Med 1978;89:157–161.
7. Rosenberg L, Hennekens CH, Rosner B, et al. Early menopause and the risk of myocardial infarction. Am J Obstet Gynecol 1981;139:47–51.
8. Stevenson JC, Crook D, Godsland IF. Influence of age

and menopause on serum lipids and lipoproteins in healthy women. Atherosclerosis 1993;98:83–90.
9. Sprecher D, McMahon R, Similo S, et al. Trends in LDL-cholesterol and apolipoprotein B in black and white girls observed at ages 9–14: effects of adiposity and sexual maturation. Unpublished, 1995.
10. Castelli WP, Anderson K. A population at risk. Prevalence of high cholesterol levels in hypertensive patients in the Framingham Study. Am J Med 1986;80(Suppl 2A):23–32.
11. Castelli WP, Doyle JT, Gordon T. HDL cholesterol and other lipids in coronary heart disease. The cooperative lipoprotein phenotyping study. Circulation 1977;55: 767–772.
12. Goldbourt U, Holtzman E, Neufeld HN. Total and high density lipoprotein cholesterol in the serum and risk of mortality: evidence of a threshold effect. Br Med J 1985;290:1239–1243.
13. Gordon T, Castelli W, Hjortland M, et al. Diabetes, blood lipids, and the role of obesity in coronary heart disease risk for women. Ann Intern Med 1977;87:393–397.
14. Matthews KA, Meilahn E, Kuller LH, et al. Menopause and risk factors for coronary heart disease. N Engl J Med 1989;321:641–646.
15. Hong MK, Romm PA, Reagan K, et al. Effects of estrogen replacement therapy on serum lipid values and angiographically defined coronary artery disease in postmenopausal women. Am J Cardiol 1992;69:176–178.
16. Kannel WB. Metabolic risk factors for coronary heart disease in women: perspective from the Framingham Study. Am Heart J 1987;114:413–419.
17. Kannel WB. High-density lipoproteins: epidemiologic profile and risks of coronary artery disease. Am J Cardiol 1983;52:9B–12B.
18. Brunzell JD, Albers JJ, Chait A, et al. Plasma lipoproteins in familial combined hyperlipidemia and monogenic familial hypercholesterolemia. Metabolism 1983;24:147–155.
19. Castelli WP. Epidemiology of triglycerides: a view from Framingham. Am J Cardiol 1992;70:3H–9H.
20. Schaefer EJ, Lamon-Fava S, Cohn SD, et al. Effects of age, gender, and menopausal status on plasma low-density lipoprotein cholesterol and apolipoprotein B levels in the Framingham Offspring Study. J Lipid Res 1994;35:779–792.
21. Lapidus L, Bengtsson C, Hallstron T, et al. Obesity, adipose tissue distribution and health in women—results from a population study in Gothenburg, Sweden. Appetite 1989;13:25–35.
22. Manninen V, Elo MO, Frick MH, et al. Lipid alterations and decline in the incidence of coronary heart disease in the Helsinki Heart Study. JAMA 1988;260:641–651.
23. Manninen V, Tenkanen L, Koskinen P, et al. Joint effects of serum triglycerides and LDL cholesterol and HDL cholesterol concentrations on coronary heart disease risk in the Helskinki Heart Study—implications for treatment. Circulation 1992;85:37–45.
24. Austin MA, Breslow JL, Hennekens CH, et al. Low-density lipoprotein subclass patterns and risk of myocardial infarction. JAMA 1988;260:1917–1921.
25. Friedewald WT, Levy RI, Fredrickson DS. Estimation of the concentration of low-density lipoprotein cho-

lesterol in plasma, without use of the preparative ul-
tracentrifuge. Clin Chem 1972;18:499–502.

26. Kannel WB. Lipids, diabetes, and coronary heart disease: insights from the Framingham Study. Am Heart
J 1985;110:1100–1107.

27. Garcia M, McNamara P, Gordon T, et al. Morbidity and
mortality in diabetics in the Framingham population:
sixteen year follow-up study. Diabetes 1974;23:
105–111.

28. Reaven GM. The role of insulin resistance and hyperinsulinemia in coronary heart disease. Metabolism
1992;41(Suppl 1):16–19.

29. Kannel WB. Status of risk factors and their consideration in antihypertensive therapy. Am J Cardiol 1987;
59:80A–90A.

30. Sempos CT, Cleeman JI, Carroll MD, et al. Prevalence
of high blood cholesterol among US adults. An update
based on guidelines from the second report of the National Cholesterol Education Program Adult Treatment Panel. JAMA 1993;269:3009–3014.

31. Manson JE, Colditz GA, Stampfer MJ, et al. A prospective study of obesity and risk of coronary heart disease
in women. N Engl J Med 1990;322:882–889.

32. Daly P, Solomon C, Manson J. Risk modification in the
obese patient. In: Manson JE, Ridker PM, Gaziano JM,
et al., eds. Prevention of myocardial infarction. New
York: Oxford University Press, 1996:203–230.

33. Logue E, Smucker W, Bourguet C. Identification of obesity: waistlines or weight? J Fam Pract 1995;41:357–363.

34. Folsom AR, Kaye SA, Sellers TA, et al. Body fat distribution and 5-year risk of death in older women. JAMA
1993;269:483–487.

35. National Task Force on the Prevention and Treatment
of Obesity. Long-term pharmacotherapy in the management of obesity. JAMA 1996;276:1907–1915.

36. Després J-P, Moorjani S, Lupien PJ, et al. Genetic aspects of susceptibility to obesity and related dyslipidemias. Mol Cell Biochem 1992;113:151–169.

37. Morrison J, Sprecher D, McMahon R, et al. Obesity and
high-density lipoprotein cholesterol in black and
white 9- and 10-year-old girls: The National Heart,
Lung and Blood Institute Growth and Health Study.
Metab Clin Exp 1996;45:469–474.

38. Office of Smoking and Health. Reducing the health
consequences of smoking. Atlanta: US Center for Disease Control, 1989.

39. Willett WC, Green A, Stampfer MJ, et al. Relative and
absolute excess risks of coronary heart disease among
women who smoke cigarettes. N Engl J Med 1987;317:
1303–1309.

40. Glantz S, Parmley W. Passive smoking and heart disease. JAMA 1995;273:1047–1053.

41. Werner RM, Pearson TA. Secondhand smoke as a cause
of atherosclerotic disease. JAMA 1998;279:157–158.

42. Willett W, Stampfer MJ, Bain C, et al. Cigarette smoking, relative weight, and menopause. Am J Epidemiol
1983;117:651–658.

43. Moffatt RJ, Owens SG. Cessation from cigarette smoking: changes in body weight, body composition, resting metabolism, and energy consumption. Metabolism 1991;40:465–470.

44. Williamson DF, Madans J, Anda RF, et al. Smoking

cessation and severity of weight gain in a national cohort. N Engl J Med 1991;324:739–745.

45. Hall SM, Ginsberg D, Jones RT. Smoking cessation and
weight gain. J Consult Clin Psychol 1986;54:342–346.

46. Warner KE, Goldenhar LM, McLaughlin CG. Cigarette
advertising and magazine coverage of the hazards of
smoking. A statistical analysis. N Engl J Med 1992;326:
305–309.

47. Palmer JR, Rosenberg L, Shapiro S. "Low yield" cigarettes and the risk of nonfatal myocardial infarction in
women. N Engl J Med 1989;320:1569–1573.

48. Eaton CB, Lapane KL, Garber CA, et al. Sedentary
lifestyle and risk of coronary heart disease in women.
Med Sci Sports Exerc 1995;27:1535–1539.

49. Reaven PD, McPhillips JB, Barrett-Connor EL, et al.
Leisure time exercise and lipid and lipoprotein levels
in an older population. J Am Geriatr Soc 1990;38:
847–854.

50. Reaven PD, Barrett-Connor E, Edelstein S. Relation
between leisure-time physical activity and blood pressure in older women. Circulation 1991;83:559–565.

51. Leon A, Connett J, Jacobs D, et al. Leisure-time physical activity levels and risk of coronary heart disease
and death. JAMA 1987;258:2388–2395.

52. Rodriguez B, Curb D, Burchfiel C, et al. Physical activity and 23-year incidence of coronary heart disease morbidity and mortality among middle-aged men. The Honolulu heart program. Circulation 1994;89:2540–2544.

53. Greendale GA, Bodin-Dunn L, Ingles S, et al. Leisure,
home, and occupational physical activity and cardiovascular risk factors in postmenopausal women. The
Postmenopausal Estrogens/Progestins Intervention
(PEPI) Study. Arch Intern Med 1996;156:418–424.

54. Lemaitre RN, Heckbert SR, Psaty BM, et al. Leisure-
time physical activity and the risk of nonfatal myocardial infarction in postmenopausal women. Arch Intern
Med 1995;155:2302–2308.

55. Pate RR, Pratt M, Blair SN, et al. Physical activity and
public health. A recommendation from the Centers for
Disease Control and Prevention and the American College of Sports Medicine. JAMA 1995;273:402–407.

56. Hunter SMD, Frerichs RR, Webber LS, et al. Social status and cardiovascular disease risk factor variables in
children: The Bogalusa Heart Study. J Chronic Dis
1979;32:441–449.

57. Lapidus L, Bengtsson C. Socioeconomic factors and
physical activity in relation to cardiovascular disease
and death. A 12 year follow up of participants in a population study of women in Gothenburg, Sweden. Br
Heart J 1986;55:295–301.

58. Matthews KA, Kelsey SF, Meilahn EN, et al. Educational attainment and behavioral and biologic risk factors for coronary heart disease in middle-aged women.
Am J Epidemiol 1989;129:1132–1144.

59. Haynes SG, Feinleib M, Kannel WB. The relationship
of psychosocial factors to coronary heart disease in the
Framingham Study. III. Eight-year incidence of coronary heart disease. Am J Epidemiol 1980;111:37–58.

60. Bush TL, Barrett CE, Cowan LD, et al. Cardiovascular
mortality and non-contraceptive use of estrogen in
women: results from the Lipid Research Clinics Program Follow-up Study. Circulation 1987;75:1102–1109.

61. Bush TL, Criqui MH, Cowan LD, et al. Cardiovascular disease mortality in women: results from the Lipid Research Clinics Follow-up Study. In: Eaker E, Packard B, Wenger N, et al., eds. Coronary heart disease in women. New York: Haymarket-Doyma, Inc., 1987:106–111.

62. Barrett-Connor E. The menopause, hormone replacement, and cardiovascular disease: the epidemiologic evidence. Maturitas 1996;23:227–234.

63. Stampfer MJ, Willett WC, Colditz GA, et al. A prospective study of postmenopausal estrogen therapy and coronary heart disease. N Engl J Med 1985;313:1044–1049.

64. The Writing Group for the PEPI Trial. Effects of estrogen or estrogen/progestin regimens on heart disease risk factors in postmenopausal women. The Postmenopausal Estrogen/Progestin Interventions (PEPI) Trial. JAMA 1995;273:199–208.

65. Schrott HG, Bittner V, Vittinghoff E, et al. Adherence to National Cholesterol Education Program Treatment goals in postmenopausal women with heart disease. The Heart and Estrogen/Progestin Replacement Study (HERS). The HERS Research Group. JAMA 1997;277:1281–1286.

66. Henderson BE, Ross RK, Paganini-Hill A, et al. Estrogen use and cardiovascular disease. Am J Obstet Gynecol 1986;154:1181–1186.

67. Grodstein F, Stampfer MJ, Manson JE, et al. Postmenopausal estrogen and progestin use and the risk of cardiovascular disease. N Engl J Med 1996;335:453–461.

68. Expert Panel on Detection, Evaluation, and Treatment of High Blood Cholesterol in Adults. Summary of the second report of the National Cholesterol Education Program (NCEP) Expert Panel on Detection, Evaluation, and Treatment of High Blood Cholesterol in Adults (Adult Treatment Panel II). JAMA 1993;269:3015–3023.

69. National Cholesterol Education Program. Report of the Expert Panel on Blood Cholesterol Levels in Children and Adolescents. Bethesda, MD: US Dept of Health and Human Services, Public Health Service, National Institutes of Health, National Heart, Lung and Blood Institute, 1991.

70. The Scandinavian Simvastatin Survival Group. Randomised trial of cholesterol lowering in 4,444 patients with coronary heart disease: the Scandinavian Simvastatin Survival Study (4S). Lancet 1994;344:1383–1389.

71. Grady D, Rubin SM, Petitti DB, et al. Hormone therapy to prevent disease and prolong life in postmenopausal women. Ann Intern Med 1992;117:1016–1037.

72. Katan MB. Diet and high density lipoproteins. In: Miller N, Miller G, eds. Clinical and metabolic aspects of high density lipoproteins. Amsterdam: Elsevier, 1984:103–131.

73. Clifton PM, Noakes M, Nestel PJ. Gender and diet interactions with simvastatin treatment. Atherosclerosis 1994;110:25–33.

74. Kohlmeier M, Stricker G, Schlierf G. Influences of "normal" and "prudent" diets on biliary and serum lipids in healthy women. Am J Clin Nutr 1985;42:1201–1205.

75. Zanni EE, Zannis VI, Blum CB, et al. Effect of egg cholesterol and dietary fats on plasma lipids, lipoproteins, and apoproteins of normal women consuming natural diets. J Lipid Res 1987;28:518–527.

76. Grundy SM, Nix D, Whelan MF, et al. Comparison of three cholesterol-lowering diets in normolipidemic men. JAMA 1986;256:2351–2355.

77. Lewis B, Hammett F, Katan M, et al. Towards an improved lipid-lowering diet: additive effects of changes in nutrient intake. Lancet 1981;2:1310–1313.

78. Cobb MM, Teitlebaum H, Risch N, et al. Influence of dietary fat, apolipoprotein E phenotype, and sex on plasma lipoprotein levels. Circulation 1992;86:849–857.

79. Mata P, Alvarez SL, Rubio MJ, et al. Effects of long-term monounsaturated- vs polyunsaturated-enriched diets on lipoproteins in healthy men and women [see comments]. Am J Clin Nutr 1992;55:846–850.

80. Barnard RJ. Effects of life-style modification on serum lipids. Arch Intern Med 1991;151:1389–1394.

81. Brownell KD, Stunkard AJ. Differential changes in plasma high-density lipoprotein-cholesterol levels in obese men and women during weight reduction. Arch Intern Med 1981;141:1142–1146.

82. La Rosa JC, Hunninghake D, Bush D, et al. The cholesterol facts. A summary of the evidence relating dietary fats, serum cholesterol, and coronary heart disease. A joint statement by the American Heart Association and the National Heart, Lung, and Blood Institute. The Task Force on Cholesterol Issues, American Heart Association. Circulation 1990;81:1721–1733.

83. Bouchard C. Genetics of obesity in humans: current issues. CIBA Foundation Symposium 1996;201:115–117, 188–193.

84. Caro JF, Sinha MK, Kolaczynski JW, et al. Leptin: the tale of an obesity gene. Diabetes 1996;45:1455–1462.

85. Schwartz M, Brunzell J. Regulation of body adiposity and the problem of obesity. Arterioscler Thromb Vasc Biol 1997;17:233–238.

86. Safer D. Diet, behavior modification, and exercise: a review of obesity treatments from a long-term perspective. South Med J 1991;84:1470–1474.

87. Wood PD. Physical activity, diet, and health: independent and interactive effects. Med Sci Sports Exerc 1994;26:838–843.

88. Fletcher G. The value of exercise in preventing coronary atherosclerotic heart disease. Heart Dis Stroke 1993;2:183–187.

89. Blair S. Dose of exercise and health benefits. Arch Intern Med 1997;157:153–154.

90. Garrow J. Treatment of obesity. Lancet 1992;340:409–413.

91. Roncari D. Obesity and coronary heart disease. Can Med Assoc J 1992;146:1106–1112.

92. Hubert HB, Feinleib M, McNamara PM, et al. Obesity as an independent risk factor for cardiovascular disease: a 26-year follow-up of participants in the Framingham Heart Study. Circulation 1983;67:968–977.

93. Krummel D, Etherton TD, Peterson S, et al. Effects of exercise on plasma lipids and lipoproteins of women. Proc Soc Exp Biol Med 1993;204:123–137.

94. La Rosa JC. Management of postmenopausal women who have hyperlipidemia. Am J Med 1994;96:19S–24S.

95. Oldridge NB, Guyatt GH, Fischer ME, et al. Cardiac rehabilitation after myocardial infarction. Combined ex-

perience of randomized clinical trials. JAMA 1988;260: 945–950.

96. O'Connor GT, Buring JE, Yusuf S, et al. An overview of randomized trials of rehabilitation with exercise after myocardial infarction. Circulation 1989;80:234–244.

97. Lavie CJ, Milani RV. Effects of cardiac rehabilitation and exercise training on exercise capacity, coronary risk factors, behavioral characteristics, and quality of life in women. Am J Cardiol 1995;75:340–343.

98. Cauley JA, Kriska AM, LaPorte RE, et al. A two year randomized exercise trial in older women: effects on HDL-cholesterol. Atherosclerosis 1987;66:247–258.

99. Boyden T, Parmenter R, Rotkis T. Effect of exercise training on plasma cholesterol, HDL-C, ApoA1, sex steroids levels of early post-menopausal women. In: Eaker E, Packard B, Wenger N, et al., eds. Coronary heart disease in women. New York: Haymarket-Doyma, Inc., 1987:160–163.

100. Pfeffer M, Sacks F, Lemuel A, et al. Cholesterol and recurrent events: a secondary prevention trial for normolipidemic patients. Am J Cardiol 1995;76: 98C–106C.

101. Tonkin AM. Management of the Long-term Intervention with Pravastatin in Ischaemic Disease (LIPID) study after the Scandinavian Simvastatin Survival Study (4S). Am J Cardiol 1995;76:107C–112C.

102. Downs JR, Beere PA, Whitney E, et al. Design and rationale of the Air Force/Texas Coronary Atherosclerosis Prevention Study (AFCAPS/TexCAPS). Am J Cardiol 1997;80:287–293.

103. La Rosa JC, Applegate W, Crouse JR, et al. Cholesterol lowering in the elderly. Results of the Cholesterol Reduction in Seniors Program (CRISP) pilot study. Arch Intern Med 1994;154:529–539.

104. Peters TK, Muratti EN, Mehra M. Efficacy and safety of fluvastatin in women with primary hypercholesterolaemia. Drugs 1994;2:64–72.

105. Stampfer MJ, Hennekens CH, Manson JE, et al. Vitamin E consumption and the risk of coronary disease in women. N Engl J Med 1993;328:1444–1449.

106. Goldbaum GM, Kendrick JS, Hogelin GC, et al. The relative impact of smoking and oral contraceptive use on women in the United States. JAMA 1987;258: 1339–1342.

107. Bjornson W, Rand C, Connett J, et al. Gender differ-

ences in smoking cessation after 3 years in the Lung Health Study. Am J Public Health 1995;85:223–230.

108. Flegal KM, Troiano RP, Pamuk ER, et al. The influence of smoking cessation on the prevalence of overweight in the United States. N Engl J Med 1995;333:1165–1170.

109. Smoking cessation: information for specialists. Rockville, MD: US Department of Health and Human Services, Agency for Health Care Policy and Research, 1996.

110. Pirie PL, Murray DM, Luepker RV. Gender differences in cigarette smoking and quitting in a cohort of young adults. Am J Public Health 1991;81:324–327.

111. US Department of Health and Human Services. The health benefits of smoking cessation. Rockville, MD: US Department of Health and Human Services, Public Health Service, Centers for Disease Control, Center for Chronic Disease Prevention and Health Promotion, Office on Smoking and Health, 1990.

112. The Smoking Cessation Clinical Practice Guidelines Panel and Staff. The Agency for Health Care Policy and Research Smoking Cessation Clinical Practice Guideline. JAMA 1996;275:1270–1280.

113. Kawachi I, Colditz GA, Stampfer MJ, et al. Smoking cessation and time course of decreased risks of coronary heart disease in middle-aged women. Arch Intern Med 1994;154:169–175.

114. Cavender J, Rogers W, Fisher L, et al. Effects of smoking on survival and morbidity in patients randomized to medical or surgical therapy in the Coronary Artery Surgery Study (CASS): 10-year follow-up. J Am Coll Cardiol 1992;20:287–294.

115. Kawachi I, Colditz GA, Stampfer MJ, et al. Smoking cessation in relation to total mortality rates in women. A prospective cohort study. Ann Intern Med 1993;119: 992–1000.

116. Manson JE, Stampfer MJ, Colditz GA, et al. A prospective study of aspirin use and primary prevention of cardiovascular disease in women. JAMA 1991;266:521–527.

117. Fuster V, Dyken ML, Vokonas PS, et al. Aspirin as a therapeutic agent in cardiovascular disease. Special Writing Group. Circulation 1993;87:659–675.

118. Walsh BW, Schiff I, Rosner B, et al. Effects of postmenopausal estrogen replacement on the concentrations and metabolism of plasma lipoproteins. N Engl J Med 1991;325:1196–1204.

SECTION VI.

Program Implementation and Function

Designing and Implementing a Prevention Cardiology Program

Dennis L. Sprecher, JoAnne Micale Foody, and Robert F. Hunter

INTRODUCTION

Recent changes in the delivery of health care in the United States and new scientific evidence strongly supporting the role of preventive interventions in the maintenance of health have focused much-needed attention and efforts on cardiovascular prevention programs. The field of cardiology is making a gradual transition from a technology-driven, intervention-oriented perspective to a preventive perspective. As new evidence is becoming available that preventive measures effect a considerable decrease in the incidence of both primary and secondary cardiac events and mortality, there is widespread acknowledgment that health care providers must initiate preventive strategies in the management of their patients. Additionally, as physicians and health care providers are faced with an increasingly limited health care dollar, they must focus attention on strategies to reduce health care costs through the reduction of hospitalizations, procedures, and clinical events. There are new financial incentives and fiscal imperatives to keep people disease-free. These factors provide new motivation for an organization to implement preventive interventions that manage the patient with or without coronary heart disease (CHD) in a cost-effective manner.

In 1995, our organization began a preventive cardiology program whose goals are to provide a multidisciplinary approach to the management of risk factors in the patient with CHD. As envisioned, our program is interdepartmental, nurse- and physician's assistant-based, algorithm-driven, cost-centered, and outcome-evaluated. In this chapter we will discuss the mission and strategy of our program as well as review the major studies and scientific evidence on which our strategies are based. Recent developments in the delivery of health care have had a dramatic effect on the conceptualization and implementation of this program. We will address these developments as well as programmatic issues in the actual implementation of the program. Finally, we will discuss potential future directions for the field of preventive cardiology and the possible impact of coordinated clinical programs such as our own.

BACKGROUND

In the United States alone, CHD claims the lives of 500,000 men and women each year. The prevalence of CHD and congestive heart failure (CHF) has increased during the past decade. During the same period, technical advances in the field of cardiology have vastly improved. These technical advances, although providing improvements in care, have come at a significant cost. Annual cardiovascular health care expenditures in the United States currently exceed $100 billion, largely resulting from hospitalizations and revascularization procedures (1). Increasing costs in medical care have led to cost shifting and a reevaluation of clinical outcomes, cost-effectiveness, and health care delivery systems. Highlighting this paradigm shift in health care delivery is the contrast between current health care dollars spent for cardiovascular intervention procedures and preventive or lifestyle interventions. For every dollar spent on cardiovascular disease in this country, only 6 cents is spent on out-of-hospital medical therapy and on reinforcing healthy lifestyles (1).

History

Preventive cardiology has only come into its own in the last several years in response to new evidence that medical interventions do in fact alter the course of cardiovascular disease and new imperatives in health care resource allocation. The preventive cardiology field has been fragmented. It has traditionally been driven by cardiac rehabilitation and has been exercise-based and diet-based. Rehabilitation programs, specifically targeting those CHD patients after coronary artery bypass grafting (CABG) surgery, percutaneous transluminal coronary angioplasty (PTCA), or myocardial infarction (MI), were initially focused on exercise but have expanded during the past decade to include diet, cholesterol reduction, and, to a lesser extent, the management of obesity. Cardiac rehabilitation interventions have been outlined by the American Association of Cardiovascular and Pulmonary Rehabilitation (AACPR) and the American College of Sports Medicine (ACSM). These organizations evolved from separate traditions from the American Heart Association (AHA) and the American College of Cardiology (ACC). Lipids and lipoproteins have customarily been in the realm of internal medicine, endocrinology, and, to a lesser extent, cardiology, whereas hypertension has traditionally been in the realm of nephrology and internal medicine with again cardiology to a much lesser extent. Thrombosis and extracoronary atherosclerotic processes have been governed by vascular medicine. As mounting evidence suggests that cardiovascular illness is the result of multiple disease processes acting unfavorably on the progression of atherosclerosis, cardiologists must become better versed in all aspects of this process. A collaborative effort to reduce cardiovascular risk would be more clinically cost-effective.

Clinical Studies

Until recently, the literature did not support protecting patients through cholesterol reduction (2). Early primary prevention trials tested the hypothesis that a decrease in total cholesterol leads to a decrease in cardiovascular events. Three early studies—the Oslo (3), the World Health Organization Primary Prevention Trial (4), and the Upjohn trial (5)—all demonstrated a decrease in total cholesterol and CHD events (Fig. 21.1).

In the early 1980s, two additional large-scale primary prevention trials were conducted: the Lipid Research Clinics—Coronary Primary Prevention Trial (LRC-CPPT) (6) and the Helsinki

Heart Study (HHS) (7). The LRC-CPPT was a randomized, double-blind placebo-controlled trial of diet plus cholestyramine versus diet and placebo. This landmark study conclusively showed that reducing cholesterol by diet and a pharmacologic regimen reduced the risk of CHD in men with hypercholesterolemia. Specifically, a 10% to 15% reduction in serum cholesterol may result in a 20% to 30% reduction in risk for CHD. The HHS was a double-blind, placebo-controlled, primary prevention trial that randomized men without CHD to receive either placebo or gemfibrozil. Overall, a 34% reduction in the incidence of CHD was observed. Importantly, the HHS identified a subgroup of patients with high risk for cardiac events. This group was characterized by a low-density lipoprotein cholesterol (LDL-C) to high-density lipoprotein cholesterol (HDL-C) ratio of more than 5 and triglycerides (TGs) more than 200 mg/dL, and patients in this group experienced a 71% reduction in CHD event rate with treatment. These studies demonstrated significant reductions in lipids and an associated decrease in CHD events. They provide clear evidence of the clinical benefits associated with the primary prevention of CHD.

During the last two decades, several large, randomized controlled trials have assessed the effect of cholesterol reduction in the prevention of both primary coronary events and subsequent CHD events among CHD patients. With the development of hydroxymethylglutaryl-CoA (HMG-CoA) reductase inhibitors, greater LDL-C reductions were attainable than with other agents. Three large-scale trials were conducted to evaluate the effect of LDL-C lowering on clinical events. The West of Scotland Coronary Prevention Study (WOSCOPS) (8) was a primary prevention trial; both the Scandinavian Simvastatin Survival Study (4S) (9) and the Cholesterol and Recurrent Events (CARE) Study (10) were secondary prevention trials. The CARE study was designed to examine the effects of LDL-C lowering in CHD patients who had normal or only minimal elevations in LDL-C. All three of these lipid-lowering trials achieved a significant reduction in clinical events. Reductions in nonfatal and fatal CHD events of between 24% and 42% were observed in patients treated with statins (Figs. 21.2–21.4).

Early trials of lipid-lowering therapy demonstrated cardiovascular benefit but were not of

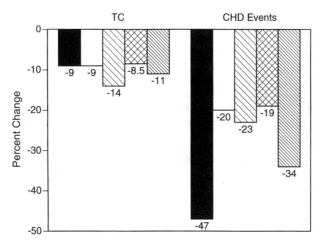

Figure 21.1.   Early primary prevention trials: overview. Solid bars, Oslo: diet and smoking cessation (N = 1,232; *P* = .02); open bars, WHO: clofibrate (N = 15,745, *P* < .05); wide diagonal-striped bars, Upjohn: colestipol (N = 3,806; *P* < .05); cross-hatched bars, LRC-CPPT: cholestyramine (N = 3,806; *P* < .05); narrow diagonal-striped bars, HHS: gemfibrozil (N = 4,081; *P* < .02). (Adapted from Levine G, Keaney JJ, Vita J. Cholesterol reduction in cardiovascular disease: clinical benefits and possible mechanisms. N Engl J Med 1995;332:512–521.)

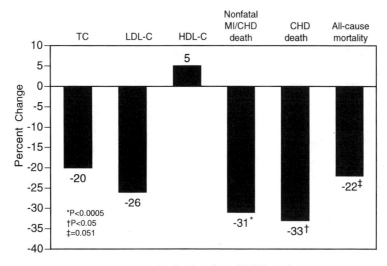

Figure 21.2.   West of Scotland Coronary Prevention Study: effect of lipid-lowering on coronary events in primary prevention trial in men. There were 6596 men, between 45 and 64 years of age, who participated in a 5-year trial on the effects of pravastatin to reduce plasma lipids. Mean baseline at the beginning of the trial for total cholesterol (*TC*) was 272 mg/dL and for low-density lipoprotein cholesterol (*LDL-C*) 192 mg/dL. *HDL-C,* high-density lipoprotein cholesterol; *MI,* myocardial infarction; *CHD,* coronary heart disease. (Reprinted with permission from Shephard J, Cobbe SM, Ford I, et al. Prevention of coronary heart disease with pravastatin in men with hypercholesterolemia. N Engl J Med 1995;333: 1301–1307.)

sufficient power to show a reduction in total mortality. The 4S study, a secondary prevention study, decisively resolved this issue. It showed a significant 30% reduction in total mortality and a 42% reduction in coronary mortality in 4444 CHD patients randomized to receive lipid-lowering therapy or placebo for an average of 5.4 years. Especially important was a 37% reduction in revascularization procedures and a 34% reduc-

tion in hospital days (Fig. 21.5). Importantly, these improvements were seen early, only 1 to 2 years after the initiation of therapy.

Furthermore, a cost analysis of the 4S trial data was conducted to determine the economic impact of lipid-lowering therapy. Fewer hospitalization (1403 versus 1905) and shorter hospital stays occurred in those patients receiving simvastatin, resulting in a 34% decrease in hospital

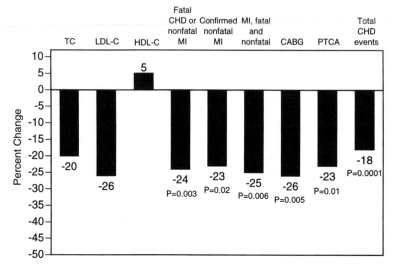

Figure 21.3. Cholesterol and Recurrent Events Study: effect of lipid-lowering on coronary events in secondary prevention trial in men and women. There were 4159 subjects, between 21 and 75 years of age, who participated in a 5-year trial on the effects of pravastatin to reduce plasma lipids. Mean baseline at the beginning of the trial for total cholesterol (*TC*) was less than 209 mg/dL and for low-density lipoprotein cholesterol (*LDL-C*), 139 mg/dL. *HDL-C,* high-density lipoprotein cholesterol; *MI,* myocardial infarction; *CHD,* coronary heart disease; *CABG,* coronary artery bypass graft surgery; *PTCA,* percutaneous transluminal coronary angioplasty. (Adapted from Sacks FM, Pfeffer MA, Moye LA, et al. The effect of pravastatin on coronary events after myocardial infarction in patients with average cholesterol levels. Cholesterol and Recurrent Events Trial Envestigators. N Engl J Med 1996;335:1001–1009.)

CARE: Event Rates

Reductions observed in:	%	P
Fatal CHD or nonfatal MI*	24	0.003
Confirmed nonfatal MI	23	0.02
MI, fatal and nonfatal	25	0.006
CABG	26	0.005
PTCA	23	0.01
Total CHD events	18	0.0001

Figure 21.4. Cholesterol and Recurrent Events Study (CARE): event rates. *MI,* myocardial infarction; *CHD,* coronary heart disease; *CABG,* coronary artery bypass graft surgery; *PTCA,* percutaneous transluminal coronary angioplasty.

days (*P* < .0001). There was also a 32% reduction in hospitalization for acute CHD events. The reduction in hospitalization costs during the study would correspond to a reduction of $3872 per patient. When these savings are applied to the cost of simvastatin for the 5-year study period, the effective cost was reduced to $0.28/day; it increases to $0.41/day for the entire 5 years when the costs of routine lipid measurements are included (Fig. 21.6). The significant findings from the 4S trial pointed to an impressive relation between clinical and economic considerations. In general it appears that reductions in LDL-C are positively

associated with reductions in CHD events, hospitalization rates, and health care costs (11).

Recent advances in vascular and molecular biology have suggested that medical interventions to arrest the atherosclerotic process must address not only obstruction but also plaque stabilization, which may prove to be even more important. Interestingly, therapy that lowers cholesterol by 20% results in a significant decrease in cardiovascular events within 1 to 2 years. However, the angiographic changes in stenoses associated with these impressive clinical event reductions are remarkably insignificant, on the order of 1% to 2% (e.g., 0.2 mm) (12, 13). Stabilization of high-risk plaques appears to account for the impressive reduction in cardiovascular events (14, 15), and aggressive modification of risk alters endothelial dysfunction, an early change in the course of atherosclerosis. Lowering LDL-C, estrogen replacement therapy, and smoking cessation all act to improve endothelial function. The major effects of lipid-lowering therapy appear to be related to stabilization of high-risk plaques and improvement in abnormal endothelial function.

There are other risk-reduction strategies with similar ability to improve the outlook for patients with CHD. Angiotensin-converting en-

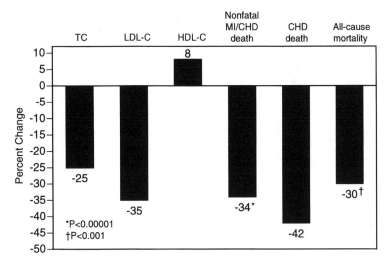

Figure 21.5.   Scandinavian Simvastatin Survival Study (4S): effect of LDL-C lowering on coronary events in secondary prevention trial in men and women. There were 4444 subjects (80% men, 20% women), between 35 and 70 years of age, who participated in a 5-year trial on the effects of simvastatin to reduce plasma lipids. Mean baseline at the beginning of the trial for total cholesterol (*TC*) was 261 mg/dL and for low-density lipoprotein cholesterol (*LDL-C*), 188 mg/dL. *HDL-C*, high-density lipoprotein cholesterol; *MI,* myocardial infarction; *CHD,* coronary heart disease. (Adapted from Scandinavian Simvastatin Survival Study Group. Randomised trial of cholesterol lowering in 4444 patients with coronary heart disease: the Scandinavian Simvastatin Survival Study (4S). Lancet 1995;345:1274–1275.)

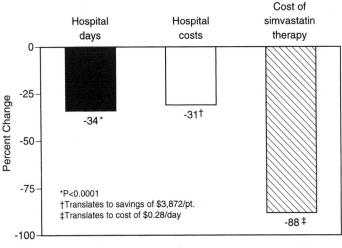

Figure 21.6.   Scandinavian Simvastatin Survival Study (4S): clinical and economic benefits of treatment over 5-year period. *LDL-C,* low-density lipoprotein cholesterol; *CHD,* coronary heart disease. (Reprinted with permission from Pederson T, Kjekhus J, Berg K, et al. Cholesterol lowering and the use of healthcare resources. Results of the Scandinavian Simvastatin Survival Study. Circulation 1996;93:1796–1802.)

zyme inhibitor therapy after MI in patients with symptomatic and asymptomatic left ventricular failure, β-blockers in the post-MI patient, aspirin therapy, and antihypertensive treatment all show reductions in mortality and morbidity in the CHD patient.

Unfortunately, most patients in the health care system do not receive comprehensive risk-reduction therapies. Despite all the research in vascular and molecular biology, despite well-designed clinical trials showing a decrease in cardiovascular events, despite consensus panels and statements emphasizing the importance of preventive strategies, most patients do not receive the risk-reduction therapies proven to prolong life and reduce morbidity.

RISK FACTOR MANAGEMENT

The concept of risk as it applies to medicine is firmly entrenched in clinical medicine and public perception. Based on data from numerous epidemiologic studies and clinical trials, a summary of 21 risk factors of cardiovascular disease (CVD) was made by the 27th Bethesda Conference in 1996. It is beyond the scope of this chapter to review the literature on risk factors for cardiovascular disease. However, it is important for clinicians in the field of preventive cardiology to develop a framework from which to evaluate and apply new data on clinical interventions. We propose that the clinician be guided by three factors: the strength of the scientific data, the ability of the clinician or therapies to modify the risk factor, and finally the cost-effectiveness of intervention. To illustrate, we will review two specific, modifiable risk factors and their cost-effectiveness.

Cholesterol Reduction

Both diet and drug therapy are successful in the reduction of LDL-C, and both result in reduction in cardiac events (16). Diet has been viewed as notoriously difficult to implement and monitor. Despite the challenges presented by diet modification, it appears that the overall reduction in cardiac events during the last 20 years has been in part the result of reductions in per capita fat intake (from approximately 40% of total calories to approximately 33% of daily calories). These reductions have been brought about by continued campaigns waged by the health care establishment. After initial consultation with a physician, a patient can achieve a mean reduction of cholesterol of approximately 5% through diet. Careful scrutiny of the data suggests that only a small percentage (less than 10%) of the population achieves more than a 10% reduction in cholesterol. The vast majority realizes only 5% to 10% reductions in cholesterol, and another 10% realize virtually no long-term improvement in cholesterol levels. This is the result of both genetic heterogeneity in the responsiveness of cholesterol to diet as well as large variations in compliance. New genetic tests (e.g., apoprotein (Apo) AIV and Apo E isoforms) (17) may aid in the identification of those best served by dietary instruction and modification. Data instruments to assess behavior and preferences may also be helpful in discerning which patients have the greatest chance of maintaining a diet lower in calories or overall fat content (18).

Drug therapy has been previously discussed, and all evidence suggests that reduction of LDL-C to the target levels recommended by the National Cholesterol Education Program–Adult Treatment Panel (NCEP–ATP) are easily accomplished by application of diet and medication (drug therapy) by the physician, resulting in a significant reduction in cardiac events, and are cost-effective.

Cigarette Smoking

The data concerning the deleterious effects of cigarette smoking are overwhelming. According to the Coronary Artery Surgery Study (CASS) (19), cigarette smokers with CHD realized a 50% reduction in the risk for recurrent cardiac events with discontinuation of the habit. Today, about 25% of adults in the United States smoke cigarettes, and approximately 40% of patients with CHD smoke cigarettes. Sixty percent of those with CHD who smoke (24% of patients with CHD) discontinue the habit after an MI with only a comment from their physician. Only another 10% to 15% terminate their habit with general cigarette cessation programs (4% to 6% of patients with CHD) (20). Given these statistics and the low rate of success of smoking interventions in the general population, are these interventions an economically reasonable use of health care resources?

Two analyses have addressed the cost-effectiveness of smoking interventions (21, 22). Cummings and colleagues (21) assessed the cost-effectiveness of counseling smokers to quit. Based on the assumptions that counseling would increase the cessation rate by 2.7%, that 10% of patients who quit would relapse, and that counseling would cost $10 in physicians' time and $2 in printed materials, the cost-effectiveness ratio of physicians' counseling was found to be $705 to $988 per year of life saved for men and $1204 to $2058 per year of life saved for women, depending on the patient's age at intervention. The incremental cost of a $30 follow-up visit was $421 to $5051 per year of life saved for men and $772 to $9259 per year of life saved for women.

Oster and colleagues (22) analyzed the cost-effectiveness of nicotine gum as an adjunct to physicians' counseling against smoking. Their analysis calculated that the incremental cost of nicotine gum therapy per year of life saved was

$4113 to $6465 for men and $6880 to $9473 for women, depending on age at intervention. Despite the difficulties of implementing a smoking cessation program and poor results in the general population, smoking remains a highly cost-effective medical intervention.

The question of which patients are most appropriate for medical intervention and which will have the largest benefit of therapy is in large part based on cost-effectiveness of the interventions. The decision tree for prevention will additionally be based on the prevention program in place. Our approach is to consider all patients with coronary artery disease at particularly high risk and to enroll them in a program in which various other risk factors are identified and an overall risk is estimated.

The cost strategy, assuming a capitated environment, hinges on the estimated yearly rate of cardiac events (MI, CABG, PTCA, etc.) in the population treated. For a general population of men between the ages of 45 and 65 years, the general incidence of MI is 0.6% as identified by the Framingham Study (23). However, in the presence of CHD, this incidence rate increases 10-fold to more than 6%. In an otherwise healthy subject with four or more risk factors for CHD, the incidence of MI is approximately 4% per year. A simplistic approach to cost analysis would be to consider a continuum of risk for the development of cardiac events in a patient population ranging from less than 1% to 6% per year. The larger the burden of risk in a given population, the larger and more cost-effective would be a series of interventions.

Of particular note in the development of our prevention program is the value of a computer-based database used at various critical points in patient management; in patient, nurse, and physician feedback; and in cost-effectiveness and outcomes analysis. The cost of a computer system and the development of a database to serve both clinical and research needs of the prevention program may make the cost of a program prohibitive; however, we should emphasize the value of the database as a mandatory part of the program. Only with a robust database can we adequately manage large volumes of patients in a cost-effective manner, provide valuable feedback to health care providers, and measure quality and outcomes of the program.

Cost-effectiveness analysis improves clinical practice and aids in the development of clinical guidelines and health policy on a larger level and in the development of individual prevention programs. This is accomplished by providing information about the value of alternative health interventions in specific high-risk populations. It should not be considered the sole basis for resource allocation, but serves as a guide.

Various forms of cues or reminders have been used to identify patients in need of preventive services. We have designed our clinical database to assist in issues of patient compliance as well as physician and nurse follow-up. It has been demonstrated that cholesterol values identified as abnormal by the laboratory computer were more likely to lead to follow-up treatment than those values not described as abnormal (24). In general, cue and reminder systems appear to improve the implementation of preventive services by assisting both the nurse and physician in using preventive strategies (25–29).

More sophisticated computer-based clinical decision making and clinical support systems have had more equivocal results. Johnston et al. (30) concluded that the success of a computer-based clinical support system was variable but did improve physician performance in four of six studies designed to enhance the quality of preventive care.

Our computer monitoring systems provide data for individual and organizational feedback and reinforcement and improve the potential for success. Computerized records in a preventive setting facilitate quality assurance and management efforts to provide performance data and to reinforce organizational and provider behavior.

Quality assurance programs are readily applicable to primary and secondary prevention programs, and the assessment of quality is more accurately performed with a database that monitors key measures of quality. As proposed by Foody et al. (31) according to Task Force 8 of the Bethesda Conference, quality should be measured by 10 key indicators (Table 21.1).

PROGRAM CONCEPTS

We have attempted to design a program based on sound clinical practice guided by current scientific evidence that reduces risk in a clinically

Table 21.1. Key Measures for Quality of Preventive Care

1. Smoking status should be documented in all patients with coronary heart disease (CHD), cerebrovascular disease (CVD), or peripheral vascular disease (PVD).
2. Organizations should have a smoking cessation program available for patients and their families.
3. All eligible patients should have documentation of a physician offer of advice and self-help materials to stop smoking.
4. All patients with CHD, CVD, or PVD should have a fasting lipoprotein profile documented within the first 3 months after onset of disease if the patient is deemed appropriate for pharmacologic intervention.
5. All patients with CHD, CVD, or PVD should be offered nutritional evaluation and counseling at the time of diagnosis.
6. All patients with CHD, CVD, or PVD who have an LDL-C level of more than 130 mg/dL after nutritional therapy should be prescribed, as documented, lipid-lowering medication if appropriate.
7. All patients with CHD, CVD, or PVD should be assessed and provided with exercise counseling or prescription at the time of diagnosis if appropriate.
8. Aspirin therapy should be offered to all eligible patients. If aspirin is not indicated, the contraindication should be documented in the medical record.
9. All patients with CHD, CVD, or PVD should have two blood pressure measurements recorded at every visit.
10. If an average of three blood pressure measurements is equal to or greater than 140 mm Hg systolic or 90 mm Hg diastolic, lifestyle and pharmacologic therapy treatment plans should be offered and documented at the time of diagnosis.

effective manner, as well as being cost-effective. Our program design and its ongoing development is based on nine key concepts (Table 21.2). These concepts were conceptualized from available scientific data, effectiveness of interventions, and economic considerations.

Dedicated Prevention Unit

The reason for referral to a dedicated prevention unit rather than having the primary local contact provide such services is several-fold. First, the prevention nursing staff can allocate the time necessary to treat behavior-related factors. This relatively large time commitment redirected to the unit can free up the physician to spend more time with diagnostic issues. Second,

the physician extender can initially evaluate the patient, revisit as often as necessary, and use the phone to remind patients about compliance. Thus, the prevention unit becomes focused on outcomes and can be more effective than the approach typically observed in the more traditional setting. Further, by cultivating a team under the direction of specialists with up-to-date expertise in the various risk factor areas, the clinic can promote and deliver cutting edge treatment.

The arguments against a dedicated unit includes the patient's perception of fragmented care and the inconvenience of a referral to a separate geographic area. This is time consuming and less appealing for the medical care consumer. If preventive specialty diagnostics and treatment can be brought immediately into the primary physician's office, this may be a feasible and appropriate compromise in which the needs of both the physician and the patient are advanced.

The challenge for the primary care physician is to provide preventive interventions to an appropriate subset of patients. Preventive cardiology is only one area of prevention. Continued scrutiny of the high cost of medical care has limited preventive measures to those patients identified as being at high risk. This has been emphasized by the American College of Physicians, which suggests that cholesterol measurement and treatment be strictly reserved for those with current vascular disease or who are at very high risk for its development (32).

For this and other reasons, our group decided to treat all CHD patients with one or more risk factors, as well as those without CHD who have at least two to three risk factors, or more than 2% annual risk, in a dedicated prevention unit. We propose that a specialized unit can provide these services very economically and should produce well above an average 20% risk reduction.

Table 21.2. Key Concepts in the Design of a Preventative Cardiology Clinic

Risk factor modification
Physician's assistant–based staffing
Multidisciplinary physician management
Algorithm-driven treatment
Outcome-based analysis
Dedicated prevention unit
Behavior modification

Multidisciplinary Physician Involvement

Patient care is supervised by physicians. Members of the physician staff are assigned to a particular clinic.

Each physician is assigned two nurse-practitioners or physician's assistants. The current staff is composed of three cardiologists, one endocrinologist–diabetologist, one vascular medicine specialist, one hypertension nephrologist, and one general internist. Physician staffing can be determined on the basis of the particular population being treated as well as institutional resources.

In addition to patient care, the staff physicians are integrally involved in the management of the program. These generalists and specialists have reached a consensus on the goals of the program, set baseline algorithms, and identified data elements to be collected. Their backgrounds include extensive experience in clinical practice, teaching, and research. Physician diversity and broad experience of the physician staff provides a strong base for program development.

Physician's Assistant–based Staffing

Staffing of a prevention unit is similar to most general internal medicine or cardiology clinics. Patients are seen by either a nurse or physician's assistant as well as a physician. Current reimbursement guidelines do not allow for a solely nurse- or physician's assistant–based visit. Ultimately, we envision that an effective, clinically sound preventive program would principally use physician's assistants as the main health care provider. A preventive clinic provides an ideal environment for physician's assistants. Physician's assistants have been shown to be more consistent and more accurate in providing routine care, and they are less expensive than general internists. Given a limited budget for the performance of multiple tasks and interventions, the costs savings achieved through the use of physician's assistant staffing can be translated into additional interventions.

RISK FACTOR MODIFICATION

Controversy surrounds the effectiveness and value of reducing a single risk factor versus intervening on multiple risks. Meta-analyses of the treatment of hypertension indicate that a 17% reduction in CHD end points occurs when blood pressure is controlled in hypertensive subjects. The Framingham data have shown greater benefits when older hypertensive patients (older than 50 years) were examined 10 years after prescribed treatment. The risk of death caused by CVD was 60% lower in treated versus untreated subjects (33). Yet, it has been suggested that the concomitant presence of hyperlipidemia is perhaps central to the overall impact of hypertension (34, 35). Once lipids are corrected, blood pressure control may not be as critical in terms of incremental reduction in risk.

When programs have focused efforts on multiple risk factor targets rather than on single predominant risk factor target, the benefit achieved has only minimally exceeded those achieved through modification of a single risk factor. Combined programs targeting cigarettes, lipids, and exercise are reported to produce no more than a 40% benefit (13). Most participants indeed have more than one risk factor; however, the incremental benefit of modification of these multiple risk factors remains unclear.

Given the large risk reduction achieved by cholesterol reduction, we have chosen to focus predominantly on cholesterol and use adjunctive therapies secondarily for the modification of other risk factors in our patients with CHD. This is not to say that other risk factors are less important in the assessment of risk; however, cholesterol reduction provides a medically feasible cost-effective intervention.

In addition to aggressive modification of lipids, the clinic focuses on a strategy to identify additional risk factors in the patient with CHD. A short summary of dietary goals as well as dietary information is provided to patients. Each patient completes a food frequency questionnaire in the interval between visits. The overall fat:saturated fat percentage of total daily calories is assessed at each visit through the completion and analysis of the Gladys Block questionnaire (31) using data provided by the patient.

Supervised nutritional counseling has been documented to lower cholesterol levels by 5%. Dietary manipulation in conjunction with drug therapy produces a reduction in cholesterol beyond that of drugs alone (36). We believe that efforts targeting dietary modification remain valuable. The best means of achieving this behavioral modification, however, remain unclear. We believe that teaching culinary arts will prove to be more effective than the traditional didactic approach.

Algorithm-driven Treatment

Cardiovascular disease prevention in some respects is an ideal application for algorithm treatment plans. When treating CVD, prevention is complex and involves multiple body systems and diseases such as hypertension, diabetes, coronary artery disease, and cerebrovascular as well as peripheral vascular disease. Baseline algorithms for the diagnosis and management of hypertension, hyperlipidemia, diabetes, and vascular disease have been developed from standard clinical practice guidelines provided by the NCEP, Joint National Commission V (JNCV), ACC, and AHA. Defined pathways for elevated cholesterol and blood pressure values (37) are available to permit algorithm-driven, nurse-run programs (38–41). Similar pathways for diabetes and postmenopausal hormone replacement therapy have been developed. These algorithms add to the clinical efficiency of a preventive program.

Behavior Modification

Treatments that require long-term behavior modifications are extremely difficult to maintain unless there is continued behavior intervention (42). Questionnaires can be filled out on all major compliance items, including medication usage, diet, weight control, cigarette cessation, and exercise. Behaviorists or psychologists are useful adjuncts to the clinic operation. Counseling becomes a crucial intervention in a population at risk. The effectiveness of behavior modification is difficult to assess. Outcomes analysis will focus on quantitative markers for behavior modification initially and then move toward psychosocial profiles and health status scores ultimately. For example, cotinine is a marker for cigarette use (43), and red blood cell membranes can be assessed for fatty acid composition (44). Metabolic assessments can be made for exercise activity (45).

Focus on Outcomes

The positive effects of cholesterol reduction have clearly been established. However, the transferability of these results to a clinical setting remains a critical question. If third-party payers are going to reimburse organizations, if primary care physicians are going to refer patients, or if organizations are going to fund these programs in a capitated environment, we must answer this question.

By collecting data on all patients who come through the program as well as monitoring their progress, we can develop an extensive database that leads to outcome measures and, as a consequence, refinement of the process. Whenever possible, data are collected using scientific methods, quality control, and uniform data collection techniques. Parts of the program that do not have clear benefit can be discontinued. The program's algorithms will be validated or adjusted on the basis of actual patient data collected and analyzed in a real-life practice setting.

Cost-Effectiveness

It is essential that programs like this operate in a cost-effective manner. The program can operate efficiently and at a low cost because of its reliance on computers for repetitive tasks, use of physician's assistants, and careful view on outcomes to define those clinical measures and interventions that are most effective. Many of these components in an overall health care system overlap the traditional domains of primary and specialty care. However, the narrow focus on issues that are treatable and relevant to CVD make such a program valuable for both the generalist and the specialist. The cost-effective nature of this clinical approach, however, rests on the characteristics of the target population.

Active Research Program

Preventive cardiology is a dynamic field. As such, a prevention unit, in our estimation, must provide the framework and the ability to conduct significant clinical research in the area of clinical efficacy, health care outcomes, and management strategies. By designing a program that collects data on its population and that compiles a robust clinical data set easily accessible to the clinician, clinical research can proceed in an efficient manner. The research component of a prevention clinic is likely to incur significant cost; however, these costs, at least initially, are necessary for self-assessment and ultimately for the advancement of the field of prevention.

PROGRAMMATIC ISSUES

The programmatic issues can be broken down into five general areas: patient flow through the program, clinical database, resources required, patient recruitment, and financial considerations. This section will focus on the general rather than the specifics and will serve to provide a framework on which to establish a program in preventive cardiology.

Patient Flow

Referral patterns for cardiac patients are similar at most institutions. In general, patients are referred to a preventive cardiology unit from one of four general referral sources. First, patients can be referred by a partner from any of several different departments within the organization, including internal medicine, endocrinology, cardiology, and hypertension and nephrology. Second, the patient can be referred after an acute episode or a recent cardiac procedure, i.e., CABG, angioplasty, transplantation, or vascular surgery. The third source would be general internists or other physicians outside the institution. The fourth source of patients is through self-referral.

Our major source of referrals are in-house cardiologists who have identified the patient as one who would benefit from risk factor modification. Referring cardiologists generally determine the lipid profile, blood pressure, cigarette use, postmenopausal estrogen use, and body mass index before referring the patient to the prevention program. Currently, a critical pathway for the management of lipids and modification of risk in cardiac patients does not exist for application by the referring staff, but it is envisioned that one will eventually be developed. In general, patients referred to the clinic have at least three risk factors. These risk factors include LDL-C more than 130 mg/dL (3.36 mmol/L), HDL-C less than 35 mg/dL (0.91 mmol/L), male age more than 45 years, female age more than 55 years, diabetes mellitus, blood pressure more than 140/90 mm Hg, and cigarette use. The Framingham database (46) is useful in establishing a risk stratification schema.

Before the patient's appointment, a letter describing the program and reviewing instructions for laboratory measurements is sent to all new patients. Relevant data abstraction tools including an 11-page medical and family history questionnaire and a 7-page nutritional assessment form (Gladys Block [31]) are included in the mailing.

At the initial visit, all forms are reviewed for completeness, and the data are scanned into the patient database. Patients then complete a nurse or physician's assistant visit, and a care plan, which is based on data obtained from the patient-completed questionnaire, the medical history, and the examination, is presented to the staff physician. In general, these care plans are developed from the application of the series of algorithms developed for clinic use. The algorithms have a series of different phenotypes (e.g., increased LDL-C or increased blood pressure) with a specific treatment (both pharmacologic and otherwise), a series of goals (potentially targeted toward the initial and follow-up visits), and laboratory assays for day of visit and for follow-up visits.

The patient flow is similar for our follow-up visits. Information on compliance with medication (i.e., pills missed per week for each risk factor category), dietary and exercise compliance, and cigarette use or date of discontinuation. We use these follow-up visits to motivate and educate. A return visit date is decided and recorded on the data form.

Resource Requirements—Facilities, Space, and Personnel

Individual and group processing of patients should be feasible within the space of the clinic. In general, the following space requirements aid in the efficient flow of patients through the clinic.

1. A phlebotomy room (approximately 400 sq ft), which should include a desktop centrifuge, phlebotomy chair, 4°C refrigerator, −20°C freezer, and general supplies including tubes and syringes for drawing blood.
2. A reception desk supported with a computer for appointment scheduling, laboratory retrieval, and database entry.
3. Two conference rooms or offices for patient counseling by dietitians.
4. Four clinical examination rooms.
5. One waiting room that can accommodate 10 to 15 people.

Each examination room has an examination table, wall ophthalmoscope, blood pressure monitor with three different-sized cuffs, and a laptop computer. Physician's assistants perform the initial evaluation of patients. The staff physician reviews the recommended treatment approach determined by the physician's assistant.

This entire process on a new patient should not take more than 2 hours. For former patients it should take less than 45 minutes. Other valuable additions to the clinical operation include an electrocardiography machine, office space for the physicians and physician's assistants, x-ray film viewing box, and medical record viewing area. The total space requirement for such a clinic is approximately 2500 sq ft. This also allows for some storage and a filing area. The addition of exercise space for rehabilitation, educational areas, or other rooms dedicated to alternative critical pathways would invariably increase the space needs. Personnel needs include the following:

1 Physician who will oversee the physician's assistants
2–3 Physician's assistants
1 Data coordinator
2 Dietitians
1 Phlebotomist
1 Receptionist/secretary/scheduler

Clinical and Research Database

The database is an integral part of the program. The organization's central appointment system populates the clinic database with patient demographics. A patient-specific questionnaire is created by means of the database and mailed to the patient. The night before the appointment, the computer generates a patient-specific data entry form. On the day of the visit findings from the visit are entered, and a patient summary note is produced to assist the physician and nurse in treating the patient. In addition, a clinical note of the visit is generated for inclusion in the patient's chart. The visit results, dietary assessment, laboratory results, and medications are recorded in the same database. Finally, the computer system generates approximately 90% of a comprehensive letter to the referring physician and a patient letter, as well as a detailed monograph on the patient's cardiovascular risk factors.

Significantly, the database used by the program was designed by physicians, nurses, admin-

istrators, front-desk personnel, biostatisticians, and support personnel. It has been expressly designed to meet the research mission, as well as the clinic needs, of the program. It provides a robust source of clinical information from which to monitor program success, aids in the identification of subsets of patients at clinically significant increased risk, and finally provides a base from which to perform clinical research trials.

Patient Recruitment and Marketing

A successful recruitment and marketing strategy hinges on the ability to assess the community needs and to formulate a plan with specific objectives. In a tertiary care facility such as ours, four sources of patients referred to the program have been identified. Each major referral population requires a specific marketing strategy tailored to its specific needs and objectives. With the assistance of the organization's marketing department, a comprehensive marketing plan was developed and implemented.

Financial Considerations

There are two major financial aspects of the program, traditional budgeting and cost analysis. Budgeting for the program follows traditional budget practices and is the same method used by all programs at this institution. Revenues were estimated on the basis of patient volume projections, personnel and other expenses allocated, and a contribution margin was calculated. Figure 21.7 shows patient recruitment during the first 48 weeks of the program along with our initial volume goals.

We show volume to illustrate two points. Prevention programs at this time initially do not make a return on investment. Physician and other operating expenses are higher than general internal medicine clinics, and these programs require more ancillary support than specialty clinics (nursing, secretarial, data management, and supervisory support).

The second financial aspect of the program concerns cost-effectiveness. Cost-effectiveness analysis is a widely used method of determining the value of a health intervention (47). Using well-established methods, both screening and treatment programs can be evaluated in terms of the cost-effectiveness of the intervention (10, 48).

Definitive cost analyses in the field of preven-

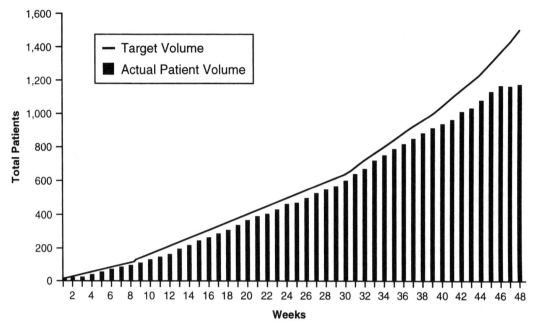

Figure 21.7. Patient volume in preventive cardiology clinic. Projected and actual patient volumes are shown for the first 48 weeks after implementing our program in preventive cardiology.

tive cardiology have been done by Goldman et al. (47). Task Force 6 of the 27th Bethesda Conference, chaired by Goldman, discussed the fundamentals of cost-analysis as it applies to preventive cardiology. The Task Force concluded that screening programs for hypertension and treatment programs for smoking cessation, hypertension, aspirin, and cholesterol-lowering were cost-effective. As was mentioned above, from a financial perspective these programs are at best a break-even endeavor. For these programs to be effective, they must demonstrate that they are cost-effective for the organization. Using the principles and methods of cost-effectiveness, program directors will be able to provide their organizations with a method of analyzing the program not from the micro departmental or program level but from the macro or overall organizational perspective. Using a hypothetical intervention costing $2000 per year and producing a 50% reduction in the risk of MI, CABG, and other events in 10,000 patients during 5 years, their example calculated an approximate cost per year of life saved of $11,500. If instead the cost per year per patient were reduced to $600, the same method could show a cost savings of $500 per life saved.

Like many aspects of preventive cardiology,

cost-effectiveness analysis has enormous possibilities for study and application. It is reasonable to conclude that cost-effectiveness is a legitimate method of definitively establishing the financial viability of preventive cardiology programs.

CONCLUSION

Recent changes in resource allocation and new evidence demonstrating the unequivocal efficacy of medical intervention in the prevention of cardiac events have focused attention on the growing field of preventive cardiology. We have provided a brief overview of the establishment, implementation, and programmatic issues that we have faced in developing a preventive cardiology program at the Cleveland Clinic Foundation.

References

1. American Heart Association. Heart and stroke facts: 1994 statistical supplement. Dallas, TX: American Heart Association, 1994.
2. Oliver M. Doubts about preventing coronary heart disease. Multiple interventions in middle aged men may do more harm than good. Br Med J 1992;304:393–394
3. Leren P. The Oslo diet-heart study. Eleven-year report. Circulation 1970;42:935–942.
4. WHO cooperative trial on primary prevention of ischaemic heart disease using clofibrate to lower serum

cholesterol: mortality follow-up. Report of the Committee of Principal Investigators. Lancet 1980;2:379–385.

5. Lithell H, Vessby B, Boberg J, et al. The effects of colestipol when combined with clofibrate in the treatment of severe hyperlipidemia. Short-term and long-term studies. Atherosclerosis 1980;37:175–186.

6. Lipid Research Clinics Program. The Lipid Research Clinics Coronary Primary Prevention Trial Results. II. The relationship of reduction in incidence of coronary heart disease to cholesterol lowering. JAMA 1984;251: 365–374.

7. Frick MH, Elo O, Haapa K, et al. Helsinki Heart Study. Primary-prevention trial with gemfibrozil in middle-age men with dyslipidemia. N Engl J Med 1987;317: 1235–1245.

8. Shepherd J, Cobbe SM, Ford I, et al. Prevention of coronary heart disease with prevastatin in men with hypercholesterolemia. N Engl J Med 1995;333:1301–1307.

9. Scandinavian Simvastatin Survival Study Group. Randomised trial of cholesterol lowering in 4444 patients with coronary heart disease: the Scandinavian Simvastatin Survival Study (4S). Lancet 1994;344:1383–1389.

10. Pfeffer M, Sacks F, Lemuel A, et al. Cholesterol and recurrent events: a secondary prevention trial for normolipidemic patients. Am J Cardiol 1995;76:98C–106C.

11. Pederson T, Kjekshus J, Berg K, et al. Cholesterol lowering and the use of healthcare resources. Results of the Scandinavian Simvastatin Survival Study. Circulation 1996;93:1796–1802.

12. Watts G, Lewis B, Brunt J, et al. Effects on coronary artery disease of lipid-lowering diet, or diet plus cholestyramine, in the St. Thomas' Atherosclerosis Regression Study (STARS). Lancet 1992;339:563–569.

13. Haskell W, Alderman E, Fair J, et al. Effects of intensive multiple risk factor reduction on coronary atherosclerosis and clinical cardiac events in men and women with coronary artery disease. The Stanford Coronary Risk Intervention Project (SCRIP). Circulation 1994;89:975–990.

14. Levine G, Keaney JJ, Vita J. Cholesterol reduction in cardiovascular disease: clinical benefits and possible mechanisms. N Engl Med 1995;332:512–521.

15. Philbin E, Pearson T. How does lipid lowering therapy rapidly reduce ischemic events? J Myocardial Ischemia 1994;6:13–18.

16. Law M, Wald N. An ecological study of serum cholesterol and ischaemic heart disease between 1950 and 1990. Eur J Clin Nutr 1994;48:305–325.

17. McCombs R, Marcadis D, Ellis J, et al. Attenuated hypercholesterolemic response to a high-cholesterol diet in subjects heterozygous for the apolipoprotein A-IV-2 allele. N Engl J Med 1994;331:706–710.

18. Rosenthal SL, Knauer-Black S, Stahl MP, et al. The National Cholesterol Education Program pediatric guidelines: behavioral considerations. J Deviated Behav Pediatr 1992;13:2188–2189.

19. Cavender J, Rogers W, Fisher L, et al. Effects of smoking on survival and morbidity in patients randomized to medical or surgical therapy in the Coronary Artery Surgery Study (CASS): 10-year follow-up. CASS Investigators. J Am Coll Cardiol 1992;20:287–294.

20. Stafford R, Becker C. Cigarette smoking and atherosclerosis. In: Fuster V, Ross R, Topol E, eds. Atherosclerosis and coronary artery disease. Philadelphia: Lippincott-Raven, 1996:303–321.

21. Cummings S, Rubin S, Oster G. The cost-effectiveness of counseling smokers to quit. JAMA 1989;261:75–79.

22. Oster G, Huse D, Delea T, et al. Cost-effectiveness of nicotine gum as an adjunct to physican's advice against cigarette smoking. JAMA 1986;256:1315–1318.

23. Sytkowski PA, Kannel WB, D'Agostino RB. Changes in risk factors and the decline in mortality from cardiovascular disease. The Framingham Heart Study [see comments]. N Engl J Med 1990;322:1635–1641.

24. Reed R, Jenkins P, Pu TA. Laboratory's manner of reporting serum cholesterol affects clinical care. Clin Chem 1994;40:847–848.

25. Davidson R, Fletcher S, Retchin S, et al. A nurse-initiated reminder system for the periodic health examination. Implementation and evaluation. Arch Intern Med 1984;144:2167–2170.

26. Cheney C, Ramsdell J. Effect of medical records' checklist on implementation of periodic health measures. Am J Med 1987;83:129–136.

27. Harris R, O'Malley M, Fletcher S, et al. Prompting physicians for preventative procedures: a five-year study of manual and computer reminders. Am J Prev Med 1990;6:145–152.

28. McDonald C. Protocol-based computer reminders, the quality of care and the non-perfectibility of man. N Engl J Med 1976;295:1351–1355.

29. Williams B. Efficacy of a checklist to promote preventive medicine approach. J Tenn Med Assoc 1981;74: 489–491.

30. Johnston M, Langton K, Haynes R, et al. Effects of computer-based clinical decision support systems on clinician performance and patient outcome. A critical appraisal of research. Ann Intern Med 1994;120: 135–142.

31. Foody JM, Hunter B, Sprecher DLS. ed. Organization and design of a preventative cardiology clinic. In Robinson K, Preventive Cardiology Clinic Operations. Armonk, NY: Futura, 1998, in press.

32. American College of Physicians. Guidelines for using serum cholesterol, high density lipoprotein cholesterol, and triglyceride levels as screening tests for preventing coronary heart disease in adults. Ann Intern Med 1996;124:515–517.

33. Shea S, Cook EF, Kannel WB, et al. Treatment of hypertension and its effects on cardiovascular risk factors: data from the Framington Heart Study. Circulation 1985;71:22–30.

34. Sytkowski P, D'Agostino R, Belanger A, et al. Secular trends in long-term sustained hypertension, long-term treatment, and cardiovascular mortality. The Framingham Heart Study 1950–1990. Circulation 1996;93:697–703.

35. Chobanian A. Adaptive and maladaptive responses of the arterial wall to hypertension: the 1989 Corcoran Lecture. Hypertension 1990;15:666–674.

36. Grundy S. Lipids, nutrition, and coronary heart disease. In: Fuster V, Ross R, Topol E, eds. Atherosclero-

sis and coronary artery disease. Philadelphia: Lippincott-Raven, 1996:45–68.

37. National Cholesterol Education Program. Report of the expert panel on blood cholesterol levels in children and adolescents. Bethesda, MD: US Dept of Health and Human Services, Public Health Service, National Institutes of Health, National Heart, Lung and Blood Institute, 1991.

38. Reichgott MJ, Pearson S, Hill MN. The nurse practitioner's role in complex patient management: hypertension. J Nat Med Assoc 1983;75:1197–1204.

39. Blair T, Bryant F, Bocuzzi S. Treatment of hypercholesterolemia by a clinical nurse using a stepped-care protocol in a nonvolunteer population. Arch Intern Med 1988;148:1046–1048.

40. Weinberger M, Kirkman M, Samsa G, et al. A nurse-coordinated intervention for primary care patients with non–insulin-dependent diabetes mellitus: impact on glycemic control and health-related quality of life. J Gen Intern Med 1995;10:59–66.

41. Taylor C, Houston-Miller N, Killen J, et al. Smoking cessation after acute myocardial infarction: effects of a nurse-managed intervention. Ann Intern Med 1990; 113:118–123.

42. van Elderen-van Kemenade T, Maes S, van den Broek Y. Effects of a health education programme with telephone follow-up during cardiac rehabilitation. Br J Clin Psychol 1994;33:367–378.

43. Pre J. Markers for smoking. Pathol Biol (Paris) 1992;40:1015–1021.

44. Theret N, Bard J, Nuttens M, et al. The relationship between the phospholipid fatty acid composition of red blood cells, plasma lipids, and apolipoproteins. Metabolism 1993;42:562-568.

45. Young J. Exercise prescription for individuals with metabolic disorders. Practical considerations. Sports Med 1995;19:43–45.

46. Anderson K, Wilson P, Odell P, et al. An updated coronary risk profile: a statement for health professionals. Circulation 1991;83:356–362.

47. Goldman L, Weinstein M, Goldman P, et al. Cost-effectiveness of HMG-CoA reductase inhibition for primary and secondary prevention of coronary heart disease. JAMA 1991;265:1145–1151.

48. Pearson T, McBride P, Miller N, et al. Task Force 8. Organization of preventative cardiology services. J Am Coll Cardiol 1996;27:1039–1047.

Program Standards and Organizational Issues

Paul M. Ribisl, Louise Morrin, and Sharon Lefroy

There has been a proliferation of cardiac rehabilitation programs in the past 10 years, and indications are that this growth will continue. The reduction in cardiovascular mortality has led to an increased prevalence of coronary heart disease (CHD) and a subsequent increase in the demand for cardiac-related services. This need will continue to grow and will be driven, in part, by changing demographics and clinical advancement. Furthermore, the rising demand for services will occur in an environment of health care reform including restructuring and fiscal restraint. Shorter hospital length of stays for coronary artery bypass grafting surgery and acute cardiac events have created a need for the postdischarge education and support that cardiac rehabilitation provides. New and established programs face the challenge of delivering an integrated, cost-effective approach for managing and preventing cardiac disease. This chapter provides guidance to the program director and the medical director regarding the key issues related to the organization and administration of the cardiac rehabilitation program, in particular the implementation of new programs and the continuing viability of existing programs. There are excellent references available that provide extensive information on guidelines for cardiac rehabilitation programs, in particular the *Guidelines for Cardiac Rehabilitation Programs* published by the American Association of Cardiovascular and Pulmonary Rehabilitation (AACVPR) (1) and the U.S. Department of Health and Human Services' *Clinical Practice Guideline for Cardiac Rehabilitation* (2). The reader is encouraged to refer to these publications for more in-depth information.

ORGANIZATIONAL ISSUES

Program Initiation

The initiation of a cardiac rehabilitation program in a community requires careful planning if success is to be ensured. During the past 20 years, the cardiac rehabilitation staff of the Wake Forest Cardiac Rehabilitation Program has been involved in the development of more than 50 new community programs in North Carolina. The Ottawa Heart Institute Prevention and Rehabilitation Centre has operated phase I through IV programs for 15 years and has formed partnerships to offer cardiac rehabilitation services in community facilities. In our experience, the initiation of a new program involves three initial steps: preliminary planning procedures; patient referral system within the community; and organizational and administrative procedures.

PRELIMINARY PLANNING PROCEDURES

The first step in the preliminary planning is to develop a small nucleus of key individuals who act as a steering committee to determine the scope and nature of the program and to decide on program direction. These individuals should be committed to a comprehensive (multiple intervention) approach to cardiac rehabilitation, and they should have the necessary characteristics (training, credibility, respect) to influence the development of the program within the community. At the very least, this nucleus should include a physician to represent the medical aspects, a cardiac rehabilitation specialist with a vision of the comprehensive nature of the program, and a hospital administrator to advise on the administrative aspects of program development. Subsequently, a board of directors should be assembled who would contribute their expertise in the further development and management of the program. Added to the nucleus would be experts in the fields of finance, marketing, patient care, and legal issues. The board of directors would be expected to meet on a regular basis to provide continued direction to the program. When forming the administrative structure of the program, a program management model should be considered to provide autonomy of budget and staffing.

New programs are also implemented in partnership with existing programs or as extensions of well-established rehabilitation programs. In this case, a joint steering committee should be formed including the program director or a delegate from the existing program and the medical director, program director, cardiac rehabilitation specialist, and facility administrator of the proposed program. From the outset, the responsibilities of the parent organization and the new facility must be clearly outlined in a contractual agreement, including any monetary commitments.

PATIENT REFERRAL SYSTEM
WITHIN THE COMMUNITY

The development of an adequate patient referral system within the community is an often neglected but important factor influencing the eventual success of the program. Because an inadequate referral base is a common cause of program failure, the first step should be an accurate identification of true patient potential. Hospital census data can be reviewed for frequency of cardiovascular-related admissions. Physician focus groups can be assembled to introduce the concept of the cardiac rehabilitation program, receive feedback on the proposal, and determine the physicians' possible interest in referring patients to the program. A word of caution: only a small percentage (10% to 20%) of all eligible patients are eventually enrolled in phase II and III programs because of various reasons related to the physicians (failure to refer through lack of awareness, time, interest, or belief in rehabilitation), to the patients themselves (disinterest, inconvenience, cost, and so forth) or to the program (lack of program flexibility). Medical community rapport is vital for ensuring referrals to the program, and we have found that early efforts at establish-

ing rapport are effective. This would include an introduction of the concept of the proposed program to the local medical society—before any public announcements are made—to inform the medical community first and then to provide an open forum for reactions and suggestions before plans are too well developed to accommodate change. Two essential points must be emphasized to the referring physicians: first, that the program is safe and effective, and second, that the program is an extension of the referring physician's own care and supervision, not a replacement. In our experience, those programs that fail to convince the community physicians on these issues are unlikely to succeed. With managed, capitated health care, the primary care physicians have become the gatekeepers for rehabilitation and secondary prevention programs. The strongest predictor of cardiac rehabilitation participation is the intensity and enthusiasm of the primary physician's recommendation to the patient (3). Efforts spent at informing primary physicians and cardiologists about the safety and benefits of cardiac rehabilitation will strengthen the referral base. The favorable outcomes of cardiac rehabilitation must be communicated not only to physicians, but also to providers, funders, and consumers.

ORGANIZATIONAL AND
ADMINISTRATIVE PROCEDURES

The organizational and administrative procedures form the blueprint for the program. Before opening the program, a manual of operations should be developed by the staff. This document should outline the policies and procedures and provide details on the operation of the program. We have developed such a set of guidelines in North Carolina (4) and have used them in training personnel for emerging phase II, III, and IV programs. Topics included in such a manual are personnel, facilities and equipment, finance and budget, insurance and billing, patient files and records, program evaluation, and procedures for assessment, prescription, therapy, and follow-up. Several of these topics have been included in this chapter as well as in other chapters in this book. Treatment of these topics also can be found in additional references (4–8). We have concentrated on the North American experience; however, interested readers should consult the World Health

Organization (WHO) document on *Rehabilitation After Cardiovascular Diseases* (9) for further information on establishing rehabilitation programs, particularly in developing countries.

Personnel, Facilities, and Equipment

A vital step in the organizational process is the identification of the personnel, facilities, and equipment to be used in the program. These topics are addressed in detail in several other sources (5, 10, 11), and the reader is referred to these for in-depth discussions. The purpose here is to identify the basic principles and outline the program needs in these areas.

PERSONNEL

More than any other factor, the success of a cardiac rehabilitation program depends on the quality of the personnel who comprise the team. At the outset, it should be emphasized that the team should be multidisciplinary in nature to effect the desired outcomes in each patient. Although the size of the staff and their qualifications may vary considerably from one program to another, depending on the size of the program and the nature of the services offered, two central figures must be identified in the developmental stages of program development: the medical director and the program director. These individuals are responsible for the key decisions in hiring other personnel, as well as for providing guidance in developing policies and procedures.

The minimum personnel (as opposed to the ideal number of personnel) and the specific competencies required for the implementation of a multi-intervention program depend on the nature of the program; however, specific recommendations have come from several sources, including national organizations such as the AACVPR (5), American College of Sports Medicine (ACSM) (12), American Heart Association (AHA) (13), state and provincial agencies (14, 15), and others (8). In general, these guidelines provide specific recommendations for the qualifications of personnel, including education, training, experience, licensing, and certification. The personnel and their qualifications that are listed in Tables 22.1 and 22.2 may be considered as a general consensus of these recommendations.

Each program should have a manual of operations that includes all the policies and procedures for the program's operation. A written staff policy is desirable, and it should address the following issues (8):

1. Description of the multidisciplinary team.
2. Identification of their requirements regarding education, experience, certification, and licensure.
3. Description of the essential personal qualities for each position.
4. Continuing education and staff meeting participation.
5. Timetable and guide for evaluation of staff performance.

Certification and Licensure of Personnel

In addition to the hiring of qualified personnel for reasons of quality control, the issue of liability must also be considered (16). In most cases, the state requires that all personnel involved in the practice of medicine (physicians, nurses, physical therapists) or psychology (psychologists) be licensed. However, few states require certification or registry of other personnel, such as exercise specialists or dietitians. Nevertheless, the hiring of the most highly qualified persons would likely reduce the liability risk, and the only nationally recognized certification program for personnel involved in exercise application of preventive and rehabilitative programs is offered by the ACSM. (Information is available from Certification Director, American College of Sports Medicine, PO Box 1440, Indianapolis, IN 46206-1440.) The ACSM offers two certification tracks: the Health and Fitness Track (preventive) and the Clinical Track (rehabilitative). The clinical track is most relevant to rehabilitation and is summarized in Table 22.1. The ACSM is also proceeding with the creation of a registry for Clinical Exercise Physiologists (CEP). The CEP program would have a broader clinical base than the current Exercise Specialist certification in that it would cover all clinical populations. The pilot for the CEP registry is targeted for 1998 with possible implementation in 1999. Although these certifications represent an excellent standard of skill and knowledge, many programs do not mandate certification as a condition of employment. North Carolina is the only state where it is legislated as a pre-requisite. In addition to the requirements and responsibilities outlined in Table 22.1, ideal characteristics of cardiac rehabilitation team members include an ability and enthusiasm to learn, a nonterritorial approach,

Table 22.1 Cardiac Rehabilitation Personnel: Responsibilities

Exercise Test Technologist (ETT)	Preventive/Rehabilitative Exercise Specialist (ESP)	Preventive/Rehabilitative Program Director
The primary responsibility of the ETT is in the administration of an exercise test. In addition to an appropriate knowledge base, the ETT must also demonstrate competence in (1) preliminary patient screening, (2) administering tests and recording data, (3) implementing emergency procedures, (4) summarizing test data, and (5) communicating test results to exercise specialists, program directors, and physicians.	The ESP is responsible for leading exercises for persons who have medical limitations, including cardiorespiratory and related diseases. The ESP should possess the knowledge and skills of the ETT, be able to design an exercise prescription based on the necessary clinical and exercise test results, lead a program of exercise and conditioning, assist in patient education, and interact and communicate effectively with the patient, as well as with the other members of the multidisciplinary team.	Program directors are the key to the success of any rehabilitative program because they have the major organizational and administrative responsibilities within the program. The scope of their duties includes: planning and initiating new programs as well as reorganizing and upgrading existing programs; hiring; staff development through training and continuing education; and supervision of all program personnel. The program director should possess the knowledge and competencies of the ETT and ESP. In addition to the practical skills required for exercise testing, prescription, and leadership, program directors are responsible for program development, including the training and monitoring of the ETTs and ESPs during exercise testing and training. Program directors are often responsible for additional duties, including financial matters (funding, budget, third-party reimbursement), liability, medical/community rapport, marketing, and public relations duties associated with the program.

Table 22.2. Cardiac Rehabilitation Personnel: Qualification

Medical Director	Program Director	Registered Nurse	Exercise Specialist	Nutritionist	Psychologist	Vocational Rehabilitation (VR) Counselor	Additional Personnel
Cardiologist, internist, or other physician licensed to practice in the jurisdiction; experienced in rehabilitative care, graded exercise testing, exercise prescription. The medical director is responsible for all policies and procedures related to medical services and emergencies.	Bachelor's degree in allied health field; experienced in coordination of staff and trained in multiintervention strategies, counseling, educational programs, and all technologies applied to cardiac rehabilitation. The program director is responsible for organizational and administrative aspects of the program and for developing program policies and procedures. The program director should be certified in advanced cardiac life support (ACLS).	Licensed to practice in jurisdiction; experienced in cardiac rehabilitation and emergency procedures; certified in ACLS. The nurse is responsible for patient assessments, developing a plan of care, monitoring patient progress, maintaining medical records, and assisting with medical emergencies. The nurse also acts as an adjunct to the medical director.	Bachelor's degree in exercise science; experienced in exercise testing, prescription, leadership, and supervision; certified in basic life support (BLS). The exercise specialist is responsible for designing and supervising the cardiac exercise therapy sessions in consultation with the medical director.	Bachelor's degree in nutrition; experienced in therapeutic dietetics, especially in areas related to cardiovascular disease (i.e., lipid disorders, hypertension, obesity, and diabetes); registered dietitian (ADA). The nutritionist is responsible for the dietary assessment, prescription, and therapeutic plan for patients in the program.	Licensed to practice in the jurisdiction as a psychologist or psychiatrist; experienced in psychological assessment, counseling, and administration of health behavioral interventions for cardiac rehabilitation patients. The psychologist is responsible for the psychological aspects of the program as well as for consulting with the staff on patient management.	Master's degree in rehabilitation counseling; experienced in vocational assessment, vocational counseling, employer relations, vocational rehabilitation services. The VR counselor also provides vocational assistance to patients regarding work or return-to-work, and advises the staff on rehabilitative matters.	Some programs may be large enough to have additional personnel who have the expertise to provide special services to the patients. These often include the following positions: physical therapist, health educator, occupational therapist, and pharmacist.

an ability to function in a team, a strong clinical sense, and an empathetic nature.

Responsibilities and Qualifications of Personnel

Core competencies for cardiac rehabilitation professionals have been identified by the AACVPR (1), yet these are not universally adopted in all programs. The personnel, responsibilities, and qualifications recommended in Table 22.2 can be considered a consensus of several national, state, and provincial organizations. In addition to the professional staff who provide the multiple intervention services to the patients, all programs require administrative staff to assist with secretarial duties, bookkeeping, billing, and records. Some programs may be large enough to have additional personnel who have the expertise to provide special services to the patients. These may include a social worker, health educator, occupational therapist, or pharmacist. Final personnel decisions are based on local standards of care as well as on such program issues as size and scope of the program, location, budget, and availability of health care professionals. Of primary concern are patient safety and program effectiveness; neither should be compromised in decisions related to personnel.

At the Ottawa Heart Institute, a contact person, or case manager, is identified for each participant. The responsibilities of the contact person are to 1) complete the initial intake assessment including medical history, coronary risk factor profile, and psychosocial concerns; 2) identify the cardiac rehabilitation and secondary prevention issues and, in conjunction with the patient, establish client-centered goals; 3) highlight areas of particular concern that require further evaluation by the medical director; 4) refer the participant to appropriate program services; and 5) review interim and final "progress reports" with clients and establish strategies for long-term lifestyle change. The role of the contact person is performed by any of the following disciplines: a cardiac rehabilitation nurse, physical therapist, vocational counselor, dietitian, or social worker. Each discipline brings a unique set of skills to the role, yet carries out the core responsibilities. We have found this contributes to the development of core skills and knowledge in all disciplines and limits the referral to specialty services to those clients with a definitive need.

FACILITIES AND EQUIPMENT

The facilities and equipment used for the rehabilitation program should be adequate to meet the stated mission of the program and also should comply with guidelines for patient safety established elsewhere by the AACVPR (5), ACSM (12), AHA (10), and the Joint Commission on Accreditation of Healthcare Organizations (JCAHO) (16).

Facility

Facility needs will differ, depending on whether programs are offered at the convalescent (in-hospital phase), early ambulatory and therapeutic (outpatient phase), or long-term program (maintenance phase) level. In any case, the facility should be located conveniently and be readily accessible to both the staff and the participants; otherwise, recruitment of personnel (medical staff in particular) and compliance of patients could be jeopardized. Adequate and affordable parking and access within the facility are important. In addition to the space used for the exercise therapy sessions, office and work space must be provided for administrative personnel and for other interventional components of the program (i.e., space for patient evaluation and counseling). Other considerations include availability of convenient hours of operation if the facility is shared with other groups or programs, adequate space to meet present needs and potential growth, and finally, cost of rental. In our experience, hours of operation should be geared toward the patient population served. Younger, employed clients tend to prefer early morning, noon, or early evening hours to accommodate work schedules. Older, retired or unemployed clients usually prefer morning or early afternoon hours. The more physically limited clients, who have lower energy reserves, will often prefer the early afternoon, finding it more difficult to complete their self-care routines and transportation to the program in time for morning classes and appointments. We have had very limited interest in weekend services, other than special time-limited courses and primary prevention programs.

The recently published work by the ACSM, *The ACSM Health/Fitness Facilities Standards and Guidelines* (11), is the most thorough set of guidelines currently available on the proper standards for facilities that offer exercise programs. These standards have been based on accepted legal, scientific, and operational tenets and cover programming, safety, staffing, facility, and equipment for exercise areas as well as other areas such as lockers, parking, and so forth. Adherence to these standards and guidelines should not only enhance the quality of the program but also minimize the risk of liability associated with negligent behavior (16).

Equipment

The equipment needs are dictated in large part by the program mission, design, and size, as well as by the location of the facility (hospital, outpatient clinic, university, YMCA). Detailed recommendations regarding specific equipment needs cannot be included here but can be found elsewhere (4, 5, 10, 12, 17). Although consideration must be given to the equipment needed for the administrative and multiple intervention (dietary, psychological, vocational, and educational) components of the program, the equipment required for the exercise-related activities (graded-exercise testing and training) is the most extensive as well as the most costly. Briefly, considerations for the latter should include the following:

1. Graded Exercise Testing. If graded exercise testing is conducted as part of the program then the following will be needed:

   Ergometers for specialized testing needs of patients who have specific disabilities or vocational applications (motor-driven treadmill, electronic or manual bicycles, and arm ergometers).

   Electrocardiogram (ECG) and oscilloscope should be multichannel to ensure evaluation of all leads during exercise testing.

   Blood pressure (BP) monitoring equipment (stethoscope and sphygmomanometer) are needed to monitor the hemodynamic response.

   Anthropometric equipment (scale, tape, and skinfold calipers) is needed to assess ideal body weight based on body mass index as well as percent fat; additional equipment is needed to assess body composition for hydrostatic weighing or bioelectrical impedance analysis, but it is not essential.

2. Exercise Program. Most inpatient exercise programs usually require a form of ECG telemetry monitoring and BP measurement to monitor exercise therapy safely. In addition, appropriate audiovisual materials and aids facilitate the educational component. The early ambulatory outpatient and maintenance programs should incorporate exercise equipment that is consistent with the identified level of risk of the patient population. In general, the equipment could include lower extremity devices (treadmills, bicycles, stair climbers, or a walking area), upper extremity devices (arm ergometers, rowing machines), and combined upper and lower extremity equipment (swimming pool, arm and leg ergometers, air walkers, and cross-country ski machines). Resistance training has become an important adjunct to conventional aerobic training, and increasing evidence has shown its value in improving muscle strength and aerobic capacity in cardiac patients (18–20). Choice of resistance equipment will be dictated by the patient's ability and risk stratification. Equipment available includes stretch elastic bands, cuff and hand weights, free weights and dumbbells, wall pulleys, and multistation weight machines. Monitoring of patients can be accomplished with ECG telemetry or spot checks with a defibrillator. The higher the risk level of the patients, the more closely they should be monitored. The need for continuous ECG monitoring is discussed in another section of this chapter.

3. Emergency Procedures. The risk of a life-threatening event is increased during exercise testing or training, making patient safety a primary concern. The recommended equipment and supplies required for a cardiovascular emergency are well documented elsewhere (5) and are treated only briefly here. The equipment and supplies required for a cardiovascular emergency include defibrillator and monitor; airway equipment, oxygen, breathing bag, and suction equipment; and intravenous fluids, intravenous sets and stand, syringes and needles, adhesive tape, and intravenous drugs.

Finance and Budget

At this point, much of the information needed to develop the program budget has been acquired. Program budgets vary widely, depending on whether programs are held within a hospital, university, YMCA, or free-standing facility such as a wellness center. Sample budgets for such programs can be found elsewhere (4, 6, 17). Nevertheless, the first step is to develop a business plan that can be presented to the administrators or board of directors.

THE BUSINESS PLAN

The business plan should contain pertinent information such as the program mission with goals and objectives, the patient population to be served, an organizational chart including personnel, the program services to be offered, and an outline of policies and procedures. A market assessment often is included to ensure an adequate market base for supporting the program and to ascertain whether competition will affect this potential. In addition, a proposed budget should be included that identifies potential sources of income and anticipated expenses. Finally, an implementation plan should outline the developmental stages and expected completion dates. A note should be made here of the role of "volunteer" programs. Many cardiac rehabilitation programs rely on the help of qualified professional volunteers. These programs may not exist if it were not for the efforts and contributions of their volunteer "staff." We believe that to ensure long-term program viability and credibility, volunteer staffing should be limited in time. After demonstration of the value of cardiac rehabilitation, committed funding is a necessity.

THE BUDGET

The budget included in the business plan should reveal a careful study of all anticipated income and expenses. Most new programs require start-up costs that must be incorporated into the budget planning. The start-up costs depend, in part, on where the program is to be housed and how much new equipment must be purchased or rented. If an existing facility and equipment can be shared with other programs, then these costs will be significantly less. Regardless, the start-up costs should be covered with separate funding that does not jeopardize the financial stability of the program during the initial development phase. Often this one-time funding can be obtained by seed money, a start-up grant, or through a separate fund-raising effort. The remaining years should be based on more stable sources of revenue. Although budgets usually are developed for a given fiscal year, the business plan should include an initial start-up budget as well as a 5-year budget plan that demonstrates a progressive movement toward a balanced budget after the first few years of adjustment.

Revenues

The major portion of program revenues most likely will come from third-party reimbursement by insurance carriers (usually 80%), with a lesser portion being supplemented through patient fees (usually 20%). It is therefore critical that reimbursement policies of the most common insurance carriers in the community be reviewed in anticipation of this primary source of income. It is important to determine the extent to which program services are covered under these policies because the financial outlook of the program will depend more on this source of revenue than on any other single factor. One reason is that the majority of patients who enter a rehabilitation program have incurred significant medical expenses before their referral, and most are unlikely to have the ability to cover the full cost of the program. In the best-case scenario, a major medical policy will cover approximately 80% whereas the patient is responsible for the 20% balance. Because not all patients have a major medical policy, a lesser degree of third-party support can be expected. Because of the increasing numbers of older patients being referred to programs, Medicare's reimbursement policy for program services should be examined carefully and then incorporated into all revenue projections, along with a realistic estimation of the proportion of Medicare patients in the total patient population.

Additional Sources of Revenue Additional funds to support program operations and fund new initiatives may be generated through the provision of cardiovascular wellness and disease prevention programs and services. In addition to generating revenue, other benefits to this strategy include enhanced public relations and public image, improved corporate relations, and increased patient referrals to the health care facility and medical staff (21). Services may be provided within the health care facility, space permitting, or within a health club as part of a corporate joint venture. Programs may also be aligned with occupational health services in the worksite, thereby potentially contributing to lowered costs related to absenteeism and expensive medical care for employers. Examples of cardiovascular programs and services with potential for income generation include the following:

- Behavioral modification and lifestyle management services including smoking cessation, fitness, nutrition, weight loss, and stress management courses and clinics.
- Cardiovascular risk appraisal and follow-up.
- Fitness assessments and exercise prescriptions.

- Nutritional analysis and consultation.
- Executive health services.
- Worksite assessment and health promotion services.
- Cardiac maintenance programs for rehabilitation graduates.
- Lecture series.
- Cardiopulmonary resuscitation courses (22).
- Cardiovascular disability assessment and work hardening.
- Educational seminars and training workshops for professionals or the lay public.

Unfortunately many health care facilities' attempts at operating such services have failed to achieve the expected level of revenue production. To generate a profit, a comprehensive business plan must be established. Direct costs, including labor, equipment, and supply expenses, should be considered, as well as overhead costs such as administrative, clerical, and building expenses. Competitors' prices and services and community interest should be reviewed to determine the appropriate level of markup and program feasibility. Segmentation of the target audience into groups such as women and those at high risk of cardiovascular disease can help improve competitive advantage through the provision of services not provided elsewhere. The business plan should identify the health care facilities' strengths to establish program priorities and avoid the problems inherent in overdiversification. Advertising costs can be considerable; therefore, careful thought should go into selecting an effective communication medium and channels and in designing the message. Prevention and rehabilitation services also form a popular platform for a hospital foundation's fundraising efforts.

Canadian Financing of Cardiac Rehabilitation
Health care funding in Canada is obtained from five different sources, including the federal, provincial and local governments, the Workmen's Compensation Board, and private sources, with the relative importance of the source varying according to the province (23). Provinces provide the majority of funding for health care institutions such as hospitals. In general, cardiac rehabilitation programs in Canada do not generate revenue and require a funding source. A cardiac rehabilitation program housed within a hospital environment may be funded from the institution's global provincially based budget but may face stiff competition from other departments for maintaining and expanding resources. Nonprofit cardiac rehabilitation centers located outside of hospitals may have separate funding from the provincial government. Many Canadian programs are partially supported through fund-raising, revenue-generating activities, charitable donations, membership fees, and support from alumni and external organizations to maintain sufficient operating funds and for new capital equipment acquisitions (24).

Expenses

Start-up costs should be determined separately and, whenever possible, fully funded before the program starts. When this is not possible, these expenses can be prorated over several years. The major expense item in most programs with a heavy service component, such as cardiac rehabilitation, is personnel. The minimal personnel required in a multiple intervention program has been identified (5) and depends on whether the program is inpatient, early ambulatory, or maintenance in nature. Few programs are large enough to support full-time personnel in each position, and most staff members are therefore employed part-time, some with their major job responsibilities elsewhere. The nature of the program also dictates the type of facility required and the expenses associated with the facility, such as overhead and maintenance costs. Other expenses to consider are supplies, equipment, staff development, insurance, and miscellaneous costs. Although a balanced budget should be the ultimate financial goal, it is prudent to make a modest profit so that a reserve fund can be established to cover unexpected expenses or emergencies. This amount is not fixed, but a reserve of 10% to 20% of the gross expenses is desirable for most programs. Table 22.3 illustrates a sample budget from a cardiac rehabilitation program that includes phases II and III. This is a budget prepared with the assumption of an enrollment of approximately 50 patients in the rehabilitation program for 1 year, with each patient given laboratory evaluations at entry and at 3, 6, and 12 months. The income and expenditure figures approximate those of representative programs in North Carolina in 1990.

It is recommended that other sources of income be sought to supplement the program budget. Below are reasonable figures for the addition of a phase IV maintenance program for program

Table 22.3.   Sample Budget for Cardiac Rehabilitation Program

Revenues

GXTs (50 patients × 4 GXTs/yr × $300/evaluation)	$ 60,000
Exercise therapy (50 patients × $150/mo. × 12 months)	90,000
Nutritional evaluation (50 patients × $100/initial evaluation)	5,000
Psychological evaluation (50 patients × $100 initial evaluation)	5,000
Total revenues at a 90% collection rate	$160,000

Expenditures

Program director (full-time)	$40,000
MD (supervise 150 exercise sessions $100/session)	15,000
MD (supervise 200 GXTs @ $50/evaluation)	10,000
Administrative assistant (full-time)	15,000
Exercise coordinator (1/4 time)	5,000
Exercise leaders (5 × 150 sessions @ $10)	7,500
GXT personnel (200 GXTs @ $25/GXT)	5,000
Nutritionist (1/5 time)	5,000
Psychologist (1/8 time)	7,500
Total Personnel	$110,000
Supplies and expenses (GXTs, exercise program, administrative)	$ 15,000
Rental fees and overhead	10,000
New equipment expense	5,000
Travel	4,000
Reserve fund (10% of income)	16,000
Total other	$ 50,000
Total Expenditures	$160,000

Table 22.4.   Comparison of Phase II Reimbursement Plans

Service (Full Fee)	HMO #1	HMO #2	BC/BS	Medicare
Laboratory Evaluations ($520 × 2)	$1040	$1000	$832	$380
Dietary Evaluation/Consult ($100)	$100	$90	$80	$0
Psychological Evaluation/Consult ($125)	$125	$115	$100	$0
Exercise Therapy (36 × $22 = $792)	$792	$792	$634	$403
Total Coverage of Plan ($2057)	$2057	$1997	$1646	$783
Percent Coverage of Fees	100%	97%	80%	38%

graduates (n = 25) with charges for an annual graded-exercise testing (GXT) and laboratory evaluation plus a fixed annual fee for the exercise program. In addition, an executive evaluation program of only one evaluation per week would yield the income for 50 additional evaluations.

Maintenance Program	
Annual fee for exercise program (25 patients @ $500/year)	$12,500
GXT and laboratory evaluations (25 @ $300)	7,500
Executive evaluations (50/year (@ $300)	15,000
Extra income	$30,000

These projections are somewhat conservative and could be increased with aggressive marketing. The increased income also could mean the difference between financial success and failure.

MANAGED CARE AND CAPITATION

An increasingly important concern in the development of the budget is the impact of managed care and capitation on program revenues. A decade ago, managed care was practically nonexistent in cardiac rehabilitation; however, in 1997 it was estimated that approximately 85% of the American workforce was enrolled in some form of managed care, up from 77% in 1996 (25). Although a variety of options are available under FFS (fee-for-service) plans such as Blue Cross/Blue Shield and other insurers, the majority of managed care is offered through either an HMO (health maintenance organization) or PPO (preferred provider organization) in which capitation is used to control costs. Future projections are for capitation payment plans to fully replace FFS payment plans by the year 2000 (26). A recent analysis by Hall (27) suggests that the only way that cardiac rehabilitation will survive in the new managed care environment is for programs to track patient outcomes and use effective behavior change to arrest disease progression and manage health care costs effectively. At the present time, the best advice for program directors is to be proactive concerning the reimbursement policies of the major providers in your community. The HMOs will not come to you to negotiate fees; therefore, you will need to contact them and present your plan for managing their patients most

cost-effectively. In our own community, we used this approach with the two HMOs serving the majority of our patients and were able to negotiate full coverage of our university-based phase II cardiac rehabilitation program for 3 months. A comparison of the coverage by these two HMOs versus BC/BS Major Medical and Medicare is presented in Table 22.4. It can be seen that both HMOs cover all costs except a small copayment on consults, whereas BC/BS covers 80% and Medicare covers only 38% of costs for 3 months of phase II cardiac rehabilitation. This program includes a laboratory evaluation on entry and after 3 months, plus dietary and psychological evaluations and consults and 36 sessions of exercise therapy.

OPERATIONS ISSUES

Since the previous edition of this book, cardiac rehabilitation is also viewed as a platform for delivery of secondary prevention services. The critical components of an effective cardiac prevention and rehabilitation program are exercise training, risk factor modification, medical surveillance and emergency support, education, and psychosocial support (28). This combination of strategies forms a "multifactorial" intervention and provides the patient with a menu of services to meet individual needs. The U.S. Department of Health and Human Services reports in their Cardiac Rehabilitation Clinical Practice Guidelines on the outcomes of more than 400 scientific studies of cardiac rehabilitation (2). When exercise is combined with aggressive risk factor reduction, progression of CHD can be slowed and even reversed in some subjects. The evidence clearly demonstrates the benefit of comprehensive, multifactorial cardiac rehabilitation services for optimal patient and program outcomes. Service delivery models should be multifactorial and patient-centered and based on coronary risk factor assessment, risk stratification, and patient goal-setting.

Applying Principles of Risk Stratification and Admission Criteria

Cardiac rehabilitation programs apply the principles of risk stratification to place patients into differing risk categories according to specific criteria. These criteria are also used in the development of patient criteria for admission to phase II and III programs.

RISK STRATIFICATION

Stratification of patients according to level of risk has become necessary to program development. The reasons are twofold: first, the safety of the patient is paramount, and risk stratification provides guidance for the level of patient supervision and monitoring; and second, reimbursement for services depends on the risk level for each patient.

The risk levels and characteristics presented in Table 22.5 have been developed by the AACVPR (5) and are based on the most recent data available in the literature. This information can be obtained from the patient's medical history, clinical course, and related information that should be requested as part of the patient's medical record on referral to the program. These guidelines also should be used to determine the nature of patient supervision and the frequency of monitoring.

Table 22.5.   Guidelines for Risk Stratification[a]

Risk Level	Characteristics
Low	Uncomplicated clinical course in a hospital
	No evidence of myocardial ischemia
	Functional capacity $\geq$ 7 METs
	Normal left ventricular function (EF $\geq$ 50%)
	Absence of significant ventricular ectopy
Intermediate (Moderate)	ST-segment depression > 2 mm flat or downsloping
	Reversible thallium defects
	Moderate to good left ventricular function (EF 35% to 49%)
	Changing pattern of or new development of angina pectoris
High	Prior MI or infarct involving $\geq$ 35% of left ventricle
	EF < 35% at rest
	Fall in exercise SBP or failure of SBP to rise > 10 mmHg on GXT
	Persistent or recurrent ischemic pain $\geq$ 24 hr after hospital admission
	Functional capacity $\leq$ 5 METs with hypotensive BP response or $\geq$ 1 mm ST-segment depression
	Congestive heart failure syndrome in hospital
	$\geq$ 2 mm ST-segment depression at peak heart rate $\leq$ 135 bpm
	High-grade ventricular ectopy

[a]AACVPR Guidelines for cardiac rehabilitation programs. Champaign, IL: Human Kinetics Books, 1991.

PATIENT ADMISSION CRITERIA

The criteria for admission to a phase II or III program should be decided by the medical director, and they depend on several issues, including the mission of the program, the availability of resources, and the reimbursement policy of the third-party carriers in the community. Patients who have one or more of the following diagnoses commonly are admitted to rehabilitation programs (5):

Myocardial infarction (MI).

Angina pectoris (AP).

Postoperative cardiovascular surgery (coronary artery bypass grafting surgery, valvular, and so forth).

Positive GXT or obstructive coronary disease by angiogram.

Percutaneous transluminal coronary angioplasty (PTCA) with or without AP or MI.

Dysrhythmias.

Hypertension with low functional capacity (less than 7 metabolic equivalents [METs]).

Pacemaker.

Chronic obstructive pulmonary disease, renal disease, or diabetes with low functional capacity and dietary or psychological therapy needs (as required).

In addition to traditional subsets of patients listed above, eligibility should be expanded to include coronary patients without residual ischemia, compensated heart failure, cardiomyopathies, non–ischemic heart disease, cardioverter/defibrillator implantation, and cardiac transplantation. On the basis of their comprehensive review, the panel of the Agency for Health Care Policy and Research (AHCPR) and the National Heart, Lung and Blood Institute (NHLBI) concluded that cardiac rehabilitation services are an essential component of the contemporary management of patients with multiple presentations of CHD and with heart failure (2). Improving access to services for currently underserviced groups such as women, racial minorities, and individuals of low-socioeconomic status should be a factor in program development. These groups are at higher risk for subsequent cardiac events or have an increased prevalence of risk factors for CVD (29, 30).

Before admission, it is important that patients' conditions be stable and that they enter the program as early as possible to ensure the likelihood of success. Patients are more likely to be receptive to the lifestyle recommendations of the cardiac rehabilitation staff if contact is made in close proximity to the event (e.g., MI, AP, coronary artery bypass grafting surgery, PTCA). Although no fixed rules exist, patients who have an uncomplicated medical course commonly enter a phase II program within 3 weeks of discharge. Admission to phases III and IV depends on progress and should be decided by the multiple intervention team.

Multifactorial Approach

Cardiac rehabilitation is a multifactorial process that includes exercise training, education and counseling regarding risk reduction and lifestyle changes, and use of behavioral interventions (2). These services can be delivered by a multidisciplinary team or coordinated through a case-management system of care. Both models emphasize a client-centered, goal-oriented approach that results in an individualized rehabilitation plan.

TEAM APPROACH

Under a team approach, various disciplines are allocated specific responsibilities related to their skills, knowledge, and area of expertise. Although there may be overlap and changing roles, each discipline is responsible for delivering one or more component of the multifactorial services. After completion of the initial assessment, which may involve some or all team members, the multidisciplinary members of the cardiac rehabilitation team should meet to address specific pathologic, psychological, nutritional, physiologic, and vocational concerns and to develop a rehabilitative plan. The team approach provides a coordinated effort to the formation of the rehabilitative plan, synthesizing the recommendations from each discipline. By sharing their interpretations with one another, the team develops a unified approach to dealing with the special needs of each patient, including a comprehensive education program and exercise prescription, as well as additional services tailored to patient needs, including weight loss strategies, lipid management, smoking cessation techniques, measures to decrease stress and improve psychological well-being, and vocational counseling (31).

CASE-MANAGEMENT SYSTEM

An alternate system for delivery of multifactorial services is the case-management approach, which entails coordination of a patient's multidisciplinary treatment plan by a single primary care provider. Individuals who commonly provide such comprehensive services include nurses, exercise physiologists, and physical therapists, although professionals providing specialized services, such as dietitians, social workers, psychologists, and vocational counselors who acquire more comprehensive skills and demonstrate the core competencies, could also provide primary care services. Individuals wishing to provide direct primary care to cardiac rehabilitation patients should possess common professional and clinical competencies regardless of their academic discipline. These have been outlined in detail in a position statement of the AACVPR to identify and promote common practice expectations (32). Case-managers are assigned to a specific group of patients (a caseload) and comprehensive risk reduction plans are formulated for every participant, including the establishment of reasonable goals. Results of the comprehensive evaluation are communicated to the patient and referring physician, and referrals are made to other health professionals as indicated. Contact with participants can be in face-to-face interviews or by phone, mail, or e-mail. Generally, there is a combination of direct and indirect contacts, scheduled on a regular basis, including initial intake assessment; formulation of a risk reduction plan with specific target outcomes including an exercise program; review of progress and goal attainment; planned or informal educational sessions; monitoring of client health status; interim and final evaluations of risk factors, functional capacity, and psychosocial status; and an exit interview to implement a long-term plan for risk reduction and maintenance of positive lifestyle changes. This approach has proven to be effective in risk factor modification and reduction in cardiovascular morbidity. The Stanford Coronary Risk Intervention Program (SCRIP) study showed that under a nurse case-managed multifactorial risk reduction program combined with exercise and lipid-lowering therapy the rate of luminal narrowing of the coronary arteries was favorably altered and hospitalizations for clinical cardiac events were significantly reduced (33). Similarly, a physician-directed, nurse-managed, home-based case management system resulted in increased functional capacity, improved lipid profiles, and increased smoking cessation as compared with usual care (34). At the Ottawa Heart Institute, the multidisciplinary team approach has evolved to incorporate a form of case-management in the contact person role, described earlier in this chapter.

Goal Setting and Individualized Programs

The work of Bandura (35, 36), Girdano (37), and others can be used to develop a program of behavior change to help the patient that is based on "outcome" theory. The following represent the major criteria:

1. Identify the problem and turn it into a positive outcome.
2. Break down the outcome into manageable target outcomes.
3. Establish belief that the outcomes, when achieved, will produce the desired results.
4. Identify the resources to learn the necessary skills.
5. Develop an appropriate plan of action.

Ideally, this approach should be used at the initial patient visit and then be updated routinely throughout the patient's course of recovery.

In addition, contemporary cardiac rehabilitation programs should incorporate tailored modifications and motivational strategies to enhance participant interest and adherence to the rehabilitation and risk factor modification plan as outlined by Franklin et al (28). These include assessing the patient's "readiness" for change (38), providing services that are designed to optimize adherence and reduce barriers, keeping goals short term and attainable, recruiting spouse support for the program, and archiving for the patient his or her recorded goal achievements. A sample of an initial action plan is provided in Figure 22.1.

Reports to Referring Physicians and Progress Notes

After the rehabilitative team has met to determine the plan for each patient, this information should be shared with the patient as well as with the patient's referring physicians. It is essential to maintain timely and informative communication between the program and the referring physicians.

Referring physicians need to be informed of the status and progress of their patients in a timely fashion because they have entrusted the program and its staff with that patient's rehabilitation. Failure to keep physicians informed may jeopardize this relationship and ultimately affect future referrals.

REPORTS TO REFERRING PHYSICIANS

Once the rehabilitative plan has been prepared for each patient it should be sent to the patient's referring physician as soon as possible for review. The information contained in the report should be of immediate interest; because of its multidisciplinary nature it often will contain a more comprehensive and thorough evaluation of the patient's lifestyle and risk factors than previously has been conducted. In addition, the referring physician may have concerns about the plan that would need to be addressed with the program staff as soon as possible.

An example of an initial assessment and rehabilitative plan for a new patient in a rehabilitative program is presented in Table 22.6. This example contains a brief review of patient history; an updated cardiovascular risk profile; a summary of the GXT and exercise prescription, along with nutritional, psychological, and vocational assessments; and interventional recommendations. The concluding remarks provide a concise summary of the rehabilitative plan. Enclosed with such a report would be a cover letter from the medical or program director and a more detailed GXT report, including appropriate ECG tracings, as well as a more extensive hematologic report (complete blood count, lipid profile).

PROGRESS NOTES

During the course of a patient's stay in a rehabilitation program, progress notes should be maintained on the patient and the pertinent information should be shared with the referring physician. At the very least, routine reports should go out to the referring physician at the time of repeat evaluations. The guidelines within North Carolina (4) recommend that patients be reevaluated at 3, 6, and 12 months and annually thereafter for patients who remain with a program more than 1 year. The extent of the evaluation varies among programs, but Table 22.7 contains an example of the type of progress notes and summary report that we use in the Wake Forest Cardiac Rehabilitation Program. These

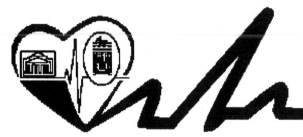

Entry
Heart Health
Risk Profile

Fri, Oct 3, 1997

Health Factor	Your Score	Desirable Level	Action Tips	Notes
Age	39		Risk rises gradually with age; start early to keep all other health factors at desirable level	
Gender	male		Males and post menopausal woman are at higher risk. Keep all other health factors at desirable level.	
Family History of CHD	Yes	No	If yes: • Keep all other factors at desirable level.	
Personal History of CHD or other CVD	Yes	No previous history	• Keep all other health factors at desirable level. • See physician regularly. • Notify physician of any changes in symptoms or new symptoms. • Take medication if prescribed.	
Smoking	quit	None	• Make decision to quit, cut down • Switch to "lighter" cigarettes and determine a "Quit Date" • Make careful preparation for quitting • Ask family and friends for their support	
Blood pressure	104/62	Less than 140/90	• Achieve recommended weight • Exercise regularly at moderate rate • Do not add salt to food • Limit salty snacks and other fast foods • Limit alcohol consumption to 2 or less drinks/day • Drink no more than 4 cups of coffee or caffeine containing beverage/day • Take medication if prescribed	

Figure 22.1. Patient coronary risk profile report and action plan. *CHD,* coronary heart disease; *CVD,* cardiovascular disease; *BMI,* body mass index; *LDL,* low-density lipoprotein; *HDL,* high-density lipoprotein. *continued*

Physical Inactivity	507 kcal/wk (60 min/wk) components: moderate	Exercise regularly 1000–2000 Kcal/wk	• Make active choices in daily living Aim to be active at least 4 to 5 times each week • Choose an activity you enjoy, and find friends to do it with • Develop your exercise program with guidelines from your physiotherapist
Obesity	Weight (kg): 120.7 (265.54 lbs) Height (cm): 176 Calculated BMI: 39 Calculated Goal Weight Range (BMI:27–25): 83.6–77.4 kg (183.92–170.28 lbs)	Body mass index less than 27	• Identify a realistic weight loss goal (10 lb or 4.5 kg) • Strive to lose 1–2 lbs (1kg)/week • Eat 3 meals every day (avoid binge eating and over-eating) • Follow a regular exercise program, aim for 2000 kcal/week of physical activity • Limit snacks to 2–3 per day • Choose low fat, high fiber foods
Food Source	80: Looking good, but there are a few things you can improve.	>81	• Try different types of breads & cereals • Eat all kinds of vegetables & fruits • Choose low-fat dairy products • Remove all visible fat from meats or poultry before cooking • Check with dietitian for guidance • Savor food without adding fats • Avoid deep fried foods
Total Blood Cholesterol	6.4	Less than 4.5 mmol/L	• See Action Tips for Food Score • Savor your food without adding fats • Get regular areobic exercise • Achieve/Maintain recommended wt • Take medication if prescribed
LDL Cholesterol	4.2	Less than 2.2 mmol/L	• See Action Tips for Total Blood Cholesterol
HDL Cholesterol	0.85	More than 1.0 mmol/L	• Avoid smoking • Get regular aerobic exercise • Achieve/maintain recommended wt • Take medication if prescribed
Triglycerides	3.08	Less than	• Achieve/maintain recommended wt

Figure 22.1—*continued.*

	1.8 mmol/L	• See Action Tips for Food Score • Limit alcohol to less than 2 drinks/day • Limit sugars and sources of sugars in diet • Limit servings of fruit to 3/day • Take medication if prescribed
Diabetes	4.8	Blood Glucose less than 6.1 mmol/L	• See Action Tips for Food Score • Achieve/maintain recommended weight • Follow a regular exercise program • Avoid sugars/sources of sugars • Limit fruit to 3 servings a day • Take medication if prescribed • See physician and dietitian for further guidance
Psychosocial factors		Successful coping	• Nurture and build supportive relationships • Practice relaxation and positive thinking techniques • Learn to recognise and manage your stress triggers and your reaction to them

Figure 22.1—*continued*.

Table 22.6. Cardiac Rehabilitation Program Initial Patient Summary

I. History

Mr. Smith is a 67-year-old man with a history of exertional angina and documented three-vessel disease. Coronary angiography revealed 90% occlusion of the left anterior descending coronary artery, 95% occlusion of the circumflex coronary artery, and severe diffuse disease in the right coronary artery.

A. Discharge diagnosis

  1. Three-vessel coronary artery disease
  2. Angina

B. Present medications

  1. Atenolol 50 mg OD
  2. Transderm Nitro OD
  3. Pravachol 40mg BID
  4. Enteric-coated ASA 325mg OD
  5. Nitrolingual 0.4 mg, metered dose spray, PRN

C. Drug allergies

  1. None

II. Cardiovascular risk profile   Exercise response

Age	67 years		
Family history	0 relatives	$\dot{V}O_2max$	4.7 METs
Smoking status	nonsmoker	Resting heart rate	61
SBP/DBP	120/74 mm Hg	Electrocardiogram	
Height	70 inches	Resting	Normal
Weight	208.5 lb	Exercise	+ for ischemia
BMI	29.9 kg/m^2		@ 3.8 METs
Obesity	27.7% fat	FEV_1	73.8% (ABN)
Cholesterol	247 mg/dL	Activity habits	Inactive

continued

Table 22.6. Cardiac Rehabilitation Program Initial Patient Summary

HDL-C	33 mg/dL		(354 kcal/wk)
TC/HDL-C ratio	7.5	Stress and tension	Under control
LDL-C	162 mg/dL		
Triglycerides	232 mg/dL		
Glucose	149 mg/dL		

III. Graded exercise test and exercise prescription

The patient achieved a $\dot{V}O_2$max of 4.7 METs on a treadmill ramp protocol. Maximum heart rate achieved was 134 beats per minute. The exercise ECG revealed onset of significant ST depression at 3.8 METs and a heart rate of 110 beats per minute, reaching a maximum of 2.5 mm downsloping ST depression. The patient experienced typical angina during exercise, the discomfort starting at 3.8 METs. Nitroglycerin was administered and it relieved the chest pain.

Recommendations: The exercise prescription for this patient has been developed to maintain exercise below the ischemic threshold and increase caloric expenditure to facilitate weight loss.

Frequency	5–7 times per week
Intensity	50–60% of the heart rate reserve
	97–104 beats per minute
	2.5–3 METs
Duration	60 minutes
Type	Walking @ 2.5 mph

IV. Lipid management

Lipid profile is total cholesterol, 247 mg/dL; HDL-C, 33 mg/dL (ratio, 7.5); LDL-C, 162 mg/dL; triglycerides, 232 mg/dL; and glucose, 149 mg/dL. The patient was started on Pravachol 40 mg BID 3 months ago and total cholesterol, LDL-C, and triglycerides remain above the desirable level.

Recommendation: The patient has been advised to discontinue the Pravachol and started on Lipitor 40 mg OD. Blood work will be repeated in 6 weeks.

V. Nutrition assessment

This patient weighs 208 pounds (BMI = 30 kg/m^2) and has a weight loss goal of 2 lb per week, or 8 lb in 1 month. The 7-day food record revealed an average daily intake of approximately 2500 calories, high in animal fats and low in vegetables, often skipping breakfast and end-loading calories at the end of the day.

Recommendations: 1) Weight loss of 2 lb/week, 8 lb within 1 month; 2) Balanced prudent diet at 1800 calories distributed evenly throughout the day (3–6 small meals); 3) Recommended diet includes reduction in animal fats (choosing low-fat cheese, skinless poultry, lean meats, skim milk) and addition of useful foods to include more soluble fiber, omega-3 fatty acids and antioxidants (oat bran, lentils, fatty fish, fruits and vegetables); 4) Exercise program with goal of 2000 kcal/week energy expenditure.

VI. Psychosocial evaluation

This patient's evaluation data portray a rather passive person who is moderately depressed in reaction to life's changes that have occurred subsequent to his cardiovascular problems. This patient engages in a moderate degree of denial concerning his cardiovascular condition. His health-related behavior seems to be greatly affected by marital systems dynamics. This patient's wife seems to be overbearing and she monitors her spouse's life, particularly in reference to his health status. This marital system factor is likely to be a significant variable affecting this patient's reaction to cardiac rehabilitation intervention. There are no indications of serious affective disturbance or any thought-processing disturbance in this protocol.

Recommendations: This patient does not want ongoing psychological intervention at this time, but it is felt that he might benefit from family-level counseling if he does not make adequate progress in the normal course of the cardiac rehabilitation program.

VII. Vocational assessment

This patient is retired, has no plans to return to work, and, therefore, no vocational intervention is needed.

VIII. Concluding remarks

Cardiac rehabilitation care plan

1. Moderate level exercise program, 3-days/wk with the Wake Forest Cardiac Rehabilitation Program and 2–4 days/week at home
2. Lipid management: Lipitor 40 mg OD
3. Weight-reducing, low-fat, low-cholesterol diet, 1800 cal/day
4. Repeat evaluation in 3 months

SBP/DBP = systolic blood pressure over diastolic blood pressure; BMI = body mass index; HDL-C = high-density lipoprotein cholesterol; TC = total cholesterol; LDL-C = low-density lipoprotein cholesterol; $\dot{V}O_2$max = maximal oxygen uptake; METs = metabolic equivalents; FEV$_1$ = forced expiratory volume in 1 second; OD = once a day; BID = twice a day; ABN = abnormal; PRN = as required.

Table 22.7. Cardiac Rehabilitation Program

Progress Notes
Name:Mr. Smith   Date of Entry: 98/02/18

GOALS AT ENTRY	(GOAL)	ENTRY	3 MO	6 MO	12 MO
1. Weight loss: 34 lb	(174 lb/ BMI≤25)	208(30)	200(29)	192(28)	
2. Normalize TC/HDL ratio	(<4.5)	5.8	5.5	5.3	
3. Normalize Triglycerides	(<140 mg%)	260	164	135	
4. Improve functional capacity	(>8 METs)	5.6	7.2	8.1	

Progress Notes:

3 months: Mr. Smith has made great progress in his weight loss goal in the first 3 months. He has lost 8 pounds and joined the weight control group. His lipid profile has improved with a reduction in both the TC/HDL-C ratio and triglycerides. He has done well in the exercise program, increasing his exercise capacity by 29%. Mr. Smith will continue in the weight control group and in the exercise program to help with his weight and lipid control.

6 months: Mr. Smith continues to make good progress toward his goals. He has lost an additional 8 pounds and continues to attend the weight control group. With the exercise and weight loss, his lipid profile has further improved. His functional capacity increased to 8.1 METs, a 45% increase over the initial level. Mr. Smith will continue in the program and work toward his goals. Repeat evaluation in 6 months.

12 months:

progress notes are taken during feedback sessions held between the patient and a staff member who reviews that patient's progress based on the most recent evaluation report and then negotiates a continuing plan with the patient.

Patient Education

Patient education can play an integral role in the success of any cardiac rehabilitation program, provided that it is done properly. A primary reason for patient education is to assist the patient with appropriate behavior change. Although we know that knowledge and understanding do not automatically infer compliance, in many cases they can provide a sound theoretical basis for efforts to help patients change their behavior. The patient education program should include family members when possible, and it can be conducted in part at the program site as well as through home assignments.

Program Content

The content of the patient education program varies, depending on the background of the patient and on the phase of rehabilitation. Ordinarily, the phase I (in-hospital) program emphasizes issues of self-care and a general knowledge of warning signs and symptoms, medications, and risk factors. The phase II (posthospital or immediate exercise intervention) program reinforces previous concepts and makes applications to daily living. The phase III (extended outpatient) program

should help the patient maintain positive behavior changes in lifestyle.

Some of the topics to consider are the following:

Phase I: Anatomy and physiology of the heart and vascular system.
Pathophysiology of a heart attack and the healing process.
Warning signs and symptoms.
Medications.
Activity progression during the recovery process.
Safety considerations.

Phases II and III: Management of risk factors through lifestyle modifications of smoking, diet, stress management, and exercise behaviors.
Vocational considerations and return to work.
Medications and surgical intervention.
Sexual activity.
Exercise testing and exercise prescription.
Psychosocial issues in recovery.

Methods of Delivery

The method of delivery of the education program is determined by the patient educator or the multidisciplinary staff. The common methods include books, pamphlets, newsletters, staff lectures, guest speakers, audiocassettes and videocassettes, interactive training programs, and group discussions. Contemporary technologies such as the Internet, CD-ROM educational programs, and computerized interactive learning modules have provided alternative methods of meeting the patient's education needs. A variety of methods will encourage an individualized approach and promote active participation in the educational process. There is a vast amount of information now available to the public on management of cardiovascular diseases, nutrition theories and diet recommendations, and exercise guidelines. The cardiac rehabilitation staff can also function to clarify this information and place it in appropriate context for the patient.

Exercise Program Delivery

Exercise training continues to be the cornerstone of cardiac rehabilitation. To develop a safe, realistic, and effective exercise program for a patient, the exercise specialist conducts a detailed assessment, including exercise limitations (e.g., cardiac symptoms, musculoskeletal conditions, claudication symptoms); pre event and post event exercise habits; and the patient's aerobic capacity and physiologic responses to exercise as determined by exercise testing. There are well-established guidelines for exercise testing and prescription for cardiac patients from the ACSM (39, 40) and the AACVPR (1) that provide further detail. Exercise program operational issues that will be addressed here include delivery models, use of ECG monitoring and safety of exercise rehabilitation.

SUPERVISED VERSUS HOME EXERCISE

The traditional model of cardiac rehabilitation exercise programs includes supervised group exercise, held one to three times per week for a duration of 60 to 90 minutes per session for a predetermined time ranging from 3 to 18 months. Completing the time-designated program is the usual criterion for discharge to the community. Exercise groups vary in size from 5 to 30 or more individuals, depending on the risk level of the participants, their stage of recovery, and their need for monitoring. The majority of cardiac rehabilitation programs operate under this model, which has been the service delivery that has been studied in several clinical trials demonstrating a positive impact of exercise on functional capacity (41, 42), cardiac symptoms (42, 43), and coronary risk re-

duction (44, 45). Supervised programs provide the ability for surveillance of the increasingly complex patients being referred to cardiac rehabilitation, facilitate delivery of education, and enhance social support. This approach has proven to be cost-effective, safe, and efficacious (2); however, it is associated with an increased cost and extended travel time (46).

An alternative to the traditional model of weekly sessions in a closely monitored, structured group format needs to be offered to improve access to cardiac rehabilitation services, further increase cost-effectiveness, support early return-to-work initiatives, and meet patients' desires for independence and flexibility. Home-based exercise rehabilitation for low-risk patients, which is medically directed, has comparable safety and efficacy to supervised group programs (46). Similarly, successful risk reduction programs for smoking cessation and hyperlipidemia have been provided through a home-based, case-managed system (33, 34). A rehabilitation plan is formulated with the patient, including an exercise program, yet carried out by the patient independently at home. A variety of techniques may be used to facilitate monitoring and communication such as telephone contact, mail, fax, e-mail, Internet, and telephonic ECG monitoring (46). At the Ottawa Heart Institute, participants are offered a home-based program as an alternative to the supervised exercise sessions. The home-program participants attend five small group sessions at the Heart Institute during a 6-month period. The initial two sessions consist of review of exercise assessment, stress test results, and exercise prescription and recommendations; instruction in self-monitoring (symptoms, rating of perceived exertion, pulse rate); teaching warm-up and cool-down principles and exercise options; and a "trial" of the exercise prescription to determine a realistic starting point and plan for progression. Participants complete activity log sheets and return for three follow-up sessions, which include an exercise session, interim and final evaluations, review of progress, and introduction of alternative exercise modalities (strength training, calisthenics, stationary equipment). Outcome analysis revealed equal benefits for our home program and supervised class participants in improvement in functional capacity, coronary risk factor reduction, and most health-related quality-of-life parameters (47).

CONTINUOUS VERSUS INTERMITTENT ELECTROCARDIOGRAPHIC MONITORING

An issue that remains controversial is whether patients enrolled in an exercise training program should have continuous or intermittent ECG monitoring. The argument in favor of continuous ECG monitoring is that the safety and effectiveness of the program is enhanced. The arguments against continuous ECG monitoring are that it is costly and ineffective, and it may lead to a patient's dependence on monitoring when independence and self-monitoring skills are primary goals of rehabilitation programs.

In an early review of complications encountered in exercise training of cardiac patients, Haskell (48) reported that programs with continuous ECG monitoring had only one-fourth the sudden death rate of programs that did not monitor. Further analysis of the characteristics of these programs revealed that, in the monitored programs, patients were supervised more closely and they also exercised at a lower intensity. In contrast, a more recent review by Van Camp and Peterson (49), which included four times as many patients as Haskell's study, revealed no statistically significant differences in serious cardiac event between programs with continuously monitored ECG and intermittently monitored patients. Although no random, controlled clinical trial exists to provide a definitive answer to this question, a recent American Medical Association (AMA) poll revealed that a majority of cardiovascular experts still believe that ECG monitoring is essential to the safety and efficacy of exercise programs for cardiac patients (50). This approach has been challenged by Greenland and Pomilla (51), who analyzed the financial aspects of continuous monitoring and concluded that it would cost approximately $1 million in ECG monitoring for a period of 8 years in the hope of preventing just one serious cardiac event.

Given the lack of experimental support for continuous ECG monitoring of patients, it would seem appropriate to determine who should be monitored and how the risks of complications can be reduced. Recommendations regarding ECG monitoring of exercise training have been produced by the AHA (10), American College of Cardiology (ACC) (52), American College of Physicians (ACP) (53), AACVPR (1), WHO (9), and ACSM (39). The ACC criteria for ECG monitoring of cardiac rehabilitation exercise training are shown in Table 22.8. This is a select group of patients who are at high risk, and the medical director should make the judgment regarding the long-term monitoring of these patients, balancing costs versus safety and efficacy of the exercise therapy. It is clear from the table that although safety and efficacy are of primary importance in the planning and implementation of a cardiac rehabilitation program, there is not a clear mandate for continuous ECG monitoring of all patients. Continuous monitoring must be selective and based on proven criteria of high risk. For the majority of others, judicious use of intermittent monitoring and occasional continuous monitoring of select patients would seem to be a prudent compromise.

In Canada, where reimbursement is not linked to the use of ECG monitoring, continuous, or even intermittent, monitoring is less prevalent. Self-monitoring suffices for many low-risk patients exercising at home, in community facilities, and even in hospital-based programs. When telemetry monitoring is available, it is used for a discrete number of sessions, and its indication is then reevaluated. Less costly alternatives such as heart rate monitors are feasible to assess exercise intensity violators and individuals unable to self-monitor heart rate.

SAFETY OF EXERCISE REHABILITATION

Risk in the General Population

Because of the attention that an exercise-related cardiac arrest or death receives in the popular press, the risks often are exaggerated. Although there is a risk of arrest or death during vigorous exercise in both healthy and diseased populations, the true risk is quite low, especially in the former. In fact, the risk of sudden cardiac arrest in the general population is approximately one arrest per 565,000 hours of vigorous exercise (10), whereas the risk of death during vigorous exercise is only about one death per year for every 15,000 to 20,000 healthy men (54). Another consideration is the transient nature of the risk, for although the risk may be higher during the actual period of exercise, it is substantially lower for the remainder of the day. In addition, being physically active affords a certain degree of protection because the overall risk of cardiac arrest for physically active men is only 5 events/10^8 person-hours compared with 18 events/10^8 person-hours in sedentary men (12).

Table 22.8. Characteristics of Patients Most Likely to Benefit From Continuous ECG Monitoring During Cardiac Rehabilitation

1. Severely depressed left ventricular function (ejection fraction $< 30\%$)
2. Resting complex ventricular arrhythmia
3. Ventricular arrhythmias appearing or increasing with exercise
4. Decrease in SBP with exercise
5. Survivors of sudden cardiac death
6. Survivors of MI complicated by CHF, cardiogenic shock, or serious ventricular arrhythmias
7. Severe CAD and marked exercise-induced ischemia (ST-segment depression ≥ 2 mm)
8. Inability to self-monitor heart rate because of physical or intellectual impairment

Risk in Cardiac Patients

The risk of cardiovascular complications during exercise is understandably greater among cardiac patients than among the general population, with cardiac arrest being estimated as being more than 100-fold higher during or soon after exertion in patients who have CHD (55). A major survey of outpatient cardiac rehabilitation programs (49) revealed an incidence rate of one cardiac arrest per 111,996 patient-hours, one MI per 293,990 patient-hours, and one death per 783,972 patient-hours of exercise. It should also be emphasized that the majority of patients who experience cardiac arrests are successfully resuscitated in supervised programs with effective emergency procedures.

In an attempt to determine the possible factors associated with cardiac arrest in exercising cardiac patients, Hossack and Hartwig (56) analyzed 25 arrests that occurred during a 13-year period in a sample of 2464 patients enrolled in a supervised exercise program. They found that although the arrest group demonstrated a higher functional capacity than those who did not experience an event, a greater percentage of the arrest victims also exhibited more serious coronary lesions, greater ischemia during GXT, and poorer adherence to the prescribed heart rate training range.

In an effort to provide recommendations on how the incidence of complications can be reduced in outpatient cardiac exercise sessions, given the higher risk of cardiac events in these patients, Franklin (57) made a number of suggestions, shown in Table 22.9.

Emergency Procedures

In spite of the relatively low incidence of cardiovascular complications during exercise testing and exercise training, when these events do occur in medically supervised programs, the successful resuscitation rate is high, estimated by Haskell (58) as being approximately 90%. In addition to the suggestions already listed for reducing the incidence of events, the most effective defense is a well-trained staff and a well-designed emergency plan.

STAFF QUALIFICATIONS AND TRAINING

The most recent recommendations of the AACVPR (1) regarding certification are that all staff who relate to patient care should be certified in basic life saving and all nonphysician staff who are medically responsible for patients during exercise testing or training be certified in advanced cardiac life support (ACLS), as designated by the AHA (59). In addition to these certified personnel, a further recommendation from AACVPR is that at least one person with current ACLS certification and medicolegal authority to provide such care shall be present whenever directly supervised exercise is provided for high- and intermediate-risk patients. The medical director of a program also is responsible for ensuring that certified staff are in attendance during the operation of the program and that an appropriate emergency plan has been developed.

Table 22.9. Recommendations for Reduction of Complications During Exercise in an Outpatient Program

1. Ensure medical clearance and follow-up, including serial exercise testing
2. Provide on-site medical supervision
3. Establish an emergency plan
4. Use continuous or intermittent ECG monitoring
5. Emphasize appropriate warm-up and cool-down procedures
6. Promote patient education
7. Emphasize strict adherence to prescribed training pulse rates
8. Reduce exercise intensity in "high-risk" patients
9. Maintain supervision during the recovery period
10. Modify recreational game rules and minimize competition
11. Adapt the exercise to the environment

EMERGENCY PLAN

A formal, written emergency plan should be developed that is specific to each program, and it should include the entire facility (gyms, laboratories, lockers and showers, and offices). Because programs often have ongoing activities in more than one site, an effective means of rapid communication must be established to make the emergency team immediately available, because success rates of resuscitation are closely related to the duration between the time of the event and the implementation of emergency procedures. Included in the emergency plan should be an explanation of how the emergency plan is activated, the personnel required, and a detailed description of the specific assignments of each staff member. This would include those directly involved in conducting the resuscitation effort as well as those who have other responsibilities, such as handling other patients in the area and coordinating the effort with the local emergency medical service team for transport of the patient to a medical facility after stabilization. The procedures as well as the equipment involved in the management of a cardiac arrest are explained in detail in the ACLS guidelines (59). In addition, a listing of the necessary emergency equipment, an emergency cart checklist, and sample forms for physician standing orders, the documentation of an emergency, equipment maintenance and calibration records, and a mock code documentation can be found in the AACVPR guidelines (5).

MOCK DRILLS

The importance of mock drills cannot be overestimated. Even the most carefully detailed emergency plans, supported by extensive emergency supplies and equipment, are wasted if the plan is not practiced routinely and the equipment is not in working order. One way to ensure that the plan will be properly executed is to conduct mock drills on a regular basis, followed up by an evaluation and documentation of the drill, as well as holding a daily review of the emergency medications, equipment, and supplies. The frequency of these mock drills has not been established but should be no less than once a month and more often if warranted either by the postdrill evaluations or changes in personnel. Another consideration is the assignment of staff members to their respective roles before the start of the program. A convenient method is the distribution of pins or tags that list the assignments; this ensures that all roles are covered each day and serves as a reminder to the staff member of the specific role for the day.

Program Evaluation

Like all contemporary medical interventions, cardiac rehabilitation services will require documentation of their efficacy and cost-effectiveness to program directors, hospital administrators, HMOs, government agencies, and health insurers. Outcome analysis is an essential component of this process and should include clinical patient-related outcomes, health-related quality-of-life, program-critical indicators, and economic outcomes. This topic is presented in detail elsewhere in this book (chapter 4), and this information will not be replicated here. The reader is also referred to the AACVPR guidelines (1) and Outcome Tools Resource Guide (60). Compiled by the AACVPR Outcomes Committee, the resource guide is a synopsis of the tools currently available for measuring outcomes in cardiac rehabilitation, categorized into health-related tools (morbidity, mortality, and quality of life), clinical tools (physical, psychological, and social functions), and behavioral tools (diet and health education).

A plan for outcome assessment should be incorporated into the implementation strategy of any new program. Likewise, within established cardiac rehabilitation programs, new subprograms (e.g., women's groups, vegetarian or nutrition programs, home-based programs) should not be implemented without an outcome analysis plan. Decisions regarding what to assess should be done prospectively, and methodologies for data collection and analysis should be designed. Tools and tests used should be standardized, with documented validity and reliability. The choice of outcome tools will be dictated by the services the program provides, the objectives of the program, the ease of administration and analysis, and the information requirements of program administrators and governing bodies. Outcomes should be assessed at program intake, at discharge from the program, and, because the maintenance of adaptive behavior change is a critical measure of program success, at a period after program completion, ideally at least 1 year after entry (1). In addition, interim assessment will also provide information on the rate of change and ideal length of programs and important feedback to the patient on progress and goal-attainment.

Outcome measurement is not an optional, but rather an essential, component to program operations. A regular reporting of outcomes, for example quarterly, will facilitate monitoring of service utilization, managing patient care, improving administrative efficiency, and supporting evidence-based decision making and planning.

Standards and Guidelines

From a legal viewpoint, Herbert and Herbert (16) state that "standards of practice might be regarded as benchmark behaviors or actions that are, at least in theory, universally exhibited by properly trained and experienced professionals." Often, only one set of professional guidelines is likely to exist when a single association speaks for those professionals. Unfortunately, in the field of cardiac rehabilitation, several groups have developed separate guidelines for professionals engaged in the various activities associated with cardiac rehabilitation programs. Although it is not feasible to present these standards here in any detail, the characteristics of each set of standards are addressed. Clearly, standards of care in cardiac rehabilitation are needed for several reasons. They can be said to do the following:

1. Provide clear directions for practitioners.
2. Ensure patient safety and program effectiveness.
3. Assist in the evaluation of methods.
4. Promote progress through research.

DEVELOPMENT OF NATIONAL STANDARDS OF CARE IN CARDIAC REHABILITATION

National standards of care in the field of cardiac rehabilitation had not been developed until 1991 with the AACVPR's publication, *Guidelines for Cardiac Rehabilitation Programs* (5). Before that, the only published guidelines for cardiac rehabilitation programs were those adopted by the Greater Los Angeles Affiliate of the AHA in 1978, entitled *Guidelines for Cardiac Rehabilitation Centers,* and the state of North Carolina's Department of Human Resources in 1984, entitled *Rules Governing The Certification of Cardiac Rehabilitation Programs.* These were subsequently revised and approved in 1990. Subse-

quently, in 1995, the U.S. Department of Health and Human Services and the Agency for Health Care Policy and Research in conjunction with the National Heart, Lung and Blood Institute published *Cardiac Rehabilitation Clinical Practice Guidelines* (2). This guideline provides broad recommendations based on evaluation of the scientific evidence pertaining to the various components of cardiac rehabilitation.

Before the publication of such guidelines, which are comprehensive in nature, include all phases of cardiac rehabilitation, and incorporate the multidisciplinary nature of cardiac rehabilitation, other professional organizations published more narrowly focused guidelines on GXT and exercise prescription.

AMERICAN COLLEGE OF SPORTS MEDICINE

In 1975, the ACSM published the first edition of its *Guidelines for Exercise Testing and Prescription.* These guidelines recently have been revised in the fifth edition (39). The original guidelines focused primarily on exercise testing and exercise prescription for cardiac patients and the general and specific learning objectives for the personnel responsible for conducting GXTs and for implementing the exercise prescription. The most recent edition covers other areas in more detail, including an expansion to include preventive programs, both health/fitness and clinical tracks of personnel certification, and recommendations concerning behavioral change and administration. In addition, in 1994, the ACSM released a position stand on exercise for patients with coronary artery disease, which concluded that most patients with coronary artery disease should engage in individually designed exercise programs to achieve optimal physical and emotional health.

AMERICAN HEART ASSOCIATION

In 1972, a committee on exercise for the AHA produced a monograph, *Exercise Testing and Training of Apparently Healthy Individuals: A Handbook for Physicians;* subsequently, in 1975, the same committee developed a second handbook, *Exercise Testing and Training of Individuals With Heart Disease or at High Risk for Its Development;* both documents addressed the issues of exercise testing and training but failed to deal with the multidisciplinary efforts associated with cardiac rehabilitation programs. In 1979, the AHA published a collection of reprints from *Circulation* under the title *The Exercise Standards Book.* There were four separate articles that dealt with adult exercise testing laboratories, exercise testing equipment, cardiovascular exercise treatment programs, and supervised cardiovascular exercise maintenance programs. In 1986, the AHA, in conjunction with the ACC, published the "Guidelines for Exercise Testing" in the *Journal of the American College of Cardiology.* This dealt specifically with the use of GXTs in the medical management of patients who had cardiovascular disease. Additional guidelines from the AHA, published in 1990 in *Circulation,* were an update of previous standards and were entitled "Exercise Standards: A Statement for Health Professionals From the American Heart Association" (10). This report provides detailed standards and guidelines for exercise testing and training of persons free of clinical manifestations of cardiovascular disease and those with known cardiovascular disease. These standards and guidelines coincide with a position statement published in the same issue of *Circulation,* "Clinical Competence in Exercise Testing" (13), to assist in the assessment of physician competence on a cardiovascular procedure-specific basis. Two years later, the AHA released a second "Position Statement on Exercise: Benefits and Recommendations for Physical Activity Programs for All Americans" (61). This documented the scientifically proven benefits of exercise and the implementation and promotion of physical activity by various key groups and stakeholders. Cardiac rehabilitation and its multifactorial approach was emphasized in a 1994 AHA position statement, which stated that "cardiac rehabilitation is standard care that should be integrated into the overall treatment plan of patients with [coronary artery disease]" (62). In keeping with the contemporary concept of cardiac rehabilitation programs as secondary prevention service providers, another AHA statement on "Preventing Heart Attack and Death in Patients With Coronary Disease" will provide programs with a guide to comprehensive coronary risk reduction including the risk intervention, desired outcome or goal, and recommended implementation strategies (63). This guideline to optimal risk factor management is nicely summarized in a one-page table and serves as an easy reference guide for clinical practice.

AMERICAN ASSOCIATION OF CARDIOVASCULAR AND PULMONARY REHABILITATION

In 1991, the AACVPR published its *Guidelines for Cardiac Rehabilitation Programs* (5). These guidelines were the first comprehensive national guidelines that contained recommendations for the multidisciplinary approach to cardiac rehabilitation. These were updated in 1995 (1) and form an authoritative, detailed publication addressing the structure and organization of cardiac rehabilitation programs, including staffing requirements, record keeping, documentation, facilities and equipment, management of emergencies, and outcome assessment. Revision of these guidelines is underway, with a targeted release date in 1998. Because these are the most recent guidelines and standards available and because they address the multidisciplinary aspects of cardiac rehabilitation, it would seem prudent for programs today to adopt them as completely as possible.

U.S. DEPARTMENT OF HEALTH AND HUMAN SERVICES

In late 1995, clinical practice guidelines for cardiac rehabilitation were developed by a multidisciplinary, private sector panel comprised of health care professionals and consumer representatives sponsored by the Agency for Health Care Policy and Research and the National Heart, Lung and Blood Institute. An explicit science-based methodology was used along with expert clinical judgment to develop specific statements on comprehensive, long-term cardiac rehabilitation. These clinical practice guidelines recommend that comprehensive rehabilitation programs be the standard of care and include individualized exercise training lasting at least 12 weeks; counseling for stress management, smoking cessation, and heart-healthy nutrition; and education on coronary risk factor and lifestyle management. This extensive review has provided the most comprehensive foundation for evidence-based practice in cardiac rehabilitation (2) and as such is an invaluable tool for groups proposing new or expanded programs.

CANADIAN CARDIOVASCULAR SOCIETY

In 1991 (64) the Canadian Cardiovascular Society published a consensus report on the management of post-MI patients, with an update released in 1995 (65). These guidelines contained 15 rehabilitation-related recommendations in the areas of exercise, risk factor and lifestyle modification, management of dyslipidemias, and psychosocial factors.

NORTH CAROLINA ASSOCIATION OF CARDIOVASCULAR AND PULMONARY REHABILITATION

Few states have become involved in the adoption of specific standards and guidelines for programs within that state. In 1984, North Carolina became the first state to adopt a set of certification procedures for outpatient programs of cardiac rehabilitation. These procedures, *Rules Governing the Certification of Cardiac Rehabilitation Programs* (15), were adopted by the Department of Human Resources and were ratified by the General Assembly. Each cardiac rehabilitation program in North Carolina requires an extensive certification assessment within the first few months of its operation, and then an abbreviated recertification review is conducted in alternate years. The rules were developed by staff members of the existing programs and were based on the existing standards of the AHA and ACSM. The 1990 rules are available from the North Carolina Department of Human Resources, Division of Facility Services—Licensure Section, 701 Barbour Drive, Raleigh, NC 27603.

HEART AND STROKE FOUNDATION OF BRITISH COLUMBIA AND YUKON

British Columbia became the first province in Canada to formulate guidelines for cardiac rehabilitation programs in 1997. Specific recommendations for program candidates, risk stratification, intake assessment, exercise prescription, staff requirements, and safety and emergency procedures are outlined for phase II, III, and IV programs. The ACSM and AACVPR guidelines are considered to be companion documents to the British Columbia guidelines (14).

BENEFITS OF STANDARDS AND GUIDELINES

Many benefits can be accrued from the development and the eventual adoption of guidelines and standards of care for programs of cardiac rehabilitation. These include, among others, an upgrade in quality of patient care; increased program effectiveness because of a comprehensive, multidisciplinary approach; quality assurance; improved emergency procedures and patient safety; and reduced liability and risk of litigation.

Critical Factors for Continuing Success

Despite the growing interest in cardiac rehabilitation, professionals working in the field should not become complacent in assuming that adhering to guidelines assures program success. Careful planning and regular program evaluation are vital to continued viability. The key organizational and management factors that contribute to long-term program success are responsiveness to needs identified through outcome assessment by strategic planning, program development, and restructuring; maximizing access to program services including traditionally underserved groups; informing the public, primary care physicians, hospital administrators, health insurers, and government sectors as to the need, benefit, and cost-effectiveness of the cardiac rehabilitation program; providing a menu of multifactorial cardiac rehabilitation services and not restricting the program to exercise alone; incorporating strategies that improve patient motivation and long-term adherence to lifestyle modifications; and developing the cardiac rehabilitation program into a structured secondary prevention service that includes exercise programming, lipid management, and other risk factor modification components. The profile of cardiac rehabilitation programs can be increased by active involvement in research, peer-reviewed publications, wide-reaching media mentions, participation in national and international cardiac rehabilitation organizations and projects, and academic affiliations such as training of allied health professionals and university appointments for staff. Within communities, cardiac rehabilitation services should be integrated into the comprehensive care of cardiac patients, and coordination of phase I–IV components should provide a seamless continuum of care.

References

1. American Association of Cardiovascular and Pulmonary Rehabilitation. Guidelines for cardiac rehabilitation programs. 2nd ed. Champaign, IL: Human Kinetics, 1995.
2. Wenger N, Froelicher E, Smith L, et al. Cardiac rehabilitation. Clinical Practice Guideline No. 17. Rockville, MD: US Department of Health and Human Services, Public Health Service, Agency for Health Care Policy and Research, and the National Heart, Lung and Blood Institute, 1995.
3. Ades P, Waldmann M, McCann W, et al. Predictors of cardiac rehabilitation participation in older coronary patients. Arch Intern Med 1992;152:1033–1035.

4. Cardiac Rehabilitation Staff. Organizational guidelines for cardiac rehabilitation programs in North Carolina. Winston–Salem, NC: Wake Forest University, 1990.

5. American Association of Cardiovascular and Pulmonary Rehabilitation. Guidelines for cardiac rehabilitation programs. Champaign, IL: Human Kinetics, 1991.

6. Wilson P, Fardy P, Froelicher V. Cardiac rehabilitation, adult fitness, and exercise testing. Philadelphia: Lea & Febiger, 1981.

7. Peterson LH, ed. Cardiovascular rehabilitation. A comprehensive approach. New York: Macmillan Publishing, 1983.

8. Pashkow F, Pashkow P, Schafer M. Successful cardiac rehabilitation. Loveland, CO: Heartwatcher Press, 1988.

9. Report of a WHO Expert Committee. Rehabilitation after cardiovascular diseases, with special emphasis on developing countries. WHO Technical Report Series, No. 831, 1993, Geneva.

10. Fletcher GF, Froelicher VF, Hartley LH, et al. Exercise standards: a statement for health professionals from the American Heart Association [special report]. Circulation 1990;82:2286–2322.

11. American College of Sports Medicine. The ACSM health/fitness facilities standards and guidelines. Champaign, IL: Human Kinetics, 1992.

12. American College of Sports Medicine. Guidelines for exercise testing and prescription. 4th ed. Philadelphia: Lea & Febiger, 1991.

13. Clinical competence in exercise testing. A statement for physicians from ACP/ACC/AHA task force on clinical privileges in cardiology. Journal of American College of Cardiology 1990,16(5): 1061-1065.

14. Guidelines for cardiac rehabilitation programs in British Columbia. Vancouver, BC: Heart and Stroke Foundation of BC and Yukon, 1997.

15. Division of Facility Services. Rules governing the certification of cardiac rehabilitation programs. Raleigh, NC: North Carolina Department of Human Resources, 1990.

16. Herbert DL, Herbert WG. Legal aspects of preventative and rehabilitative exercise programs. 2nd ed. Canton, OH: Professional Reports Corp, 1989.

17. Patton RW, Grantham WC, Gerson RF, et al. Developing and managing health/fitness facilities. Champaign, IL: Human Kinetics, 1989.

18. Stewart K, Mason M, Kelemen M. Three year participation in circuit weight training improves muscular strength and self-efficacy in cardiac patients. J Cardpulm Rehabil 1988;8:292–296.

19. McCartney N, McKelvie R, Haslam D, et al. Usefulness of weightlifting training in improving strength and maximal power output in coronary artery disease. Am J Cardiol 1991;67:939–945.

20. Kelemen M. Resistance training safety and essential guidelines for cardiac and coronary prone patients. Med Sci Sports Exerc 1989;21:675–677.

21. Sol N. Revenue benefits of health promotion. In: Sol N, Wilson P, eds. Hospital health promotion. Champaign, IL: Human Kinetics, 1989:63.

22. Aguiar C. Overall benefits of health promotion to hospitals. In: Sol N, Philip K, eds. Hospital health promotion. Champaign, IL: Human Kinetics, 1989:71.

23. Sutherland R, Fulton J. Health care: a description of health care in Canada. The Health Group, Ottawa, Canada, 1992.

24. Profiles of six cardiac rehabilitation programs in Canada. Canadian Association of Cardiac Rehabilitation: second annual symposium proceedings. Ottawa, Canada, 1992.

25. Mercer/Foster Higgins National Survey of Employer-Sponsored Health Plans. New York: William M. Mercer, 1997.

26. Jordan B. Contracting: financial and service matrix. In: Ott R, Tanner T, Henderson B, eds. Managed care and the cardiac patient. St. Louis: Mosby, 1995.

27. Hall L. Will my cardiac rehabilitation program survive in the new managed-care era? The road map will be drawn by measuring outcomes. J Cardpulm Rehabil 1998;18:9–16.

28. Franklin B, Hall L, Timmis G. Contemporary cardiac rehabilitation services. Am J Cardiol 1997;79:1075–1077.

29. Balady G, Fletcher B, Froelicher E, et al. Cardiac rehabilitation programs: a statement for healthcare professionals from the American Heart Association. Circulation 1994;90:1602–1610.

30. Cannistra L, Balady G, O'Malley C, et al. Comparison of the clinical profile and outcome of women and men in cardiac rehabilitation. Am J Cardiol 1992;69: 1274–1279.

31. Dafoe W, Huston P. Current trends in cardiac rehabilitation. Can Med Assoc J 1997;156:527–532.

32. Southard D, Certo C, Comoss P, et al. Core competencies for cardiac rehabilitation professionals. J Cardpulm Rehabil 1994;14:87–92.

33. Haskell W, Alderman E, Fair J, et al. Effects of intensive multiple risk factor reduction on coronary atherosclerosis and clinical cardiac events in men and women with coronary artery disease: the Stanford Coronary Risk Intervention Project (SCRIP). Circulation 1994;89:975–990.

34. DeBusk R, Miller N, Superko H, et al. A case-management system for coronary risk factor modification after acute myocardial infarction. Ann Intern Med 1994;120:721–729.

35. Bandura A. Social learning theory. Englewood Cliffs, NJ: Prentice-Hall, 1977.

36. Bandura A. Self-efficacy: toward a unifying theory of behavioral change. Psychol Rev 1977;84:191–215.

37. Girdano DA, Dusek DE. Changing health behavior. Scottsdale, AZ: Gorsuch Scarisbrick, 1988.

38. Prochaska J, DiClemente C. Common processes of change in smoking, weight control, and psychological distress. In: Shiffman S, Wills T, eds. Coping and substance abuse. San Diego: Academic Press, 1985:345–363.

39. American College of Sports Medicine's guidelines for exercise testing and prescription. 5th ed. Baltimore: Williams & Wilkins, 1995.

40. American College of Sports Medicine position stand: exercise for patients with coronary artery disease. Med Sci Sports Exerc 1994;26:i-v.

41. Foster C, Pollock M, Anholm J, et al. Work capacity and left ventricular function during rehabilitation after myocardial revascularization. Circulation 1984;69: 748–755.

42. Froelicher V, Jensen D, Genter F, et al. A randomized

trial of exercise training in patients with coronary artery disease. JAMA 1984;252:1291–1297.

43. Ehsani A, Heath G, Hagberg J, et al. Effects of 12 months of intense training on ischemic ST-segment depression in patients with coronary artery disease. Circulation 1981;64:1116–1124.

44. Kallio V, Hamalainen H, Hakkila J, et al. Reduction in sudden deaths by a multifactorial intervention programme after acute myocardial infarction. Lancet 1979;2:1091–1094.

45. Schuler G, Hambrecht R, Schlierf G, et al. Regular physical exercise and low-fat diet: effects of progression of coronary artery disease. Circulation 1992;86:1–11.

46. DeBusk R, Haskell W, Miller N, et al. Medically directed at-home rehabilitation soon after uncomplicated acute myocardial infarction: a new model for patient care. Am J Cardiol 1985;55:251–257.

47. Morrin L, Mayhew A, Reid R, et al. Home vs. supervised exercise programs: do participant characteristics and outcomes differ [abstract]? J Cardpulm Rehabil 1997;17:354.

48. Haskell WL. Cardiovascular complications during exercise training of cardiac patients. 1978;57:920–924.

49. Van Camp SP, Peterson RA. Cardiovascular complications of outpatient cardiac rehabilitation programs. JAMA 1986;256:1160–1163.

50. Diagnostic and therapeutic technology assessment (DATTA): coronary rehabilitation services. JAMA 1987;258:1959–1962.

51. Greenland P, Pomilla PV. ECG monitoring in cardiac rehabilitation: is it needed? Physician Sportsmed 1989;17:75–82.

52. Parmley W. Position report on cardiac rehabilitation: recommendations of the American College of Cardiology on cardiovascular rehabilitation. J Am Coll Cardiol 1986;7:451–453.

53. American College of Physicians, Health and Policy Committee. Cardiac rehabilitation services [position paper]. Ann Intern Med 1988;109:671–673.

54. Thompson P. The safety of exercise testing and participation. In: American College of Sports Medicine's resource manual for guidelines for exercise testing and prescription. Philadelphia: Lea & Febiger, 1988: 273–277.

55. Cobb LA, Weaver WD. Exercise: a risk for sudden death in patients with coronary heart disease. J Am Coll Cardiol 1986;7:215–219.

56. Hossack KF, Hartwig R. Cardiac arrest associated with supervised cardiac rehabilitation. J Cardiac Rehabil 1982;2:402–408.

57. Franklin BA. Safety of outpatient cardiac exercise therapy: reducing the incidence of complications. Physician Sportsmed 1986;14:235–248.

58. Haskell WL. Safety of outpatient cardiac exercise programs: issues regarding medical supervision. In: Franklin BA, Rudenfire M, eds. Clinics in sports medicine. Philadelphia: WB Saunders, 3(2): 455-469, 1984.

59. American Heart Association. Textbook of advanced cardiac life support. Dallas, TX: American Heart Association, 1987.

60. American Association of Cardiovascular and Pulmonary Rehabilitation outcome tools resource guide. Middleton, WI: American Association of Cardiovascular and Pulmonary Rehabilitation.

61. Fletcher G, Blair S, Blumenthal J, et al. Statement on exercise: benefits and recommendations for physical activity programs for all Americans.. A statement for health professionals by the Committee on Exercise and Cardiac Rehabilitation of the Council on Clinical Cardiology, American Heart Association. Circulation 1992;86:340–344.

62. Balady G, Fletcher B, Froelicher E, et al. Cardiac rehabilitation programs: a statement for healthcare professionals from the American Heart Association. Circulation 1994;90:1602–1610.

63. Smith S, Blair S, Criqui M, et al. Preventing heart attack and death in patients with coronary disease. Circulation 1995;92:2–4.

64. Fallen EL, Armstrong P, Cairns J, et al. Report of the Canadian Cardiovascular Society's consensus conference on the management of the postmyocardial infarction patient [review]. Can Med Assoc J 1991;144: 1015–1025.

65. Fallen E, Cairns J, Dafoe W, et al. Management of the postmyocardial infarction patient: a consensus report—revision of 1991 CCS guidelines. Can J Cardiol 1995;11:477–486.

Program Models for Cardiac Rehabilitation

William A. Dafoe, Sharon Lefroy, Fredric J. Pashkow, Peg L. Pashkow, Kathy A. Berra, William L. Haskell, Hank L. Brammel, and George Gey

As discussed in chapter 1, cardiac rehabilitation consists of all the activities that help a cardiac patient achieve the best possible physical, medical, and social potential. Cardiac rehabilitation programs have developed in various settings, such as health care institutions, home-based programs, and community-based and industry-based programs. Each model has certain core elements that are important for a cardiac rehabilitation program, but much diversification exists considering various administrative structures that may predate the program. The models that follow represent some of the various ways that cardiac rehabilitation can be delivered. Since the previous edition of this text, program models have evolved to reflect the incorporation of both primary and secondary prevention.

Part A. Institution-based
William A. Dafoe and Sharon Lefroy

Cardiac rehabilitation programs that are established in new or existing health care institutions need to address a number of important issues. Other details regarding general issues can be found in chapter 22. This section addresses the concept of a cardiac rehabilitation program in an institution that uses the University of Ottawa Heart Institute as one particular model.

THE UNIVERSITY OF OTTAWA HEART INSTITUTE PREVENTION AND REHABILITATION PROGRAM

The University of Ottawa Heart Institute Prevention and Rehabilitation Program (HIPRC) is a multidisciplinary prevention and rehabilitation program that began in 1983. Figure 23.1 outlines all the different facets of the various prevention and rehabilitation programs. The Heart Institute is a freestanding structure devoted to the prevention, investigation, treatment, and rehabilitation of persons with cardiovascular disease. It is physically attached to the Ottawa Civic Hospital, a large tertiary care center. The physical structure includes 125 beds, a surgical and medical intensive care unit (ICU), and a day care unit for short-stay referrals from other hospitals. The cardiac operating rooms, catheterization suites, noninvasive laboratories, outpatient clinics, radiological facilities, pharmacy services, and the prevention and rehabilitation center are all housed in the same building.

Physical Description

The physical facilities of HIPRC are located on the second floor of the Heart Institute, providing ready access for inpatients and outpatients alike. There is a large open area surrounded by a four-lane walking and jogging track. Exercise equipment includes bicycle and rowing ergometers, a treadmill, free weights, and a multistation gym for strength training. Other physical therapy and occupational therapy equipment is available for cardiac patients who have other neurologic or orthopedic problems. A control desk is used for telemetry units, participant exercise records, and the resuscitation equipment. Emergency and cardiac arrest alarm systems summon medical personnel from within the building, should the need arise. Offices, change rooms, and a conference room are located around the periphery of the track area. A separate area, entitled *Heart*

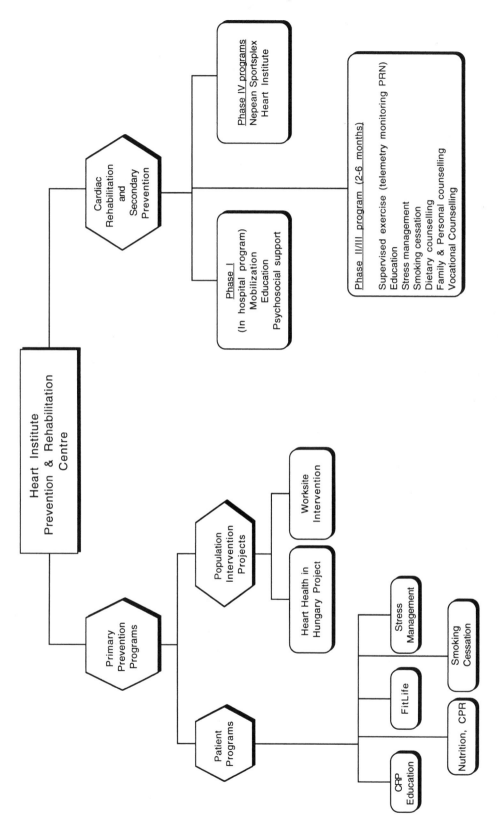

Figure 23.1. University of Ottawa Heart Institute Prevention and Rehabilitation Program.

Check, is responsible for all of the various primary prevention programs.

Prevention and Rehabilitation Team

The HIPRC team involves representatives from the phase I (in-hospital), phase II–III (outpatient program), phase IV (a maintenance program), and prevention programs. The team consists of the following disciplines: medicine, nursing, physical therapy, social work, psychology, vocational counseling, exercise physiology, occupational therapy, and dietetics. Certain staff are involved with all four phases of cardiac rehabilitation. For example, the physical therapists have rotations that involve inpatient and outpatient care. The allocation of responsibilities for the Ottawa Heart Institute team evolved during the first 2 years of the program. The process continues to be dynamic as interests change, the participants in the various disciplines change, and subprograms are modified. Areas of overlap need to be acknowledged. For example, the psychologist or the social worker may help treat a patient who has family difficulties; however, the perspective used by these different disciplines may vary.

At the outset of the program, it was important for there to be specific assignments for all staff members. The responsibilities of each member need not be absolute because there is a learning curve for the development of the program. Certain responsibilities also may depend on the type of people hired. For example, in the HIPRC program, certain team members develop interests in other program aspects. For example, the stress management program is coordinated by the psychologist and has other disciplines as co-therapists. It is important to retain a certain degree of flexibility with regard to matching different program components with the training of various disciplines. Exercise specialists have emerged from a number of different disciplines. As staff acquire experience in cardiac rehabilitation, they may wish to assume different responsibilities that may overlap with another discipline. An exercise specialist becomes proficient with respect to the interpretation of electrocardiograms, and expresses interest in assuming responsibility for telemetered interpretation. This allocation of responsibilities needs to be considered within the constraints of each organizational setting. Most hospitals have clear guidelines regarding the professions that can and cannot monitor patients.

For the first 10 years, the HIPRC team used the matrix model of administration with staff having accountability to discipline-related departments and to the program. With the restructuring of hospital departments, a new program model was formulated. The medical director is responsible for the team functioning and all aspects related to program function. An administrative management team is responsible for day-to-day program management. Evaluations of staff are a conjoint responsibility of the program director and a discipline leader.

Prevention and Rehabilitation Program
PHASE I

The phase I program consists of the mobilization and education components characteristic of most in-hospital programs. The phase I staff are now part of the HIPRC, and thus, the artificial barriers between inpatient and outpatient responsibilities have been obviated. The mobilization program commences with cardiac care unit (CCU) activities in the 1- to 2-metabolic equivalent (MET) range and ward activities in the 2- to 3-MET range. Before discharge, patients should climb one flight of stairs successfully. High-risk surgical patients are seen preoperatively by a physical therapist for preparatory training. During hospitalization there is an educational class for all appropriate surgical and medical patients. One of the most popular classes for the surgical patients is held in the rehabilitation track area. The change in setting from the ward and the introduction to the rehabilitation milieu set the stage for the next phases. On discharge, all patients receive education material and discharge teaching related to medications, appropriate activity, and signs and symptoms to watch. Should any concerns arise, a nursing care coordinator can be paged at the Heart Institute 24 hours a day.

During the phase I period, some patients require the expertise of other rehabilitation staff (e.g., vocational counselor) who may traditionally work with the outpatient program. Such participants might include those with a prolonged hospitalization, those with a number of psychosocial problems, or those with specific vocational concerns. Patients who have other rehabilitation problems, such as cerebrovascular accidents or amputations, are also seen by cardiac rehabilitation personnel. Initial general rehabilitation is provided, and once stabilized, the patient may be transferred to the regional rehabilitation center or to an appropriate community facility. Cardiac rehabilitation personnel play a key role in patient management and planning.

PHASE II/III

All patients are referred by their own cardiologist, surgeon, or family physician. In 1996, the intake procedure underwent a significant restructuring to increase the program intake, lessen the time required for evaluation, and revamp the education sessions. The new protocol requires patients to complete a questionnaire at home and then attend two educational workshops at the Heart Institute. Various outcome indicators, including risk factors and quality-of-life measurements, are measured at intake and on graduation. Patients receive a binder with educational materials and an individualized risk factor assessment. Each patient is assigned a "contact person" who functions as a case manager for the patient through the program. After the two initial workshops, patients are seen for a medical consultation. Common medical issues can include treatment for elevated lipids, dyspnea, depression, and concomitant cardiovascular problems. Any further medical evaluations are initiated at this point with appropriate consultations with the referring physician. Depending on the issues, patients may be seen by specialized cardiac rehabilitation services including dietetics, psychology, social work, or vocational counseling services.

EXERCISE PROGRAM

Exercise programs are coordinated by the physical therapy staff. After the initial evaluation, participants are assigned to an appropriate exercise class. These classes include a phase II class for recently discharged patients; a phase IIIA class for those who have complicated medical histories or who are unable to exercise at moderately high intensities; a phase IIIB class for patients with a good functional capacity; or a low-intensity class (LIC) for patients with an exercise capacity below 3 to 4 METs. The average participant attends the program for 6 months; however, the duration can be extended if the participant and contact staff person feel that further goal attainment is warranted.

Stress tests (if deemed appropriate) are performed at program entry and at discharge. Most stress tests are performed using a metabolic cart and a ramp protocol. The modified Borg scale from 0 to 10 is used for the stress test and during the exercise classes. The exercise prescription is devised using the Karvonen method with an exercise intensity from 50% to 80% of the heart rate (HR) reserve. Telemetry monitoring during exercise is used for high-risk participants according to published guidelines. Reimbursement for cardiac rehabilitation in Canada is not contingent on monitoring.

Safety aspects are addressed by the usual standards of resuscitation and emergency equipment. The hospital departments who manage all arrest carts and defibrillators take responsibility for the rehabilitation equipment. All staff must maintain basic cardiac life support (BCLS) training, and mock arrests are held regularly. Any medical problem during exercise is recorded as a "medical event." All incidents are reviewed by the medical director.

Low-risk and motivated patients may pursue a home exercise program. Because most of the exercise is at home, attendance at the Heart Institute is required only for educational workshops, a stress test, and follow-up classes at 1, 3, and 6 months. Telephone contact is maintained to monitor progress, and patients are asked to complete exercise log sheets.

EDUCATION

The education program is coordinated by the nursing staff. Participants have individual sessions to discuss specific aspects of their disease or medications. Didactic sessions, using either a lecture or video format, are presented as part of the program entry workshops. These sessions cover all aspects of risk factors, the disease process, and the components of rehabilitation. Other disciplines include education in their particular subprograms or individual counseling.

FAMILY SUPPORT

Adult family members are encouraged to come to the introductory workshops. Spouses are provided with resource material appropriate to the disease entity. Families or family members who are having significant difficulties may be seen by the team social worker or psychologist, or in consultation with the liaison psychiatrist.

PSYCHOSOCIAL ISSUES

All participants are screened at intake for psychosocial problems that may impede an effective rehabilitation program. The screening consists of an interview by the contact person at the intake workshop plus appropriate screening psychometrics. Severely depressed or suicidal patients are seen by the team liaison psychiatrist. Other patients with significant psychosocial concerns are seen by either the team social worker or psychologist. The ready access to psychological or social work expertise facilitates psychosocial counseling and evaluation. There does not appear to be a psychological hurdle or stigma to providing such help. If problems predate the cardiac event, then after an initial assessment recommendations are made for more in-depth treatment by community counselors. The psychosocial problems encompass the spectrum and can include depression, anxiety, family discord, or personality disorders. If substance abuse is a concomitant problem, then the participant is asked to complete a detoxification program before entering the cardiac rehabilitation program.

VOCATIONAL

There is one full-time vocational counselor who is part of the rehabilitation team. The vocational program follows the approach as outlined in chapter 17 on vocational issues. A number of patients are referred with a request for vocational analysis. If appropriate, a complete job analysis is arranged that involves the participant's and employer's description of the work. An on-site job visit can be arranged to quantify environmental aspects of the job and the possibility of job modification. Both physical and emotional stressors of the job are assessed.

The work capacity is assessed from recent stress tests (ideally with gas analysis), the progress in the exercise program, and a specialized work capacity test using a "weightlifting and carrying" protocol. The final evaluation includes a detailed analysis of the job, an estimate of potential risks of work return, and a final recommendation. It should be noted these recommendations are directed to the referring physician, who has the final decision about the work return.

RISK FACTOR MODIFICATION

The major risk factors are ascertained at program intake. Those patients found to be hypertensive are monitored with frequent blood pressure (BP) recordings during the exercise program. If BP is not under adequate control, the referring physician is notified. Lifestyle modification to improve BP control, such as weight loss and decreased alcohol consumption, are incorporated into the rehabilitation program.

A baseline lipid screen (including fasting total cholesterol [TC], high-density lipoprotein [HDL], and triglycerides) is obtained. Most patients are now treated with lipid-lowering agents by the time they reach the rehabilitation program. Nevertheless, certain high-risk patients still require further evaluation, such as lipoprotein(a) or homocysteine. The cornerstone of treatment for all these patients is lifestyle change, including dietary management, weight loss, and exercise. Lipids are retested at varying intervals during the program.

Any participant who is still smoking can be treated in the smoking cessation program. The program involves behavioral therapy, addictive disorders therapy, and adjunctive pharmacologic and relapse prevention. The treatment program can include additional counseling sessions, group therapy programs, or intensive self-help resources.

Diabetes, an important risk factor, is ascertained on intake either from the patient's history or from a fasting blood glucose. Blood sugars are obtained before and after exercise. An inappropriately high or low blood sugar before exercise leads to cancellation of the exercise program for that day. Appropriate lifestyle modification to help ameliorate the diabetic state is included as part of the rehabilitation program.

Obesity is determined by a measure of the body mass index (BMI). A BMI greater than 27 kg/m^2 indicates that the patient is approximately 20% above the ideal body weight. Such persons are seen for individual counseling with the dietitian, and exercise is modified to include a longer duration and lower intensity sessions.

LOW-INTENSITY PROGRAM

A number of patients are referred to the rehabilitation program who require an exercise program of relatively low intensity. Such patients may have a significantly impaired left ventricle with an ejection fraction less than 30%, a musculoskeletal or neurologic problem, or a moderate to severe claudication. In a number of cases, participants of this class are awaiting coronary artery bypass grafting surgery or possibly heart transplantation. The program for these participants is 12 months long. Educational materials applicable for heart failure patients are provided that outline the physical, psychological, social, and vocational issues associated with this condition.

PHASE IV

After 6 months on the rehabilitation program, the participant graduates with a certificate and appropriate congratulations. A few reluctant graduates exist who would like to stay in the program indefinitely. An exit interview helps to determine whether the participant would like to pursue an individualized program or enroll in one of the community programs that cater to cardiac patients. There are two sites for the phase IV program: the Heart Institute and a community center. The community program was established in 1985 at a community center, the Nepean Sportsplex, located in the west part of the city. A group of interested graduates, together with appropriate staff from the Heart Institute, formed a steering committee that eventually established this community program.

The Heart Institute trains and selects staff for the community program; reviews all potential applicants for the community program; maintains the exercise records; provides for the stress tests; and arranges for proper maintenance of the arrest cart and defibrillator. Fund-raising efforts purchased the defibrillator and exercise equipment. Each class is supervised by an exercise leader who is trained as an American College of Sports Medicine (ACSM) exercise specialist and a nurse, who is trained in advanced life support (ALS). When necessary, physicians at a nearby sports medicine clinic can provide support for emergency situations.

HEART CHECK

Heart Check is the health promotion and primary prevention component of the prevention and rehabilitation program. It provides public education and health promotion programs to the families of patients, the general public, and worksites in the Ottawa-Carleton region. Recent initiatives for population intervention involve the modification of cardiovascular risk factors in the worksite and a World Bank study in Hungary designed to increase knowledge and skills and to effect changes in the dietary habits of the population.

The various primary prevention programs are described in the following sections.

Risk Factor Assessment

Family members of cardiac patients and interested members of the general public are seen for individual assessment of cardiac risk factors. The goals of this program are as follows:

1. To quantify the levels of coronary risk by the assessment of current behaviors and measurable risks.
2. To sensitize individuals to their own modifiable risk factors and to encourage and support appropriate dietary and lifestyle changes.
3. To develop a database from which longitudinal population-based risk can be tracked.
4. To develop healthy behaviors in the community by communicating information about the role played by modifiable risk factors in the development of coronary heart disease (CHD).

The Heart Check area consists of facilities that allow patients and families to fill out questionnaires and to acquire BP, height, weight, and TC measurements. An optical scanner and appropriate computer software provide individual printouts. This facility was established with a commercial grant, and any interested person or family can receive a risk factor screen at no charge. A brief interview is held with each person to explain the computerized printout. To date, approximately 16,000 people have had their risk factors screened. The facility is relatively portable and various industries are screened on a cost-recovery basis.

An analysis of the first 2000 clients through Heart Check showed the following:

1. Risk factor screening in a tertiary care cardiac center attracts a primary prevention population.
2. Older persons with several modifiable risk factors are more likely to use this service.
3. There is a high level of interest in learning about heart disease prevention through more detailed health enhancement programs.
4. Hospital-based risk factor screening information centers should have protocols established to manage acutely symptomatic persons effectively.
5. The successful integration of a risk factor screening and education center in a tertiary care facility requires the active involvement and support of the medical health care professionals.

Smoking Cessation Program

The HIPRC smoking cessation program opened May 1993. Since this time, the program has achieved a 28% quit rate at 3 months and a 17% quit rate at 6 months. Working with other community groups, smoking cessation staff have been active in lobbying for healthy public policy in smoking-related issues, including tobacco taxation, the sale of tobacco to minors, and high school smoking policies. The program philosophy is that nicotine dependence is a medical problem that produces physical and psychological characteristics that can be identified and treated. The treatment plan emphasizes a triangular relationship of physician, patient, and counselor. This program involves four major components: behavioral therapy, addictive disorders therapy, adjunctive pharmacologic therapy, and relapse prevention. It incorporates an individual approach in which specially trained nurse counselors, with active physician support, provide intervention, information, and therapy for the patient with any level of nicotine dependence and in any stage of readiness to quit. The treatment plan for each patient may include additional counseling sessions, group therapy programs, or intensive self-help resources.

Fitlife

"Fitlife" is a primary prevention, exercise, and behavioral change program offered to the general public. This program was launched September 1993 and evolved after a needs analysis from the individuals who had come through the risk factor screening program. It comprises twice-weekly sessions for a 12-week period. During a half-day workshop and twice-weekly classes, health care professionals specializing in nutrition, exercise, and risk reduction provide participants with a personalized, step by step approach to making realistic, heart-healthy choices and reducing cardiovascular risk. The Fitlife program is intended for individuals at moderate to high risk for CHD on the basis of coronary risk factors but who are clinically free of CHD. The objectives of the Fitlife program are to accomplish the following:

- Teach program participants about the multifactorial nature of CHD, the behaviors associated with heart health, and the association of dietary and exercise habits to coronary risk.
- Provide a comprehensive coronary risk profile

and exercise readiness assessment, which includes lifestyle evaluation with special emphasis on dietary and exercise habits, serum lipid profile, and physical fitness evaluation.

- Guide program participants in realistic goal-setting for effective lifestyle modification in the areas of nutrition and physical activity.
- Lead participants in selecting a self-directed heart-healthy eating plan that meets their personal goals (e.g., cholesterol, BP reduction, or weight reduction).
- Provide a safe and personalized exercise program that is effective in safely increasing physical activity to at least 1000 kcal/wk.

Participants are advised to discuss their participation in the Fitlife program with their personal physician. On completion of the Heart Check Fitlife program, each participant's personal physician is informed about the patient's risk factor and risk behavior status. The Fitlife program is financially self-sufficient. Although established as a primary prevention program, a certain number of individuals, as part of their program evaluation, are found to have bona fide cardiac disease.

Stress Management

The Stress Management program is a group intervention involving 12 to 15 people. Classes are held for a 6-week period, one time per week, and there are typically three to four sessions per year. Each session is of 2 hours' duration and comprises a didactic presentation, a participant self-assessment strategy, a facilitated group discussion or exercise, a demonstration and group practice of a stress management skill, and a "homework" exercise for participants to complete during the subsequent week. The program is lead by a clinical psychologist on a cost-recovery basis. The guiding principle of the program is that, although many life stressors cannot be controlled, people can learn to attenuate the negative emotional, behavioral, and physical effects of stress. In this way individuals can positively affect their health, well-being, and quality of life. The focus of such an intervention is to help participants determine their stress levels, discover the relationships between stressors and stress responses, identify coping strengths and weaknesses, and learn skills to better manage the negative effects of stress by responding to stressful situations more adaptively and by ameliorating the physical, behavioral, and emotional consequences of stress to enhance health potential.

Nutrition Course: "A New Way of Eating"

The nutrition course, "A New Way of Eating," was developed at Stanford University and was introduced in 1995 in response to repeated requests from the public for information on nutrition. This workshop-style program takes a behavioral modification approach and is designed to teach skills for maintaining a low-fat, low-cholesterol diet to the general public. Highlights of the course, taught by a professional nutritionist, include a supermarket tour, a cooking demonstration, and a personal nutritional profile analysis.

Public Education

The George Seman Public Library, located in Heart Check, is a multimedia library consisting of various texts, magazines, pamphlets, cassette tapes, and video information on cardiovascular disease and heart health. Patients, staff, and the general public are able to borrow this information from the library without charge. The public is able to access a computer and software for general information on nutrition including personal nutritional analysis and low-fat recipe makeovers. Future plans include the development of an interactive learning center that will contain six to eight computers for public education purposes.

Observations on the Institutional Model

A unique set of challenges arises when a cardiac prevention and rehabilitation program is incorporated in an institution.

In such a setting, it is absolutely necessary to have control over the program budget, which functions as a cornerstone. Other departments, which have made vague commitments of support, lose their enthusiasm when financial constraints are imposed.

All sources of revenue should be considered as well as program expenditures. One often overlooked source of income is revenue generated from the stress tests required for the cardiac rehabilitation participants. Some programs have made arrangements to have all or a certain percentage of the stress test profits come back to the program. Conservatism in expenditures allows for unexpected expenses or a change in the amount of revenue. Normally, expenditures equal 75% to 85% of

guaranteed income. Other potential sources of revenue are from various adult fitness programs. Other forms of revenue that may be important include fund-raising, donations, and research grants. Medical staff may direct funds from overages to such a research program; however, such staff will want to have direct involvement in such projects. It is our experience that the largest funds are derived from industry-related projects.

For cardiac rehabilitation to flourish in a health care institution, it is important that the program and staff be well represented in the institutional hierarchy. It is important that major initiatives of the institution be supported and encouraged.

Cardiac rehabilitation in an institutional setting fosters the concept that the rehabilitation phase is a necessary and vital part of complete cardiovascular services. Being within an acute care hospital allows a number of high-risk patients to access cardiac rehabilitation services. If the institution is a teaching hospital, then cardiac rehabilitation personnel can be involved with undergraduate and graduate university programs alike.

Part B. Community-based
Fredric J. Pashkow and Peg L. Pashkow

COMMUNITY-BASED CARDIAC REHABILITATION: AN IMPORTANT ALTERNATIVE MODEL

Community-based rehabilitation refers to programs that are located and supported administratively distant from institutions. These programs can serve as the major means of providing long-term exercise rehabilitation to cardiovascular patients (1). Hämäläinen et al. (2) suggest that even modest community-based after-care efforts compare favorably with the more elaborate and expensive short intervention course in a rehabilitation center. Community-based programs often borrow or lease space in schools and recreational facilities such as YMCAs, and sometimes receive a significant amount of their funding from public sources (1). In small communities where the hospital may not have the wherewithal to provide such services, such programs may function as the only outpatient rehabilitative services available in a community (3). More frequently, they will catch the "run-off" from phase II rehabilitation programs existing within the community (2). These programs are especially appropriate for furnishing a neutral, noncompetitive alternative (4) or when there are two or more institutions that cannot individually support such a program. With increasing shortening of length of stay and serious questions about the efficacy of phase II rehabilitation for those who stratify at low risk, the community-based alternative is likely to become increasingly important (5).

THE IMPACT OF LONG-TERM CARDIAC REHABILITATION PROGRAMS

The most significant impact of long-term programs is the effect of extended exercise and education on outcome and risk factor modification. Oldridge and associates' (6) milestone review of rehabilitation determined that the reduction in the odds ratio for all-cause mortality was only 8% in those participating less than 12 weeks of cardiovascular rehabilitation, 24% in those participating 12 to 52 weeks, but 38% ($P = .004$) in those participating more than 36 months.

O'Connor and colleagues (7), in addition to demonstrating similar reductions in all-cause and cardiovascular mortality, found a highly significant (37%) reduction in the odds ratio for sudden cardiac death in the first year after rehabilitation, but a declining odds ratio in the second and third years after participation ceases (24% and 8%, respectively). Hämäläinen et al. (8) found in a controlled, prospective trial that even after 10 years the significantly lower sudden death and coronary mortality observed 3 years after myocardial infarction persisted in the intervention group compared with the control. The incidence of sudden death in the intervention group was roughly half (12.8% compared with 23.0%) that of the controls (8).

Studies show that 12 months or more of exercise are effective for control of mild hypertension (9) or in long-term weight loss maintenance (10), and even modest amounts of exercise for extended periods of time are associated with meaningful alterations in the high-density lipoprotein (HDL) levels of cardiac patients (11, 12). It appears that elderly patients seem to benefit when their exercise training is extended into the phase III environment (13, 14). Those who commit to exercise rehabilitation for very extended periods of time (minimum, 10 years) are able to maintain their exercise capacity despite increasing age and rehospitalizations for cardiac problems (15).

ROLE OF THE PHYSICIAN IN COMMUNITY-BASED PROGRAMS

In our experience, we have observed that community-based programs are most successful if they are championed by one or more physicians within the community. Physicians will often serve as the catalyst for the establishment of the program with the motive of securing rehabilitation services for their own patients (1). Physicians typically will serve as the medical advisor (required) and as an expert resource, for example, for staff in-services or as a lecturer in the educational sessions. It is important that the program be designed so that all of the participating parties derive tangible benefits from supporting such an effort. This "buy-in" process by all of the major parties concerned ensures program success (1).

The physician can help define and focus the program and should have significant input into the design of the "product" and the services offered. Exercise and education are the minimal elements of a cardiac rehabilitation program (16). What is offered beyond this, to a large extent will further specify the doctor's role. If exercise testing or cardiac telemetry monitoring are to be provided, these will have significant impact on staffing, budgeting, and selection of equipment, training, and application protocols. The physician should be involved in the determination of the admission and discharge criteria (Table 23.1). In the event that secondary prevention is integrated into the program the physician will have additional responsibility for appropriate medical supervision of this activity and facilitating communication with the patient's primary physician and cardiologist.

We advocate that all program functions conform to the standards and guidelines of the American College of Sports Medicine (17) and the American Association of Cardiovascular and Pulmonary Rehabilitation (18). Although exercise rehabilitation has proven to be extremely safe (19), the physician adviser should see that the program is properly equipped (Fig. 23.2) and staffed with the appropriate personnel—trained,

Table 23.1.   Admission and Discharge Criteria for Community-based Phase III Cardiac Rehabilitation

Admission
- Stabilized after a cardiovascular incident or have chronic stable angina
- Demonstrated potential to benefit from cardiac rehabilitation
- Referred by a physician
- Performed an exercise ECG within 3 months of admission
- Identified resources for service payment

Discharge
- Achievement of all stated goals
- Demonstration of ability to continue or maintain progress independently or in a less-structured program
- Noncompliant with respect to guidelines for safety to oneself or others
- Destabilization medically (complications or concurrent medical condition)

experienced, licensed, and certified—and that written policies and procedures regulating the safety and well-being of participants are established, followed, and critically reviewed (17). The physician serving in the role of medical advisor must be licensed in that state to practice medicine, should have medical liability coverage, and should maintain certification in advanced cardiac life support or an equivalent.

If testing is to be offered, the physician needs to be knowledgeable about the indications and contraindications for testing and familiar with the testing procedures (see chapter 5). He or she should be able to recognize electrocardiographic (ECG) and physiologic abnormalities during exercise that mandate a test should be stopped.

CARDIAC REHABILITATION IN A SEMI-RURAL COMMUNITY

Most of our experience in the development and management of community-based cardiac rehabilitation was gained with our involvement for a 10-year period in Loveland, Colorado. We found the program there similar in its origins, operations, evolution, and experience to other community-based rehabilitation programs (3, 4, 20).

Cardiac rehabilitation in Loveland begins in the hospital as soon as the patient is medically stabilized after the occurrence of an acute coronary event. This early rehabilitation process, referred to as phase I, consists primarily of educa-

tion and psychological reassurance and early progressive ambulation with a goal of self-care in activities of daily living. Just before or after discharge, the patient undergoes submaximal exercise ECG testing, with end points determined by the presence of moderate fatigue, angina, dyspnea, claudication, ECG signs of ischemia, problematic ectopy, or hemodynamic instability. This low-level exercise study has great value in assessing the patient's prognosis and potential for further rehabilitation and provides guidelines for the exercise prescription.

Patients who exhibit signs or symptoms of exercise intolerance on the exercise ECG at or below a level of 4.0 metabolic equivalents (METs) are generally referred to the phase II rehabilitation at the hospital. In Loveland, this is a closely supervised, hospital-based outpatient program that includes a high ratio of medical personnel to

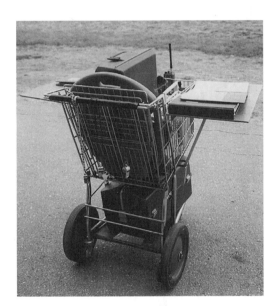

Figure 23.2. "Crash-cart" for the Loveland, Colorado, community-based rehabilitation program. The humble origin of this emergency response cart is obvious—it was donated by a local supermarket and then modified by volunteer members of the program. Note the large, ball-bearing wheels added to the rear that allow the cart to be moved quickly over rough ground. The writing surfaces on each side fold down for transfer or storage. The basket portion contains a LifePak synchronized cardioverter/defibrillator with monitor, cardiac arrest board, battery-operated suction device, oxygen and O$_2$ regulator with fittings, and a two-way radio for communication with the emergency medical service dispatcher. A drug box with medications, intravenous and intubation equipment, and so forth, is underneath. Each staff person carries an emergency whistle when patients are on the track (cart handle).

patients, continuous ECG monitoring during exercise, and a very close proximity to extensive medical support services within the facility. Patients who can safely complete greater than 4.0 METs are occasionally referred directly to phase III, though the majority currently begin with a course in phase II.

PROGRAM HISTORY

The precursor of the Loveland program was a university-based cardiac rehabilitation program developed at Colorado State University (CSU) in 1976 as a laboratory model. In 1977, the semi-rural community of Loveland established their own program, staffed by a graduate student exercise leader provided under contract from CSU and a cadre of volunteers from the local community, including people with medical, paramedical, and nonmedical backgrounds. University affiliation provided the liability coverage for staff, students, and volunteers. A nonprofit organization called Loveland HeartWatchers was incorporated, and financial support was solicited from community tax revenues and United Way. The patient participants elected a board of directors that has overall responsibility for the program and provides expertise in certain areas such as business and accounting. Within 2 years, Loveland, with a population of only 35,000, was able to support the cardiac rehabilitation program without direct affiliation with the hospital or university.

During the years, the Loveland HeartWatchers became more self-sustaining financially. Currently the cost to operate the program is $1020 per member per year. Fees to patients have not been increased in 12 years, so funds are solicited from nontraditional sources and service agencies. Patients who can not afford the $50 per month membership fee are given scholarship assistance. The program has also evolved administratively. In September of 1979, the program changed from a contract arrangement with CSU to local independent administration. The Board contracts day-to-day operations of the program to rehabilitation specialists, the "program coordinators." The professional staff of registered nurses and exercise physiologists are salaried but are required to provide their own liability insurance coverage. Volunteers have traditionally filled the role of exercise assistants and been important contributors to program success in the

past, but the role of exercise assistants has been filled in recent years by CSU students who need the clinical experience.

Members are strongly urged to attend every session the first 2 months. Those wishing to continue with the program are encouraged to attend 75% of the exercise sessions. Compliance figures have been closely monitored as one indicator of program success and average about 65%. Compliance is calculated as gross attendance divided by total number of sessions offered.

Operating in a community public school before and after student hours, the program uses classrooms, gymnasium, and an outdoor track. Originally, a nominal per diem fee was paid for the use of the school, but in 1982, the school district elected to eliminate the facility user fee, further reducing operating costs. The cost per patient is approximately $725 annually and the amount paid per patient is about $575 per year. An endowment fund has been established to provide "scholarships" to those who cannot cover all or part of their fees.

OVERVIEW OF THE COMMUNITY-BASED PHASE III PROGRAM

After an orientation that includes a physical assessment and goal setting, the basic program consists of three 60-minute exercise sessions and two 45-minute educational sessions per month. Weather permitting, the aerobic portion of the program is held outdoors, using a quarter-mile track on the school grounds. All the exercise equipment is portable so it may be moved outside when the weather permits. Each patient's exercise prescription is reviewed and revised daily during the first 2 weeks in the program. After the patient begins to condition, it is revised only once or twice per month. Exercise MET levels for both walking or jogging and biking are calculated, and this information is incorporated in progress reports, which are generated monthly or more frequently, as needed, for both patients and their physicians (Fig. 23.3).

Twice monthly square dancing classes were offered as an option to the regular aerobic activities. Such generalizations of activity are conceptually central to the program. It is thought to help patients apply their exercise prescriptions practically in their everyday lives. They are taught to use the

PROGRESS REPORT FOR:
ARNE STEMSRUD
Id: 123456789 ~ Gender: M ~ Age: 47
Report Period: 1/1/96 — 1/31/96

EVERGREEN HEARTWATCHERS
P.O. BOX 4117
EVERGREEN, CO 80437-4117
303 670-9631

Physicians   Dotson, P.D. - Newman, Zoe

Medications   ASA, 1, qd - Xanax, 1, qd

Diagnoses/Risks   Sedentary lifestyle, 10/95 - Nicotine addiction, 12/69 - MI - Inferior, 07/95

Goals   Return to work, 1/2 time, 12/95 - Increase exercise MET level, 2 METs, 12/95 - Maintain low fat diet, <20%, 12/95 - Adherance to exercise program, 85%, 12/95 - Smoking cessation, 100%, 12/95

Data Comparison			
	Current Period 1/1/96	% Change	Previous Period 12/ 1/95
# Sessions Completed	6		12
Average Weight	150.3 lbs.	0.2%	150.0 lbs.
Target Heart Rate (BPM)	128-144		128-144
Average Exercise Heart Rate	142.7	1.9%	140.0
Average MET Level	6.4	52.4%	4.2
Average Kcal's Used	101.3	6.1%	95.5
Average R.P.E.	12.2	1.7%	12.0
Primary Activity	Treadmill Walking (Speed)		Treadmill Walking (Speed)
Average Workload	3.6 Miles/hr	16.1%	3.1 Miles/hr
	5.0 % incline	150.0%	2.0 % incline

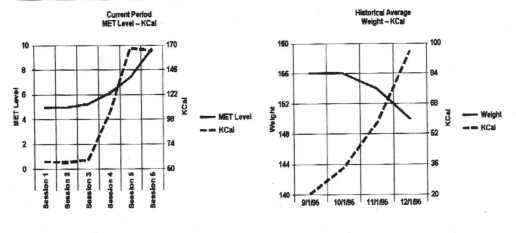

Current Period
MET Level – KCal

Historical Average
Weight – KCal

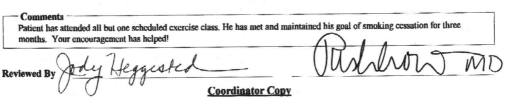

Comments
Patient has attended all but one scheduled exercise class. He has met and maintained his goal of smoking cessation for three months. Your encouragement has helped!

Reviewed By *Jody Heggested*   *Rushlow* MD

Coordinator Copy

Figure 23.3.   A representation of an end-of-period patient report. Note the graphics and individualized communications derived from the database system.

same principles and tools of exercise monitoring, mainly pulse and perceived exertion, in "real-life" functional activities. Square dancing also is important in that it allows the involvement of the spouse. Spousal participation has been identified as a potentially significant factor in the mainte-nance of compliance (21). The educational series focuses mostly on cardiovascular disease and risk factors. Since 1980, the series has been aug-mented, once each month, by the introduction of professionals from various sister disciplines who lead discussions on a wide range of subjects. The patients themselves strongly influence the selection of topics, for example, eye disorders of aging, managing arthritis, selection of footwear for exercise, and prevention of sports injuries. We have found that involvement of the local physicians also serves as an effective means of introducing and promoting the program. Quarterly cardiopulmonary resuscitation (CPR) classes are also offered to the families and friends of the members, as well as to the community at large. In addition, social and support group activities, such as breakfasts, picnics, and recognition dinners, are considered an important aspect of the program for the members and their families.

COMPUTERIZATION OF REHABILITATION RECORDS

Since the spring of 1984 the program has been using a data processing system to facilitate the management of exercise data and to reduce staff time required for the generation of reports to patients and physicians. The computer program used initially was fairly elementary, but provided sufficient experience and criteria for the development of newer generation software. The system is reviewed in some detail in chapter 26.

In continuous use since August 1985, the software provides an extensive patient database with lists of the patients' demographic data, medications, drug allergies, referring physicians, and exercise prescriptions. It also provides for acquisition of exercise data at the time of exercise. A daily log listing staff and patients, with messages about specific patients or the program, can be printed at each session. All relevant medical and exercise data can be collated and summarized for analysis and reporting. Special features are provided for communication with patients, including group and individual messages displayed at the time of sign-in and sign-out.

The Loveland program, in continuous operation since 1977, has now accumulated more than 100,000 patient-hours of participation. By using creative means of support and the computer to economize on staff hours (22), the costs of the program have been kept low, allowing patients to continue to participate beyond the time for which their insurance provides. The program's success demonstrates the feasibility and reasonable cost of supervised community-based cardiac rehabilitation for the purpose of improving quality of life through safe physical exercise conditioning, education, and mutual group support.

As Ades and colleagues (23) recently pointed out, it is no longer difficult to justify the significant costs and human effort associated with the provision of cardiac rehabilitation services in terms of a reduction in the economic burden of illness and losses from premature illness and death. In addition, regular exercise has a marked effect on overall well-being, perceived health, industrial performance, and perhaps maintenance of physical independence by the elderly, reducing their need for subordinate medical services. In community-based rehabilitation the strategy is to substantially curtail expense on the provider side by cost diffusion, sharing expenses and maximizing staff efficiency, so that the time to "break-even" for the health care consumer is closer to the here-and-now than the 5 to 10 years estimated in the most conservative of models (24). For patients interested in such group programs the community-based rehabilitation model still appears very appropriate and, in this time of cost containment, even more timely.

Part C.   Home-based

Kathy A. Berra and William L. Haskell

INTRODUCTION

Participation in formal exercised-based cardiac rehabilitation (CR) programs after myocardial infarction (MI) is associated with a substantial (20% to 25%) decrease in mortality from coronary heart disease (CHD) (1, 2). Analysis of the CR studies demonstrating a reduction in mortality indicates that the exercise component of these programs contributes significantly to this benefit (2). This reduction in mortality is comparable to benefits produced by cholesterol lowering and other post-myocardial infarction interventions such as aspirin and β-blocker therapies (3–5).

Cardiac rehabilitation programs range widely from highly structured, supervised exercise programs using continuous electrocardiographic (ECG) monitoring to casual recommendations by physicians for patients to exercise on a regular basis. Although class- or facility-based CR programs provide important services to patients, their families, and their physicians, it is estimated that only between 11% and 38% of eligible patients participate in such programs (6). This underutilization of class-based programs is evident for all categories of patients but is more prevalent among women, ethnic minorities, and the elderly (7). Reasons for underutilization are broad and complex. Program cost, convenience, gender, age, psychological and socioeconomic factors, and work status play important roles in referral as well as in participation rates (8, 9). In addition, class-based CR programs are more likely to be located in populated urban areas as opposed to rural settings. This fact alone makes facility-based programs inaccessible to many patients with CHD and makes evident the need for development of other models to deliver CR services.

Initial studies have demonstrated that home-based CR programs can play an important role in the full recovery of many patients with CHD. The major feature that is different in home-based versus class-based CR programs is the lack of direct medical supervision of the exercise program. Because this supervision, along with the capacity for immediate cardiopulmonary resuscitation by a medical professional, is not available in home-based programs, special consideration needs to be given to the safety aspects of the exercise, including proper patient selection, exercise prescription, education regarding adverse responses, and monitoring.

The purpose of this chapter is to 1) review the scientific evidence regarding the efficacy of home-based cardiac rehabilitation programs, 2) review safety data regarding home-based cardiac rehabilitation programs, 3) discuss the role of the physician in the prescription and management of home-based exercise, 4) describe the features of successful home-based exercise programs, and 5) define new models of integrated practice designed to enhance the effectiveness and safety of home-based CR for persons with CHD.

EFFICACY OF HOME-BASED REHABILITATION

There have been seven randomized controlled trials reported in the literature since 1982 that have evaluated home-based exercise in patients with CHD (10–16). Two of these trials that in-

cluded exercise therapy also evaluated multifactor risk reduction using a comprehensive nurse case-manager approach (14, 16). Populations represented in these studies included patients after myocardial infarction (MI), coronary artery bypass grafting (CABG) surgery, and percutaneous transluminal coronary angioplasty (PTCA). In these trials, patients were free of signs or symptoms of unstable cardiovascular disease before participation in the home-based exercise program. Programs included endurance exercise at 60% to 85% of peak or symptom-free heart rate determined by standard treadmill exercise testing. Five of these studies used nurse-managed telephonic ECG monitoring during some of the exercise sessions (11–15). One study used portable heart rate monitors with audible signals that alerted patients when they were above or below prescribed target heart rate limits (16). Most patients derived benefit in the form of increased exercise capacity without any evidence of an increase in cardiovascular complications as compared with patients in class-based exercise.

Another important feature of the home-based programs was that most patients were able to maintain a high rate of compliance to the exercise program. Two of the randomized trials also evaluated multifactorial risk intervention versus usual care (14, 16). For example, DeBusk and colleagues (16) demonstrated significant improvement in biochemically measured smoking cessation as well as exercise capacity and lipoprotein levels compared with usual care. Haskell and coworkers (14) demonstrated that home-based multifactorial nurse case-management of coronary risk factors for persons with CHD resulted in significant improvement in angiographically measured atherosclerosis as well as hospitalization for coronary events during 4 years of follow-up.

In addition to the randomized trials, there have been four nonrandomized trials that included home-based exercise (17–20). In all of these trials, the home-based groups derived similar benefits from exercise as compared with the more traditional group-based programs. There were no significant differences in the frequency of coronary events in the home-based versus the class-based or control groups in any of these trials.

Other reports in the literature support these controlled trials. In a preliminary report, Ades and colleagues (21) reported that telephonic monitoring of home-based exercise rehabilitation, including posttransplant patients, was safe and resulted in improvements in physical functioning compared with controls. The use of telephonic monitoring is an emerging and potentially useful technology. It provides the opportunity to increase home-based monitoring capabilities of higher risk patients who are unable to attend formal class-based rehabilitation programs. Fletcher et al. (11) reported on the use of ECG telephonic monitoring during home-based exercise in post-CABG patients. Electrocardiographic abnormalities requiring diagnostic or interventional therapies occurred in 9 of the 46 male patients. No life-threatening abnormalities were observed during the 12-week home-based program. Others (22–24) have also reported similar responses of increased functional capacity without increased incidence of coronary events during telephonic monitoring of home-based exercise in moderate to lower risk post-MI and post-CABG patients.

The scientific literature supports the concept that home-based exercise programs in selected patients without significant comorbidity, ventricular dysfunction, residual cardiac ischemia, or serious arrhythmias are safe and that patients are likely to benefit with an increase in functional capacity. Also, reductions in clinical coronary events and angiographically confirmed improvements in atherosclerosis have been seen in multifactor coronary risk reduction home-based CR programs (14).

SAFETY OF HOME-BASED CARDIAC REHABILITATION PROGRAMS

The prevention and management of serious cardiovascular complications during CR historically is the reason for the development of programs that include on-site medical supervision or continuous ECG monitoring. Safety issues also are of utmost importance in the design and implementation of home-based rehabilitation programs. There have been three important studies of the safety of medically supervised CR programs reported in the literature (25–27). All of these studies were conducted before the widespread use of thrombolytic agents and PTCA in the emergent treatment of acute MI and unstable angina pectoris; thus, their relevance to the current risk status of CR programs may be in some

doubt. Also, they were conducted before the adoption of home-based exercise training for patients with CHD.

Haskell found during the early 1970s that the overall incidence of cardiac arrest was 1 per 116,400 patient-hours of participation in supervised exercise programs (25). Van Camp and Peterson (27) analyzed data collected from 1980 to 1985 related to cardiac complications from 142 CR programs in the United States. In more than 51,000 patients enrolled in formal cardiac rehabilitation programs who exercised for greater than 2.3 million hours, 21 cardiac arrests (1 per 109,500 patient-hours) were reported, with data analyzed for 20. Successful resuscitation occurred in 17 of the 20 arrests (85%). The risk of cardiac events occurring during medically supervised exercise in these studies was influenced by clinical measures such as prior history of MI, history of congestive heart failure, ventricular tachycardia, the presence of residual ischemic myocardium, triple-vessel coronary disease, an ejection fraction less than 40%, ST depression at a heart rate of less than 120 beats per minute, peak systolic blood pressure of less than 130 mm Hg, exertional hypotension, and a functional capacity of less than 5 metabolic equivalents (METs). Other factors, such as adherence to prescribed exercise heart rate guidelines and adherence to appropriate cool-down exercises, were associated with an increased risk of a cardiac complication. To put this event rate in some perspective, a study of apparently healthy male joggers reported a death rate of 1 per 396,000 hours of exercise (28). This study also reported that those joggers who died had evidence of one or more coronary risk factors. Unfortunately, this type of information is not available for women.

No systematic study of adequate size has been conducted to establish the risk of exercise-related clinical cardiac events during home-based CR programs. In the 11 studies cited in the preceding section on the benefits of home-based CR, there were no major clinical cardiac events associated with the exercise and overall medical complications were not any higher in the home-based compared with the class-based program (10–21). None of these studies were of adequate size or duration to establish a medical complication rate that can be compared with the reports providing data for supervised CR exercise programs (25–27). However, the failure of any study to report an excess of events provides some confidence in current guidelines for identifying patients at the greatest risk for experiencing a clinical event associated with exercise and the relatively low risk imposed by low- to moderate-intensity exercise.

Identification of high-risk patients is especially important when considering home-based exercise prescriptions. The American Association of Cardiovascular and Pulmonary Rehabilitation (AACVPR) has summarized guidelines for stratification of exercise-related risk on the basis of recommendations of the American Heart Association, the American College of Cardiology, and the American College of Physicians (29). These guidelines are outlined in Table 23.2. Authoritative guidelines for patient selection criteria, frequency of monitoring, design of the exercise regimen, and methods of dealing with changes in clinical status or life-threatening emergencies (i.e., new-onset angina with ECG changes consistent with those of ischemia) have not yet been established for home-based exercise. In addition, medicolegal issues and reimbursement for telephonic services are not well defined and lack established criteria. Telephonic monitoring has important implications for home-based exercise for selected persons with CHD, but additional research is needed to establish medical and reimbursement guidelines. In a report by Sparks et al. (30), 10 patients considered to be at high risk for a cardiac complication were telephonically monitored during home-based exercise. Eight of 10 patients had symptoms during an exercise session that required emergency medical services or contact with their referring physician. The symptoms included supraventricular tachycardia, new-onset chest pain, arrhythmia, and severe shortness of breath. Although two patients died in this group, neither died during or in close proximity to an exercise session. Research needs to focus on home-based exercise and coronary risk reduction programs for moderately high-risk and high-risk patients. Many of these patients will be unable to participate in formal group programs for the same reasons listed earlier. There is a need for evidence-based guidelines for those patients with ejection fractions less than 40% and for those who are medically managed with residual ischemia.

Table 23.2.   Risk Classification of Patients for Assignment to Exercise Training Program

Low	No significant left ventricular dysfunction (i.e., ejection fraction ≥50%)
	No resting or exercise-induced myocardial ischemia manifested as angina or ST-segment displacement
	No resting or exercise-induced complex arrhythmias
	Uncomplicated myocardial infarction, coronary artery bypass grafting surgery, angioplasty, or atherectomy
	Functional capacity >6 METs on graded-exercise test 3 or more weeks after clinical event
Intermediate	Mild to moderately depressed left ventricular function (ejection fraction 31–49%)
	Functional capacity <5–6 METs on graded-exercise test 3 or more weeks after clinical event
	Failure to comply with exercise intensity prescription
	Exercise-induced myocardial ischemia (1–2 mm ST-segment depression) or reversible ischemic defects (electrocardiographic or nuclear radiography)
High	Severely depressed left ventricular function (ejection fraction ≤30%)
	Complex ventricular arrhythmias at rest or appearing or increasing with exercise
	Decrease in systolic blood pressure of >15 mm Hg during exercise or a failure to rise with increasing exercise workloads
	Survivor of sudden cardiac death
	Myocardial infarction complicated by congestive heart failure, cardiogenic shock, or complex ventricular arrhythmias
	Severe coronary artery disease and marked exercise-induced myocardial ischemia (>2 mm ST-segment depression)

Reprinted with permission from the American Association of Cardiovascular and Pulmonary Rehabilitation. Guidelines for cardiac rehabilitation programs. Champaign, IL: Human Kinetics, 1995:14.

ROLE OF THE PHYSICIAN IN HOME-BASED EXERCISE PROGRAMS

Providing comprehensive health care that is based on careful evaluation, comprehensive testing, and detailed education is a challenging role for today's physician. Home-based cardiac rehabilitation calls for all of the features of optimum health care delivery to be effective. The role of the physician is pivotal in the successful accomplishment of home-based rehabilitation along with the active involvement of other team members.

Behaviorally oriented lifestyle modification involving exercise, healthy nutrition, stress reduction, smoking cessation, and intensive therapies involving both lifestyle changes and medications for CHD risk reduction traditionally have not been stressed in medical school education. This fact, plus the tremendous time demands that exist in physician-based office practice in the era of cost containment, makes it particularly difficult for physicians to implement interventions promoting long-term behavior change. Physicians are adept at assessment and management of ischemic burden, cardiac arrhythmias, and left ventricular dysfunction. In addition, physician responsibility includes assessment of risk status for future coronary events and the intensive management of hypertension, dyslipidemia, diabetes, obesity, and smoking cessation. Equally important is the physician's advice and management in the area of stress management, nutrition, and exercise. The role of the physician is critical in establishing safe guidelines for home-based exercise, influencing compliance with exercise recommendations and educating patients about the important influence that exercise has in their recovery.

Identification of those patients at high risk for a clinical cardiac event who should be excluded from a home-based exercise program is the first important task that a physician provides in home-based program implementation. Evaluation of the patient's risk includes a careful medical history and cardiovascular-oriented physical examination, including assessment of all the major risk factors, and a symptom- or sign-limited exercise test. Table 23.3 outlines recommendations by the American College of Sports Medicine for physician supervision of clinical exercise testing. These recommendations have been discussed in more detail in sections 1 and 2 of this text.

Persons with CHD represent an enormous spectrum of disease severity as well as risk for a recurrent coronary event. Patients with CHD without diminished ventricular function, life-threatening arrhythmias, or significant comorbidity are the most appropriate patients to enroll in a home-based exercise program. This would include those with uncomplicated MI, successful revascularization, and well-preserved left ventricular function. However, with fewer than 15% to 20% of all coronary patients participating in formal supervised programs, safe home-based programs are critical. For almost all patients, except for those with unstable or severe symptoms of valvular heart disease, congestive heart failure, or cardiomyopathy, some level of physical reconditioning should be implemented.

Once the patient is considered eligible for a home-based program, the physician needs to formulate an appropriate exercise plan based on the clinical, risk, and functional status of the patient. Very specific written as well as verbal instructions need to be given to the patient regarding their individualized exercise program. These instructions should include the exercise prescription (type, intensity, duration, and frequency), any exercise(s) to be avoided (e.g., heavy lifting, running), and specific instructions regarding signs or symptoms of overexertion.

FEATURES OF HOME-BASED PROGRAMS

Important features of home-based CR programs include a comprehensive clinical evaluation including exercise testing, an exercise prescription and proscription, education regarding untoward clinical symptoms, a comprehensive risk reduction plan, and plans for systematic follow-up counseling. Risk factor goals for patients with cardiovascular disease have been established by the American Heart Association and the American College of Cardiology, as well as other nationally recognized groups such as the National Cholesterol Education Program, Adult Treatment Panel II, and the Joint National Committee on the Detection and Management of High Blood Pressure VI. Follow-up counseling includes clinical, physiologic, and behavioral measures to maximize medical and lifestyle therapies and evaluate exercise safety.

Home-based programs must be based on clinical status and responses to exercise testing, as well as measures of coronary risk factors. Nurse case-managers and other health care professionals, such as exercise physiologists and nutritionists, are well versed in exercise and risk reduction and can provide the critical link to successful home-

Table 23.3.   Medical Supervision of Clinical Exercise Testing

	Apparently Healthy Younger[c]	Older	Increased Risk[a] No Symptoms	Yes Symptoms	Known Disease[b]
A. Medical examination and clinical exercise test is recommended before					
Moderate exercise[d]	No[e]	No	No	Yes	Yes
Vigorous Exercise[f]	No	Yes[g]	Yes	Yes	Yes
B. Physician supervision recommended during exercise test					
Submaximal testing	No[e]	No	No	Yes	Yes
Maximal testing	No	Yes[g]	Yes	Yes	Yes

[a]Persons with 2 or more coronary risk factors or 1 or more signs or symptoms of coronary heart disease.
[b]Persons with known cardiac, pulmonary, or metabolic disease.
[c]Younger is ≤ 40 years for men, ≤ 50 years for women.
[d]Moderate exercise as defined by an intensity of 40–60% of $\dot{V}O_2$max; if intensity is uncertain, moderate exercise may alternatively be defined as an intensity well within the individual's current capacity, one which can be sustained for a prolonged period of time, i.e., 60 minutes, which has a gradual initiation and progression, and is generally noncompetitive.
[e]A "No" response means that an item is deemed "not necessary." No does not mean that it should not be done.
[f]Vigorous intensity is defined by an exercise intensity > 60% $\dot{V}O_2$max; if intensity is uncertain, moderate exercise may alternatively be defined as exercise intense enough to represent a substantial cardiorespiratory challenge or if it results in fatigue within 20 minutes.
[g]A "Yes" response means that an item is recommended. For physician supervision, this suggests that a physician is in close proximity and readily available should there be an emergent need.
Reprinted with permission from the American College of Sports Medicine. Guidelines for exercise testing and prescription. Baltimore: Williams & Wilkins, 25.

based programs. Systematic follow-up can provide motivation and support and answer patient questions. In addition, systematic follow-up provides a way to measure program compliance and safety.

Alternate approaches to the delivery of cardiac rehabilitation services, other than traditional supervised group interventions, can be implemented effectively and safely for carefully selected and clinically stable patients. Trans-telephonic and other means of monitoring and surveillance of patients can extend cardiac rehabilitation services beyond the setting of supervised, structured, group-based rehabilitation. These alternate approaches have the potential to provide cardiac rehabilitation services to low- and moderate-risk patients who comprise the majority of patients with stable coronary disease, most of whom do not currently participate in supervised, structured rehabilitation (6).

Most frequently, a home-based exercise program will be based on walking or stationary cycling or both. These activities are preferred because their intensity can be easily controlled, they can be performed at low intensity with the intensity gradually increased as the capacity of the patient increases, and they are low impact and reduce the risk of overuse injuries. Stationary cycling has the advantage that it can be performed in the home where other people who know the patient are available to help monitor the patient or

Table 23.4.   Revised Scale for Ratings of Perceived Exertion

0	Nothing at all	5	Strong
0.5	Very, very weak	6	
1	Very weak	7	Very strong
2	Weak	8	
3	Moderate	9	
4	Somewhat strong	10	Very, very strong Maximal

Reprinted with permission from Noble BJ, Borg GAV, Jacobs I, et al. A category-ratio perceived exertion scale: relationship to blood and muscle lactates and heart rate. Med Sci Sports Exerc 1983;15:523–528.

be of assistance in case of an emergency. Walking is an excellent activity that can be performed almost anywhere. Patients can use walking in a productive manner, such as walking to the grocery store, walking the dog, or walking to visit with other people, thus adding an important social component to their rehabilitation program.

Because the characteristic of exercise most associated with increased cardiovascular risk is exercise intensity, it is recommended that a lower intensity of exercise be traded for increased session frequency or duration. Given this approach, and the increased convenience of performing exercise at home compared with travelling to a facility, the recommendation should include 30 minutes or more of exercise on most days—ideally at least 5 days per week. Early in the program, multiple short bouts of exercise can be performed several

Table 23.5.   Daily Log for Angina

Daily Log for Angina								
No. of episodes/day								
Triggered by exercise, emotions, eating etc.								
Spontaneous								
Grade (1–4)[a]								
Duration								
Management								
Rest								
Nitroglycerin								
Other								

[a]Grade 1—Very mild symptoms (i.e., onset of symptoms, slight pressure, heaviness, tightness, burning, discomfort in the chest, neck, arms, shoulders, or back).
Grade 2—Symptoms increase in intensity or location (i.e., the pressure has increased to a grade 2 and has changed to include left arm as well as substernal area).
Grade 3—Symptoms are relatively severe at this time, patients would definitely rest and take nitroglycerin if nitrates are prescribed.
Grade 4—Symptoms increased in intensity to a point that patients would definitely stop what they are doing, rest, and take nitroglycerin if nitrates are prescribed.
From YMCArdiac Therapy, 1981. Gary Fry and Kathy Berra, Carolyn Bean Associates, San Francisco, California. Reproduced with permission of the authors.

Table 23.6.   Daily Log for Exercise Arrhythmias

Daily Log for Exercise Arrhythmias								
No. of episodes/day								
Triggers coffee, exercise, stress, etc.								
Are they associated with lightheadedness or fainting?								
Number of irregular beats per minute while exercising								
Do they also occur at rest?								
Do they resolve when you stop exercising?								

From YMCArdiac Therapy, 1981. Gary Fry and Kathy Berra, Carolyn Bean Associates, San Francisco, California. Reproduced with permission of the authors.

Table 23.7.   Weekly Log of Risk Reduction Program Participation

	Monday	Tuesday	Wednesday	Thursday	Friday	Saturday	Sunday
Blood pressure							
Weight							
Smoking (# cig/ day)							
% of calories from fat							
Minutes of exercise							
Medication side effects							
Minutes of relaxation or stress reduction/day							

From YMCArdiac Therapy, 1981. Gary Fry and Kathy Berra, Carolyn Bean Associates, San Francisco, California. Reproduced with permission of the authors.

times per day to reach a total of 30 minutes. For example, three 10-minutes sessions could be performed, one early morning, one around noon, and one in the evening. Splitting up the activity into bouts of 10 minutes or so has been shown to produce benefits similar to one 30-minute session per day in sedentary middle-aged men (31). The intensity should be set at a workload that keeps the patient symptom-free and is below the intensity at which signs or symptoms of cardiac distress (ischemia, left ventricular dysfunction, or significant arrhythmias) occurred during the most recent exercise test. In most cases, intensity can be translated into heart rate (HR) and perceived exertion (PE) guidelines. A useful 10-point scale for rating PE during exercise known as the Borg scale has been established (Table 23.4) (32).

For instance, if a patient develops symptoms of cardiac distress at a HR of 130 beats per minute and a PE of 7 during exercise testing, an exercise heart rate prescription of 90 to 100 beats per minute with a PE of 5 would be well below potentially unsafe exertion levels. Using HR and PE levels between 60% and 85% of maximal safe limits based on exercise testing can be safe for home-based exercise. At this intensity the patient would not be experiencing untoward signs or symptoms. If the test was symptom- and sign-free, then the intensity should be set at 70% to 80% of peak HR or 60% to 75% or HR reserve.

SELF-MONITORING

Self-monitoring provides a way to evaluate the presence, frequency, and severity of ischemic symptoms and arrhythmias and provides a means of measuring compliance to other risk reduction interventions. Self-monitoring tools such as the simple checklists seen in Tables 23.5–23.7 can help patients measure important physiologic responses to exercise as well as compliance to their home-based programs. Self-monitoring tools are more effective when added to the patient's medical record. Having patients bring monthly logs to their regular office visits can provide useful insights regarding needs for education as well as helping to confirm the safety of the home-based exercise prescription (Tables 23.5–23.7).

COMMUNITY-BASED PROGRAMS

Community-based cardiac exercise programs that rely on nonmedical or patient self-monitoring are an additional model that provides evidence to support home-based exercise safety and efficacy. These programs are located in Jewish Community Centers, YMCAs, community colleges, or other facilities such as health clubs. They are generally low cost, based on self-pay, and extend the exercise and educational opportunities for patients for months to years as opposed to weeks in the more formal hospital-based programs. Costs can be kept low by providing programs that involve relatively large class size and having some groups exercise without direct supervision. They also provide important social support networks.

NEW MODELS OF SECONDARY PREVENTION USING HOME-BASED APPROACHES

New models of care include the development of case-management systems, which, using physician evaluation and supervision, can be successfully carried out by well-trained health care practitioners. One model of this type, the Health Education and Risk Reduction Training (HEAR^{2}T) Program, has been developed at the Stanford Center for Research in Disease Prevention to meet the increasing needs for cost-effective coronary risk reduction programs. HEAR^{2}T is being tested at two worksites and within an independent practice organization (IPA). Within both worksites, high-risk persons are identified by means of a self-report coronary risk assessment questionnaire. Computer analysis provides nurse case-managers with information on all those who participate. Individuals considered to be at high risk are invited to a clinical risk factor screening and initial consultation. Those persons identified at highest risk for a new or recurrent cardiovascular event are invited to participate in a year-long education and risk reduction program. This program is closely linked to each participant's personal physician. All interventions, such as medications for hypertension, diabetes, and dyslipidemia, are prescribed at the discretion of the patient's physician and are monitored as to efficacy and tolerability by the nurse case-manager. Intensive lifestyle education counseling is provided on a regular basis. Participants are referred to existing community resources that can help with risk reduction, including YMCA, community college, and adult education-sponsored exercise programs; commercial weight reduction classes; stop smoking programs sponsored by the American Cancer Society; and diabetes education classes taught by the American Diabetes Association.

The IPA model is unique in that the participants are identified as being at high risk through computerized health care and laboratory databases. Primary care physicians (PCP) are then invited to participate in the program by allowing their patients to be contacted and invited to participate in the lifestyle counseling. Facilitation of medical interventions is accomplished through regular communications between the nurse casemanager and the participating PCP. These new models provide a workable, cost-effective, and safe means of providing home-based coronary risk reduction programs to large numbers of high-risk persons and patients with known CHD.

CONCLUSION

Safe and effective home-based rehabilitation is an important component in the overall management of patients with CHD. Research has demonstrated that home-based interventions can be safe and effective for low- to moderate-risk patients. Additional research is needed to determine appropriate approaches for patients at very high risk of a recurrent coronary event when a medically supervised class-based program is not available. Physician involvement in the evaluation of exercise safety and risk factor status sets the stage for intensive risk reduction behaviors by their patients. Such evaluation, coupled with detailed advice as to appropriate treatment and long-term follow-up, is critical in the implementation of successful home-based cardiac rehabilitation. Integration of case-managers for counseling and systematic follow-up adds additional safety and improves compliance to home-based programs.

Part D.   Corporate-based: Coors Brewing Company

Hank L. Brammell

INTRODUCTION

The description of the phase II cardiac rehabilitation program at the Coors Wellness Center that appeared in the first edition of this text remains valid and is reproduced below in its entirety. The process by which a patient is enrolled, evaluated, participates, and returns to work in a timely fashion is an acceptable and effective model and is recommended for those interested in doing this work in an industrial setting or those who wish to develop a program for a local industry that serves both employer and employee well. Current results of the program are discussed in the Update section at the end of the program description.

Since the first edition was published, some major changes have taken place in the Coors Brewing Company that have impacted the cardiac program. The company has moved from being self-insured and self-administered for health care costs to offering its employees the option of enrolling in one of four different health maintenance organizations (HMO). In addition, the cardiac program, which was mandatory for employees from 1982 to 1994, is now voluntary. Some of those involved in choosing the HMOs wanted to terminate the in-house cardiac rehabilitation program and leave all care in the hands of the contract providers. The program has survived that challenge but has had to come to grips with some new realities. These will be discussed in the Update section at the end of the program section. The employees who enroll in the Wellness Center program are managed as described in that section.

Health care costs in the United States continue to escalate, reaching $661 billion in 1990, or 12.2% of the gross national product (GNP) (1). Cardiovascular diseases will cost in excess of $108 billion in 1992 (2). More than 40% of the total cost burden is borne by business and industry. As a result, industrial leaders are assuming greater responsibility for efforts to reduce health care costs. At the Adolph Coors Company, these efforts began in earnest in 1981 with the opening of the Coors Wellness Center, a 25,000 sq ft remodeled supermarket located at the entrance to the valley in which the majority of Coors industries are located. Soon after the opening of the center, a phase II, early posthospitalization cardiac rehabilitation program was implemented for employees, spouses, dependents, and retirees (3). The program for the employee participant is presented in this section.

THE COMPANY

The Adolph Coors Company was founded more than 100 years ago in Golden, Colorado. The company includes more than 20 distinct businesses, with the brewing operation being the best known and accounting for the greatest sales volume. The brewery is the largest single plant of its kind in the world. There are 10,600 employees worldwide, with approximately 7,000 working in the Golden area. The work force is 78% male, 52% are classified as blue-collar production workers, and the age of the average employee is almost 44 years. The company is self-insured for health care and covers almost 34,000 lives. In 1989, cardiovascular diseases comprised the fourth most costly group of illnesses to the company, accounting for expenditures of $2.3 million. Also, cardiovascular illness accounted for the majority of high cost hospitalizations (greater than $5000), exceeding mental health and musculoskeletal conditions by a significant margin.

THE CARDIAC REHABILITATION PROGRAM

Development of the program was driven by the belief that rehabilitation, when properly practiced, is a wellness program for the person with a disabling condition (internally, the program is called Cardiac Wellness). It therefore was necessary to address a number of program components and to charge participants with attaining their best in each area. Program staff function as facilitators. The outcomes to be realized from the program are the responsibility of each participant. Self-responsibility is taught and encouraged from the outset. Program components addressed for all participants include exercise conditioning, psychosocial issues, education, and vocational concerns. Referral to other modules offered in the Wellness Center is made on an individual basis. Commonly used modules include smoking cessation, weight loss, anger reduction, stress management, and nutritional counseling.

Getting Started

The cardiac rehabilitation program staff is notified by the leave of absence coordinator when an employee is hospitalized for a cardiac event. If the employee is not hospitalized or the patient is a spouse, dependent, or retiree, notification of staff usually comes from Group Health, the company's insurance unit when a bill is received, but may also come from the patient, a family member, or other employee. As soon as the event is confirmed, letters are sent to the patient-employee, the employee's supervisor, and the attending cardiologist. These letters explain the program and create the expectation of participation (the program is mandatory for employees). If the clinical course is uncomplicated, the symptom-limited entry graded-exercise evaluation is scheduled to occur within 2 weeks of discharge from hospital (Fig. 23.4). After completion of the exercise study, the exercise prescription is written using the clearance heart rate (HR) method. The employee then meets with the program coordinator, who reviews the prescription, schedules appropriate entry interviews and Wellness Center modules, outlines the program in detail, and instructs the participant in the correct use of the exercise equipment in the center. Also, personal goals are identified for completion during the program, and a contract is negotiated and signed by the employee to achieve the goals. A brief quiz is given that identifies the employee's knowledge regarding coronary heart disease (CHD) risk factors and appropriate lifestyle modifications. Knowledge gaps identified from the quiz help to guide the staff to provide individual targeted instruction during the course of the program. Finally, the employee is given a notebook that contains five sections: welcome (Cardiac Wellness general information and participant responsibilities, consent form, medical questionnaire, medication wallet card, consent for release of information, schedule of the education classes), getting started (exercise prescription, pretest of cardiovascular disease knowledge, health improvement contract), return to work, graduation (assessment of progress toward goals, posttest of knowledge), and on your own (identification of company and community resources to assist with maintenance of changes made during the program). All employee-patient records are kept in a closed area within the Wellness Center. Specific information is shared with the employee, the program staff, and the attending physician. There is no discussion by staff of employee's medical status with disinterested or otherwise inappropriate persons.

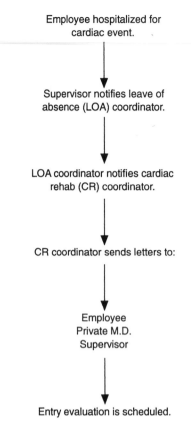

Employee hospitalized for cardiac event.

Supervisor notifies leave of absence (LOA) coordinator.

LOA coordinator notifies cardiac rehab (CR) coordinator.

CR coordinator sends letters to:

Employee
Private M.D.
Supervisor

Entry evaluation is scheduled.

Figure 23.4. The usual procedure in which an employee is enrolled in the cardiac rehabilitation program.

Exercise Conditioning

The exercise component is traditional in that formal, supervised sessions are scheduled for 3 days each week for a total of 12 weeks. Although most employees return to work in some form shortly after beginning the program, they are kept involved for the full duration to complete the educational component and to increase the likelihood of permanent lifestyle changes.

Exercises are primarily aerobic, although roughly 25% of the exercise time is devoted to strength training. Each exercise session begins with staff-led warm-up of 10 to 15 minutes. These activities emphasize improving balance, coordination, and flexibility. Individual participants are responsible for following their own prescription for the remaining 45 to 60 minutes. Aerobic exercises include walking or jogging on the elevated 1/18-mile track or on a motor-driven treadmill, or stationary cycling. Participants also can use the Nordic Trac, StairMaster, Versa-Climber, or Concept II rower. One session each week is devoted to low-impact aerobic exercise. Resistance training is performed on isokinetic devices or with free weights. Initial exercises are low weight or low resistance with frequent repetitions to emphasize muscle groups required to perform job tasks. Gradually, weight or resistance is increased until it matches the job requirement. Telemetry monitoring is available but is reserved for high-risk participants (persons with ejection fraction less than 30%, complex resting or exercise-induced ventricular arrhythmias, history of sudden cardiac death, falling systolic blood pressure (BP) with exercise, or inability to self-monitor). Most participants are able to monitor their HR accurately by palpation of the carotid or radial pulse. In those individuals who require telemetry monitoring, monitoring is discontinued as soon as clinical stability and safety are achieved and self-monitoring is instituted. Exercise prescriptions are upgraded each week.

Vocational Component

The job site visit and job evaluation are the first activities to be completed when the staff learns that an employee has had a cardiac event. The visit is made by one of the staff (physician, exercise physiologist, occupational therapist, vocational rehabilitation counselor) who reviews physical requirements, environmental factors such as temperature extremes or chemical exposures, and psychosocial issues. Finally, management willingness to modify the job tasks, at least temporarily, and to accommodate a phased return to work are assessed.

The new participant's job analysis is discussed with the program staff at the weekly cardiac rehabilitation staffing. Job-specific strength training exercises are developed and included in the supervised exercise sessions. The employee is told at the time of entry to the program that returning to work is part of the rehabilitation process and that doing so is a confirmation that life is normalizing. All return-to-work decisions are made in-house.

Most program participants will return to work while still enrolled in the rehabilitation program. When the employee is ready to return to the workplace, a meeting is held in the Wellness Center that includes the employee, the employee's supervisor, the program coordinator, and the physician. At this time, the employee's medical situation is reviewed, any job and temporary shift modifications are negotiated, and a return-to-work date is identified. Generally, a phased return is arranged in which the employee begins working 4 hours a day with 2-hour increases in the work day that occur every 1 to 2 weeks until the full shift and all job tasks are being worked. Employees who work an 8-hour shift generally will be working the full shift before those who work 10- or 12-hour shifts. The final event of the return-to-work meeting is to offer the supervisor an opportunity to have one of the rehabilitation staff make a presentation to other employees in the work unit at one of the regular unit meetings. At this meeting, held at the work site, the recovering employee's condition is discussed (with their permission), a general overview of the problem of cardiovascular disease and CHD risk factors is presented, and questions are answered.

Educational Component

Twelve weekly interactive educational programs are given for the employee and family members. Classes are presented by program staff and emphasis is placed on CHD risk factors, exercise, medical issues, and diet modification. A 2-hour trip to a local supermarket with the employee and spouse is led by the nutritionist and is designed to demonstrate practical ways to identify heart-healthy foods. The overall objective of each class is to help the persons attending assume responsibility for their own health outcomes. As a result, much emphasis is placed on how to effect meaningful change and the potential benefit to be derived from lifestyle changes.

Psychosocial Component

When the employee enters the program, an appointment is made with the counselor in Employee and Family Counseling Services who has responsibility for cardiac clients. This is a 1-hour one-on-one session in which the counselor explores the employee's mood, family or financial problems, the status of interpersonal relations at the worksite, the presence or suspicion of substance abuse, and any other issue the employee chooses to discuss. If a significant problem is identified, referral to an outside provider is rec-

ommended. Problems that can be handled in one to three sessions often are managed by the in-house counselor.

Finally, four 1-hour classes are held for the participants and spouses that focus on the role of stress in their lives and its potential impact on their disease process. A number of stress management techniques are introduced and practiced for a short time. The goal of the classes is to heighten the employees' awareness of stress and to help each participant recognize whether stress is an important problem in their lives. If stress is a significant factor that requires extended intervention, then referral is made to an outside provider.

Exit and Follow-Up

When the program is completed, a symptom-limited maximal treadmill exercise study is repeated, and the exercise prescription is upgraded for independent maintenance exercise. Most participants will continue to use the Wellness Center for exercise, and many choose to remain with the scheduled and supervised cardiac rehabilitation class. A brief quiz that deals with coronary disease, risk factors, and lifestyle changes is given to assess changes in the employee's knowledge and to help the staff evaluate the effectiveness of the education program. Progress made toward goals that were negotiated at the beginning of the program is reviewed, and new goals are set for the maintenance program. Finally, the employee is given (with some fanfare) a certificate of completion signed by the program staff and a Cardiac Wellness T-shirt.

Exercise studies are repeated 3 months after completing the program and then annually on the anniversary of the cardiac event. These evaluations include a current history, physical examination, resting and exercise electrocardiograms (ECGs), and a lipid profile. The importance of maintaining lifestyle changes is reinforced, the exercise prescription is reviewed, and referral to other Wellness Center modules is made as indicated. The results of all procedures are shared with the prescribing physician.

Program Evaluation

All program activities are evaluated by program staff on an ongoing basis. Specific program objectives have been identified that we believe are important for maintaining a high-quality program. These include the following:

1. Participants improve functional capacity 10% or more.
2. Participants know their coronary disease risk factors.
3. Participants make progress toward achieving personal goals.
4. Participants return to work in a timely fashion (8 weeks or less).
5. Participants returned to the job held at the time of the cardiac event.
6. Few participants require long-term disability.

Each objective has been assigned minimally acceptable, target, and optimal expectancies. When objectives are not met, a thorough review is made by the coordinator, deficits are defined, and corrective action is taken. Except for the long-term disability objective, the program evaluation is conducted quarterly.

PROGRAM OUTCOMES

Since the program began, 10 to 23 employees have been served each year (average, 19) and 30 to 43 total participants (average, 34) have completed the program annually. Nonemployee participants include spouses, retirees, and employees who have not had a cardiac event (e.g., cardiomyopathy, peripheral vascular disease). Although only 52% of the company's employees are production or maintenance (blue-collar) workers, 75% of the rehabilitation participants have come from these groups. Fifty-five percent of patients were employees. Eighty-five percent were men and 15% were women. The most common diagnoses were acute myocardial infarction (MI), coronary artery bypass graft surgery, and percutaneous transluminal coronary angioplasty. An occasional valve replacement and one heart transplant were represented in the program.

Before implementing the program, the previous 2 years' return-to-work experience of cardiac employees was reviewed. The average time from the cardiac event to returning to work was 7.5 months. The reason for this long delay in returning to work is not clear. It may relate in part to the attending physician not being familiar with the employees' job and delaying permission to return

to work until the clinical situation was stable and good functional status was demonstrated. It also may have been because of the company leave of absence policy, which states that an injured or ill employee will receive full pay for up to 182 days if the medical condition warrants. It was thought that this policy would be a disincentive for cardiac employees to return to work from the Wellness Center program. This has not been the case. For the life of the program, return-to-work time has averaged 2 months from the event, resulting in a significant reduction in employee replacement costs during the convalescent period. This replacement cost avoidance has averaged in excess of $268,000 annually.

In addition to an earlier return-to-work, employees have, with one exception, returned to the same job held at the time of the cardiac event. The company, therefore, has incurred almost no retraining costs. Also, there have been only two employee participants (1.8%) who were too ill at the end of the program to return to work and who were placed on long-term disability. The 10-year return-to-work rate has been 98%.

The program has been safe; there was one cardiac arrest and death of a nonemployee participant in approximately 11,000 hours of phase II participation. There have been no acute MIs, arrhythmias, or other events that required transport from the Wellness Center to hospital for immediate care. In addition, there have been no untoward events with any strength training activities.

The company calculates that the in-house cardiac rehabilitation program has resulted in significant cost savings. Each year, the cardiac rehabilitation staff conducts a survey of community costs of similar rehabilitation programs and the cost of a graded-exercise evaluation to compare with the cost of providing services in-house. In the first full 9 years of the program, community cardiac rehabilitation costs averaged $1766 (range, $1500 to $1875), whereas the cost of the Wellness Center program averaged $539 (range, $500 to $575). The graded-exercise evaluation averaged $258 in the community (range, $220 to $332) and was $76 when provided in-house (range, $50 to $108). Because the company is fully self-insured, these savings have an immediate and direct effect on health care costs. These direct savings plus the replacement employee cost avoidance have resulted in net average savings of more than $325,000 annually.

The nature of this industrial-based cardiac rehabilitation program does not permit an assessment of its impact on mortality, the incidence of repeat cardiac events, or its effect on the natural history of CHD. One would expect that an industrial-based rehabilitation program would have a reduction in cardiovascular end points similar to published trials (4, 5).

COMMENT

The experience of an early posthospitalization cardiac rehabilitation program in an industrial wellness center has been a good one for the Adolph Coors Company. The program has been safe, it has kept valued employees on the job, and it has been economically sound. We believe that long-term disability and retraining costs have been avoided. First-hand knowledge of the employees' job tasks and the use of job-specific strength training have been helpful in getting employees back to work in a timely fashion and in avoiding the need for retraining, particularly for employees whose jobs are physically demanding. Staff attendance and participation in employee unit meetings have been a valuable contact with employees for education and primary prevention activities. Furthermore, these meetings create visibility for the Wellness Center and help to allay anxieties that coworkers may have regarding colleagues with heart disease.

From a philosophical perspective, we feel that industry serves its employees and its community best when it enters into a partnership with the employee and health care providers to improve the health status of employees who have chronic illness. The goals of this partnership are to keep the employee on the job, to provide the opportunity to learn secondary prevention strategies, and to make reasonable worksite accommodations. No one is well served when a productive employee with a chronic condition is released in the hope of avoiding future catastrophic health care costs.

Business and industry, particularly self-insured companies, whose bottom line is directly influenced by any cost-saving enterprise, should be considered appropriate customers for the managers of a cardiac rehabilitation program. If not already in place, the community-based program would need to develop a strong vocational component with skill in job analysis, willingness to visit the plant, and willingness to interact with management to create a win-win situation. The win for management is earlier return to work, retention in the same job, avoidance of retraining, long-term disability costs, and lower program costs; the win for the employee is returning to work, no reduction in pay, and support from the company in making appropriate and healthful lifestyle changes. The alliance of a company with a cardiac rehabilitation provider who understands the needs of the employee and the company alike can help avoid the adversarial relationship that too often occurs among the company, the employee, and the employee's physician. Finally, once involved with a company, the cardiac rehabilitation staff could develop and offer primary prevention programming for employees as a cost avoidance activity—helping the employer avoid the high cost of catastrophic coronary events in the future.

UPDATE

The general statistics regarding the program have changed little. Through 1996, 548 persons had completed the program. Seventy-five percent were hourly wage earners, 98% of employee participants returned to the same job held at the time of their cardiac event, and 2% required training for a new position or were placed on long-term disability. The average return to work time from the onset of the event was 1.4 months. Return to work was usually to a restricted duty job as described above. Savings to the company through 1995 were substantial: more than $8.4 million. Savings came from early return to work, money saved by not having to pay replacement personnel, performing exercise studies in-house, and the lower cost of conducting the program compared with the community average. There has still been only one death during more than 20,000 hours of patient participation. We continue to conclude that the industrial-based program has been cost effective and safe.

As indicated previously, Coors has recently given up its self-insured status and has selected four HMO offerings for employees and retirees not yet eligible for Medicare. Not all of these providers were equal in their provision of cardiac rehabilitation services: two had no program at all, one would cover 20 exercise sessions (if the patient met Agency for Health Care Policy and Research guidelines for monitored exercise) but would not cover any education activities or stress management effort and has no systematic return-to-work component. The fourth provider would cover 13 exercise classes, 3 education classes, and 1 stress management session, and had no vocational effort. As indicated previously, participation in cardiac rehabilitation is no longer mandatory for employees.

As expected, enrollment in the Wellness Center program has dropped almost 50%. This has occurred in spite of an aging work force (the average employee is 47 years old). Patients come to the program because they learned of it from a coworker or they are self-referred. Provider referrals are uncommon unless the physician had previous knowledge of the program. Occasionally, program staff learns of an employee who has been off work for many months and who has not been involved in any rehabilitation effort.

The company's response has been to continue to offer the cardiac program at no cost to employees, retirees, or dependents even though the HMO refuses coverage. Although program staff has met with each of the HMO management groups, there has been little, if any, apparent filtering down of information regarding the program availability to cardiology and primary care providers. Other approaches will clearly be necessary, e.g., direct physician meetings, mailings, and Wellness Center open house for physician and their staff. Each effort should be evaluated for its impact on referrals and enrollment. In addition, a concerted internal company marketing effort to employees, supervisors, and management should be undertaken together with the external program to optimize supervisor referrals and self-referrals.

Data need to be collected regarding the number of employees who participate in cardiac rehabilitation, their return-to-work outcomes versus those not participating, changes in the long-term disability rate with HMO involvement, and any change in costs to the company regarding replacement employees, long-term disability or early retirement, or the need for retraining. The HMOs have a unique opportunity to respond to the needs of employers by providing cardiac rehabilitation programs that include a strong, appropriately aggressive vocational component in addition to the usual exercise conditioning, education, and stress management activities. Such an effort might help an HMO retain business when the annual enrollment period arrives.

Part E.   Corporate-based: The Boeing Company
George O. Gey

Worksite cardiac programs have been in existence in Seattle, Washington, since 1974 and are a spin-off from the CAPRI cardiac rehabilitation programs begun at the YMCA in Seattle in 1968 (1, 2). Our purpose has been to provide a supportive environment for employees with heart disease near a worksite where exercise could be done under medical supervision. The goals of our program are better health and continued active employment to all who would benefit (3). Our mission is "to improve the health and quality of life of employees with cardiovascular disease by providing a medically supervised program whereby employees can experience reduction of risk factors, reduction in morbidity and mortality, and improved cardiorespiratory capacity through health education and regular supervised exercise."

Our philosophy has changed during the years to keep pace with the changing clinical presentation of workers with cardiac disease (4). Cardiac arrest with exercise and large myocardial infarctions were common in the 1970s. Today, this is much less prevalent and is replaced with early angioplasty closure and chronic heart failure with atrial fibrillation. The program has been open to all employees with referral from their personal physicians. The American Association of Cardiovascular Pulmonary Rehabilitation (AACVPR) risk stratification has allowed most employees returning to work opportunities to join one of three programs: one with medical supervision for those who are at high risk for collapse during exercise; one with supervised exercise for those with coronary disease of low risk for collapse during exercise; and one with minimum supervision for those with a record of stable medical conditions and lowest risk for collapse during exercise. This has been developed during the years with success of safe, convenient, and helpful health and fitness programs for all employees. Many of our employees have had a phase I and II cardiac rehabilitation program after medical and surgical treatment for heart disease in the community and seek a phase III or IV cardiac rehabilitation program on return to work.

The corporate rehabilitation programs are at

two locations: one in Seattle, and one in Everett, where most of the workforce is located. The components of the cardiac rehabilitation program are listed in Table 23.8. The program is promoted through the use of brochures, industrial clinics on return to work, private medical referrals, Boeing newsletters, and community cardiac rehabilitation programs. The number of participants varies from year to year depending on employment, retirement, and change of job location. All of our clients have significant heart disease and are at high risk for sudden cardiac death.

Only active employees are admitted to the program. Retirees are allowed to remain in the program if they are active at the time of retirement. Retirees who have a coronary event after retirement are encouraged to participate in outside rehabilitation programs and are eligible for our health and fitness programs if they stratify at low risk. This has been found to be beneficial to both retirees and employees (5–11). There are now several cardiac rehabilitation programs available in the community in which many employees elect to participate. Logistics are a significant issue in that traffic and distant locations are an ever-present problem in the Puget Sound area. Low-risk cardiac clients are given the option of coming during off-peak traffic times to use several available health and fitness exercise rooms. The cardiac rehabilitation population number is potentially 1% of the workforce; thus, with an employee population of 100,000 in the Puget Sound area, there are 100 to 150 active participants in the cardiac rehabilitation program and more than 600 low-risk employees and retirees in the health and fitness programs.

Table 23.8.   Boeing Cardiac Rehabilitation Program Components

Referral by personal physician
Intake interviews
Review participant's occupational requirements
Provide individual program prescription
Provide medically supervised exercise
Incorporate stretching and strengthening exercises
Provide disease prevention and health education
Periodic diet review
Provide group and individual support
Provide for psychological/social issues discussion
Provide ongoing health evaluations
Perform yearly participant evaluation

Therefore, approximately one-tenth the number of high-risk cardiac patients who could benefit from the program are enrolled. The reasons for this are 1) time of shift work, 2) preference of location, 3) sick leave, and 4) activity in an outside phase I or II program after medical or surgical treatment.

Many employees are exercising at home in addition to the worksite programs. In some respects our program is like the Toronto Program with several days per month of supervised exercise, but consisting mainly of at-home exercise. There are many who participate habitually; some as long as 20 years. During 1993 and 1994, the number of visits of cardiac clients was tracked and is shown in Figure 23.5. Fluctuations in participation depend on company vacation and holiday periods throughout the year. Our staffing ratio is generally based on one staff to 20 participants, with a minimum of one physician and one nurse in addition to a specially trained physiologist part-time to advise on exercise equipment and exercise prescriptions. Some of the dynamics of our cardiac population in the rehabilitation program can be seen in Table 23.9 subsequent to reduction in the employee population into two programs in 1995. The current number of active participants is 110 in the two active sites. Turnover is about 20 per year entering and transitioning to other programs.

Exercise sessions are 1.5 hours in duration including 15 minutes of calisthenics. For more than 23 years the program has consisted of brief monitoring for heart rhythm and blood pressure determinations before and after exercise in the high-risk group. Charting hemodynamics and reporting alterations in symptoms and medications are important means of documenting fluctuating clinical cardiac medical problems. Many times, significant changes in these parameters help unmask underlying cardiac and medical problems. The experience with cardiac arrest has been minimal: only one arrest per 5 years for the past 20 years that the program has been in existence. There have been several deaths during exertion outside the medically monitored program. Most were related to overexertion and unsuspected coronary disease.

All of our participants use a heart rate monitor during exercise and have a training heart rate determined from an annual treadmill test. We have provided areas to test blood sugar levels be-

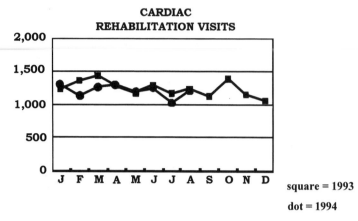

square = 1993

dot = 1994

Figure 23.5. Cardiac rehabilitation visits.

Table 23.9. Boeing Cardiac Rehabilitation Program Dynamics—October, 1993–August, 1994

	Everett	Oxbow	Renton
Total Participants			
October, 1993	70	118	55
August, 1994	58	98	54
Transferred to H&F	8	5	2
Dropped for other reasons *	9	20	2
New Participants	24	17	3
Low Risk	9	5	10
Moderate Risk	25	91	37
High Risk	8	13	5
** Undetermined	9		

* These include work schedule incompatibility, retirement, commuting, termination, long illness, financial difficulty, etc. Numbers do not indicate transfer between program sites. Risk stratification for Seattle participants has been consistent for those people who had their physicals and exercise tests at the Boeing Clinic. The numbers supplied here are "best estimate" and would not be more than one or two actuals off.
**Risk stratification not completed at date of review.

fore and after exercise and do not allow patients with insulin-dependent diabetes to exercise if their blood sugar is less than 100 mg/dL. Symptomatic hypoglycemia occurs rarely, and there have been no participants who have collapsed during or shortly after exercise as result of hypoglycemia. Participants with blood sugars less than 100 mg/dL are generally fed a light snack and can then exercise without medical incident.

Hypotension after exercise has been a common problem, but has not required emergency care. Attention to the postexertional cool-down and to overmedication with antihypertension medication has addressed this common medical problem in exercising patients with hypertension. It has been our experience that hyperten-

sive participants starting an exercise program can safely perform submaximal exercise with frequent blood pressure checks. With exercise and vasodilation, the blood pressure usually normalizes and exercise can continue. No cerebral vascular accidents (CVAs) have occurred during exercise even though our cardiac population ranges up to 80 years of age. Cerebral vascular accidents have occurred in our clients during nonexercise periods. This suggests that factors other than high systolic blood pressure are active in the cause of stroke in an exercising cardiac population. We have observed few problems using the Bruce protocol for maximally testing our population of workers both with and without documented coronary disease.

Goals for participants include achievement of a better quality of life, reduction of risk factors, reduction of medication and more appropriate medication with exercise, improved functional capacity, improved oxygen uptake, reduced anxiety, increased understanding of physical limitations and meaning of symptoms with exercise, and less morbidity and mortality. A customer satisfaction questionnaire in 1992 showed interesting results and insight to our clients' attitudes (Fig. 23.6). As with any program there are successes and failures; it shows how a sample of 56 participants felt about perceived benefits from the cardiac rehabilitation program. One observation we have made during the years the program has been in existence is that once employees participate in the program and experience benefit, they return after long absences when work and retirement take them elsewhere. Most absences

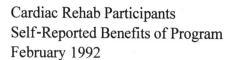

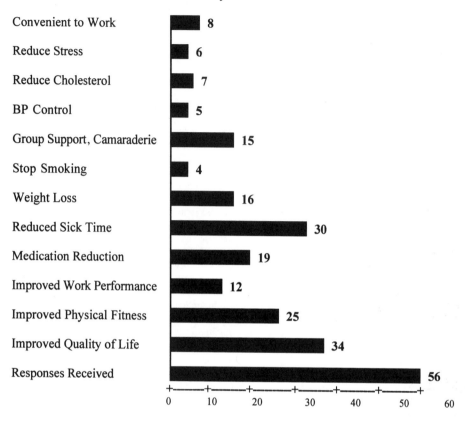

Figure 23.6.   Cardiac rehabilitation participants' self-reported benefits of programs.

are caused by nonmedical reasons. We have documented the effect of kilocalorie expenditure on our participants (12). This overall regular caloric expenditure may help explain the improvement in mortality and morbidity reported to be associated with exercise that cannot be explained on the basis of improvement of physical fitness alone. Another way to look at this is that continuing good health may be related to continuing goodly amounts of exercise, and vice-versa.

Cardiac rehabilitation is active caring for those who cannot safely exercise alone (13) or have had recent medical and surgical treatment. Continued (long-term) cardiac rehabilitation is appropriate for those who find benefit in a structured environment and regular follow-up for risk factors. Such programs are especially appropriate for those cor-

porations and businesses who have more than 20,000 employees in a single geographic location where there is interest and enthusiasm for such an endeavor. Cost benefit (4) is related to better health of each employee. It can be related to fewer illnesses, which minimized poor performance, work absences, hospitalizations, medical care, recovery periods after a morbid event, and loss of self-confidence. It may also be related to lower mortality through training of household members in cardiopulmonary resuscitation, a regular educational feature of our program. For those of us who exercise with our clients, it provides a unique opportunity to observe symptoms that occur only with exercise, and it is a splendid way of sharing healthy pursuits and aspirations to achieve a healthy lifestyle and wellness.

References

Part B.

1. Pashkow FJ, Pashkow PS, Schafer MN. Successful cardiac rehabilitation: the complete guide for building cardiac rehab programs. 1st ed. Loveland, CO: The HeartWatchers Press, 1988.
2. Hämäläinen H, Kallio V, Knuts LR, et al. Community approach in rehabilitation and secondary prevention after acute myocardial infarction: results of a randomized clinical trial. J Cardpulm Rehabil 1991;11:221–226.
3. Pashkow F, Schafer M, Pashkow P. HeartWatchers—low cost, community-based cardiac rehabilitation in Loveland, Colorado. J Cardpulm Rehabil 1986;6: 469–473.
4. Hartwig R. Cardiopulmonary research institute—CAPRI. J Cardiac Rehab 1982;2:481–483.
5. Pashkow FJ. Issues in contemporary cardiac rehabilitation: a historical perspective. J Am Coll Cardiol 1993;21:822–834.
6. Oldridge NB, Guyatt GH, Fischer ME, et al. Cardiac rehabilitation after myocardial infarction. Combined experience of randomized clinical trials. JAMA 1988;260: 945–950.
7. O'Connor GT, Buring JE, Yusuf S, et al. An overview of randomized trials of rehabilitation with exercise after myocardial infarction. Circulation 1989;80:234–244.
8. Hämäläinen H, Luurila OJ, Kallio V, et al. Long-term reduction in sudden deaths after multifactorial intervention programme in patients with myocardial infarction: 10-year results of a controlled investigation. Eur Heart J 1989;10:55–62.
9. Drimmer AM, Hibbett A, Arnold M. Exercise effect on long-term control of mild hypertension [abstract]. J Cardpulm Rehabil 1989;9:404.
10. Lavie CJ, Milani RV. Effects of cardiac rehabilitation, exercise training, and weight reduction on exercise capacity, coronary risk factors, behavioral characteristics, and quality of life in obese coronary patients. Am J Cardiol 1997;79:397–401.
11. Murray PM, Herrington DM, Davis S, et al. Modest physical training in a cardiac rehabilitation program associated with significant elevations in high density lipoprotein [abstract]. J Cardpulm Rehabil 1991;11:303.
12. Warner JG Jr, Brubaker PH, Zhu Y, et al. Long-term (5-year) changes in HDL cholesterol in cardiac rehabilitation patients. Do sex differences exist? Circulation 1995;92:773–777.
13. Williams MA, Maresh CM, Esterbrooks DJ, et al. Early exercise training in patients older than age 65 years compared with that in younger patients after acute myocardial infarction or coronary artery bypass grafting. Am J Cardiol 1985;55:263–266.
14. Williams MA, Esterbrooks DJ, Sketch MH. Extension of phase II exercise training period produces significant benefit in the older elderly participant [abstract]. J Cardpulm Rehabil 1991;11:312.
15. Vitcenda M, Einerson J. Long-term maintenance of maximal and training capacity in cardiac rehabilitation patients [abstract]. J Cardpulm Rehabil 1991;11:313.
16. Wenger NK, Froelicher ES, Smith LK, et al. Cardiac rehabilitation as secondary prevention. Clinical Practice Guideline No. 17. Rockville, MD: US Department of Health and Human Services, Public Health Service, Agency for Health Care Policy and Research and the National Heart, Lung, and Blood Institute. AHCPR Publication #96–0673, October 1995.
17. American College of Sports Medicine. Guidelines for exercise testing and prescription. 4th ed. Philadelphia: Lea & Febiger, 1991.
18. American Association of Cardiopulmonary Rehabilitation. Guidelines for cardiac rehabilitation programs. 2nd ed. Champaign, IL: Human Kinetics, 1995:2–3.
19. VanCamp S, Peterson R. Cardiovascular complications of outpatient cardiac rehabilitation programs. JAMA 1986;256:1160–1163.
20. Pescatello LS, Arnold N, Dow-Conklin D, et al. The New Britain cardiac rehabilitation program: a sixteen year evolution for illness to wellness. J Cardpulm Rehabil 1989;9:115–121.
21. Burkett PA, Rectanus EF, Bultena KS. Compliance to a phase III exercise program [abstract]. J Cardpulm Rehabil 1990;10:381.
22. Pashkow FJ. Computer-assisted program management for cardiac rehabilitation. In: Broustet JP, ed. Fifth World Congress of Cardiac Rehabilitation. Bordeaux, France: Intercept Ltd., 1993:347–356.
23. Ades PA, Pashkow FJ, Nestor JR. Cost-effectiveness of cardiac rehabilitation after myocardial infarction. J Cardpulm Rehabil 1997;17:222–231.
24. Shephard RJ. Exercise in secondary and tertiary rehabilitation: costs and benefits. J Cardpulm Rehabil 1989;9:188–194.

Part C.

1. O'Conner GT, Buring JE, Yusuf S, et al. An overview of randomized trials of rehabilitation with exercise after infarction. Circulation 1989;80:234–244.
2. Oldridge NB, Guyatt GH, Fischer ME, et al. Cardiac rehabilitation after myocardial infarction. Combined experience of randomized clinical trials. JAMA 1988;260: 945–950.
3. Yusuf S, Lessem J, Jha P, et al. Primary and secondary prevention of myocardial infarction and strokes: an update of randomly allocated controlled trials. J Hypertension 1993;11(Suppl):562–573.
4. Antiplatelet Trialists Collaboration. Collaborative overview of randomised trials of antiplatelet therapy: maintenance of vascular graft or arterial patency by antiplatelet therapy. BMJ 1994;308:1159–168.
5. Hampton JR. Secondary prevention of acute myocardial infarction with beta-blocking agents and calcium antagonists. Am J Cardiol 1990;66:3C–8C.
6. Wenger, NK, Froelicher ES, Smith LK, and Guideline Panel. Cardiac rehabilitation: clinical practice guideline. Agency for Health Care Policy and Research Publication No. 96–0672, October 1995:1.
7. Thomas RJ, Miller, NH, Lamendola C, et al. National survey of gender differences in cardiac rehabilitation programs: patient characteristics and enrollment patterns. J Cardpulm Rehabil 1996;16:402–412.
8. Oldridge NB, Ragowski B, Gottleib M. Use of outpatient rehabilitation services: factors associated with attendance. J Cardpulm Rehabil 1992;12:25–31.

9. Ades PA, Waldman ML, Polk DM, et al. Referral patterns and exercise response in the female coronary patients aged > 62 years. Am J Cardiol 1992;69:1422–1425.

10. Sivarajan ES, Bruce RA, Lindskog BD, et al. Treadmill test responses to an early exercise program after myocardial infarction: a randomized study. Circulation 1982;65:1420–1428.

11. Fletcher GF, Chiaramida AJ, LeMay MR, et al. Telephonically-monitored home exercise early after coronary artery bypass surgery. Chest 1984;86:198–202.

12. Miller NH, Haskell WL, Berra K, et al. Home versus group exercise training for increasing functional capacity after myocardial infarction. Circulation 1984;70:645–649.

13. Fletcher BJ, Dunbar SB, Felner JM, et al. Exercise testing and training in physically disabled men with clinical evidence of coronary artery disease. Am J Cardiol 1994;73:101–103.

14. Haskell WL, Alderman EL, Fair JM, et al. Effects of intensive multiple risk factor reduction on coronary atherosclerosis and clinical cardiac events in men and women with coronary artery disease: the Stanford Coronary Risk Intervention Project (SCRIP). Circulation 1994;89:975–990.

15. DeBusk RF, Haskell WL, Miller NH, et al. Medically directed at-home rehabilitation soon after uncomplicated myocardial infarction: a new model for patient care. Am J Cardiol 1985;55:251–257.

16. DeBusk RF, Houston Miller N, Superko HR, et al. A case management system for coronary risk factor modification after acute myocardial infarction. Ann Intern Med 1994;120:721–729.

17. Stevens R, Hanson P. Comparison of supervised and unsupervised exercise after coronary bypass surgery. Am J Cardiol 1984;53:1524–1528.

18. Heath GW, Maloney PM, Fure CW. Group exercise versus home exercise in coronary artery bypass graft patients: effects on physical activity habits. J Cardpulm Rehabil 1987;7:281–285.

19. Hands ME, Briffa T, Henderson K, et al. Functional capacity and left ventricular function: the effects of supervised and unsupervised exercise rehabilitation soon after coronary artery bypass surgery. J Cardpulm Rehabil 1987;7:578–584.

20. Perk J, Hedback B, Jutterdal S. Cardiac rehabilitation: evaluation of long-term programme of physical training for out-patients. Scand J Rehabil Med 1989;22:15–20.

21. Ades P, Pashkow F, Fletcher G, et al. A controlled trial of cardiac rehabilitation in the home setting: improving accessibility [abstract]. J Am Coll Cardiol 1996;27(Suppl):741.

22. Sparks KE, Sechler J, Steele R, et al. Effectiveness of trans-telephonic-monitored home exercise program [abstract]. J Cardpulm Rehabil 1990;10:372.

23. Squires RW, Miller, TD, Harn T, et al. Transtelephonic electrocardiographic monitoring of cardiac rehabilitation exercise sessions in coronary artery disease. Am J Cardiol 1991;67:962–964.

24. Shaw DK, Sparks KE, Hanigosky P. Exercise compliance and patient satisfaction: transtelephonic exercise monitoring [abstract]. J Cardpulm Rehabil 1990;10:373.

25. Haskell WL. Cardiovascular complications during exercise training of cardiac patients. Circulation 1978;57:920–924.

26. Hossock KF, Hartwig R. Cardiac arrest associated with supervised cardiac rehabilitation. J Cardiac Rehabil 1982;2:402–408.

27. Van Camp SP, Peterson RA. Cardiovascular complications of outpatient cardiac rehabilitation programs. JAMA 1986;256:1160–1163.

28. Thompson PD, Funk EJ, Carelton RA, et al. The incidence of death during jogging in Rhode Island from 1975 through 1980. JAMA 1982;247:2535–2538.

29. The American Association of Cardiovascular and Pulmonary Rehabilitation. Guidelines for cardiac rehabilitation programs. Champaign IL: Human Kinetics, 1995:14.

30. Sparks KE, Shaw DK, Vantrease J. Transtelephonic exercise monitoring of high risk cardiac patients [abstract]. J Cardpulm Rehabil 1992;12:358.

31. DeBusk, RF, Hakansson U, Sheehan M, et al. Training effects of long versus short bouts of exercise. Am J Cardiol 1990;65:1010–1013.

32. Noble BJ, Borg GAV, Jacobs I, et al. A category-ratio perceived exertion scale: relationship to blood and muscle lactates and heart rate. Med Sci Sports Exerc 1983;15:523–528.

33. American College of Sports Medicine. Guidelines for exercise testing and prescription. Media, PA: Williams & Wilkins, 1995:25.

Part D.

1. Sullivan LW. Address to the society of thoracic surgeons. Ann Thorac Surg 1991;52:410–412.

2. American Heart Association. Heart and stroke facts. Dallas, TX: American Heart Association, 1991.

3. Henritze J, Brammell HL. Phase II cardiac wellness at the Adolph Coors Company. Am J Health Promotion 1989;4:25–31.

4. Oldridge NB, Guyatt GH, Fischer ME, et al. Cardiac rehabilitation after myocardial infarction. Combined experience of randomized clinical trials. JAMA 1988;260:945–950.

5. O'Connor GT, Buring JE, Yusuf S, et al. An overview of randomized trials of rehabilitation with exercise after myocardial infarction. Circulation 1989;80: 234–244.

Part E.

1. Bruce EF, Bruce RA, Fisher LD. Comparison of active participants and drop outs in CAPRI (Cardio Pulmonary Rehabilitation Institute). Am J Cardiol 1976;37:53–60.

2. Bruce RA, Kusumi F, Frederick R. Differences in cardiac function with prolonged physical training for cardiac rehabilitation. Am J Cardiol 1977;40:597–603.

3. Fletcher BJ, Griffin PA, Lloyd A, et al. Cardiac rehabilitation in the workplace. Current concepts and methodology. AAOHN Journal 1990;38(9)440–447.

4. Barhnart L. Hospital helps Coke develop exercise program for employee with cardiac problems. OHM, 1993, 44–45.

5. Mital A, Kerman GM, Colan-Brown K. Aerobic capac-

ity of coronary heart disease (CHD) patients and its use in accommodating them in the workplace. Disabil Rehabil 1996;18:396–401.

6. Dedmon RE. Exercise prescription in an industrial fitness program. US Department of Health, Education, and Welfare, National Institute of Occupational Safety and Health Publication No. 78–169, 1978:160–177.

7. Naas R. Health promotion programs yield long term savings. Bus Health 1992;10(13):41–42, 44–47.

8. Bailey NC. Wellness programs that work. Bus Health 1990;8:28(8).

9. McDonald M. Valuing experience, how to keep older workers healthy. Bus Health 1990;8(1):35, 37–38.

10. Chua TB, Lipkin DP. Cardiac rehabilitation. BMJ 1993;306:731–732.

11. Taylor R, Kirby B. The evidence base for the cost effectiveness of cardiac rehabilitation. Heart 1997; 78:5–6.

12. Parker DL, Leaf DA, Sailer K, et al. A kilocalorie expenditure-based-work-site cardiac rehabilitation program: sustaining prognostic risk. Med Exerc Nutr Health 1994;3(5):232–239.

13. Siscovick DS, et al. The incidence of primary cardiac arrest during vigorous exercise. N Engl J Med 1984; 311(14):874–877.

Medical–Legal Liability

David L. Herbert and William G. Herbert

Recently, the United States has been engulfed in what many claim to be a litigation explosion of unprecedented proportions. At the same time there has been much concern expressed about a medical malpractice crisis in this country that many believe is eroding the foundation of medical care delivery. Although some medicolegal analysts strenuously argue that neither of these situations really exists, it must be obvious to all providers that the risks of claim and suit that arise out of patient care are greater today than at any time in our nation's history. Today, the health care system is undergoing extensive change and the impetus is cost curtailment. Without a national policy to guide this process, managed care megacorporations are forming and devising strict cost-containment policies in ways that limit hospital stays, constrain individual clinician's decisions, and narrow greatly the lists for reimbursable procedures. In this setting, health care providers face a mix of discordant issues: 1) a duty to adhere to high professional standards of care to help their patients; 2) an urge to use all technologies and procedures that might shield them from possible negligence challenges in the event of claim and suit; and 3) pressure from managed care affiliates who impose restrictive reimbursement rules and financial disincentives in the event they choose to do comprehensive patient workups. Another problem is that providers in many specialties continue to have difficulty in obtaining malpractice liability insurance coverage or coverage at reasonable rates. Although some investigators have contended that the malpractice crisis has eased somewhat, others continue to maintain that it strikes at the viability of health care provision in this nation.

The malpractice and liability problem is attributed to various complex personal and socioeconomic considerations; however, it seems that two basic beliefs may contribute to the crisis. First, it appears that there is a basic attitude in this society that if anything bad happens to anyone, it must be someone else's fault. People simply are unwilling to accept blame and responsibility for their own misfortunes. This undoubtedly leads to a search for external responsibility for those misfortunes and for the so-called deep pockets from which these persons and others seek compensation for their own misfortunes. Second, in part because of the rapid development of and progress in medicine, people now seem to expect uniformly favorable treatment of and even cure for all ills and conditions; bad results simply are thought by many not to be acceptable. People no longer go to the hospital to die but, rather, to be cured and to be treated for their conditions. This apparent expectation of cure and treatment, coupled with the tendency to look outward for responsibility for personal misfortunes, certainly contributes to the overall litigation problem in health care provision.

OVERVIEW

Although cardiac rehabilitation is a specialty health care area of relatively recent origin, the legal concerns that face the medical care provider population as a whole are clearly applicable to this particular provider area. In fact, recent judicial attention to certain aspects of rehabilitative provider care indicates increasing attention to testing, prescription, leadership, monitoring, and emergency response protocols in these programs. Litigation has touched on all these areas and certainly will continue to do so in the years to come as a large segment of the population ages and seeks more care and attention from rehabilitative health care providers. This conclusion is particularly true when one considers a number of trends that have developed recently as a function of trends in professional practice and externally imposed cost containment: 1) patients being admitted to exercise rehabilitation without recent graded-exercise evaluations; and 2) restriction of electrocardiographic-monitored and supervised exercise only for those postevent patients classified by insurance providers as being in the higher clinical risk strata, providing organized home-based exercise rehabilitation for more and more patients in the intermediate risk strata for which surveillance can only be periodic and rapid access to defibrillation and other advanced cardiac life support services is not possible.

Certain procedures in cardiac rehabilitation—particularly those associated with graded-exercise testing—seem to be particularly susceptible to claim and litigation. In part this is because of the nature of the procedure; however, this is also certainly related to the dramatic increase in the use of such practices for diagnostic and assessment purposes. As we shall see, a number of suits have been brought on the basis of untoward incidents that occurred during or immediately after such procedures. Although the results have not been uniform, at least one verdict in favor of an injured party has approached $1 million.

THE TORT SYSTEM—NEGLIGENCE AND MALPRACTICE

Noncontractual civil wrongs are resolved judicially through the tort system by an adversarial process in which competing interests are judged and damages for determined wrongs are awarded to the injured party. Negligence actions are a form of tort resolved within this system. Although incapable of precise definition, negligence is a failure to conform conduct to a generally accepted standard or duty. A cause of action in negligence is established by proof of a breach of that duty that proximately results in harm and damage to the injured party.

Malpractice is a form of negligence that traditionally is limited to actions against physicians and other health care providers. In a malpractice action, proof of the standard of care and breach thereof is established through expert witness testimony supplied at time of trial. Historically, expert witness testimony often has resulted in the expression of individualized opinions about what constitutes the standard of care under a given set of facts applied to a particular legal case. Frequently, however, such testimonial expressions provide inconsistent and often biased views about the so-called standard of care. Uncertainty sometimes results from such cases and often creates a sense of professional anxiety and confusion about the provision of patient care in light of such expressions.

As a partial result of these problems, many medical and other provider organizations have turned to the development of written standards of practice, sometimes referred to as guidelines, parameters of practice, recommendations, or even suggestions. In 1988, the American Medical Association (AMA) announced that adoption of such standards had been the top medical story for that year (1). The hope, at the time, seemed to be that written expressions about the standard of care would lead to more uniform application of standards in the delivery of patient care, improved patient outcomes, and possibly a reduced vulnerability for malpractice claims. Some within the profession feared, perhaps with good reason, that such efforts would unduly restrain practitioner prerogatives in areas in which the scientific evidence or national consensus of experts could not define the single best course of treatment for the patient. Others expressed the belief that proliferation and rigidity in professional standards was tantamount to providing blueprints for proof of negligence when some untoward and unpredictable clinical event takes place. At least one recent analysis as to the use of standards statements would seem to give support to this argument inasmuch as standards appear to be used more frequently than otherwise to attack the care that is provided. However, it also appears that those providers who follow such statements will be more successful in defending against malpractice suits than those who do not do so. In the last decade or so, some newer published consensus standards reflect efforts to reduce practitioner exposure somewhat by including information on strength of expert support for various medical management alternatives. For example, the American Heart Association's newest recommendations on Advanced Cardiac Life Support (ACLS) (2) specifies the level of agreement within the panel (class I, IIa, IIb, and III) as to how much a particular action in the ACLS algorithm is likely to help a given patient. This would appear to appropriately allow for a certain latitude in clinical judgment. It should be kept in mind that all of these written pronouncements if applicable to a given legal case can result in proof of a failure to adhere to the appropriate standard of care; sometimes, even without the need of expert witnesses, such guidelines can provide an objective basis on which to judge provider conduct. An examination of the applicable standards, in light of the obvious provider movement toward the adoption of same, should be important to those practicing in the cardiac rehabilitation field.

STANDARDS OF PRACTICE

In the field of cardiac rehabilitation, numerous professional associations have been active in the promulgation of written expressions that deal with the standard of care. A brief review of the principal standards developed by these groups should be interesting to any discussion of the medicolegal aspects of cardiac rehabilitation.

American Heart Association

The American Heart Association (AHA) was among the first to develop standards related to the provision of cardiac rehabilitation care. The original work of the AHA, first published in 1972, was updated in 1980 with the publication of *The Exercise Standards Book*. Recently, these standards have been updated. These include "Special report: exercise standards, a statement for health professionals" (3); "The AHA medical/scientific statement on exercise" (4); and "The AHA medical/scientific statement on cardiac rehabilitation programs" (5). These AHA publications are basically physician-oriented (6). Nonetheless, the implications are important for all cardiac rehabilitation practitioners, especially with regard to patient screening and evaluation, exercise testing, exercise prescription, monitoring, and supervision.

The AHA together with the American College of Cardiology (ACC) developed new and rather comprehensive practice guidelines for exercise testing procedures in mid-1997. These guidelines have application to exercise testing related to cardiac rehabilitation (7).

American College of Sports Medicine

The American College of Sports Medicine (ACSM) first developed a set of comprehensive guidelines to deal with preventive and rehabilitative exercise programs in 1975. These standards subsequently were revised in 1980, 1986, 1991, and again in 1995 and currently are contained in *Guidelines for Graded Exercise Testing and Exercise Prescription*, 5th edition (8). These standards provide comprehensive written expressions about various rehabilitative exercise activities, including exercise testing and prescription. These ACSM guidelines also specify the ACSM's consensus on the knowledge domains, skills, and abilities expected of the personnel carrying out the exercise prescription and supervision of cardiac patients in the rehabilitation setting, e.g., the certified ACSM Exercise Specialist.

Unlike the guidelines of the AHA, the ACSM guidelines provide for a multidisciplinary team approach to cardiac rehabilitation and do not necessarily require the involvement of a physician for all program activities. Compared with the guidelines of the AHA, these guidelines may, in some respects, be in conflict. Such disparities may well impact the ability of counsel to defend against any negligence claim because the injured party may cite an expanded number of breaches of the standard as a result of any conflict or ambiguity in these pronouncements.

American College of Cardiology

In 1986, the ACC developed a set of standards to deal with cardiovascular rehabilitation services. The standards are extremely broad in certain respects and attempt to approve many activities carried on in diverse settings, including those that are both formal and informal in nature, and those that are supervised or unsupervised. Pursuant to these guidelines, much is left to individual determination and discretion of the physician (9). As previously stated, the ACC and the AHA also published new guidelines for exercise testing in mid-1997 (7).

American Association of Cardiovascular and Pulmonary Rehabilitation

The American Association of Cardiovascular and Pulmonary Rehabilitation (AACVPR) published comprehensive standards of practice for cardiac rehabilitation programs in 1990 and these were revised in 1995 (10). The guidelines emphasize not only the expectations for delivery of patient care, e.g., screening, evaluation, risk stratification, exercise prescription, counseling, and education, but how programs should be organized, staffed, and assured of quality control. As a part of the AACUPR's second edition, the organization has published its own set of "Core Competencies" for cardiac rehabilitation professionals. (See Chapter 22, Program Standards and Organizational Issues.) The AACVPR competency expectations, although complementary to those of the ACSM Exercise Specialist, go well beyond the exercise area and thus would appear to hold out a much broader competency standard for cardiac rehabilitation professionals who provide more than just the exercise portion of care. The AACVPR standards are quite comprehensive and have considerable consequence for managing medicolegal risk in cardiac rehabilitation. It is noteworthy that AACVPR has been working since approximately 1994 to define a review process by which to conduct nationwide certification for cardiac rehabilitation programs. This certification may become available within the next 2 years. Once implemented, it will afford programs with one means for verifying that patient service has been delivered in conformance to the AACVPR minimum standard.

Other Groups

In recent years, two other entities also have published documents that have a bearing on the medicolegal standards in cardiac rehabilitation. One is the Agency for Health Care Policy and Research (AHCPR), which contracted with AACVPR in the early 1990s to develop an evidence-based practice guideline for cardiac rehabilitation (11). The AHCPR practice guideline specifies decision points and interventions for patient treatment with cardiac rehabilitation. The substance of the recommendations is based on expert panel consensus derived from a science-based methodology by which the published literature on cardiac rehabilitation treatment was exhaustively studied. The AHCPR guideline now has been widely circulated by the U.S. Public Health Service in print and electronic form on the Internet. In follow-up, AHCPR/AACVPR jointly charged a panel that created a quality assessment instrument by which any cardiac program's documentation could be inventoried for evidence of conformance to the AHCPR practice guideline (copies available from AACVPR, Madison, WI, 1996). The AHCPR initiative was undertaken to promote appropriate and effective cardiac rehabilitation care on a nationwide scale. However, it also will have impact on many other stakeholders including those in the legal field who need to resolve questions of standard of care and failure to meet standards.

The other entity to recently publish materials that speak to the legal standards in cardiac rehabilitation is the American Nursing Association (ANA). In the early 1990s, the ANA published its own set of competency standards and a credentialing program for nursing care in cardiac rehabilitation (12, 13). These competency requirements for cardiac rehabilitation providers, as published by ACSM, AACVPR, and ANA, are all commendable in that they demonstrate collective commitments to quality care for patients. However, these pronouncements show wide variance in defined roles and specificity stated for what should be the set of duties that are expected of the entry-level service provider who is fully qualified to act as a cardiac rehabilitation provider. In the setting of any legal claim and suit that includes challenges of practitioner competence, these inconsistencies cloud determinations of professional responsibility and make practitioners more vulnerable.

POLICIES AND PROCEDURES

Programs should develop policies and procedures for intense activities, based on applicable association statements about the standard of care, to serve as the framework within which care is to be delivered. Such documents must be developed in conjunction with medical and legal advisors and must be developed and appropriately referenced to association standards of practice. Once such policies are in place, program personnel need to become intimately familiar with them to ensure adherence to the proper provision of patient care. In the event that program policies and procedures are violated by program personnel, a finding of negligence is nearly automatic. Moreover, when such policies are violated proximately resulting in harm to program participants, proof of negligence may even come solely from the program's policies and procedures without the necessity of expert witness testimony (14).

Documentation of adherence to program policies and procedures, when based on accepted medical standards of care, should provide an acceptable level of program defensibility from successful claim and suit. Another level of program protection from claim and suit can arise out of properly trained and competent personnel in addition to appropriately acquired, maintained, and supervised equipment usage.

PERSONNEL AND EQUIPMENT

Appropriately trained and licensed or certified personnel are always part of the appropriate standard of care and, as such, part of the defensibility of any rehabilitative program. Because of the diversity of services provided in rehabilitative programs, it is clear that for certain procedures only certain personnel will be authorized to provide service for patients. In this regard, it is important to review the applicability of state statutes that apply to certain procedures within the rehabilitative area.

In virtually all states, there exists a series of statutes that defines the practice of medicine and certain allied health care provider services, as well as statutes that proscribe certain unauthorized practices. Generally, under these statutes, no one is permitted to engage in practices reserved for licensed personnel. Pursuant to these statutes, the practice of medicine, for example, is typically defined "as [the] diagnosis of an individual's symptoms to determine with what disease or illness he is afflicted, and then to determine on the basis of that diagnosis what remedy or treatment should be given or prescribed to treat that disease and/or relieve the symptoms" (9).

Persons found to engage in such practices without the appropriate license are subject to two potential consequences, one civil and one criminal. From the criminal perspective, persons found to be engaged in the unauthorized practice of medicine face the possibility of criminal prosecution that can result in the imposition of a fine or incarceration for up to 1 year. From the civil perspective, persons found to be engaged in unauthorized practice face an elevated standard of care by which their conduct would be compared against the presumed conduct of a properly licensed person acting under the same or similar circumstances. In a civil lawsuit, because of participant injury and claim, nonlicensed persons simply will be unable to meet this expected

standard of care, almost invariably resulting in a judgment of liability in favor of an injured party.

Exercise stress testing procedures within this setting, as well as exercise prescription activities for the rehabilitative patient, almost invariably are deemed to be medical in nature and, thus, probably are reserved for physician action. In certain instances, state legislative enactments or administrative pronouncements have even dictated that physicians, as opposed to other licensed or nonlicensed personnel, must perform such procedures (15). Prescription of exercise activities for persons within this setting is also probably medical in nature, just like the exclamation of a popular T-shirt offered by *The Physician in Sports Medicine Journal:* "Exercise is medicine!" Given the purpose behind the prescription (i.e., to help alleviate disease or ill health or to improve the status of a patient's health), when compared with state definitions for medical practice, such a determination in this setting is likely. Nonlicensed personnel would seem to be required to work either under the supervision of or in conjunction with a licensed provider to escape these potential concerns.

Equipment used in diverse exercise programs often is involved in claim and litigation related to exercise. Although some of these cases deal with improper design or manufacture, a good number of cases also deal with improper provider assembly, maintenance, repair, instruction, warning, or supervision. Many programs face such claims without adequate preparation and without having met the appropriate standard of care in reference to the equipment before the untoward incident that led to the claim and suit. All these potential equipment liability areas deserve close and ongoing attention so that claims and suits related to the use of same might be minimized.

INFORMED CONSENT

The provision of health care services in the rehabilitative model is medical in nature. As such, care providers must comply with the principles and practices of informed consent. Informed consent is simply the process by which patients are given information sufficient to enable them to make a decision about whether or not to undergo a particular procedure or surgical operation. Historically, through this process practitioners have been required to provide explanations of the contemplated procedure and its benefits and alternatives, as well as a statement of the material risks associated with the treatment or procedure.

Despite the historical and traditional requirements of the informed consent process, the law has been moving toward requiring more and more information disclosure in the process so that the patient might make a more informed decision about what is to be done with his or her body. The law is, in fact, moving toward the requirement of compelling the disclosure of all information sufficient for the patient to make an informed decision about treatment alternatives. This move toward more information disclosure, sometimes referred to as the patient rule, is causing some problems for practitioners in the risk disclosure aspect of the informed consent process. Because almost anything is possible, there is virtually an unlimited list of risks that could be subject to disclosure. The practical problem arises, however, in determining which possible risks within the realm of all risks should be or need to be disclosed to the patient (16).

To illustrate the dilemma as applied to a rehabilitative procedure, consider the 1985 U.S. District Court case of *Hedgecorth v. United States* (ED Mo 1985) (17). In this case, a somewhat elderly patient underwent a physician-performed graded-exercise stress test at a Veterans Administration facility. Although he previously had undergone another test shortly before this procedure, the results of that test were not obtained by the physicians at the VA center. During the performance of the VA-conducted test, the plaintiff complained of a loss of vision in his left eye and chest pain during the procedure. It was later determined that he suffered a stroke and blindness attributed to a stroke that occurred during the test. Subsequently, the plaintiff brought an action contending that the facility was responsible for his injuries because of their failure to disclose the risks of those injuries during the informed consent process. In determining these issues the court ruled that (17 [pp 631–632]):

The credible medical evidence presented at time of trial demonstrates that giving the [VA conducted] stress test to the plaintiff . . . was a deviation from the appropriate standard of care. The purpose of a stress test is, as the name

implies, to place a stress on the heart through physical exercise and thereby derive information concerning the heart's condition. Because of the nature of the test certain dangers accompany its administration. These dangers include the possibility that the patient will suffer a stroke. The patient should be warned that a stroke could result from the administration of the test, and plaintiff Lowell Hedgecorth was not warned of this danger. Thus, plaintiff . . . did not take the test with informed consent of its dangers.

Based on these findings, the court held that (17 [p 632]):

As a direct result of the negligent acts and omissions of the defendants, the plaintiff . . . suffered an infarct in the right occipital lobe of his brain. This stroke directly caused plaintiff'(s) . . . total and permanent disability.

Consequently, the court awarded the plaintiff and the plaintiff's spouse almost $1 million for the damages that he suffered.

In light of rulings like this and the law's movement toward broader disclosure as part of the informed consent process, practitioners should consult with their legal advisors to review their own practices and procedures for the informed consent process. In situations in which risks are not properly disclosed to patients and that lead to an untoward occurrence from one of those nondisclosed risks, liability likely will attach to the practitioner.

EXERCISE TESTING AND PRESCRIPTION

Exercise testing and prescription deserve special mention because of the increasing use of these testing mechanisms for the purposes of assessing patient condition or status and for determining an appropriate prescription to improve that condition or status. The dramatic increase and use of these procedures for diagnostic purposes, coupled with the increase in claim and litigation related to the same, mandate a special examination of this area of rehabilitative activity (18).

To illustrate the potential for litigation related

to this procedure, consider the 1982 case of *Tart v. McGann,* 697 F2d 75 (2d Cir 1982) (19). In this case, an airline pilot was undergoing his annual physical examination, which included among other things a graded-exercise stress testing procedure. Although he made no verbal expressions of undue fatigue during the test, he claimed to have suffered a great deal of strain during the final stage of the test. His physicians, however, continued to encourage him to complete the test. He subsequently developed a myocardial infarction and brought suit, contending that the physicians should have terminated the test before its end point.

Although the jury returned a defense verdict in this case, the defense provided a substantial settlement for the plaintiff as part of a pre-jury verdict agreement by and between the injured party and the physicians. One of the principal focuses of the entire case centered on the question of whether or not the plaintiff's facial expressions of fatigue during the test should have been sufficient to mandate that the physician terminate the test before its end point. Although the standards of the AHA were used entirely during the testimony—which did not specifically deal with such issues—the standards of the ACSM then in effect did provide information about the termination of testing procedures on the basis of undue facial expressions of fatigue, among other things. If such standards had been used in this case, an entirely different result may have been returned by the jury.

Aside from this often cited case, there have been numerous other cases related to alleged treadmill deficiencies (20); slip and fall injuries on the treadmill (21); claimed improper instruction or supervision in the use of such devices (22); and claims related to alleged improper continuation or supervision of the procedure when the test should have been terminated (19, 21).

Because of the active nature of the procedure and the obvious but remote risks associated with same, it is clear that claim and litigation will continue to occur in the rehabilitative setting with regard to these procedures in the years ahead. Practitioners would be well advised to review their own policies and procedures about same to minimize the risks of claim and suit arising from the procedure.

MONITORING ACTIVITIES

Monitoring of activities for rehabilitative patients is of some concern to professionals in the field. The concern is almost always centered on what monitoring is required for activity in the setting. Questions frequently center on the need for telemetry-monitored activities; direct-instructor supervision of on-site exercise; and the monitoring, if any, of prescribed off-site and unsupervised exercise activity. Claims and litigation related to these areas have not been substantial to date but certainly expose the program and its personnel to the potential for claim and suit (23). Despite the risks, the necessary move toward quicker and more frequently unsupervised exercise activities is certain to expose many practitioners to the potential for claim and suit in years to come.

CONCLUSION

Like the general medical field, the cardiac rehabilitative area has a number of legal concerns that may arise in the course of carrying out patient activities. Persons forearmed with a basic knowledge of the areas of difficulty, the written standards of practice available for medicolegal citation, and the law should be better prepared to provide defensible patient counseling and patient treatment.

References

1. The year in review, medicine by the book. American Medical News, January 6, 1989:1–28.
2. American Heart Association. Standards and guidelines for cardiopulmonary resuscitation (CPR) and emergency care (ECC). JAMA 1992;268: 2171–2302.
3. Fletcher GF, Froelicher VF, Hartley LH, et al. Exercise standards. A statement for health professionals. Circulation 1990;81:396–398.
4. Fletcher GF, Balady G, Blair S, et al. Statement on exercise: benefits and recommendations for physical activity programs for all Americans. Circulation. 1996;94: 857–862.
5. Balady GJ, Fletcher BJ, Froelicher ES, et al. Cardiac rehabilitation programs: a statement for healthcare professionals. Circulation 1994;90:1602.
6. Schlant RC, Friesinger GC, Leonard JJ. Clinical competence in exercise testing: a statement for physicians from the ACP/ACC/AHA Task Force on Clinical Privileges in Cardiology. J Am Coll Cardiol 1990;16: 1061–5.
7. Gibbons RJ, Balady GJ, Beasley JW, et al. ACC/AHA

guidelines for exercise testing: a report of the American College of Cardiology/American Heart Association Task Force on Practice Guidelines. J Am Coll Cardiol 1997;30:260–315.

8. American College of Sports Medicine. Guidelines for graded exercise testing and exercise prescription. 5th ed. Baltimore: Williams & Wilkins, 1995.

9. Herbert D, Herbert W. Legal aspects of preventive, rehabilitative and recreational exercise programs. 3rd ed. Canton, OH: PRC Publishing, 1993, 44718-3629, 184–186.

10. American Association of Cardiovascular and Pulmonary Rehabilitation. Guidelines for cardiac rehabilitation programs. 2nd ed. Champaign, IL: Human Kinetics, 1995.

11. Cardiac rehabilitation: clinical practice guideline No. 17. Rockville, MD: US Department of Health and Human Services, Publication No. 96–0672, 1995.

12. ANA publications, Scope of cardiac rehabilitation nursing practice. Washington, DC: American Nursing Publications, 1993.

13. 1995 Credentialing Catalog, Washington, DC: American Nurses Credentialing Center, 1995.

14. Herbert DL. Litigation and court rulings: standard of care and deviation therefrom can be established without expert testimony. Exerc Stand Malpract Report 1989;3:12.

15 Herbert DL. Is physician supervision of exercise stress testing required? Exerc Stand Malpract Report 1988; 2:6–7.

16. Herbert DL. Risk disclosure in the informed consent process: judging the adequacy of disclosure in light of the patient's need for information, an emerging trend. Exerc Stand Malpract Report 1988;2:56–57.

17. Herbert DL. Informed consent and new disclosure responsibilities for exercise stress testing: the case of *Hedgecorth v. United States*. Exerc Stand Malpract Report 1987;1:30–32.

18. Trends: dramatic increase in diagnostic testing for MI patients reported. Exerc Stand Malpract Report 1988; 2:28.

19. Edelman. The case of *Tart v. McGann:* legal implications associated with exercise stress testing. Exerc Stand Malpract Report 1987;1:21–26.

20. Herbert DL. Litigation and court rulings: suit against treadmill manufacturer dismissed. Exerc Stand Malpract Report 1990;4:11–12.

21. Herbert DL. Litigation and court rulings: treadmill fall results in defense verdict. Exerc Stand Malpract Report 1988;2:30.

22. Litigation and court rulings: participant injuries suffered while on jogging treadmill can be facility's responsibility. Exerc Stand Malpract Report 1987;1:61.

23. Herbert DL. Selected liability considerations of prescribed but unsupervised cardiac rehabilitation activities. Exerc Stand Malpract Report 1988;2:89–94.

Adherence and Motivation in Cardiac Rehabilitation

Neil B. Oldridge and Fredric J. Pashkow

ADHERENCE WITH MEDICAL THERAPEUTIC REGIMENS

Ethical Implications of Adherence and Adherence-enhancing Strategies

GENERAL DEFINITION OF ADHERENCE

Adherence is a fundamental issue in the success of any therapy (1). Adherence can be considered as "the extent to which patients comply with recommendations"; alternatively, compliance can be considered as "the extent to which patients adhere to recommendations." Either way, the concern is the extent to which the recommendations made are followed. In other words, how much of what we prescribe for patients with coronary heart disease (CHD) truly hits the target? Nonadherence with cardiovascular risk factor behavior changes is apparently so common that it has been suggested that it should be considered a risk factor for cardiovascular disease (2). Adherence with medication may be a marker for a better prognosis in patients with CHD, but more research is needed to determine whether better adherence improved outcomes (3–5). However, it is clear that changes in lifestyle associated with medical recommendations are difficult to implement and maintain (1) and that this concern applies equally to cardiac rehabilitation (6, 7). The issue of adherence addresses this difficult challenge and, more than any other issue in the field of cardiac rehabilitation, confronts the essential ethical issue of "what we do to people," the implications of their consent, and how we affect this change (8, 9).

Adherence has been identified as a major public health problem, imposing a considerable health and financial burden on the health care system (9). The interaction between patients and physicians is crucial to the achievement of adherence, but it is extremely difficult to assess the nature of this interaction and to measure its components (9–12). What is clear is that the central feature of the traditional interpretation of nonadherence, or noncompliance, is the connotation of failure on the part of the patients to follow recommendations, suggesting a pejorative effect toward patients and the implication that the physician and his or her style of communication with the patient may alter the patient's capability and inclination to adhere. However, with the increasing emphasis on the patient's role in clinical decision making, there can be little argument that the traditional interpretation is outdated and is a major obstacle to a better understanding of patient and clinician (9, 11–13).

In this chapter we focus on the issue of adherence, concentrating on the physician involved in cardiac rehabilitation. In the recently published *Cardiac Rehabilitation Clinical Practice Guideline* (14), cardiac rehabilitation is considered to consist of exercise training, behavioral interventions, counseling, and education with the goal of appropriate lifestyle modification. The Clinical Practice Guidelines expert panel took the position that adherence is not an intervention but rather an important contributor to the effectiveness of cardiac rehabilitation (14).

TRADITIONAL MEDICAL MODEL OF COMPLIANCE: A CHANGING SOCIAL AND ETHICAL ENVIRONMENT

Traditionally, medical therapies have been prescribed by the provider (active role) and then followed by the patient (passive role). This relationship between the active provider and the passive patient assumed that the provider has the best interests of the patient in mind and that the single most important motivation for this relationship is the provision of service for the patient's benefit (15). Thus, the provider functioned as a "benevolent autocrat," the patient as a "patriotic citizen" (16). Providers prescribed, the patients did as they were told. This no longer is the case.

During the past 20 years, complex changes have occurred in the social and ethical aspects of health care as well as in the well-recognized and often discussed scientific progress (11). Most significant has been the rise of consumerism, which appears to be an outgrowth of an increasingly aggressive and demanding public. In addition, whereas the "contract" for services formerly was exclusive with the recipient of the care provided, the truth is that insurers (often the government) who pay for it and those who are involved collaterally to a significant degree, such as health care institutions, have intruded into the previously exclusive bilateral relationship of the provider and the patient.

The positive aspect of this trend has been some reverse transfer of responsibility for therapeutic outcome to the patient. If the patient does not follow the recommendations of the provider, poor results are not just the "fault" of the provider alone; they must be shared. Thus, we have witnessed further evolution not only of patients' rights, but also a broadening of patients' responsibilities in the process of realizing therapeutic outcome. Data from the Medical Outcomes study suggest that there is increasing awareness that the responsibility for decision making lies somewhat more with the patient than the physician (17). The acceptance of this requires an improved understanding of at least two factors in future adherence research: 1) an increased recognition of the patient's perspective and role in medical decision making, and 2) a critical examination of the role of the physician (9).

The philosophical implication is significant. Now the bilateral relationship is better described as a "partnership," and a failure to adhere is not so much a failure of the clinician with an ensuing loss of face but the loss of an opportunity for therapeutic success in persons who are motivated by their free will. A positive aspect of this change has been the development of the concepts of self-actualization and self-efficacy, whereby a cardiac rehabilitation patient's perception of his or her ability to make positive change influences how much

effort is expended toward achievement of the desired therapeutic goals (18, 19).

A MORE CONTEMPORARY MODEL OF ADHERENCE

The ethics of adherence-enhancing research are based on the acceptance of patient–provider mutual responsibility, a correct diagnosis and treatment plan, and proof of therapeutic effectiveness. When the diagnosis is correct and the therapy demonstrably effective, patients are fundamentally responsible for their own adherent behavior. This behavior is an expression of the patient's capabilities, needs, fears, circumstances, inclinations, and wishes, in short, an entire motivational matrix. Patient behavior is further affected by their medical, social, and cultural viewpoints. This means that under a given set of circumstances, the decision not to adhere with the advice of the health professional may be justified (6, 9, 12). Although the patient has the right to refuse prescribed treatment, presuming the patient initially asked for the help, the provider has the recourse to try to improve adherence if it is poor.

The phenomenon of the doctor–patient relationship is "elusive," but a number of components have been identified as important in cardiac rehabilitation. These include communication between physician and patient, patient involvement in the decision-making process, physician awareness of patient concerns, patient satisfaction, and family involvement (1, 14). When patients have a demonstrably clear understanding about what is expected of them, they show significant conformity to those expectations, i.e., they adhere. An additional provider with specific training and skills in communication can improve the transfer of information.

Health professionals are cognizant of their responsibility to monitor and detect adherence problems and to implement straightforward and workable strategies to improve patient adherence (1, 4, 9, 13, 20–26). Although certain patient characteristics may be associated with the likelihood of poor adherence, providers are increasingly aware that the predictive accuracy of such features is not consistent enough to be extremely useful (18, 19).

A major reason for poor adherence may be deficient communication by the provider about the benefits of the intervention, and simply improving lines of communication may be a potent adherence-enhancing strategy (26, 27). Education and behavioral management counseling are patient-directed adherence strategies; the goal is to bring relevant, understandable, useful information to bear in a truthful and noncoercive fashion at a time and place when it is most likely to move positive cardiovascular health behaviors to action. This means that the objective of education and health behavior counseling is to permit the patient to make informed decisions about the prescribed therapeutic regimen.

These observations and beliefs raise the following issues: 1) What should be done about the persistently nonadherent patient? 2) What are the limits on efforts to improve adherence? 3) Are the science and the ethics of adherence-enhancing research, which may involve "deception" concerning strategy and outcome, compatible? and 4) To what extent may the provider be responsible for poor adherence?

CARDIAC REHABILITATION AS A REPRESENTATION OF SELF-RESPONSIBILITY

One major objective of cardiac rehabilitation is return to a normal, active, productive life, which is an integral part of the recovery process after any acute cardiac event (14). It requires adequate provision of information and services by appropriate professionals with proper use of available services by the patient and his or her primary supporters. In the World Health Organization definition of cardiac rehabilitation, the emphasis is placed on the patient with regard to a return to normalcy by "their own efforts" (28). Furthermore, secondary prevention in patients with CHD has become increasingly apropos in the face of evidence that corroborates the possibility of attenuation or reversal of the atherosclerotic process in association with lifestyle modification (29, 30).

The essential elements of risk factor and lifestyle modification include smoking cessation, normalization of abnormal blood lipid levels, control of systemic hypertension, initiation of stress-alleviating techniques, and conversion from a sedentary to an active lifestyle. These goals most likely can be achieved when the intervention or prescription needed to accomplish these benefits is attainable and attractive enough for long-term adherence. Because behavior change cannot work without adequate adherence, better understand-

ing of why patients do not adhere and how to encourage them to do so is needed (1, 6).

The power of an intervention is a function of its efficacy and patient adherence. The clinical significance of poor adherence must be balanced against the observation that therapeutic benefit can be achieved without real adherence or, alternatively, that substantial adherence does not guarantee therapeutic benefit. A matrix illustrating the relative relationship between therapeutic efficacy and adherence is seen in Figure 25.1. We usually assume that patients fall into the upper left cell, where adherence is high and the goals of therapy often are achieved, or, in the lower right cell, where adherence is poor and the goals of therapy are not met. In reality, patients often fall into the upper right cell, where goals are not achieved despite high adherence, or in the lower left cell, where adherence is poor but the goals are achieved.

The reasons for these apparently paradoxical associations between adherence and outcomes are not clear (31). Examples of this can be found in the Coronary Drug Project (CDP), a randomized, controlled trial of lipid-lowering medication on mortality in men with a myocardial infarction (MI) (32) and the β-Blocker Heart Attack Trial (BHAT), a randomized, controlled trial of β-blockade medication on mortality in men after an MI (33). In the CDP trial, 5-year mortality in the intervention group was 20.9% compared with 20.0% in the control group (32). When adherence to medication was considered in the CDP trial, mortality among the poor adherers (less than 80% of prescription) was higher than that of the good adherers (24.6% versus 15.0%, $P < .001$) (34). However, the 28.3% mortality among poor adherers with placebo also was significantly higher ($P < .001$) than the 15.1% mortality among the good adherers, and the lower mortality in good adherers was similar in patients regardless of random assignment (34). In the BHAT, 25-month mortality in the intervention group was 7.2% compared with 9.8% in the control group (33). When overall adherence was considered in the BHAT (35), mortality among the poor adherers (less than 75% of prescription) with either propranolol or placebo was 2.6 times higher than that of good adherers ($P < .001$). But again, mortality was higher for poor adherers than good adherers, with an odds ratio of 3.1 on

		Increased Exercise Tolerance	
		Achieved	Not Achieved
C o m p l i a n c e	High	• Achieves or maintains goals	• Inadequate exercise Rx • Inappropriate definition of adherence
	Low	• Overadequate exercise Rx • Inappropriate definition of poor compliance	• Compliance-enhancing strategy needed

Figure 25.1. Matrix illustrating the association among adherence with cardiac rehabilitation (high/low), the goal of increased exercise tolerance (achieved/not achieved), and the need for adherence enhancement.

active medication and 2.5 on placebo (35). For some reason, it appears that adherent patients have a better outcome than poorly adherent patients but that this is not solely a drug-specific effect, which suggests some other nonspecific therapeutic effects are associated with good adherence (31).

The conceptual model outlined in Figure 25.1 targets the patient, the provider, and the therapeutic intervention for possible adherence-enhancing strategies. Although a number of strategies to improve adherence with cardiac rehabilitation interventions have been suggested (6, 26, 36), adherence-enhancing strategies have received little attention in cardiac rehabilitation (21, 37). One possible reason that poor adherence has not received the attention it deserves is poor lines of communication between patient and health professionals. It has been pointed out that health care professionals sometimes make erroneous assumptions that have significant implications related to the attainment of adherence and appropriately informed consent (38, 39). These assumptions presume that 1) all cases of nonadherence are problems in need of a solution, 2) the solution to the problem of nonadherence is simply adherence, 3) all instances of adherence are nonproblematic, and 4) the locus of the problem of nonadherence is primarily the patient.

The implementation of adherence-enhancing strategies in cardiac rehabilitation thus requires both medical and ethical justification. Before attempting to alter adherence with a particular intervention, the rehabilitation professional needs to ask the following questions:

Does the disease represent a significant risk to the patient, and is the therapy likely to alter the prognosis?

Do the benefits of rehabilitation outweigh the costs and risks?

Is the patient prepared or ready to adhere to the recommendations?

Will poor adherence clearly affect the potential benefits of the rehabilitation?

There is overwhelming evidence that coronary disease is a major source of morbidity and mortality in this country (40). There also are clear indications that, for most patients, the benefits of cardiac rehabilitation outweigh the risks (14) and, although subsequent nonfatal events may not be reduced with exercise rehabilitation, that all-cause and cardiovascular mortality can be affected significantly (41, 42).

These generalizations must be applied to individual and various subsets of patients. For example, Jugdutt and associates (43) have shown that patients with severe thinning and spatial distortion of the anterior wall after MI show deterioration in all variables monitored, including exercise capacity and ejection fraction with exercise training. At the other extreme, by 6 months after an acute coronary event, low-risk patients achieve similar levels of exercise capacity, whether or not they participated in a formal exercise-rehabilitation program (44). The indication for participation in a rehabilitation program for both of these groups is for education concerning the efficacy and safety issues related to exercise, knowledge concerning the disease process and its therapy, and motivation to strive for success in secondary risk factor modification.

CARDIAC REHABILITATION AND ADHERENCE: EDUCATION, COUNSELING, BEHAVIORAL INTERVENTIONS, AND EXERCISE TRAINING

The objective of patient education as an information exchange (didactic) and health education (counseling), and modification of cardiovascular risk factors, such as cholesterol, hypertension, smoking, psychosocial concerns, and physical inactivity, is to facilitate voluntary adaptations of behavior conducive to better cardiovascular health. The number of publications addressing adherence in cardiac rehabilitation appeared to plateau after an early interest in the subject. This may have been owing to the fact that most programs last a relatively short time (12 weeks or less). However, there appears to be a renewed interest in adherence with recommendations for reducing cardiovascular risk factors, and this is consistent with the trend toward incorporating many of the services presently included in cardiac rehabilitation programs into secondary prevention settings with the objective of risk factor reduction (45–50).

Education, Counseling, and Behavioral Interventions

The *Cardiac Rehabilitation Clinical Practice Guideline* has examined data published before 1995 on education, counseling, and behavioral interventions on various outcomes (14). Using a strength-of-evidence rating scale of A (well-designed, well-conducted, controlled trials, randomized and nonrandomized, with statistically significant results consistently supporting the guideline recommendations), B (observational studies or controlled trials with less consistent results), or C (expert opinion because the scientific evidence was not consistent or controlled trials were lacking), the panel made a number of recommendations about the impact of cardiac rehabilitation on certain outcomes including smoking, hypertension, cholesterol, behavior, and exercise tolerance. There was one recommendation with an A rating (improvement in psychosocial well-being), eight recommendations with a B rating (including improved management of smoking habits, lipids, blood pressure), and two recommendations with a C rating (including no effect on exercise tolerance) (14).

EDUCATION AND COUNSELING

When compared with the didactic approach, patient education in chronic disease may have a greater effect on the degree to which patients follow therapeutic advice as measured by adherence, therapeutic progress, and healthy outcomes (26, 27). However, in a review of selected studies that looked at different education techniques specifically in cardiac rehabilitation, the authors concluded that no conclusive evidence existed to show that didactic teaching or health education was helpful after MI (51).

Why educational strategies are only partially successful or even fail completely probably involves a number of diverse reasons. The interventions may be presented prematurely or at inappropriate times; they may be too short, too long, or misunderstood. There may be lack of feedback or insufficient rewards for progress, and materials may be focused at the wrong reading level (27), or the whole educational strategy may be off the mark (52). Daltroy (37) has reported that fewer than 10% of patients were adherent with a 12-month exercise program using an education intervention on entry designed to improve adherence. Such a meager return suggests that one or several obstacles to successful communication were operating here.

We have noted an inconsistency in the quality of educational media and the patients' expectations based on what they observe in their regular day-to-day environment. This problem is a reflection of the high costs of production. Educational budgets are not commensurate with those of the commercial sector, particularly with respect to the development and production of audiovisual materials, but desktop publication of printed and visual materials (slides and video especially) may help improve quality yet keep creative costs down. Materials produced with the sponsorship of pharmaceutical companies generally are of high quality, but the impetus to produce these materials usually comes from advertising agencies who adhere mainly to the sponsor's agenda, are not integrated into other aspects of the rehabilitation program, and are supported only for a limited time. Once the promotion for the sponsoring product is finished, so is the availability of the materials. A good example is the availability of the individual pamphlets created to accompany a video or audio tape. Most rehabilitation programs have found that such materials, although lavishly produced and comparable in technical quality to what the patient sees on commercial television, are only adjunctive and, therefore, are of limited value. The danger of such materials is that physicians may use them and feel that by handing them out they completely satisfy the patients' educational requirement or that the materials may take the place of a formal rehabilitation program.

Despite this, there is a belief that there is great potential for cardiovascular health education or counseling after MI but that the challenge is to communicate, to bring relevant, comprehensible, useful information to bear at the time, and to place it where it is most likely to motivate, enable, or reinforce positive health behaviors (26).

BEHAVIORAL INTERVENTIONS

Strategies, including behavioral interventions, to modify cardiovascular risk factors, such as serum cholesterol reduction, blood pressure (BP) control, and smoking cessation, have had great impact on the observed decline in the incidence of CHD and currently are regarded as essential elements in the management of patients with known ischemic heart disease (53).

Cholesterol

Behavioral interventions such as diet to improve blood lipid levels and are recommended as components of cardiac rehabilitation (14). Lowering elevated serum cholesterol has been shown to reduce the excess risk attributable to increased serum cholesterol among survivors of MI, preventing a significant number of recurrent events (54–57.)

Angiographically reduced progression of atherosclerosis with adequate adherence to cholesterol-lowering medication and diet in patients with elevated low-density lipoprotein cholesterol (LDL-C) and documented CHD has been demonstrated in a number of randomized clinical trials (30, 58, 59). Dietary intervention trials (with or without adherence rates) for patients after MI are rare, but, again, greater adherence with treatment resulted in greater dietary improvements in the treatment group than in the control (60, 61). Although a very-low-fat, vegetarian diet and participation in a supervised setting have been associated with significant decreases in total cholesterol and LDL-C but not high-density lipoprotein cholesterol (HDL-C) (62), difficulties with long-term adherence with this kind of diet have been reported in a cardiac rehabilitation setting (63).

Hypertension

Education, counseling, and behavioral interventions, in conjunction with medication, are rec-ommended approaches to take in cardiac rehabilitation programs (14). A 6- to 8-mm Hg decrease in diastolic blood pressure (DBP) with medication has been associated with a significant 12% reduction in CHD in patients with severe hypertension, and there is a borderline significant 9% reduction in patients with moderate hypertension (64). Although it is recognized that nonadherence with treatment for hypertension is associated with significant negative consequences (65), apparently no randomized trials exist of nonpharmacologic intervention for hypertension with adherence rates in patients after an MI.

Smoking

Smoking cessation may be the single most important risk factor modification for both primary and secondary prevention of CHD (54). Although it would be unethical to carry out controlled trials of smoking cessation in secondary prevention of CHD, evidence from representative observational studies after MI demonstrate an approximate 45% to 50% quit rate for 5 to 6 years with a similar reduction in mortality (66, 67). Although a nurse-delivered, inpatient education program does not increase smoking cessation rates (68), a combined approach of education, counseling, and behavioral interventions is recommended for smoking cessation and relapse prevention in cardiac rehabilitation (14).

Stress Management and Psychosocial Well-Being

Studies of education, counseling, and behavioral interventions in cardiac rehabilitation settings provide evidence of improvement in psychological well-being and stress (14). Although the issue of coronary-prone ("Type A") behavior remains unresolved, personality plays a substantial role in the management of patients with CHD. Type A behavior is a complex covariable in its relationship to coronary disease. Although the behavior trait itself may have deleterious effects in primary prevention, in the secondary prevention population it may be associated with higher levels of intervention adherence.

In patients allocated to behavioral treatment and cardiologic counseling, the 4.5-year recurrent event rate has been shown to be significantly lower than that observed in those receiving cardiologic counseling alone (12.9% versus 21.25%) (69). Importantly, the cardiac recurrence rate was lower in those patients who adhered to the intervention for 4.5 years than in those who dropped out (13% versus 33%, *P* <.001) (69).

In a recent meta-analysis of the results of studies published before 1994, there is some suggestion that the addition of psychosocial treatments to standard cardiac rehabilitation programs may reduce mortality and morbidity and psychosocial distress (70). The results of studies published more recently are mixed, specifically in terms of cardiac events (71–73).

In a trial of stress-relieving interventions after MI, initiated when stress levels were elevated, adherence with the 1-year intervention was 88% in 128 of 229 males randomized to the experimental group (74). During the year of intervention, intervention patients had a relative risk of 0.49 for cardiac death rate compared with those not receiving the intervention (74). During the next 5 years, the relative risk decreased to 0.36 among the high-stress patients in the treatment compared with the control group (75). When a similar intervention was repeated in men and women, adherence with the intervention was 86.3% with no intervention effect on 1-year cardiac mortality in men but a higher cardiac mortality in women randomized to intervention (9.4%) than to usual care (5.0%) (72). The focus of the intervention, supportive and educational home nursing interventions for distressed patients, may have had the opposite effect to that intended by significantly focusing on the existing problems over which patients may have had little control. A large trial of rehabilitation comprising psychological therapy, counseling, relaxation training, and stress after MI was carried out for 7 weeks, with the authors' conclusion that the interventions "seem to offer little objective benefits to patients" in terms of anxiety, depression, morbidity, use of medication, or mortality (73). Apparently 27% of the patients randomized to the intervention group failed to "attend" any intervention session (73), and the results observed in this trial have been ascribed either to an inadequate intervention or to the fact that many patients did not require this kind of intervention (76).

On the other hand, a recent randomized trial of stress management and exercise training with a 5-year follow-up found that 95.3% of the 107 patients completed the 4-month intervention (71). When compared with the control group, the stress management intervention was associated with a relative risk for cardiac events (death, nonfatal MI, and revascularization procedures) of 0.26 (95% confidence intervals, 0.07–0.90, *P* < .03), and the exercise intervention was associated with a nonsignificant lower relative risk of 0.68 (71).

Despite relatively high adherence rates with the prescribed interventions, these observations reinforce the need to examine further the effects of psychological interventions in both men and women with CHD as they may respond in different ways.

Exercise Tolerance

Cardiac rehabilitation education, counseling, and behavioral interventions are not recommended for improving exercise tolerance (14).

Exercise Training

Exercise training is the other major component of cardiac rehabilitation that was evaluated in the *Cardiac Rehabilitation Clinical Practice Guideline* (14). Using the same strength-of-evidence rating scale of A, B, and C as explained earlier in the chapter, the panel made a number of recommendations about outcomes with cardiac rehabilitation exercise training as a sole intervention. There were four recommendations with an A rating (including improved exercise tolerance), eight recommendations with a B rating (including no or an inconsistent effect on smoking habits, lipids, blood pressure), and one recommendation of an inconsistent effect on body weight with a C rating (14). The overall conclusion by the panel is that cardiac rehabilitation services are most beneficial when provided as a comprehensive package but with individualization of services according to the need to modify cardiovascular risk factors (14).

Cholesterol

Although multifactorial cardiac rehabilitation has a positive impact on reducing blood cholesterol levels, exercise training as a sole intervention is not recommended for lipid modification because of its inconsistent effects on lipid and lipoprotein levels (14). In a randomized trial of exercise in survivors of MI, LaRosa and coworkers (77) reported that, although adherence was "adequate" in 73% of the exercise patients (n = 110) and in 69% (n = 113) of the control group, there were no differences in blood cholesterol levels between the exercise and the control patients. This observation has been substantiated recently (78) with the additional observation that participation for more than 1 year increased HDL-C more than participation for only 3 months (79).

HYPERTENSION

Exercise training as a sole intervention has only a modest effect on lowering BP because medication, frequently not controlled for, is a major confounding variable (14). Although there is little evidence in patients with CHD, in those studies that have demonstrated some effect of exercise training in persons with hypertension, adherence with the intervention ranged from approximately 80% to 98%, with decreases of approximately 10 mm Hg in systolic blood pressure (SBP) and 8 mm Hg in DBP (80). This decrease in BP is similar to that reported with medication.

SMOKING

Exercise training as a sole intervention has little or no effect on smoking cessation (14). In one trial, the conclusion was that there were no differences between the exercise and no exercise groups for smoking cessation or prevention of relapse, although smokers in the training group reported smoking significantly fewer cigarettes (81).

EXERCISE TOLERANCE

Cardiac rehabilitation exercise training consistently has been shown to improve objective measures of exercise tolerance without significant complications or other adverse outcomes (14). Of 35 randomized controlled trials of exercise training, 30 demonstrated significant improvements in exercise tolerance with the proviso that continued exercise training is necessary to maintain the improvement observed (14).

ADHERENCE WITH CARDIAC REHABILITATION

Adherence with exercise rehabilitation after documentation of CHD has been the focus in and included as a component of more-comprehensive reviews of adherence with exercise and physical activity (6, 7, 26, 82, 83). Two major groupings of factors have been associated with adherence and dropout rate in cardiac rehabilitation exercise programs (Table 25.1): patient characteristics and intervention factors, such as the type of program (e.g., individualized or group), program problems (e.g., staff, facilities,

convenience factors), and communication (6, 7, 26, 83, 84).

Much data on adherence with exercise after MI are derived from randomized trials that primarily study efficacy or from nonexperimental reports and quasi-experimental studies. The information available frequently suffers, therefore, from methodological limitations. These include a lack of theoretical basis, unsuitable measures or end points, strictly observational and correlational data, inconsistent definition of adherence, and other potential biases, including sampling problems such as self-selection, uncontrolled confounding variables, and incomplete follow-up. Despite these design limitations and the fact that the available data do not especially increase our understanding of adherent and nonadherent behavior, there is useful and clinically relevant information for the practicing cardiac rehabilitation professional.

Factors that appear most predictive of dropout from cardiac rehabilitation have been identified and are summarized in Table 25.1. It appears though that dropping out from a supervised program does not necessarily mean a behavioral change failure because a considerable number of dropouts continue with their successful behavior modifications (85).

Because many of the common reasons for dropout are avoidable, there is a need for adherence-enhancing strategy research to optimize the probability for all patients—not just those who are highly motivated—to realize the potential benefits of cardiac rehabilitation. This emphasizes the need to examine factors associated with the professional who provides the service and the technique of intervention, although most data published to date have focused on more inflexible patient characteristics.

Rates of Dropout

Adherence in cardiac rehabilitation generally is considered to follow a negatively accelerating curve with a relatively larger dropout rate early, followed by a decreasing dropout rate with time (Fig. 25.2). The mean 2- to 3-month dropout rate from exercise participation in recent reports was 20% to 30%, increasing to approximately 40% and 50% at 6 and 12 months, respectively (6, 7), paralleling the observations of a decreasing attendance in supervised exercise rehabilitation (44,

Table 25.1. Factors Associated with Dropout From Cardiac Rehabilitation Programs and Suggested Means of Correction

Patient Characteristic	Suggested Primary Means of Correction
Smoking	Cessation: nicotine withdrawal, behavior modification
Obesity	Diet: behavior modification
Physical inactivity	Exercise: behavior modification
Low self-motivation	Psychological counseling and support
Lack of interest	Education, special events
Lack of spousal support	Counseling, education
Symptoms	Exercise prescription adjustment, refer to MD
Medical instability	Return to MD, close supervision and monitoring
Job-related factors	Intercession with employer, job change
Intervention Factors	
Individual/group	Refer to appropriate program model
Staff	Staff selection, education, training
Inconvenient location	Transportation facilitation (e.g., car pools)
Inconvenient time	Flexible scheduling

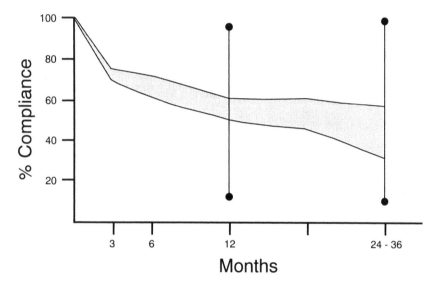

Figure 25.2. A typical adherence curve derived from studies of cardiac rehabilitation, including randomized clinical trials and investigations with random assignment to an exercise regimen. Minimum and maximum reported adherence rates at 12 and 24-36 months are indicated.

86). Long-term follow-up of exercise behavior is variable with dropout reported as high as 90% at 12 months (37) and as low as 0% during 4.5 years (87), and less than 20% during 5 years in hospital programs (88) to greater than 80% with heavier exercise during 6 to 9 years (89). Other trials have reported intermediate rates of 45% to 70% dropout during 3.5 to 4.5 years (84, 90).

The huge variation in reported adherence rates has to do with the definition of adherence, the socioeconomics of the population being studied, program location, available hours, and so on. These various factors, once identified, con-

stitute obstacles to program success and need to be addressed collectively and on an individual basis (36). Individualization of the problem is important as it has been reported that although fewer than 10% of patients were attending supervised sessions at 11 months, 78% reported doing some exercise on their own (37). This supports observations that, in some instances of dropout from supervised exercise programs, the behavior change is maintained at some other location more convenient or preferable to the patient (85).

Although the dropout rates may seem high, the adherence rates in some of the trials are higher than might be expected. Consider the fact that 55% or more of these volunteer patients adhere with long-term behavior change programs in which they are asked to spend as many as 4 years of their lives carrying out the exercise recommendations, which are often quite complex and not necessarily enjoyed by all, often at a location at some considerable distance from their homes, and often at relatively inconvenient times of the day for patients with families. We are struck by the fact that as many patients actually adhere to the demands of clinical trials as well as they do.

Reasons for Dropout

As first suggested by Bruce (91), the reasons for dropout from cardiac rehabilitation can be divided into the avoidable and unavoidable. Approximately 40% of dropouts occurred for avoidable reasons, and of the unavoidable reasons, medical dropout accounted for almost 60% (19, 84, 91, 92). This will be even higher in specific subsets of patients, for example, postangioplasty, in which, in our experience (F.J.P.), early dropout almost always represents angioplasty failure. Awareness of the reasons for dropout may have important immediate and potentially significant consequences for program planning because many of the avoidable reasons for dropout often are more amenable to change than patient characteristics.

Patient Characteristics and Interventions

Despite the methodological shortcomings of many of the studies found in the literature, certain characteristics are predictive of dropout from cardiac rehabilitation (Table 25.1), although, as stated earlier, the predictive accuracy of such features is not consistent enough to be extremely useful (18, 19). Factors that significantly influence adherence include the patient's knowledge, previous levels of adherence, confidence in the ability to follow recommendations, perception of health and the benefits of the treatment or behavior, availability of social support, and the complexity of the intervention (1). The characteristics of CHD patients most consistently associated with high incidence of dropout from supervised programs are smoking, blue-collar trade, obesity, low self-motivation, angina pectoris, spousal nonsupport, and sedentary lifestyle (6, 7).

The improvement expected with exercise training is a function of duration and intensity of exercise (93, 94). Although patients who participate in cardiac rehabilitation for a year improve more than those who participate for a more typical 3 months (79), the relationship between adherence and exercise intensity may be more complex than previously thought. For example, and as expected, higher adherence has been shown to be associated with lower intensity exercise and lower adherence with higher intensity exercise during a 2-year period (86). On the other hand, there also is recent evidence, in healthy older adults, that higher adherence, also at 2 years, is associated with higher intensity, home-based exercise interventions than with either similar intensity, group-based programs or lower intensity, home-based programs (95).

Women, when compared with men, are not referred as frequently (14, 96) and have been shown to either adhere as well (97) or not as well (98, 99). It has been reported that women younger than 45 years of age and on Medicaid/Title 19 have a mean attendance of only 18% and as such are a high-risk group who would benefit from strategies to enhance the use of cardiac rehabilitation services (99). This low attendance rate in younger women on Medicaid/Title 19 (n = 40) was not confirmed in a study of patients on Medicaid (n = 36) in which attendance was 92%, but in that study there were only 7 women and their age is not provided (100). It may well be that the women in our study (99) had homemaking and other responsibilities that the predominantly male population in the study by Friedman et al. (100) did not have, making it more difficult for them to attend regularly.

Patient health distress is negatively associated with exercise adherence (17). Although the relationship between adherence and patient self-efficacy is unclear (86, 101), improvement in health-related quality of life (HRQL) is associated with better adherence rates (102). Substantiating these observations on HRQL and adherence, we have preliminary results from our randomized trial of rehabilitation and HRQL (103) that both baseline HRQL and change in HRQL were significantly lower in poor compared with good adherers. These observations of health distress and poor adherence and greater improvement in HRQL among better adherers provide additional reasons for more research on adherence-enhancing strategies.

Adherence-enhancing Strategies

One basic approach to enhancing adherence may be to recommend low-intensity exercise such as walking. Lee and colleagues (86) have demonstrated that patients have higher attendance rates with low-intensity exercise recommendations than with higher intensity recommendations. This is an important observation because, although the low-intensity exercise may not have as marked an effect on cardiorespiratory fitness (86, 93), there is evidence that low-intensity exercise can substantially improve metabolic fitness, thereby reducing CHD risk (93, 94, 104, 105).

Potential adherence-enhancing strategies have been identified, and these include reinforcement control, stimulus control, and cognitive or self-control procedures (1, 6). Although health education strategies have a potentially important role in adherence enhancement (26), few investigations have been carried out in cardiac exercise rehabilitation with different adherence-enhancing strategies as the dependent variable. To our knowledge, only two exercise studies have investigated adherence-enhancing strategies in cardiac rehabilitation (21, 37). Daltroy (37) used an educational intervention that included telephone counseling for patient and spouse and found no difference in adherence between that group and the comparison group. In a study of contracting to improve adherence, we have demonstrated that those participants who signed an agreement to adhere and who then used self-monitoring techniques showed a 65% adherence rate, compared with the 42% rate seen in the control group and the 20% rate for the experimental group who declined to sign the contract agreement (21).

The transtheoretical model posits that there are stages that people move through as they intentionally consider a behavior change and then initiate and maintain that behavior change (106). Identification of the stage an individual is at may provide clues as to how the individual is likely to adhere to a given treatment and should provide a paradigm for exercise adherence-enhancing strategies that are associated with a particular stage (107). This model has been used in older adults with a cardiac diagnosis to study exercise behavior with the conclusion that exercise time is directly associated with the ordering of the stages; 0 minutes of exercise per week with patients in the precontemplation and contemplation stages, 67 minutes with patients in the preparation stage, 155 minutes in patients in the action stage, and 234 minutes in patients in the maintenance stage (108). This suggests that it may be possible to identify stage-specific adherence-enhancing strategies.

Adherence with effective lifestyle behavior-change treatments is associated with greater improvement (1). With the evidence that cardiac rehabilitation services are beneficial (14) but that there is relatively poor adherence to exercise recommendations in routine clinical practice (109), significantly more research needs to be initiated to identify which current adherence-enhancing strategies are most successful and also to identify new and successful strategies.

CARDIAC REHABILITATION IN THE FUTURE

There is an increasing awareness of the need to combine CHD prevention and rehabilitation efforts. The call for restructuring of the delivery of cardiac rehabilitation services has to a considerable degree been driven by the managed care forces in the health care system with a need to consider not only health effectiveness but also cost-effectiveness. This will require reevaluation of both the components and the delivery of cardiac rehabilitation services (45–50). There is evidence to support the effective and safe implementation of alternatives such as home programs, with or without telephonic and other ways of monitoring patients, that will extend the cost-effective delivery of cardiac rehabilitation services beyond traditional supervised, group-based rehabilitation programs (14). For example, the effectiveness and safety of home-based exercise programs have long been demonstrated (44, 110), however, without extensive implementation. Home-based nurse management, using a case-management approach, has been shown to be effective in clinical trials both in patients with MI (111) and catheterization-documented CHD (30), as well as in routine clinical practice in large private practice cardiology groups (49). In the former trial (111), cumulative dropout at 12 months was 15.4% in the special intervention group and 11.6% in the usual care group; smoking cessation rates, LDL-C levels, and exercise tolerance had each improved significantly more in the special intervention group than in the usual care group, suggesting more effective modification of coronary risk factors. In the latter trial (30), significantly more intervention than usual care patients had decreased their consumption of calories from fat and their intake of cholesterol, and were adhering to their lipid medication with significantly greater improvements in their lipid profile; significantly more intervention patients than usual care patients were exercising regularly with significantly greater exercise tolerance levels. After bypass surgery, telephonic monitoring of home-based walking and cycling exercise demonstrated no adverse effects (112). This presumably will result in a reduction of the impact of CHD by encouraging greater use of effective strategies by a more diverse pool of patients including presently underserved populations.

Effective programs must provide relevant services for those patients who need them at a time when they are needed most. With appropriate patient referral, an individualized approach (45) could maximize the likelihood of more optimal use and adherence by patients who need a particular service, for example, smoking cessation for smokers, diet for hyperlipidemic or overweight patients, and exercise for those with inadequate exercise tolerance. Individualization of rehabilitation services is essential and should be a highly cost-effective approach.

The "idea of a 'right' to health should be replaced by that of a moral obligation to preserve one's own health . . . the next major advances in the health of the American people will be determined by what the individual is willing to do for himself [or herself] and for society at large" (113). The emphasis on patients carrying out the recommendations with less supervision in less-structured environments will require that even greater attention be paid to the issues of adherence and the development of adherence-enhancing strategies. It will be increasingly incumbent on the physician to accept the active role of the patient in the decision-making process, to be willing to provide the patient with appropriate information, and to be aware of adherence-enhancing strategies and their potential effectiveness.

THE PHYSICIAN AND ADHERENCE

In the face of nonadherent patient behavior, the physician needs to answer the following questions: 1) Have I made the right diagnosis? 2) Has the recommended therapy been shown to do more good than harm? and 3) Is the patient fully informed and freely consenting to participate in the therapeutic or preventive intervention? If the answer to any of these questions is "no," then the nonadherent behavior is expected and explained, but corrective action is fruitless until the violated principle is rectified (6, 114).

Sackett goes on to recommend the following five steps for the detection and improvement of low adherence (114). First, identify patients who have dropped out of treatment. The importance of this cannot be emphasized enough. The most common form of nonadherence with long-term therapies is complete dropout from care. Most rehabilitation programs have poor systems for tracking and follow-up. We know that a significant number of patients who have dropped out of an 8- to 12-week program and who continue to show improvement by 1 year are indistinguishable from those who participated fully. Does their nonadherence represent a true failure of the program?

Second, identify patients who, despite program participation, have not achieved the goals of therapy. Distinguish between patients who demonstrate arrested progress on the basis of medical complexity—a potentially serious sign—and those who show lack of achievement because of adherence that is low or zero. The latter are targets for adherence-enhancing strategies.

Third, be sure that the regimen prescribed is vigorous enough to achieve the goal if the participants are reasonably adherent. In the rehabilitation milieu, one of the most common causes of deficient progress has to do with inadequate achievement of target heart rates for sufficient time to produce a conditioning response. This often is related to inaccuracy in the measurement of pulse rate during exercise or frequent interruption of aerobic exercise to change exercise modalities, resulting in the pulse returning to normal repeatedly during exercise.

Fourth, identify the subgroup of patients who show low adherence. Although this seems inherently obvious in the rehabilitation environment, patients may be very subtle in their ability to "ride the shovel" and appear adherent when they really are not. We have noticed that large discrepancies between heart rates during prescribed exercise activity and a concomitant level of activity during graded-exercise testing suggest some shortcutting. It could represent an abbreviation of the prescribed distance or leaning on the rails of the treadmill. We advocate the use of perceived exertion scales, such as the Borg scale (115), in conjunction with the reporting of achieved heart rate, to help control this.

Last, the adherence-enhancing strategies should be applied in sequence. These include increasing attention and supervision. The improved mortality among patients in rehabilitation programs should come as no surprise given the higher intensity and frequency of contact with knowledgeable rehabilitation professionals during exercise (41). This contact inevitably leads to earlier recognition and resolution of problems before they become critical. The patient sees this and the experience reinforces the validity of rehabilitation involvement.

Can the program be simplified? If the patient cannot achieve an appropriate training rate with treadmill, aerobic dance, biking, rowing, and pulleys, would he or she be better served to be placed on a simple walking regimen? If the patient is failing to reduce weight, lower cholesterol, quit smoking, and control hypertension, would it be acceptable to concentrate on just one issue until progress has been made? Referral of the patient to other health professionals such as psychologists, vocational counselors, and the like may reduce pressure on the rehabilitation staff to succeed with the resolution of every management problem.

Behavioral strategies such as positive reinforcement are simple and can be extremely successful. Ironically, people being what they are, we frequently cannot motivate our patients to walk 1 mile to save their lives, but they will walk a hundred miles for a T-shirt. The formalization of adherence negotiations in the form of written contracts can be very effective (21, 26, 116), and there is positive evidence from 10 of 11 trials that financial incentives can improve patient adherence (117).

The physician has a special role for motivating patients and for encouraging adherence (1). Studies have shown that the mere discussion of the problem during the course of a clinical visit and the verbal validation of the need to initiate change lead to a higher likelihood of success in achieving the desired health behavior (118). As we inferred earlier, the physician's responsibility for patient adherence seems to be related inversely to the extent that the patient participates in making choices concerning his or her health, and physicians who do not involve patients in essential decisions assume considerable responsibility for therapeutic outcomes and place themselves in a potentially compromising ethical position (119).

Education of the patient, so often deferred entirely by physicians or given over to other providers in the rehabilitation program, is fundamentally the responsibility of the physician. The information communicated must be truthful and any attempts at behavioral change must be noncoercive (119). As we have alluded to earlier in this chapter, education has two components: information transfer sufficient to make informed decisions, and for the motivated patient who wishes to act on that knowledge, instruction in behavioral skills that helps to achieve the desired goals (119). A common problem with physicians is the use of language that is too vague or technical, which contributes tangibly to nonadherence (120).

In the ideal patient–physician relationship, in which adherent behavior is intended by both parties, there exists an ethic of freedom, mutual understanding, responsibility, and satisfaction (119). Although the physician has the right to expect the patient to adhere with recommended treatments and therapies, nonadherence does not relieve the physician from further responsibility for the patient (8, 121). The physician should not expect the patient to remember the recommendations made. In the Medical Outcomes Study, as many as 35% of the patients did not remember being given recommendations about regular exercise, and whether or not they recalled being given the recommendation, fewer than 25% of the 1305 patients adhered to the exercise recommendation (109).

In the event of repeated nonadherence the physician should reassess the diagnosis, the appropriateness of the therapeutic strategy, and the patient's capability to adhere. If no modifications can be made, then the physician essentially has two alternatives: 1) accept the nonadherence and provide as much assistance as possible—in essence, changing from a "curing" to a "caring" mode; or 2) withdraw from care. The latter should be based on the premise that the physician has finite limits to his or her resources and time and that an alternative provider may prove more effective. The option of alternative providers should be offered to the patient and the withdrawal from care should be nonpunitive.

Exercise rehabilitation, although extraordinarily safe, is not entirely benign, particularly for specific subsets of patients (14), and it is only recently that the efficacy of cardiac rehabilitation after an acute coronary event has been clarified (41, 42). It is fundamentally the physician's responsibility to see that the patient is fully informed concerning the risks and benefits of such therapy. Patient preference with respect to these benefits and risks must be discussed and integrated into decisions regarding the prescribed therapy.

In addition to the medical considerations, the economics of rehabilitation services have become increasingly important (122). What is the best dollar value for a given patient? A fully monitored, institutional-based program or a home-based program with telephone supervision? The physician should have a comprehensive understanding of the medical and socioeconomic circumstances of each patient and should be able to provide appropriate guidance and direction. Should this responsibility be delegated, it is mandatory that the physician be sure that the professional who fulfills this important role is suitably trained, qualified, and certified.

A FINAL WORD

We know from our own lives that the success of lifestyle modification depends on the decision to adhere to the modification; thus, low adherence with lifestyle-altering regimens constitutes the major impediment to achieving significant impact. One major question that concerns lifestyle management of risk factors in cardiac rehabilitation is whether poor adherence is a result of inadequate communication by the health professional. This chapter has attempted to demonstrate the association between adequate adherence and the increased likelihood of achieving the benefits of cardiac rehabilitation services. Simultaneously, we must recognize that adherence with the health behavior change initiated in cardiac rehabilitation programs needs to be, and can be, improved. Strategies that emphasize health behavior counseling to improve communication and to increase patient motivation and self-responsibility must be a high priority of the cardiac rehabilitation physician.

References

1. Miller NH, Hill M, Kottke T, for the Expert Panel on Compliance. The multilevel compliance challenge: recommendations for a call to action. A statement for healthcare professionals. Circulation 1997;95:1085–1090.
2. Luepker RV. Patient adherence: a "risk factor" for cardiovascular disease. Heart Stroke 1993;2:418–421.
3. Hays RD, Kravitz RL, Mazel RM, et al. The impact of patient adherence on health outcomes for patients with chronic disease in the Medical Outcomes Study. J Behav Med 1994;17:347–360.
4. Fawcett J. Compliance: definitions and key issues. J Clin Psychiatry 1995;56(Suppl 1):4–8.
5. McDermott MM, Schmitt, B, Wallner E. Impact of medication nonadherence on coronary heart disease outcomes. A critical review. Arch Intern Med 1997; 157:1921–1929.
6. Oldridge NB. Cardiac rehabilitation exercise programme: compliance and compliance-enhancing strategies. Sports Med 1988;6:42–55.
7. Oldridge N. Compliance with cardiac rehabilitation services. J Cardpulm Rehabil 1991;11:115–127.
8. Jonsen AR. Ethical issues in compliance. In: Haynes R, Taylor D, Sacket D, eds. Compliance in health care. Baltimore: Johns Hopkins University Press, 1979:113–120.
9. Donovan JL. Patient decision making. The missing ingredient in compliance research. Int J Technol Assess Health Care 1995;11:443–455.
10. Hulka BS. Patient-clinician interactions and compliance. In: Haynes RB, Taylor DW, Sackett DL, eds. Compliance in health care. Baltimore: Johns Hopkins University Press, 1979:63–77.
11. Trostle J. Medical compliance as an ideology. Soc Sci Med 1988;27:1299–1308.
12. Donovan J, Blake DR. Patient non-compliance: deviance or reasoned décision-making? Soc Sci Med 1992;34:507–513.
13. Morris LS, Schulz RM. Medication compliance: the patient's perspective. Clin Ther 1993;15:593–606.
14. Wenger NK, Froelicher ES, Smith LK, et al. Cardiac rehabilitation. Clinical Practice Guideline No. 17. Rockville, MD: US Department of Health and Human Services, Public Health Service, Agency for Health Care Policy and Research, and the National Heart, Lung and Blood Institute. AHCPR Publication No. 96–0672, 1995:1–202.
15. Zembaty JS. A limited defense of paternalism in medicine. In: Mappes TA, Zembaty JS, eds. Biomedical ethics. 2nd ed. New York: McGraw-Hill, 1981:60–66.
16. Guccione AA. Ethical and legal limits to professional dominance. Top Geriatr Rehabil 1988;3:62–73.
17. DiMatteo MR, Sherbourne CD, Hays RD, et al. Physicians' characteristics influence patients' adherence to medical treatment: results from the Medical Outcomes Study. Health Psychol 1993;12:93–102.
18. Oldridge N. Cardiac rehabilitation, self-responsibility, and quality of life. J Cardpulm Rehabil 1986;6:153–156.
19. Oldridge NB, Rogowski BL. Self-efficacy and in-patient cardiac rehabilitation. Am J Cardiol 1990;66:362–365.
20. Andrew GM, Oldridge NB, Parker JO, et al. Reasons for

dropout from exercise programs in post-coronary patients. Med Sci Sports Exerc 1981;13:164–168.

21. Oldridge NB, Jones NL. Improving patient compliance in cardiac exercise rehabilitation: effects of written agreement and self-monitoring. J Cardiac Rehabil 1983;:257–262.

22. Simpson M, Buckman R, Stewart M, et al. Doctor-patient communication: the Toronto consent statement. Br Med J 1991;303:1385–1387.

23. Delbanco T. Enriching the doctor-patient relationship by inviting the patient's perspective. Ann Intern Med 1992;116:414–418.

24. Gorlin R. Must cardiology lose its heart? J Am Coll Cardiol 1992;19:1635–1640.

25. Sotile WM, Sotile MO, Ewen GS, et al. Marriage and family factors relevant to effective cardiac rehabilitation: a review of risk factor literature. J Sports Med Training Rehabil 1993;4:115–128.

26. Burke L, Dunbar-Jacob J. Adherence to medication, diet, and activity recommendations: from assessment to maintenance. J Cardiovasc Nurs 1995;9:62–69.

27. Mazzuca SA. Does patient education in chronic disease have therapeutic value? J Chronic Dis 1982;35:521–529.

28. World Health Organization Expert Committee. Rehabilitation of patients with cardiovascular disease. Technical Report Series No. 270. Geneva: World Health Organization, 1964.

29. Ornish D, Brown SE, Scherwitz LW, et al. Can lifestyle changes reverse coronary heart disease? The Lifestyle Heart Trial. Lancet 1990;336:129–133.

30. Haskell WL, Alderman EL, Fair JM, et al. Effects of intensive multiple risk factor reduction on coronary atherosclerosis and clinical cardiac events in men and women with coronary artery disease. The Stanford Coronary Risk Intervention Project (SCRIP). Circulation 1994;89:975–990.

31. Horwitz RI, Horwitz SM. Adherence to treatment and health outcomes. Arch Intern Med 1993;153:1863–1868.

32. Coronary Drug Project Research Group. Clofibrate and niacin in coronary heart disease. JAMA 1975;231:360–381.

33. Beta-blocker Heart Attack Trial Research Group. A randomized trial of propranolol in patients with acute myocardial infarction: I. Mortality results. JAMA 1982;247:1710–1714.

34. Coronary Drug Project Research Group. Influence of adherence to treatment and response of cholesterol on mortality in the Coronary Drug Project. N Engl J Med 1980;303:1038–1041.

35. Horwitz RI, Viscoli CM, Berkman L, et al. Treatment adherence and risk of death after a myocardial infarction. Lancet 1990;336:542–545.

36. Pashkow FJ, Pashkow P, Schafer M, eds. Successful cardiac rehabilitation: the complete guide for building cardiac rehab programs. 1st ed. Loveland, CO: HeartWatchers Press, 1988:253-256.

37. Daltroy LH. Improving cardiac patient adherence to exercise regimens: a clinical trial of health education. J Cardpulm Rehabil 1985;5:40–49.

38. Coy JA. Philosophical aspects of patient noncompli-

ance: a critical analysis. Top Geriatr Rehabil 1989;4:52–60.

39. Coy JA. Autonomy-based informed consent: ethical implications for patient noncompliance. Phys Ther 1989;69:826–832.

40. Smith CJ. Risk-reduction therapy: the challenge to change. Circulation 1996;93:2205–2211.

41. Oldridge NB, Guyatt GH, Fischer ME, et al. Cardiac rehabilitation after myocardial infarction. Combined experience of randomized clinical trials. JAMA 1988;260:945–950.

42. O'Connor GT, Buring JE, Yusuf S, et al. An overview of randomized trials of rehabilitation with exercise after myocardial infarction. Circulation 1989;80:234–244.

43. Jugdutt BI, Michorowski BL, Kappagoda CT. Exercise training after anterior Q wave myocardial infarction: importance of regional left ventricular function and topography. J Am Coll Cardiol 1988;12:362–372.

44. DeBusk RF, Haskell WL, Miller NH, et al. Medically directed at-home rehabilitation soon after clinically uncomplicated acute myocardial infarction: a new model for patient care. Am J Cardiol 1985;55:251–257.

45. Wenger NK. Modern coronary rehabilitation. New concepts in care. Postgrad Med 1993;94:131–141.

46. Merz CNB, Rozanski A. Remodeling cardiac rehabilitation into secondary prevention programs. Am Heart J 1996;132:418–427.

47. Froelicher VF, Herbert W, Myers J, et al. How cardiac rehabilitation is being influenced by changes in healthcare delivery. J Cardpulm Rehabil 1996;16:151–159.

48. Franklin BA, Hall L, Timmis GC. Contemporary cardiac rehabilitation services. Am J Cardiol 1997;79:1075–1077.

49. Gordon NF, Haskell WL. Comprehensive cardiovascular disease risk reduction in a cardiac rehabilitation setting. Am J Cardiol 1997;80:69H–73H.

50. Dafoe W, Huston P. Current trends in cardiac rehabilitation. Can Med Assoc J 1997;156:527–32.

51. Greenland P, Chu J. Efficacy of cardiac rehabilitation services with an emphasis on patients after myocardial infarction. Ann Intern Med 1988;109:650–653.

52. Morley D, Ribisl PM, Miller HS. A comparison of patient education methodologies in outpatient cardiac rehabilitation. J Cardpulm Rehabil 1984;4:434–439.

53. 27th Bethesda Conference. Matching the intensity of risk factor management with the hazard for coronary disease events. J Am Coll Cardiol 1996;27:957–1047.

54. Forrester JS, Merz CNB, Bush TL, et al. Efficacy of risk factor management. J Am Coll Cardiol 1996;27:991–1006.

55. Roberts WC. Effects of lipid lowering on coronary plaque and coronary events. Am J Cardiol 1997;80:8H–9H.

56. Grundy SM. Cholesterol and coronary heart disease. Arch Intern Med 1997;157:1177–1184.

57. Merz CNB, Rozanski A, Forrester JS. The secondary prevention of coronary artery disease. Am J Med 1997;102:572–581.

58. Brown G, Albers JJ, Fisher LD, et al. Regression of coronary artery disease as a result of intensive lipid-lowering therapy in men with high levels of apolipoprotein B. N Engl J Med 1990;323:1289–1298.

59. MAAS Investigators. Effect of simvastatin on coronary atheroma: the Multicenter Anti-Atheroma Study (MAAS). Lancet 1994;344:633–638.

60. Karvetti R. Effects of nutrition education. J Am Diet Assoc 1981;79:660–667.

61. Singh RB, Rastogi SS, Verma R, et al. Randomized controlled trial of cardioprotective diet in patients with recent acute myocardial infarction: results of one year follow-up. Br Med J 1992;304:1015–1019.

62. Barnard ND, Scherwitz LW, Ornish D. Adherence and acceptability of a low-fat, vegetarian diet among patients with cardiac disease. J Cardpulm Rehabil 1992;12:423–431.

63. Franklin TL, Kolasa KM, Griffin K, et al. Adherence to a very-low-fat diet by a group of cardiac rehabilitation patients in the rural Southeastern United States. Arch Fam Med 1995;4:551–554.

64. Hennekens CH, Satterfield S, Herbert PR. Treatment of elevated blood pressure to prevent coronary heart disease. In: Higgins MW, Luepker RV, eds. Trends in coronary heart disease mortality. The influence of medical care. New York: Oxford University Press, 1988: 103–108.

65. Sanson-Fisher RW, Clover K. Compliance in the treatment of hypertension. A need for action. Am J Hypertens 1995;8:82S–88S.

66. Perkins J, Dick TBS. Smoking and myocardial infarction: secondary prevention. Postgrad Med J 1985;61: 295–300.

67. Hermanson B, Omenn GS, Kronmal RA, et al. Beneficial six-year outcome of smoking cessation in older men and women with coronary artery disease. Results from the CASS registry. N Engl J Med 1988;319:1365–1369.

68. Rigotti NA, McKool KM, Shiffman S. Predictors of smoking cessation after coronary artery bypass graft surgery. Results of a randomized trial with 5-year follow-up. Ann Intern Med 1994;120:287–293.

69. Friedman M, Thoresen CE, Gill JJ, et al. Alteration of type A behavior and its effect on cardiac recurrences in post myocardial infarction patients: summary results of the recurrent coronary prevention project. Am Heart J 1986;112:653–665.

70. Linden W, Stossel C, Maurice J. Psychosocial interventions for patients with coronary artery disease. Arch Intern Med 1996;156:745–752.

71. Blumenthal JA, Jiang W, Babyak MA, et al. Stress management and exercise training in cardiac patients with myocardial ischemia. Effects on prognosis and evaluation of mechanisms. Arch Inter Med 1997;157: 2213–2223.

72. Frasure-Smith N, Lesperance F, Prince RH, et al. Randomised trial of home-based psychological nursing intervention for patients recovering from myocardial infarction. Lancet 1997;350:473–479.

73. Jones DA, West RR. Psychological rehabilitation after myocardial infarction: multicentre randomised controlled trial. Br Med J 1997;313:1517–1521.

74. Frasure-Smith N, Prince R. The ischemic heart disease life stress program: impact on mortality. Psychosom Med 1985;47:441–445.

75. Frasure-Smith N. In-hospital symptoms of psycholog-

76. Mayou R. Rehabilitation after heart attack. Br Med J 1997;313:1498–1499.

77. LaRosa JC, Cleary P, Muesing RA, et al. Effect of long-term moderate physical exercise on plasma lipoproteins. Arch Intern Med 1982;142:2269–2274.

78. Warner JG, Brubaker PH, Zhu Y, et al. Long-term (5-year) changes in HDL cholesterol in cardiac rehabilitation patients. Do sex differences exist? Circulation 1995;92:773–777.

79. Brubaker PH, Warner JG, Zhu Y, et al. Comparison of standard- and extended length participation in cardiac rehabilitation on body composition, functional capacity, and blood lipids. Am J Cardiol 1996;78:769–773.

80. Hagberg JM. Physical activity, physical fitness, and blood pressure. In: Leon AS, ed. Physical activity and cardiovascular health. A national consensus. Champaign, IL: Human Kinetics, 1997:112–119.

81. Taylor C, Houston-Miller N, Haskell W, et al. Smoking cessation after acute myocardial infarction: the effects of training. Addict Behav 1988;13:331–335.

82. Dishman RK. Epilogue and future directions. In: Dishman RK, ed. Exercise adherence. Its impact on public health. Champaign, IL: Human Kinetics, 1988:417–426.

83. King AC, Blair SN, Bild DE, et al. Determinants of physical activity and interventions in adults. Med Sci Sports Exerc 1992;24:S221–S236.

84. Oldridge NB, Donner AP, Buck CW, et al. Predictors of dropout from cardiac exercise rehabilitation. Ontario Exercise-Heart Collaborative Study. Am J Cardiol 1983;51:70–74.

85. Oldridge NB, Spencer J. Exercise habits and perceptions before and after graduating or dropout from supervised cardiac exercise rehabilitation. J Cardpulm Rehabil 1985;5:313–319.

86. Lee JY, Jensen BE, Oberman A, et al. Adherence in the Training Levels Comparison Trial. Med Sci Sports Exerc 1996;28:47–52.

87. Marra S, Paolillo V, Spadaccini F, et al. Long-term follow-up after a controlled randomized post-myocardial infarction rehabilitation programme: effects on morbidity and mortality. Eur Heart J 1985;6:656–663.

88. Hedback B, Perk J. Five-year results of a comprehensive rehabilitation programme after myocardial infarction. Eur Heart J 1987;8:234–242.

89. Prosser G, Carson P, Phillips R. Exercise after myocardial infarction: long-term rehabilitation effects. J Psychosom Res 1985;29:535–540.

90. Wihelmsen L, Sanne H, Elmfeldt D, et al. A controlled trial of physical training after myocardial infarction. Prev Med 1975;4:491–508.

91. Bruce E, Frederick R, Bruce R, et al. Comparison of active participants and dropouts in CAPRI cardiopulmonary rehabilitation programs. Am J Cardiol 1976; 37:53–60.

92. Cannistra LB, O'Malley CJ, Balady GJ. Comparison of outcome of cardiac rehabilitation in black women and white women. Am J Cardiol 1995;75:890–893.

93. Haskell WL. Health consequences of physical activity:

understanding and challenges regarding dose-response. Med Sci Sports Exerc 1994;26:649–660.

94. Haskell WL. Physical activity, lifestyle, and cardiovascular health. In: Leon AS, ed. Physical activity and cardiovascular health. A national consensus. Champaign, IL: Human Kinetics, 1997:16–24.

95. King AC, Haskell WL, Young DR, et al. Long-term effects of varying intensities and formats of physical activity on participation rates, fitness, and lipoproteins in men and women aged 50 to 60 years. Circulation 1995;91:2596–2604.

96. Ades PA, Waldmann ML, McCann WJ, et al. Predictors of cardiac rehabilitation participation in older coronary patients. Arch Intern Med 1992;152:1033–1035.

97. Cannistra LB, Balady GJ, O'Malley CJ, et al. Comparison of the clinical profile and outcome of women and men in cardiac rehabilitation. Am J Cardiol 1992;69:1274–1279.

98. Oldridge NB, LaSalle D, Jones NL. Exercise rehabilitation of female patients with coronary heart disease. Am Heart J 1980;100:755–757.

99. Oldridge NB, Ragowski B, Gottlieb M. Use of outpatient cardiac rehabilitation services. Factors associated with attendance. J Cardiopulm Rehabil 1992;12:25–31.

100. Friedman DB, Williams AN, Levine BD. Compliance and efficacy of cardiac rehabilitation and risk factor modification in the medically indigent. Am J Cardiol 1997;79:281–285.

101. Robertson D, Keller C. Relationships among health beliefs, self-efficacy, and exercise adherence in patients with coronary artery disease. Heart Lung 1992;21:55–63.

102. Jeng C, Braun LT. The influence of self-efficacy on exercise intensity, compliance rate and cardiac rehabilitation outcomes among coronary artery disease patients. Prog Cardiovasc Nurs 1997;12:13–24.

103. Oldridge N, Guyatt G, Jones N, et al. Effects on quality of life with comprehensive rehabilitation after acute myocardial infarction. Am J Cardiol 1991;67:1084–1089.

104. Despres J-P, Lamarche B. Low-intensity exercise training, plasma lipoproteins and the risk of coronary heart disease. J Intern Med 1994;236:7–22.

105. Bouchard C. Physical activity and prevention of cardiovascular diseases: potential mechanisms. In: Leon AS, ed. Physical activity and cardiovascular health. A national consensus. Champaign, IL: Human Kinetics, 1997:48–56.

106. Prochaska J, DiClemente C. The transtheoretical model. Homewood, IL: Dow Jones-Irwin, 1984.

107. Marcus BH, Simkin L. The stages of exercise behavior. J Sports Med Phys Fitness 1993;33:83–88.

108. Hellman EA. Use of the stages of change in exercise adherence model among older adults with a cardiac diagnosis. J Cardpulm Rehabil 1997;17:145–155.

109. Kravitz RL, Hays RD, Sherbourne CD, et al. Recall of recommendations with adherence to advice among patients with chronic medical conditions. Arch Intern Med 1993;153:1869–1878.

110. Miller NH, Haskell WL, Berra K, et al. Home versus group exercise training for increasing functional capacity after myocardial infarction. Circulation 1984;70:645–649.

111. DeBusk RF, Miller NH, Superko HR, et al. A case-management system for coronary risk factor modification after acute myocardial infarction. Ann Intern Med 1994;120:721–729.

112. Fletcher GF, Chiaramida AJ, LeMay MR, et al. Telephonically-monitored home exercise early after coronary artery bypass surgery. Chest 1984;86:198–202.

113. Knowles JH. Responsibility for health. Science 1977;198:16.

114. Sackett DL. A compliance practicum for the busy practitioner. In: Haynes RB, Taylor DW, Sackett DL, eds. Compliance in health care. Baltimore: Johns Hopkins University Press, 1979:286–294.

115. Borg G, Ottoson D. The perception of exertion in physical work. Dobbs Ferry, NY: Sheridan House, 1986.

116. Miller LJ. The formal treatment contract in the inpatient management of borderline personality disorder. Hosp Community Psychiatry 1990;41:985–987.

117. Giuffrida A, Torgerson DJ. Should we pay the patient? Review of financial incentives to enhance patient compliance. Br Med J 1997;315:703–707.

118. Nett LM. The physician's role in smoking cessation. A present and future agenda. Chest 1990;97(Suppl 2):28S–33S.

119. Eraker SA, Kirscht JP, Becker MH. Understanding and improving patient compliance. Ann Intern Med 1984;100:258–268.

120. Ley P. Doctor-patient communication: some quantitative estimates of the role of cognitive factors in noncompliance. J Hypertens Suppl 1985;3:551–555.

121. Thomasma DC. Beyond medical paternalism and patient autonomy: a model of physician conscience for the physician-patient relationship. Ann Intern Med 1983;98:243–248.

122. Oldridge NB. Outcome assessment in cardiac rehabilitation. Health-related quality of life and economic evaluation. J Cardiopulm Rehabil 1997;17:179–194.

Newer Technology in Cardiac Rehabilitation

Fredric J. Pashkow

HIGH TECHNOLOGY IN CARDIOVASCULAR MEDICINE

The influence of high technology in medicine is no greater anywhere than in the subspecialty of cardiovascular disease. This headlong rush to push the limits of the technological "envelope" encompasses the diagnostic as well as therapeutic, the electronic as well as biologic, and the invasive as well as noninvasive aspects of cardiovascular care (1). Since 1963, when coronary angiography became available for patients, more cardiovascular diagnostic and therapeutic interventions have been introduced than during all the previous years in the history of cardiovascular medicine. To a significant degree, the technology explosion is related both to the development of a safe and reliable means for the visualization of the coronary circulation, which inevitably led to the most significant palliative therapy for advanced coronary disease, coronary artery bypass graft surgery, and to the systematic development of powerful drugs for the control of hypertension, heart failure, and ischemia. For the most part, however, present and future innovations are contingent on the further development of tiny, waferlike chips that have the ability to store large amounts of information. These chips, called *microprocessors*, are now more complex than the miniaturized printed circuit boards they once were. They are virtual computers, capable of handling millions of bits of information routinely, so that real-time, noninvasive imaging of the heart with high-frequency sound, for example, is not only feasible but became commonplace in the mid-1980s (2).

The application of high technology in cardiovascular medicine has, until recently, been focused largely on the high-visibility areas of car-

diology—those in which a "quick fix" to the huge problem of coronary heart disease might be found. The search for a "magic bullet"—be it a laser "plaque-blaster," a new "clot-busting" enzyme, or a magic elixir ("not a real drug, doctor, please")—has been preeminent in the minds of the public, cardiologists, and medical industry (1). The latter has been especially ardent because whatever provides the greatest return on the dollar attracts the most attention. Thus, the term *high-tech* has been equated with the word *expensive* in the minds of many (3, 4).

This is a misconception that potentially obstructs the use of many available and worthwhile high-tech applications in cardiac rehabilitation and prevention. Because of the phenomenon of "trickle down," by which technology becomes less expensive as more is produced and competitive forces come to bear, what once was considered exotic is now widely available at lower cost. The microcomputer is a good example. When programmers first began working with computerization of rehabilitation records in 1983, the processor we used had 256K (K = kilobyte or one thousand bytes) of random access memory (RAM), and storage was on 400K floppy disks. Today, we use machines that typically operate with 16 MB (MB = one megabyte or one million bytes) of RAM with data storage on inexpensive hard drives that typically hold 1000 MB (or 1 GB = gigabyte, or one billion bytes) of data.

Another misconception is that high technology involves only sophisticated imaging or interventional therapies delivered through catheters (1). The reality is that cardiac rehabilitation, although relatively "low-tech" in its overall approach, can benefit most in areas in which traditional techniques are time-consuming, (i.e., costly to implement or limited in their success) (5). Another example would be the use of interactive educational technology for modification of coronary risk factors (6, 7).

Kashyap (8) has pointed out that modern technological advances such as coronary angiography, angioplasty, coronary artery bypass graft surgery, or pacemaker insertion can ameliorate the effects of heart disease in the elderly, but such advances are costly (9). Although the most effective cost-reduction strategy lies in prevention of atherosclerosis and its complications, it is not certain that these data apply directly to the older population (8).

In this chapter I review a selection of high-tech applications that have had or will have some significant application in cardiac rehabilitation. I will focus on the more direct application of high technology in cardiac rehabilitation services and only mention in passing the important and increasing use of sophisticated technologies for the performance of essential aspects of the rehabilitative process (for example, the application of nuclear and ultrasound imaging as an essential part of the methodology of risk stratification). I also discuss the further development of existing and future technologies.

Patient-monitoring Systems

Patient monitoring was one of the first technological applications to see widespread use in cardiac rehabilitation. In several areas of this book the application of this technology, its historical background, and the current implications of its use have been discussed in detail from the medical and economic points of view. It is reviewed briefly from the technology perspective here.

The use of electronic monitoring really had its origins with the parallel beliefs that exercise after an acute coronary event may be of significant risk (10, 11) and that untoward events can be predicted by the presence of frequent or "complex" ventricular ectopy (12). We subsequently have learned that exercise rehabilitation is safe for the majority of patients (13) and that the occurrence of ventricular ectopy is a relatively poor predictor of subsequent events (14). By this time, however, electrocardiographic (ECG) monitoring has become tied to reimbursement for rehabilitative services and, therefore, mandatory for programs that hope to qualify for compensation.

In the meantime, technology has improved progressively and the cost, as noted generally, has come down (4). Technology currently exists to provide telemetric monitoring, using radio transmission in lieu of wires, that is lightweight, durable, and waterproof. Base stations that contain microprocessors are now available that automatically monitor predefined criteria and report the occurrence of potentially serious dysrhythmias. There are other important uses of ECG monitoring during exercise in addition to the detection of arrhythmia. The measurement of accurate heart rates (HRs) during various exercise activities seems rudimentary and trivial but is actually difficult to perform accurately by most other means. This is essential for the tracking of progress (15) and for the calculation of caloric expenditure if this is an important part of the patient's program (16).

In the last several years, cardiologists have seen the refinement of telephonic monitoring technologies that can be used at a site distant from the base station to establish monitoring in the home environment (17–19). Telephonic exercise monitoring provides simultaneous transmission of voice and ECG signals during exercise therapy (20, 21). The application of this technology is controversial with respect to exercise-rehabilitation safety and the legal issues that concern appropriate response to patient emergencies (20). Telephonic exercise monitoring appears to be efficacious and cost-effective; moreover (22), for purposes of observing for conformity to the prescribed exercise regimen, monitoring training progress, and compliance to exercise (23), such systems work well (16).

Computerized Cardiac Rehabilitation Records

Until now, most cardiologists generally have encountered microprocessors as an integrated element in some high-tech imaging equipment (an imaging processor) or in bedside monitoring or stress testing systems. Some clinicians have familiarity with fiscal information programs for insurance or billing purposes, laboratory data-retrieval systems, or, more rarely, multimedia teaching systems. Despite their potential benefits, digital medical records systems and applied databases have infrequently been applied in clinical practice.

As the medical record becomes overloaded with information, the need for clinically focused programs capable of tracking and organizing large volumes of data has become increasingly important (24–26). These information-management database programs usually start out in the minds of the clinical providers as an electronic (but otherwise relatively traditional) medical record. It is hoped that they evolve to provide highly organized, relational, information-management systems (27, 28). Once available, their programs can interface with software that was mentioned earlier, providing a totally different approach to the concept of systems development. Such programs, although uncommon, are becoming increasingly available (5, 25, 29).

The motivating factor in the development of these programs for cardiac rehabilitation was the large volume of data that required manipulation and storage, and the frustration and time required to process this information manually for the generation of reports. Cardiac rehabilitation has large informational-management requirements. For example, a patient who exercises in a rehabilitation program has multiple-field data entries at the time of check-in and checkout (blood pressure [BP], weight, pulse, and so on). The patient typically participates in a half-dozen exercises in which the time, distance, resistance, pulse rate, and several other pieces of data may be recorded for each activity. Patients usually exercise 12 to 15 times per month, so the dimensions of the data-tracking problem can be appreciated.

Related directly to the issues of cost containment and efficiency of program operation are management of patient records and staff-to-patient and staff-to-physician communications (5, 30). The issue is not one of just increased record-keeping efficiency per se, but also the design and use of systems to provide an administrative framework consistent with the highest professional standards, to maximize the opportunity for positive staff and patient reinforcement, and ideally, to encourage compliance and long-term modification of lifestyle and behavior. The technical capability to provide such systems at reasonable cost is now at hand (5, 25, 28, 31).

Computerized information ("database") management systems have become more of a reality for cardiac rehabilitation with the development of relatively small, powerful personal computers

often referred to as PCs (5). These computers can be coupled to relatively large (2 GB and up) storage drives to provide systems eminently capable of handling patient records for even the largest cardiac rehabilitation programs.

The ability to organize, categorize, and rapidly retrieve medical and exercise information is the first and most obvious advantage of computerized information-management systems (32). They also provide an opportunity to improve administrative efficiency and increase staff time available for direct patient care by eliminating time-consuming and tedious manual data transfer (33). Such systems, when thoughtfully designed, however, can integrate nicely with other aspects of good patient-management and provide an opportunity for reiterative education, enhanced patient communications, and positive reinforcement on incremental progress, leading to improved patient compliance and better long-term outcome (34). For example, software can be modified to provide feedback interactively to the patient about specific information, such as BP, rate-response to exercise, and cholesterol levels, and to follow progress over time and relate this to the patient's individualized goals.

COMPUTER SYSTEMS DESIGNED SPECIFICALLY FOR CARDIAC REHABILITATION MANAGEMENT

When designing or buying such an information-management system the database software must accommodate all the essential information yet allow for easy input (35). Ideally, the database portion of the program should be accessible even when the computer is "busy" with another task, especially if access to certain patient information at particular times may be medically necessary. Operationally, the program should be simple enough so that staff can learn to use it without extensive training and patients can learn to post at least a portion of their own data (Fig. 26.1). The latter provides an opportunity for instant feedback and the enhanced patient communication and positive reinforcement alluded to previously.

Conceptually, information-management programs for cardiac rehabilitation should consist of three parts. The first part is the actual database. These files must include baseline specifications (e.g., file listings of patient demographic information, patient diagnoses, different exercises available). The second part handles individual pa-

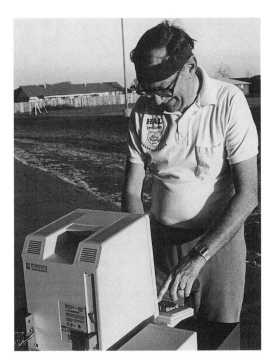

Figure 26.1. A patient entering exercise data on a cart-mounted Macintosh computer during an exercise session.

tient records in which information is accumulated, organized, calculated, and stored on a continuing basis. The third part is the report function. What program developers have realized is that this third part of the information-management system has power beyond mere summary, storage, and listing. It allows for a higher level of information use—one that can be relational or even discriminatory. This provides the means by which the application can raise program quality, efficiency, and productivity, motivate patients and staff, facilitate communication, and encourage adherence.

The system should be designed to facilitate the generation of reports (see Fig. 23.3), particularly to patients as well as to physicians, in such a way that it economizes staff time. Finally, the system should be designed so that records can be archived periodically to provide a coherent audit trail that would satisfy health insurers and government quality assurance and utilization reviewers. In short, the software most suitable to fulfill the rehabilitation program's needs is the prime requisite and the hardware necessary to run it is secondary.

EXPERIENCE WITH A DATABASE MANAGEMENT SYSTEM

System Development

Lesser (24) has pointed out that although the acquisition and maintenance of patient medical records lend themselves well to computerization, there were few, if any, descriptions of successful implementations of computerized medical records in a noninstitutional setting, at least through the mid-1980s. More on this subject is becoming available (26), but our experience suggests that such technology has been infrequently applied in the cardiac rehabilitation setting.

Beginning in the summer of 1985, we have been involved in the development and deployment of such a patient record and data management system in a community-based rehabilitation setting (5, 30). The software has evolved extensively over the past decade. Two versions of the program were developed, one for Apple Macintosh and another for IBM-compatible PCs. The Macintosh version was designed specifically to be patient-interactive. The patient-interactive aspect of the program was carefully thought out, and the appropriate hardware configuration was considered in great detail. One technical specification required was significant "user friendliness," because the patients themselves would interact with the device at each exercise session (Fig. 26.1). O'Leary and associates (36) have pointed out that activity that involves a personal computer can be a valuable modality in the rehabilitation of older adults, but access is a key issue. Portability, the type and availability of additional software programs, and cost were also prerequisites. Such system configurations can use off-the-shelf equipment and cost less than $2,000. It is sufficiently powerful to allow for real-time access by the staff to the computer during the time that patients actually are exercising, and it can provide the staff immediate entry to such information as diagnoses, medication allergies, and current medications. Whoever enters the data, whether patient or staff, has the option of logging the information as the individual exercise activities are completed (or all at once after the exercise session).

Macintosh Versus IBM and IBM-Compatibles

Although each PC has relative strengths and weaknesses, during the past few years each has become more like the other. The Macintosh high-contrast display screen accommodated oversized type-fonts with black characters on a light background. A "mouse" facilitated the rapid input of data, and the integration of the video screen with the central processor allowed it to be mounted on a mobile cart so that it could be moved to wherever the exercise activities took place. The same computer software program could be adapted to accommodate phase II to phase IV exercise programs. Patient acceptance of the Macintosh system was excellent (30).

Although the IBM-compatible operating (OS) systems lacked the patient-interactive qualities of the Macintosh version until the introduction of Windows '95, it always appealed more to hospital and information-management administrators. With large numbers of standard business analysis and statistical programs available, the IBM standard was more suitable for hospitals with integrated systems or for persons interested in research. The MS-DOS operating software of the IBM-compatible systems required more training than the Macintosh user-interface. The Windows operating system, however, now offers many of the "user friendly" features of the Macintosh OS, including pull-down menus, large fonts, and so on. The IBM-compatible systems, however, are only just starting to provide the "plug-and-play" low-cost audio and graphics integration capability of the Macintosh.

Experience with the Information Management System

Such software can provide an extensive patient database and can produce instant facsimiles of patient demographic data, medications, drug allergies, referring physicians, exercise prescriptions, a daily log that lists staff in attendance at each session, and a display of generic group or individual messages at the time of sign-in and sign-out. All relevant medical and exercise data can be collected, collated, and summarized for analysis and reporting. When HRs are out of target range for a prescribed activity, this information can be stored in a report assembled for the supervising staff member at the end of the session. A hard copy summary of that session (i.e., who attended, what happened during the session, what messages were communicated to the patients during the sign-in and sign-out process) can be produced for legal documentation. The patient population can be summarized relationally, or an up-to-date medical and exercise profile can be generated at any time including during the exercise session. Multiple end-of-period reports with graphical figures can be produced, providing documentation of performance, compliance, and achievement (see Fig. 23.3) (33). With the more recent emphasis on outcomes (37), such a database becomes a foundation for long-term analysis of experience (28).

A review of 5 years' experience indicates that all this can be accomplished at less than half the cost of manual processing for a comparable time, with much more detailed reporting of the information (5). In addition, manual handling of the data eliminates the opportunity for patient interactivity, reinforcement of educational concepts, and the fail-safe documentation of notable occurrences during the exercise sessions and introduces the possibility of data-entry error.

COMPUTERS AND REHABILITATION RECORDS: OTHER CONCERNS

As with any other technology used in the rehabilitation or wellness environment, the application of computers has ethical and legal ramifications (38, 39).

Reliability

Reliability pertains to hardware and software as well as to the operational routine used in the application of the computerized system. The system must be maintainable in an adequate and reasonable time frame. If vital patient information cannot be accessed on demand because of technical failure, patient safety may be jeopardized.

Privacy and Access

With increasing computerization of potentially sensitive personal records, privacy has become a growing issue. A proper balance must be achieved between confidentiality of patient information and shared access to records by health care personnel (38). Each person who has access to the computer should be assigned a unique code (40). Ideally, the computer should be able to recall who has "signed-on" during a given time. Certain files should be protected from entry by nonprofessional staff. Programs designed to upload data to mainframe systems for storage or further processing, such as billing or administrative analysis, should not transfer information that may be sensitive.

Archive and Backup

The system should be designed so that data may be archived and backed up appropriately. Archival copies differ from routine backups in that once generated, the archival copy provides a permanent record and thereafter is not altered. In addition to the obvious reason of records integrity, good archives and backups can provide excellent documentation for legal and quality assurance purposes (39). This also can provide a coherent audit trail and should satisfy insurers and government quality assurance and utilization reviewers.

Adequate hardware and a reasonable routine are required for this important task. Although streaming-tape backup is popular in industry, backup with removable large disks (50 MB to 1.5 GB) is less expensive and the devices can see dual service as a hard drive. Floppy disks actually may work well for a rehabilitation program archive in that data from one period, for example 1 month, is easily stored on one diskette. Experts suggest that a different backup copy be made on 2 or 3 successive days and that these backups be stored in different locations (31). Should the previous day's data be lost or proven faulty, no more than 1 or 2 days' worth of data entry will need to be reconstructed (25).

Timmons (35) has also reviewed the topic of computer use in cardiac rehabilitation and provided recommendations for hardware and software design.

Other Important and Potential Applications of Computers in Rehabilitation

Risk Factor Inventory and Analysis Programs

Another important use of personal computers in the rehabilitation environment is in the area of primary and secondary cardiovascular risk screening. Although these systems perform some of the same tasks as the more comprehensive rehabilitation management systems described previously, the primary functions of this type of software are to test the person and calculate risks for subsequent events, to highlight potential problem areas, and to refer participants for management of identified problems. Most of these software programs require that the participant complete a questionnaire, sometimes including a medical history or clinical test data, and then the computer performs an analysis and produces a printed report. These reports often are elaborated with graphs and carefully selected verbiage. Although the technology is helpful in organizing information and performing the calculations of risk, we find that this tool requires a fair amount of participant education by our staff for the patient-client to derive any benefit. These programs probably will find more application when they are coupled to interactive learning technology (7, 41).

Computer-assisted self-interviewing for dietary assessment is a potentially valuable application (41). Many obstacles to gathering data can be overcome with computer-assisted self-interviewing. Computers can conduct personalized, in-depth interviews without a trained interviewer, provide standardized data collection with appropriate levels of inquiry, automate data entry, encourage subjects to review and correct inconsistent data, and ensure that responses are complete (41). Such an approach may prove to be appropriate for use in populations in which literacy is low and in ethnic minorities. A prototype diet-history program has been designed to improve cognitive support and capture information on usual diet (41). Scripts are based on recorded interviews with dietitians and interviewers. At the end of the interview, participants are given information on how their reported nutrient intakes compare with current recommendations for their age and sex. The prototype has been tested in focus groups of mixed age, sex, ethnicity, and education with encouraging results (41). Such programs could be integrated with one of the nutritional analysis programs that are becoming more widely available. Nutritional education could then be tailored to the individual characteristics of those whose diet-histories have been recorded. Other, similar nutritional education systems have been successfully implemented (42).

"Expert" Systems

Until now, I have discussed computer systems that provide automation and organization of information to improve the traditional written record (24). The ability of these systems to incorporate formulas for the calculation of exercise prescriptions is included, but even if automated, still remains under the direct control of the user (33). Software programs now exist that provide medical direction or alter exercise prescriptions on an algorithmic basis. Such software, referred to as an *expert system,* is very likely to be increasingly applied. We are in the process of completing a working prototype of a system in which such software is contained within a kiosk that can be deployed in the community to provide *automated cardiovascular training* (CardiACT Kiosk).

One specific type of artificial intelligence, called "neural networks," has been successfully applied in several areas of cardiology including interpretation of ECGs and imaging. The neural network is capable of identifying relations in tracked data and in modifying itself based on learning and experience (43). The identification of who should review the clinical appropriateness of the algorithm and the reliability of the system, similar to the issues of efficacy and safety that apply to pharmaceuticals and other medical devices, is controversial and still the subject of debate (38).

EDUCATION AND MOTIVATION

A related high-tech application that will have an important future impact on cardiac rehabilitation programs is patient education (6). Sophisticated audiovisual devices that use CD-ROM (compact disk read-only memory) optical data disks or laser disks can now be integrated easily with microcomputers at reasonable cost (44). This technology provides the opportunity for highly dynamic, interactive learning experiences for patients and the expansion of the learning process to include goal-setting with continuous tracking of achievement (45). It also may provide the individualized reinforcement and motivation needed to accomplish and maintain the prescribed lifestyle modifications. Again, as with the computerized database systems, it is important to focus on overall program quality and content and not be seduced by the glitter of the hardware (33). These devices, if improperly selected, can squander funds that are becoming scarce for rehabilitation and risk factor education programs (34).

Probably the greatest change we will witness related to the impact of PCs in the field of cardiac rehabilitation and preventive cardiology will be the access to information provided through the Internet (46, 47). Although the Internet has already become a cliché to many physicians, the reality is that it provides a means of access so that patients can now search libraries of information that were virtually impossible for the average person to ac-

cess even a scant few years ago (48). This is already having an impact on how patients and their families seek out information (49). Although a large number of credible sources such as the American Heart Association are already established on the World Wide Web, sites promoting unproved or potentially harmful advice are common.

Thus, the widespread availability of information is a double-edged sword. On the one hand it can be empowering, helping patients gain insight into their illness, motivating them to make lifestyle changes and to adhere to their medical program, and alleviating fear and doubt about the future. On the other hand, it can undermine the patient's confidence in currently recommended conventional dietary and exercise therapy or mislead them into trying alternative therapies that are still incompletely proven despite conjectural claims or poor quality studies that are offered for corroboration. When this happens it is not the fault of the technology—although the medium may be the message (self-directed health care is, in fact, the future), in this case, the medium is also just the messenger.

Monitoring Risk Factor Modification

Adherence in cardiac rehabilitation has been discussed in some detail in chapter 25. Several recent technological innovations are now available that go beyond the issue of education and can help in the monitoring of patient compliance during efforts at risk factor modification. The ability to provide more accurate estimates of compliance may prove to be adherence enhancing. In addition, such technologies make it easier to observe objectively what previously could only be "measured" by using self-reporting methods (50). This is especially true of difficult-to-alter behaviors such as cigarette smoking.

Before discussing the exotic, however, we must mention what is one of the simplest and least expensive, yet most forgotten, devices in many rehabilitation programs—the scale. The scale provides simple documentation of compliance to weight reduction, it is an important ingredient in all lipid-modifying regimens, and when used in combination with a stopwatch and measurement of known distance, it provides a tool that allows for calculation of caloric expenditure.

We should also mention other important measures of fatness. The waist-to-hip ratio (WHR) is derived simply by dividing the girth measurement of the waist by that of the hips. The WHR has a demonstrated association with the occurrence of coronary atherosclerosis (51), and when elevated, it is associated with a less favorable lipid and lipoprotein profile in both men and women (52). Peirus and colleagues (53) observed that intra-abdominal fat deposition constitutes a greater cardiovascular risk than obesity alone.

Body mass index calculated from mass displacement using underwater weighing is the "gold standard" for the measurement of body fat, but two indirect methods have been popularized in recent years—one using skinfold measurements with calipers and the other using measures of body impedance. Estimations of percent body fat with the impedance method appears to have little advantage over the use of skinfold calipers (54, 55), but one recent study suggests that for a population of diverse age and gender, bioelectrical impedance may be a more precise method than body mass index calculated from skinfold measurements (56).

The issue of ECG monitoring has been discussed in detail elsewhere with regard to patient safety including mention in this chapter as an example of applied technology. The aspect of ECG recording that is relevant to note here is the provision of highly accurate measures of HRs during exercise—useful not only for their physiologic value but for the documentation of adherence. This does not require sophisticated recording capability; however, the devices should measure HR accurately. Watch devices such as those marketed by Polar, which record the HR successively during exercise and then can download the entire aggregate of recorded rates into the computer via a modem connection, may be entirely sufficient for this purpose.

All such successive objective measures can provide valuable indicators of patient adherence, however, and can help staff in developing individually tailored patient education programs (50). Two examples of newer technologies for monitoring adherence to risk factor modification include carbon monoxide measurement with a handheld device and portable cholesterol analyzers.

CARBON MONOXIDE MEASUREMENT

Traditionally, smoking has been an extremely difficult behavior to monitor, relying entirely on patient and family reporting. Cheating is notorious. The carbon monoxide (CO) index is easily

measured with a handheld, battery-operated instrument with an electrochemical sensor that samples expired alveolar air and provides a direct means of reading CO content. Normal range for nonsmokers generally is 0 to 12 ppm (50). Studies show that carboxyhemoglobin levels can be estimated reliably by measuring the concentration of CO in breath (57), that smokers can be reliably discriminated from nonsmokers (58), and that it compares favorably with two well-established, validated techniques, serum thiocyanate and blood carboxyhemoglobin levels (59).

PORTABLE CHOLESTEROL ANALYSIS

The measurement of cholesterol for screening purposes has been discussed widely in the literature, particularly with respect to the implementation of the National Cholesterol Education Program guidelines (60, 61). Relatively portable and inexpensive devices developed primarily for screening purposes have proved to be reliable (62, 63) and are particularly suited for follow-up of cholesterol levels in the rehabilitation setting as long as the analyzing technique is controlled closely and the results are monitored carefully (64). Recently, in addition to the measurement of total cholesterol, triglycerides and HDL-C appear to be measured reliably with these portable systems (63).

Thus, although cardiac rehabilitation and preventive programs are inherently "soft technology" and rely mostly on the tried and true approach of exercise and dietary change rendered by highly motivating and caring people, multiple technologies are potentially valuable for more effective and efficient delivery of the services.

References

1. James TN. Cascades, collusions, and conflicts in cardiology [editorial]. JAMA 1988;259:2454–2455.
2. Collins SM, Skorton DJ. Computers in cardiac imaging. J Am Coll Cardiol 1987;9:669–677.
3. Hlatky MA, Greenfield JC. Technologic innovation and care of elderly patients with cardiovascular disease: how will the diagnosis-related group system respond? Am J Med 1990;88:1N–2N.
4. Laupacis A, Feeny D, Detsky AS, et al. How attractive does a new technology have to be to warrant adoption and utilization? Tentative guidelines for using clinical and economic evaluations. Can Med Assoc J 1992;146: 473–481.
5. Pashkow FJ. Computer-assisted program management for cardiac rehabilitation. In: Broustet JP, ed.

Fifth World Congress of Cardiac Rehabilitation. Bordeaux, France: Intercept Ltd., 1993:347–356.

6. Ronan J, Weisberg M, Perloff J, et al. Cardiovascular teaching techniques: planning and presenting effective instruction—alternative technologies of teaching in cardiovascular medicine. October 10–11, 1985. J Am Coll Cardiol 1986;8:465–484.

7. Consoli SM, Ben Said M, Jean J, et al. Interactive electronic teaching (ISIS): has the future started? J Hum Hypertens 1996;10:S69–S72.

8. Kashyap ML. Cardiovascular disease in the elderly: current considerations. Am J Cardiol 1989;63:56H–59H.

9. Ryan TJ, Graham TPJ, Annas GJ, et al. 21st Bethesda conference: ethics in cardiovascular medicine. Task Force III: perspective on the allocation of limited resources in cardiovascular medicine. J Am Coll Cardiol 1990;16:17–23.

10. Haskell W. Cardiovascular complications during exercise training of cardiac patients. Circulation 1978;57:920–924.

11. Wenger N, Gilbert C, Skoropa M. Cardiac conditioning after myocardial infarction. An early intervention program. Cardiac Rehabil 1971;2:17–22.

12. Kostis JB, Byington R, Friedman LM, et al. Prognostic significance of ventricular ectopic activity in survivors of acute myocardial infarction. J Am Coll Cardiol 1987;10:231–242.

13. VanCamp S, Peterson R. Cardiovascular complications of outpatient cardiac rehabilitation programs. JAMA 1986;256:1160–1163.

14. Pashkow FJ, Schweikert RA, Wilkoff BL. Exercise testing and training in patients with malignant arrhythmias. In: Holloszy J, ed. Exercise and sport sciences reviews. Baltimore: Williams & Wilkins, 1997;25:235–270.

15. American College of Sports Medicine. Guidelines for exercise testing and prescription. 5th ed. Philadelphia: Lea & Febiger, 1995.

16. Rogers F, Juneau M, Taylor CB, et al. Assessment by a microprocessor of adherence to home-based moderate-intensity exercise training in healthy, sedentary middle-aged men and women. Am J Cardiol 1987;60:71–75.

17. Taylor CB, Kraemer HC, Bragg DA, et al. A new system for long-term recording and processing of heart rate and physical activity in outpatients. Comput Biomed Res 1982;15:7–17.

18. DeBusk RF, Haskell WL, Miller NH, et al. Medically directed at-home rehabilitation soon after clinically uncomplicated acute myocardial infarction: a new model for patient care. Am J Cardiol 1985;55:251–257.

19. Sparks KE, Sechler J, Steele R, et al. Effectiveness of trans-telephonic-monitored home exercise program [abstract]. J Cardpulm Rehabil 1990;10:372.

20. Shaw DK. Transtelephonic exercise monitoring: medico-legal and other considerations. Exerc Stand Malpract Report 1991;5:81, 84–86.

21. Shaw DK, Sparks KE, Jennings H Sr, et al. Cardiac rehabilitation using simultaneous voice and electrocardiographic transtelephonic monitoring. Am J Cardiol 1995;76:1069–1071.

22. Ades P, Pashkow F, Fletcher G, et al. A controlled trial of cardiac rehabilitation in the home setting: improving accessibility [abstract]. J Am Coll Cardiol 1996;27 (Suppl A):150A.

23. Shaw DK, Sparks KE, Hanigosky P. Exercise compliance and patient satisfaction: transtelephonic exercise monitoring [abstract]. J Cardpulm Rehabil 1990;10:373.

24. Lesser MF. Computerized records in clinical cardiology. J Am Coll Cardiol 1986;8:941–948.

25. Shepard RB, Blum RI. Cardiology office computer use: primer, pointers, pitfalls. J Am Coll Cardiol 1986;8:933–940.

26. Wyatt JC. Clinical data systems, part 3: development and evaluation. Lancet 1994;344:1682–1688.

27. Wingert K. Electronic medical records: the next generation. Hosp Pract 1995;30:30I–30J, 30L.

28. Lauer MS, Fortin DF. Databases in cardiology. In: Topol E, ed. Textbook of cardiovascular medicine. Philadelphia: Lippincott-Raven, 1998:1083–1105.

29. Tierney WM, Overhage JM, McDonald CJ. Toward electronic medical records that improve care [editorial; comment]. Ann Intern Med 1995;122:725–726.

30. Pashkow F, Schafer M, Pashkow P. HeartWatchers—low cost, community-based cardiac rehabilitation in Loveland, Colorado. J Cardpulm Rehabil 1986;6:469–473.

31. Wyatt JC. Clinical data systems, part 2: components and techniques. Lancet 1994;344:1609–1614.

32. Wyatt JC. Clinical data systems, part 1: data and medical records. Lancet 1994;344:1543–1547.

33. Pashkow FJ. Specialized data-base systems for cardiology. Physicians Comput 1987;5:32–35.

34. Wenger NK. Future directions in cardiovascular rehabilitation. J Cardpulm Rehabil 1987;7:168–174.

35. Timmons DR. The role of computers in cardiac rehabilitation. In: Hall LK, Meyer GC, eds. Cardiac rehabilitation: exercise testing and prescription. Champaign, IL: Life Enhancement Publications, 1988: 157–171.

36. O'Leary S, Mann C, Perkash I. Access to computers for older adults: problems and solutions. Am J Occup Ther 1991;45:636–642.

37. Pashkow P. Outcomes measures. In: Hillegass EA, Sadowsky HS, eds. Essentials of cardiopulmonary physical therapy. Philadelphia: WB Saunders, 1998: in press.

38. Miller RA, Schaffner KF, Meisel A. Ethical and legal issues related to the use of computer programs in clinical medicine. Ann Intern Med 1985;102:529–537.

39. Pashkow FJ. Legal aspects of computer applications in cardiac rehabilitation. Exerc Stand Malpract Report 1989;3:41–43.

40. White R. Computer security: an introduction for the medical practitioner. Urol Clin North Am 1986;13:119–128.

41. Kohlmeier L, Mendez M, McDuffie J, et al. Computer-assisted self-interviewing: a multimedia approach to dietary assessment. Am J Clin Nutr 1997;65(Suppl 4):1275S–1281S.

42. Brug J, Steenhuis I, van Assema P, et al. The impact of a computer-tailored nutrition intervention. Prev Med 1996;25:236–242.

43. Itchhaporia D, Snow PB, Almassy RJ, et al. Artificial neural networks: current status in cardiovascular medicine. J Am Coll Cardiol 1996;28:515–521.

44. Millman A, Lee N. ABC of medical computing. CD ROMS, multimedia, and optical storage systems. BMJ 1995;311:675–678.

45. Consoli SM, Ben Said M, Jean J, et al. Evaluation of a computer assisted training program for hypertensive patients. Arch Mal Coeur Vaiss 1994;87:1093–1096.

46. Pallen M. Guide to the Internet. Logging in, fetching files, reading news. BMJ 1995;311:1626–1630.

47. Pallen M. Guide to the Internet. The World Wide Web. BMJ 1995;311:1552–1556.

48. Doyle DJ. Surfing the Internet for patient information: the personal clinical web page [letter]. JAMA 1995; 274:1586.

49. Widman LE, Tong DA. Requests for medical advice from patients and families to health care providers who publish on the World Wide Web. Arch Intern Med 1997;157:209–212.

50. Shankar K, Mihalko-Ward R, Rodell DE, et al. Methodologic and compliance issues in postcoronary bypass surgery subjects. Arch Phys Med Rehabil 1990;71: 1074–1077.

51. Thompson CJ, Ryu JE, Craven TE, et al. Central adipose distribution is related to coronary atherosclerosis. Arterioscler Thromb 1991;11:327–333.

52. Anderson AJ, Sobocinski KA, Freedman DS, et al. Body fat distribution, plasma lipids, and lipoproteins. Arteriosclerosis 1988;8:88–94.

53. Peiris AN, Sothmann MS, Hoffmann RG, et al. Adiposity, fat distribution, and cardiovascular risk. Ann Intern Med 1989;110:867–872.

54. Jackson AS, Pollock ML, Graves JE, et al. Reliability and validity of bioelectrical impedance in determining body composition. J Appl Physiol 1988;64:529–534.

55. Eckerson JM, Stout JR, Housh TJ, et al. Validity of bioelectrical impedance equations for estimating percent fat in males. Med Sci Sports Exerc 1996;28:523–530.

56. Roubenoff R, Dallal GE, Wilson PW. Predicting body fatness: the body mass index vs estimation by bioelectrical impedance [published erratum appears in Am J Public Health 1995 Aug;85(8 Pt 1):1063]. Am J Public Health 1995;85:726–728.

57. Wald NJ, Idle M, Boreham J, et al. Carbon monoxide in breath in relation to smoking and carboxyhaemoglobin levels. Thorax 1981;36:366–369.

58. Ebert RV, McNabb ME, McCusker KT, et al. Amount of nicotine and carbon monoxide inhaled by smokers of low-tar, low-nicotine cigarettes. JAMA 1983;250: 2840–2842.

59. Galvin KT, Kerin MJ, Williams G, et al. Comparison of three methods for measuring cigarette smoking in patients with vascular disease. Cardiovasc Surg 1994;2: 48–51.

60. Cleeman JI, Lenfant C. New guidelines for the treatment of high blood cholesterol in adults from the National Cholesterol Education Program. From controversy to consensus. Circulation 1987;76: 960–962.

61. Goodman DS. The National Cholesterol Education Program: guidelines, status, and issues. Am J Med 1991;90:325–355.

62. Bradford RH, Bachorik PS, Roberts K, et al. Blood cholesterol screening in several environments using a portable, dry-chemistry analyzer and fingerstick blood samples. Lipid Research Clinics Cholesterol Screening Study Group. Am J Cardiol 1990;65:6–13.

63. Marotta G, Auletta P, Liguori M, et al. The utilization of dry chemistry methods in a campaign to identify risk factor of cardiovascular diseases. Epidemiol Prev 1994;18:230–236.

64. Naughton MJ, Luepker RV, Strickland D. The accuracy of portable cholesterol analyzers in public screening programs. JAMA 1990;263:1213–1217.

Appendix A

Tables of Energy Requirements for Activities of Daily Living, Household Tasks, Recreational Activities, and Vocational Activities

William A. Dafoe

The following tables and figures display the energy requirements for various activities in which a cardiac patient may wish to partake.

The tables list various activities in alphabetical order and outline the range of energy requirements in metabolic equivalents, or METs, where 1 MET is equivalent to 3.5 mL of oxygen per kilogram body weight per minute. The energy requirements have been abstracted from the references (1–15). The reference by Ainsworth et al. (1) provides an extensive list of activities and their energy costs. The second and third columns of these tables represent the minimum and maximum METs, respectively, for each task. Factors like mental stress, as well as isometric and environmental effects, may place a superimposed stressor on the normal physiologic demands of a given activity. These factors should be considered with the energy costs to determine the appropriateness and safety of resuming various tasks. A more complete discussion is outlined in chapter 8, Exercise Prescription Development and Supervision.

The figures that accompany each table show bar graphs of the minimum and maximum energy requirements for each activity. The actual range of energy costs for each activity is denoted by the black bars. These figures serve as a useful guideline for appropriate patient activities. The peak and functional range of safe activities can be derived from the stress test and placed on each figure for individual patients.

For example, assume that a patient is able to accomplish 7 METs on a stress test with ischemic changes at 6 METs. An appropriate training intensity is established as 4 to 5 METs. Thus, activities within the 4- to 5-MET range may produce a training effect if performed for sufficient duration. Activities generally should be kept below the 5-MET range with a peak reaching no more than 6 METs when ischemic changes occur. Figure A.1 illustrates how a graph of the activities of daily living might be used for this patient.

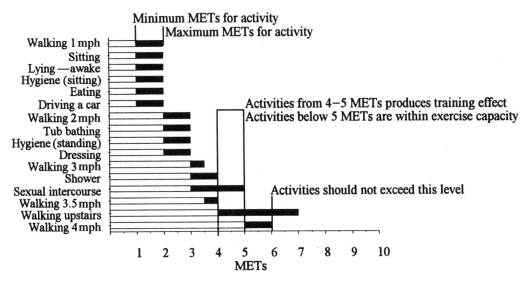

Figure A.1. An example using a patient with ischemia occurring at 6 METs after a stress test.

Table A.1. Energy Costs—Activities of Daily Living

Task	METs Min	METs Max	Comments
Dressing	2	3	
Driving a car	1	2	
Eating	1	2	
Hygiene (sitting)	1	2	Shaving, brushing teeth, combing hair
Hygiene (standing)	2	3	
Lying—awake	1	2	
Sexual intercourse	3	5	
Shower	3	4	Vasodilation, toweling → possible angina
Sitting	1	2	
Tub bathing	2	3	Vasodilation, toweling → possible angina
Walking 1 mph	1	2	Increased with a grade or against wind
Walking 2 mph	2	3	Increased with a grade or against wind
Walking 3 mph	3	3.5	Increased with a grade or against wind
Walking 3.5 mph	3.5	4	Increased with a grade or against wind
Walking 4 mph	5	6	Increased with a grade or against wind
Walking upstairs	4	7	

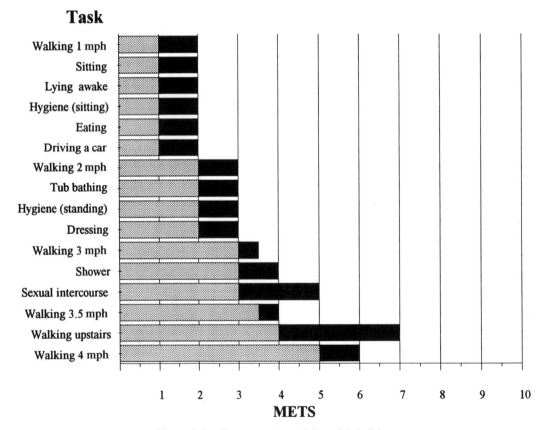

Figure A.2. Energy costs—activities of daily living.

Table A.2. Energy Costs—Household Tasks

Task	METs Min	METs Max	Comments
Beating carpets	4	5	
Bed making	2	6	5–6 METs—stripping and making beds
Carpentry	3	7.5	
Carry 18 lb upstairs	7	8	
Carry 20–44 lb	4	5	
Carry 45–64 lb	5	6	
Carry 65–85 lb	7	8	
Carrying suitcase	6	7	
Cleaning floors	3	5	
Cleaning windows	3	4	
Clothes washing (machine)	2	5	4–5 METs—loading and unloading
Cooking (standing)	2	3	
Dusting	2	4	
Floors—cleaning, wax	4	5	
Food prep (standing)	2[a]	—	
Gardening—heavier	3	5	Planting trees or shrubs, hoeing, raking
Gardening—light	2	4	Watering, planting, light weeding
Grass cutting—push handmower	5	7	
Grass—push power mower	3	5	
Grass—riding mower	2	3	
Grocery shopping	2	3	1–7 METs carrying heavy groceries
Grocery—unpack	1.7	3.1	
Hanging clothes	3	4	
Housework—general	3	4	
Ironing	2	4	
Laundry	2	2.5	Folding or hanging clothes while standing, put in dryer
Mopping floors	3	4	
Move furniture	4	8	Varies according to weight of furniture
Painting	4	5	Possible angina with arms above head
Playing with children (sitting)—light	2.5	3	
Playing with children (standing)—light	2.8	3.5	
Playing with children (running)	4	5	
Polish floors	3	4	
Polish furniture	1	2	
Raking leaves	3	5	
Remodeling	4	5	
Scrub pots	1.5	2.7	
Scrubbing (kneeling)	3	4	
Shoveling 16 lb/10 min	9	10	
Snow shoveling—self-paced lift throw	6.7	7.6	Varies with rate, type of snow
Snow shoveling—self-paced push throw	6.7	7.2	Varies with rate, type of snow
Storm windows—install	6	7	
Sweeping indoors	1	2.5	
Sweeping outdoors	4	5	Garage, sidewalk
Vacuuming	2.9	3.6	
Wash car	6	7	
Wash floor	3	4	Wash and wax
Wash windows	3.1	5	
Wash dishes	2	3	

[a]This MET value is given only as an average, not as a range.

Task

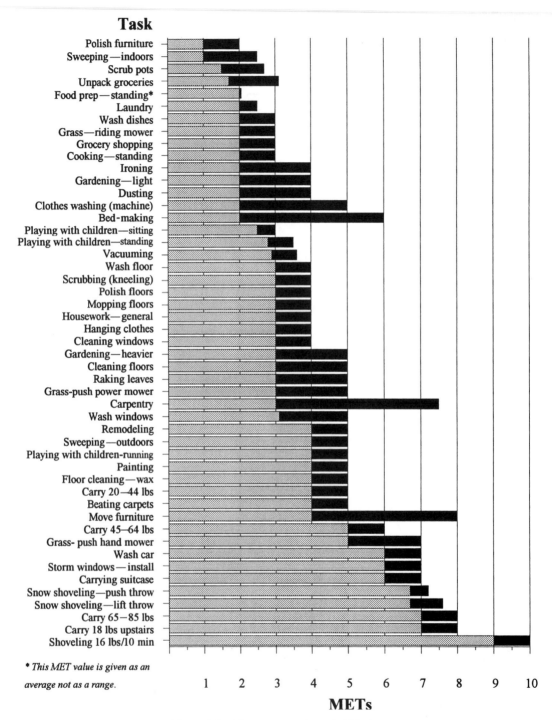

Figure A.3. Energy costs—household tasks.

Table A.3. Energy Costs—Recreational Activities

Task	METs Min	METs Max	Task	METs Min	METs Max
Archery	3	4	Lacrosse	6	13
Backpacking—45 lb	6	11	Motorcycling	2.5	7
Badminton	4	9	Musical instrument	2	4
Ballet	6	7	Orienteering	8	12
Baseball—competitive	5	6	Paddleball	8	12
Baseball—noncompetitive	4	5	Painting	3	5
Billiards	2	3	Raquetball	8	12
Body building	3	7	Reading	1	2
Bowling	2	4	Ringette	5	13
Boxing	6	12	Rope jumping 80/min	8	10
Broomball	5	9	Rope jumping 120–140/min	11	12
Calisthenics	3	8	Rowing 10 mph	2.8	3.4
Canoeing—2–5 mph	2	8	Rowing 15 mph	3.5	5.1
Card playing	1	2	Rowing 20 mph	5	7.4
Carry 20–44 lb	4	5	Running 12 min/mile	8	9
Carry 45–64 lb	5	6	Running 11 min/mile	9	10
Chop wood	7	17	Running 9 min/mile	10	11
Climbing—mountain	7	10	Sailing—small boat	2	5
CPR	2.3	5.7	Sawing	2.9	3.9
Cricket	3	7.5	Scuba diving	5	10
Croquet	2	3.5	Sewing	1	2
Curling	4	6	Sewing—machine	2	3
Cycling	2	4	Shuffleboard	2	3
Cycling 5 mph	2	3	Skating—figure	4	10
Cycling 6 mph	3	4	Skating—roller	5	11
Cycling 8 mph	4	5	Skiing—cross country 3 mph	6	7
Cycling 10 mph	5	6	Skiing—cross country 4 mph	8	9
Cycling 12 mph	7	8	Skiing—cross country 5 mph	9	10
Cycling 13 mph	8	9	Skiing—downhill	5	9
Dance—aerobic	4	9	Skiing—water	5	7
Dancing—folk	3	7	Sledding—tobogganing	4	8
Dancing—square	5	7	Snowshoeing	8	12
Dancing—ballroom	4	5	Soccer—noncompetitive	5	8
Dancing slow	3	4	Squash—competitive	5	12
Fencing	6	10	Squash—social	8	9
Fishing—from a boat	2	4	Swimming—backstroke	7	8
Fishing—fly	3	4	Swimming—breaststroke	8	9
Football—touch	7	10	Swimming—crawl	9	10
Frisbee	3	5	Swimming—slow	4	5
Gardening—digging	5	6	Table tennis	3	5
Golf—cart (riding)	2	3	Television	1	2
Golf—cart (pulling)	3	4	Tennis—singles	4	9
Golf—carrying clubs	4	5	Tennis—doubles	4	8
Gymnastics	5	10	Volleyball	3	8
Hand drilling	2.7	4.6	Walking 1 mph	1	2
Hiking	3	7	Walking 2 mph	2	3
Hockey—ball	3	5	Walking 3 mph	3	3.5
Hockey—field	7	8	Walking 3.5 mph	3.5	4
Hockey—ice	7	8	Walking 3.6 mph with	4.6	6.0
Horseback—gallop	8	9	1-lb weights		
Horseback—trot	6	7	Walking 4 mph	5	6
Horseback—walk	3	4	Woodworking	2	
Horseshoes	2	3	Wrestling	9	10
Hunting—small game	3	7	Yoga[a]	4	—
Hunting—large game	3	14			
Judo	6	12			
Karate	8	12			
Kayaking	7	11			
Knitting	1	2			

[a]This MET value is given only as an average, not as a range.

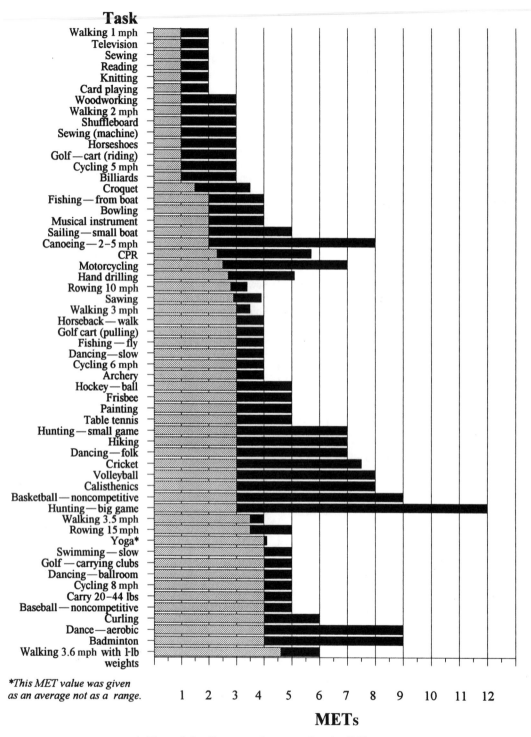

Figure A.4.   Energy costs—recreational activities.

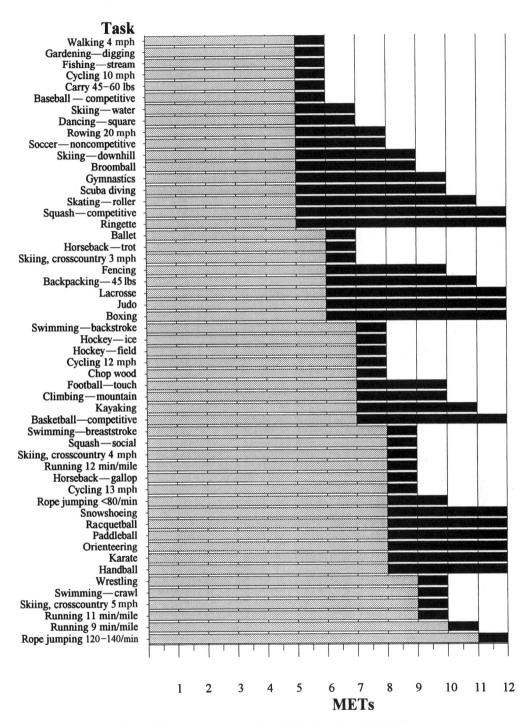

Figure A.4. Energy costs—recreational activities—*continued.*

Table A.4.   Energy Costs—Vocational Activities

Task	METs Min	METs Max	Comments
Assembly-line work	3	5	
Auto repair	2	3	
Bakery	2	4	
Bartending	2	3	
Bricklaying	3	4	
Carpentry	3	7.5	
Carry 18 lb upstairs	7	8	
Carry 20–44 lb	4	5	
Carry 45–64 lb	5	6	
Carry 65–85 lb	7	8	
Cement—mixing	3	4	
Chopping—wood (slowly)	7	17	Slowly → 7 METs; quickly → 17 METs
Coal mining	6	7	
Desk work	1.5	2	
Digging—ditches	7	8	
Drill press—lathe	3	4	
Farm work—light	1.5	4.5	Milking, feeding animals
Farm work—heavier	5	8	Bailing hay, cleaning barn, forking straw
Filing	2	3	
Firefighter	8	12	
Hand tools	2	3	
Handyman	5	6	
Janitorial—light duties	2	3	
Ladder—climb	4	5	
Lift—44 lb/10 min	7	8	Floor to waist
Lift 100 lb	7	10	
Machine assembly	3	4	
Masonry	4	5	
Painting	4	5	
Paperhanging	4	5	
Planing—hardwood	8	9	
Plastering	3	4	
Push—heavy objects	7	8	
Push cart—75 lb	4	5	
Radio/TV repair	2	3	
Sawing—hardwood	6	8	
Sawing—power	3	4	
Sawing—softwood	5	6	
Shoveling—light	5	6	
Shoveling 10 lb/min	6	7	
Shoveling 14 lb/min	7	9	
Shoveling 16 lb/min	9	12	
Tailoring	2.5	4.0	
Tools—heavy	5	6	Jackhammer, drills
Tools—very heavy	7	8	Pick, shovel
Tractor plowing	4	5	
Trucking	3	4	
Typing	1.5	2	
Welding—light/mod load	3	4	
Wheelbarrow—50–100lb	3	4	
Wood—splitting	6	7	

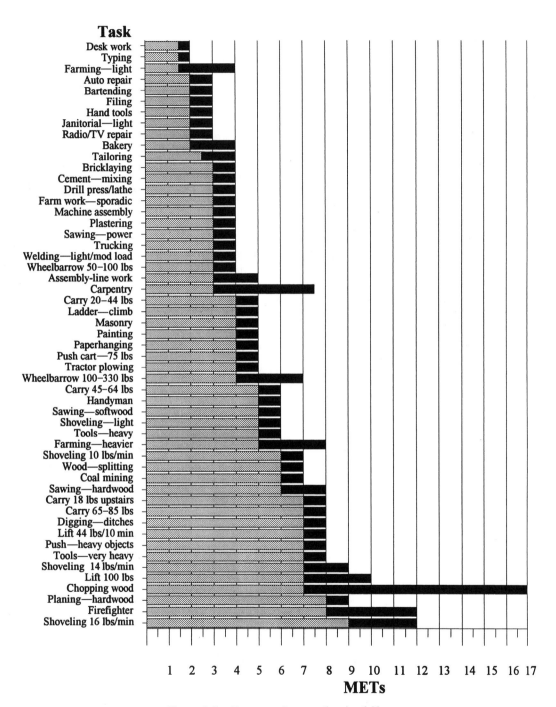

Figure A.5.   Energy costs—vocational activities.

References

1. Ainsworth BE, Haskell WL, Leon AS, et al. Compendium of physical activities: classification of energy costs of human physical activities [see comments]. Med Sci Sports Exerc 1993;25:71–80.
2. Aronov DM, Rosykhodzhajeva GA. Energy expenditure and cardiovascular response to daily activities in patients with coronary heart disease of different functional classes. J Cardpulm Rehabil 1992;12:56–62.
3. Bassett DR, Smith PA, Getchell LH. Energy cost of simulated rowing using a wind-resistance device. Physician Sportsmed 1984;12:113–118.
4. Foster C, Thompson NN. Functional translation of exercise test responses to recreational activities. J Cardpulm Rehabil 1992;11:373–377.
5. Friedman DB, Ramo BW, Gray GJ. Tennis and cardiovascular fitness in middle-aged men. Physician Sportsmed 1984;12:87–91.
6. Graves JE, Martin AD, Miltenberger LA, et al. Physiological responses to walking with hand weights, wrist weights, and ankle weights. Med Sci Sports Exerc 1988;20:265–271.
7. Haskell WL, Brachfeld N, Bruce RA, et al. Task Force II: determination of occupational working capacity in patients with ischemic heart disease. J Am Coll Cardiol 1989;14:1025–1034.
8. Jette M, Sidney K, Blumchen G. Metabolic equivalents (METS) in exercise testing, exercise prescription, and evaluation of functional capacity [review]. Clin Cardiol 1990;13:555–565.
9. Mital A, Kumar GM, Colon BK. Aerobic capacity of coronary heart disease (CHD) patients and its use in accommodating them in the workplace. Disabil Rehabil 1996;18:396–401.
10. Morgans LF, Scovil JA, Bass KM. Heart rate responses during singles and doubles competition. Physician Sportsmed 1984;12:64–72.
11. Rosiello RA, Mahler DA, Ward JL. Cardiovascular responses to rowing. Med Sci Sports Exerc 1987;19:239–245.
12. Sheldahl LM, Wilke NA, Dougherty SM, et al. Effect of age and coronary artery disease on response to snow shoveling. J Am Coll Cardiol 1992;20:1111–1117.
13. Squires WG, Hartung GH, Pratt CM, et al. Metabolic cost and electrocardiographic changes in cardiac patients during cardiopulmonary resuscitation practice. J Cardpulm Rehabil 1982;2:313–317.
14. Walter PR, Porcari JP, Brice G, et al. Acute responses to using walking poles in patients with coronary artery disease. J Cardpulm Rehabil 1996;16:245–250.
15. Wilke NA, Sheldahl LM, Dougherty SM, et al. Energy expenditure during household tasks in women with coronary artery disease. Am J Cardiol 1995;75:670–674.

Appendix B

Recommendations for Participation in Sports for Patients with Various Cardiac Abnormalities

William A. Dafoe and Teresa M. Rudkin

The 26th Bethesda Conference, titled "Recommendations for Determining Eligibility for Competition in Athletes with Cardiovascular Abnormalities," was held on January 6, 1994, under the auspices of the American College of Cardiology. The purpose of the conference was to develop "prudent consensus recommendations regarding the eligibility of athletes for competition in sport." The authors stress that there is little definitive data that participation in competitive activities necessarily hastens a cardiovascular death that otherwise would have occurred, or conversely, that avoidance will prolong life. The recommendations were not formulated with cardiac rehabilitation patients in mind, but it was recognized that physicians might use this information combined with clinical judgment for recreational athletic activity. Competitive sports place unique demands on the individual: difficulties for self-monitoring for cardiac difficulties and discontinuing the activity, high levels of aerobic demand, combined dynamic and static components, risk of bodily collision, an increased risk if syncope occurs, and possible exposure to extreme environmental conditions with possible alterations in blood volume changes and electrolytes. The ethical, legal, and practical issues regarding medical decision making for competitive athletes is beyond the scope of this appendix, and the clinician involved in decision making for competitve athletes should refer to the full text. Some salient points from the Bethesda conference that have relevance for cardiac rehabilitation are as follows:

1. The athlete-patient is highly motivated to participate in sports and in a number of cases will assume almost any risk to keep on playing.
2. Additional diagnostic evaluations may be required taking into account the sport and the patient's condition.
3. The type of level of competition and the importance of the event to the patient needs to be considered.
4. There are responsibilities of the athlete-patient, which include weighing the risks and benefits of participation in competitive activities and the effects of any adverse outcomes on family and fellow athletes.
5. In general, the medical evaluation should be provided only to the patient and family unless permission is given to provide it to others. However, the legal aspects of disclosure of information and confidentiality are unresolved with regard to the competitive athlete and the potential of harm to others.
6. The athlete-patient should be provided with as many options as possible and the possibilities for minimizing risks.

This appendix presents a precis of the recommended activities according to various medical conditions. Individual recommendations within each category are still required. For example, "curling" and "cricket" are listed as low dynamic activities, but relatively high cardiovascular intensities can still be achieved.

Adapted from the 26th Bethesda Conference.
Recommendations for determining the eligibility for competition in athletes with cardiovascular abnormalities. J Am Coll Cardiol 1994;24:845–1899.

Table 1B Classification of Sports (Based on Peak Dynamic and Static Components During Competition)

	A. Low Dynamic	B. Moderate Dynamic	C. High Dynamic
I. Low Static	Billiards Bowling Cricket Curling Golf Riflery	Baseball Softball Table tennis Tennis (doubles) Volleyball	Badminton Cross-country skiing (classic technique) Field hockey[a] Orienteering Race walking Racquetball Running (long distance) Soccer[a] Squash Tennis (singles)
II. Moderate Static	Archery Auto racing[a,b] Diving[a,b] Equestrian[a,b] Motorcycling[a,b]	Fencing Field events (jumping) Figure skating[a] Football (American)[a] Rodeoing[a,b] Rugby[a] Running (sprint) Surfing[a,b] Synchronized swimming[b]	Basketball[a] Ice Hockey[a] Cross-country skiing (skating technique) Football (Australian rules)[a] Lacrosse[a] Running (middle distance) Swimming Handball
III. High Static	Bobsledding[a,b] Field events (throwing) Gymnastics[a,b] Karate/judo[a] Luge[a,b] Sailing Rock climbing[a,b] Waterskiing[a,b] Weight lifting[a,b] Windsurfing[a,b]	Body building[a,b] Downhill skiing[a,b] Wrestling[a]	Boxing[a] Canoeing/kayaking Cycling[a,b] Decathlon Rowing Speed skating

[a]Danger of bodily collision.
[b]Increased risk if syncopy occurs.

Table 2B Alphabetical Categorization of Sports and Their Athletic Classification

Sport	Class	Sport	Class	Sport	Class
Archery	IIA	Football (American)	IIB[a]	Running (sprint)	IIB
Auto racing	IIA[a,b]	Gymnastics	IIIA[a,b]	Sailing	IIIA
Badminton	IC	Handball	IIC	Skiing—cross-country	IC
Basketball	IIC[a]	Ice Hockey	IIC[a]	(classic technique)	
Billiards	IA	Judo	IIIA[a]	Skiing—cross-country	IIC
Bobsledding	IIIA[a,b]	Karate	IIIA[a]	(skating technique)	
Body building	IIIB[a,b]	Kayaking	IIIC	Skiing—downhill	IIIB[a,b]
Bowling	IA	Lacrosse	IIC[a]	Soccer	IC[a]
Boxing	IIIC[a]	Luge	IIIA[a,b]	Speed skating	IIIC
Canoeing	IIIC	Motorcycling	IIA[a]	Squash	IC
Cricket	IA	Orienteering	IC	Surfing	IIB[a,b]
Curling	IA	Race walking	IC	Synchronized swimming	IIA[b]
Cycling	IIIC[a,b]	Racquetball	IC	Table tennis	IB
Decathlon	IIIC	Riflery	IA	Tennis (doubles)	IB
Diving	IIA[a,b]	Rodeoing	IIB[a,b]	Tennis (singles)	IC
Equestrian	IIA[a,b]	Rockclimbing	IIIA[a,b]	Volleyball	IB
Fencing	IIB	Rowing	IIIC	Waterskiing	IIIA[a,b]
Field events (jumping)	IIB	Rugby	IIB[a]	Weight lifting	IIIA[a,b]
Field events (throwing)	IIIA	Running (long	IC	Windsurfing	IIIA[a,b]
Field hockey	IC[a]	distance)		Wrestling	IIIB[a]
Figure skating	IIB[a]	Running (middle distance)	IIC		

[a]Danger of bodily collision.
[b]Increased risk if syncope occurs.

Contents

Congenital Heart Defects

Coronary Artery Diseases

Myocardial Diseases

Arrhythmias

Systemic Hypertension

Acquired Valvular Heart Disease

[a]In the absence of Wolff-Parkinson-White syndrome.

How to Use the "Recommendation" Icons

The highlighted areas indicate competitive sports in which the athlete with a given cardiac abnormality is able to participate safely according to the 26th Bethesda Conference.

For example:

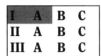

Patient cannot
participate in
IA classified
sports only.

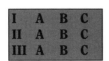

Patient can
participate in
sports of all
classifications.

None

Patient cannot
participate safely
in any
competitive sports.

Have a pacemaker
implanted before
participation in
sports. Avoid
sports with risk
of bodily contact.

CONGENITAL HEART DEFECTS

Coarctation of the Aorta
Untreated
- **If the following conditions exist:**
  - absence of large collateral or severe aortic root dilation
  - normal exercise test and small pressure gradient at rest ($\leq$ 20 mm Hg between upper and lower limbs)
  - peak systolic pressure $\leq$ 230 mm Hg with exercise

- **If the following conditions exist:**
  - a systolic arm/leg gradient > 20 mm Hg
  - exercise-induced hypertension with a systolic blood pressure > 230 mm Hg

Treated
- **During the first year after repair:**
  Six months after repair, if:
  - pressure gradient at rest $\leq$ 20 mm Hg between upper and lower limbs
  - normal peak systolic blood pressure during exercise and at rest

- **After the first year after repair, if:**
  - continue to be asymptomatic
  - have normal blood pressure at rest and at exercise

- **With evidence of significant aortic dilation, wall thinning, or aneurysm formation**

Cyanotic Congenital Cardiac Disease
Unoperated
  Individualized exercise prescription recommended

Postoperative palliated
- **If the following conditions are met:**
  - arterial saturation above ~80%
  - symptomatic arrhythmias are not present
  - there is no symptomatic ventricular dysfunction
  - have near-normal physical working capacity

Recommendations

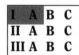

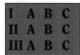

Avoid sports with
risk of collision

Except not power
lifting

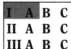

Ebstein's Anomaly
Unoperated
- **If mild Ebstein's anomaly and the following:**
  - no cyanosis
  - nearly normal heart size
  - no evidence of arrhythmia

I	A	B	C
II	A	B	C
III	A	B	C

- **With tricuspid regurgitation of moderate severity and no evidence of arrhythmia on ambulatory ECG monitoring**

I	A	B	C
II	A	B	C
III	A	B	C

- **With severe abnormalities**

None

Surgically repaired
- **If:**
  - mild or absent tricuspid regurgitation
  - heart size not substantially increased
  - no arrhythmias

I	A	B	C
II	A	B	C
III	A	B	C

Elevated Pulmonary Vascular Resistance
Note: At risk for sudden death during intense sporting activities
- **When pulmonary artery peak systolic pressure ≤ 40 mm Hg**

- **When pulmonary artery peak systolic pressure > 40 mm Hg**
  Full evaluation and exercise prescription are required for athletic participation

I	A	B	C
II	A	B	C
III	A	B	C

Individual exercise prescription

Marfan's Syndrome
- **With aortic root dilation**

I	A	B	C
II	A	B	C
III	A	B	C

No sport with risk of collision

- **With no aortic root dilation and:**
  - no mitral regurgitation
  - no family history of premature sudden death
  - echocardiographic measurements every 6 months

I	A	B	C
II	A	B	C
III	A	B	C

No sport with risk of collision

- **With associated valvular aortic regurgitation**

See section on aortic regurgitation. No sport with risk of collision

Patent Ductus Arteriosus
Untreated
- **With small patent ductus**

I	A	B	C
II	A	B	C
III	A	B	C

- **With moderate-to-large patent ductus causing left ventricular enlargement**
  - must undergo surgical repair before unrestricted participation in competitive sports

None

- **With large patent ductus and severe pulmonary hypertension**
  - similar to Eisenmenger syndrome

See section on elevated pulmonary vascular resistance

Closed
- **With all of the following:**
  - no symptoms
  - no pulmonary hypertension
  - no ventricular enlargement

I	A	B	C
II	A	B	C
III	A	B	C

3 months after repair

- **With residual pulmonary artery hypertension** — See elevated pulmonary vascular resistance

---

Septal Defects

Atrial septal defects, untreated
- Small defect with no pulmonary hypertension

	A	B	C
I			
II			
III			

(all cells shaded)

- Defect with significant pulmonary hypertension and/or right-to-left shunt

	A	B	C
I			
II			
III			

(IA shaded)

- Severe Eisenmenger class with marked cyanosis and large right-to-left shift

None

See section on arrhythmia and valvular dysfunctions

- Symptomatic supraventricular, *or*
- Ventricular arrhythmia, *or*
- Significant mitral regurgitation

Atrial septal defect, treated
- With no associated cardiac dysfunction

	A	B	C
I			
II			
III			

(all cells shaded)

See sections on elevated pulmonary vascular resistance and ventricular dysfunctions

- With *any* of the following cardiac dysfunctions:
  - associated pulmonary hypertension
  - arrhythmia with symptoms
  - myocardial dysfunction

Ventricular septal defect, untreated
- Small or moderate size

	A	B	C
I			
II			
III			

(all cells shaded)

See section on elevated pulmonary vascular resistance

- Large right-to-left shunt

- Large defects

	A	B	C
I			
II			
III			

(IA shaded)

Ventricular septal defect, treated (greater than 6 months after repair)
- With no residual defect and no symptoms
- With small residual defect *with:*
  - no pulmonary hypertension *and*
  - no arrhythmias or myocardial dysfunction

	A	B	C
I			
II			
III			

(all cells shaded)

- With residual moderate or large defect

	A	B	C
I			
II			
III			

(IA shaded)

See sections on elevated pulmonary vascular resistance or ventricular dysfunction after cardiac surgery

- With mild-to-moderate pulmonary hypertension or ventricular dysfunction

- With persistent, severe pulmonary hypertension

None

See section on arrhythmia

- With significant arrhythmia

Stenosis—Congenital Valvular

The severity is determined by the peak instantaneous systolic pressure gradient at rest (with normal cardiac output)

Aortic valve, untreated
- **With mild aortic stenosis (< 20 mm Hg) and:**
  - normal ECG
  - normal exercise tolerance
  - no history of exercise-related chest pain, syncope, or arrhythmia associated with symptoms
- **With moderate aortic stenosis (21–49 mm Hg): if have mild or no left ventricular hypertrophy and none of conditions listed above**

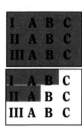

- **With severe aortic stenosis (> 50 mm Hg)**

None

Aortic valve, treated
- **With residual mild, moderate, or severe stenosis**

See recommendation for untreated aortic stenosis

- **With moderate to severe aortic regurgitation**

See guidelines for valvular dysfunctions

Pulmonary valve, untreated
- **With peak systolic gradient, < 50 mm Hg and both:**
  - normal right ventricular function
  - no cardiac symptoms

- **With peak systolic gradient > 50 mm Hg**

Pulmonary valve, treated
- **With normal ventricular function and no cardiac symptoms:**
  - if balloon valvoplasty, can begin sports ~ 1 month after
  - if operation, can begin ~ 3 months after

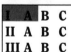

- **With a persistent peak systolic gradient > 50 mm Hg**

- **With severe pulmonary incompetence characterized by marked right ventricular enlargement**

Use individual assessment

Tetralogy of Fallot—Postoperative
- **If the following conditions are met:**
  - normal or near-normal right heart pressure
  - only mild right ventricular volume overload
  - no rhythm abnormality on ambulatory ECG or exercise testing
  - no evidence of a significant left-to-right shunt

- **If have any of the following:**
  - marked pulmonary regurgitation
  - residual right ventricular hypertension (peak systolic right ventricular pressure ≥ 50% systemic pressure)
  - rhythm abnormalities

Transposition of the Great Arteries
Postoperative Mustard or Senning operation
- **If there is:**
  - no significant cardiac enlargement
  - no atrial flutter or ventricular arrhythmia
  - no syncope
  - normal exercise test

	A	B	C
I	**A**	B	C
II	**A**	B	C
III	A	B	C

Congenitally corrected
- **If there are none of the following:**
  - no cardiomegaly
  - no evidence of arrhythmia on ambulatory ECG or exercise testing
  - no other cardiac abnormalities (VSD, pulmonary stenosis, AV valve abnormalities)
- Patient should be periodically assessed to monitor the development of arrhythmia and to determine deterioration of cardiac function

	A	B	C
I	A	B	C
II	A	B	C
III	A	B	C

Fontan operation—operated
- **All patients**

	A	B	C
I	**A**	B	C
II	A	B	C
III	A	B	C

- **If have the following:**
  - normal or near-normal ventricular function
  - normal or near-normal oxygen saturation
  - near-normal exercise tolerance

	A	B	C
I	**A**	B	C
II	**A**	B	C
III	A	B	C

Postoperative arterial switch
- **Six months after surgery, if each of the following exists:**
  - normal heart size
  - no residual defects
  - normal exercise test
  - absence of arrhythmia associated with symptoms

	A	B	C
I	A	B	C
II	A	B	C
III	A	B	C

- **If more than mild hemodynamic abnormalities or ventricular dysfunction**
  - exercise test is normal

	A	B	C
I	A	B	C
II	**A**	B	C
III	A	B	C

Ventricular Dysfunction After Cardiac Surgery (for Congenital Heart Disease)
- **Normal or near-normal ventricular function**

	A	B	C
I	A	B	C
II	A	B	C
III	A	B	C

- **With mildly depressed ventricular function**

	A	B	C
I	A	B	C
II	A	B	C
III	A	B	C

- **With moderately depressed ventricular function**

	A	B	C
I	**A**	B	C
II	A	B	C
III	A	B	C

CORONARY ARTERY DISEASES

Coronary Artery Disease in Kawasaki's Disease
- **With no coronary involvement or with documented resolution of any previous aneurysms**

	A	B	C
I	A	B	C
II	A	B	C
III	A	B	C

- **With minor residual abnormalities after resolution of coronary aneurysms**

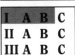

	A	B	C
I	A	**B**	C
II	A	B	C
III	A	B	C

- **With persistent coronary artery aneurysm or stenosis**

I **A** B C
II A B C
III A B C

- **With evidence of intermittent myocardial ischemia**

None

Myocardial Bridging of an Epicardial Artery
- **With no evidence if myocardial ischemia at rest or during exercise**

I **A B C**
II **A B C**
III **A B C**

- **With evidence of myocardial ischemia**

I **A** B C
II A B C
III A B C

Cardiac Transplant Recipients
- **Without advanced coronary artery disease and with normal exercise tolerance for age**

I **A B C**
II **A B C**
III **A B C**

- **Without advanced coronary artery disease with reduced exercise capacity for age**

Sports according to patient's exercise capacity

- **With documented coronary artery disease**

I **A** B C
II A B C
III A B C

MYOCARDIAL DISEASES

Hypertrophic Cardiomyopathy
Note: The relative risk for sudden death by virtue of participating in competitive athletics is largely unknown. At present, it is not possible to stratify risk for individuals with hypertrophic cardiomyopathy (see full text in JACC, 1994).
- **Patients < 30 years old: only selected low-risk patients may participate in IA sports**
  - This includes patients with or without symptoms
  - This includes patients with left ventricular outflow obstruction
  There is a higher risk for patients with arrhythmias

I **A** B C
II A B C
III A B C

- **Selected patients > 30 years with *none* of the following cardiac complications:**
  - ventricular tachycardia on ECG
  - family history of sudden death due to hypertropic cardiomyopathy
  - history of syncope
  - severe hemodynamic abnormalities (e.g., dynamic left ventricular outflow gradient ≥ 50 mm Hg)
  - exercise-induced hypotension
  - mitral regurgitation, enlarged left atrium, paroxysmal atrial fibrillation
  - evidence of abnormal myocardial perfusion

Individual exercise prescription

Myocarditis
- **After onset of clinical manifestations**

None

For at least 6 months

- **When ventricular function and cardiac dimensions have returned to normal and no ventricular ectopic activity or sustained supraventricular tachycardia are present**

I **A B C**
II **A B C**
III **A B C**

Pericarditis

| None |

Until there is no
evidence of active
disease

Other Myocardial Diseases:

▶ **Arrhythmogenic right ventricular dysplasia**
▶ **Idiopathic dilated cardiomyopathy**
▶ **Primary restrictive cardiomyopathies**
▶ **Systemic diseases with cardiac involvement (e.g., sarcoidosis)**

| None |

Until there is more
information available

ARRHYTHMIAS

Atrial Fibrillation (in the absence of Wolff-Parkinson-White syndrome)

Note: If on anticoagulants, avoid sports with danger of collision
● **Patients without structural disease:**
  • Who maintain ventricular rate comparable to that of appropriate sinus
    tachycardia during physical activity with or without therapy

● **Patients with structural disease:**

  • Who maintain ventricular rate comparable to that of appropriate sinus
    tachycardia during physical activity with or without therapy:

Can participate in
sports consistent
with the limitations
of the structural
heart disease.

Atrial Flutter (in the absence of Wolff-Parkinson-White syndrome)

Note: If on anticoagulants, avoid sports with danger of collision
● **Patients without structural disease:**
  • Who maintain a ventricular rate comparable to that of appropriate sinus
    tachycardia during physical activity while receiving pharmacologic treatment

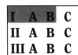

Warning: rapid 1:1
conduction may still
occur

● **Patients without structural disease:**
  • who have been without atrial flutter 3–6 months with or without treatment

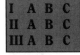

● **Patients with structural heart disease:**
  • who have not had an episode of atrial flutter after 6 months

Atrioventricular Junctional Escaped Beats/Rhythms

● **With normal or structurally abnormal hearts:**
  • in whom bradycardic rate increases appropriately by physical activity
● **With symptoms of impaired consciousness clearly attributable to
  arrhythmia but asymptomatic after 3–6 months of treatment**

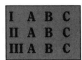

● **With treated symptomatic tachycardia/bradycardia syndrome or
  inappropriate sinus tachycardia that has been asymptomatic 3–6 months**

I A B C
II A B C
III A B C

● **With syncope or near syncope**

Should not particip-
ate in sports in which
momentary loss of
consciousness may
be hazardous

● **With pacemaker**

Should not partic-
ipate in any sports
in which there is
danger of collision

Complete Left Bundle Branch Block
● **Older athletes with acquired left bundle branch block**

Follow recommen-
dations of complete
right bundle branch
block

● **With normal HV interval and a normal AV conduction response to pacing**

● **With an abnormal AV conduction characterized by an HV interval > 90 ms or a His-Purkinje block**

Complete Right Bundle Branch Block
● **Asymptomatic and:**
  - without ventricular arrhythmia
  - no development of AV block with exercise
  This also applies to athletes with associated left-axis deviation

---

Complete Heart Block
Congenital
● **With structurally normal heart and normal cardiac function and all of the following:**
  - no history of syncope or near syncope
  - a narrow QRS complex
  - ventricular rates at rest > 40–50 beats/min increasing with exertion
  - no or only occasional premature ventricular complexes
  - no ventricular tachycardia during exertion

● **With ventricular arrhythmia, symptoms of fatigue, near syncope or syncope, or with an abnormal hemodynamic status**

Acquired

Congenital Long QT Interval Syndrome
● **With prolonged QT or QTU interval syndrome**
  These patients are at risk for sudden death with activity

None

Disturbances of Sinus Node Function

See atrioventricular
junctional escape
beats/rhythms

First-degree AV Block
● **If the following conditions apply:**
  - asymptomatic
  - no evidence of structural heart disease
  - first-degree AV block does not worsen with exercise

● **If underlying heart disease is present**
  The nature and severity of the underlying heart defect can independently
  dictate alternative restrictions

Follow the recomm-
endations of the
heart defect present

Nonparoxysmal AV Junctional Tachycardia
● **Patients with no symptoms and without structural disease who:**
  • maintain controlled ventricular rate that increases and slows appropriately in relation to the level of activity with or without therapy

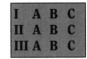

● **Patients with no symptoms and either:**
  • structural heart disease
  • incompletely controlled ventricular rates

(If the nature of the structural defect allows)

Premature Atrial Complexes

Premature Ventricular Complexes
● **Without structural heart disease and**
  • have premature ventricular complexes at rest, during exercise and exercise testing

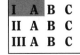

● **Without structural heart disease but:**
  • premature ventricular complexes increase in frequency during exercise or exercise testing to the extent that they produce symptoms of impaired consciousness, significant fatigue, or dyspnea
● **With structural disease and either:**
  • with premature ventricular complexes with or without exercise
  • complexes suppressed by drug therapy

Supraventricular Tachycardia
● **Asymptomatic with reproducible supraventricular tachycardia**
  • recurrences are prevented with therapy or episodes are 5 to 10 seconds that do not increase in duration
● **With successful catheter or surgical ablation and are symptomatic and no inducible arrhythmia**

● **With syncope or near syncope**
● **Significant palpitations secondary to arrhythmia**
● **Have significant structural heart disease**
Should not participate in competitive sports until they have been treated and have no recurrences for ≥ 6 months.

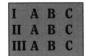

Type 1 Second-degree (Wenckebach) AV Block
● **With no structural heart disease and no worsening of AV block with exercise or recovery**

I	A	B	C
II	A	B	C
III	A	B	C

● **With structural heart disease and no worsening of AV block with exercise or recovery**

Follow the recommendations according to the structural abnormality

● **Asymptomatic but AV block initially worsens with exercise or recovery**

I	A	B	C
II	A	B	C
III	A	B	C

Type 2 Second-degree (Mobitz) AV Block

Follow recommendations for acquired complete heart block

Ventricular Flutter and Ventricular Fibrillation
- If there are no episodes of ventricular flutter or ventricular fibrillation for 6 months with treatment

  This recommendation applies in the presence or absence of structural heart disease

I	A	B	C
II	A	B	C
III	A	B	C

Ventricular Preexcitation (Wolff-Parkinson-White Syndrome)
- Without structural heart disease, history of heart palpitations, or tachycardia

  In younger age groups < 20 years, a more in-depth evaluation is recommended

I	A	B	C
II	A	B	C
III	A	B	C

- With syncope or near syncope
- With episodes of atrial flutter/fibrillation whose maximal ventricular rate at rest without therapy > 240 beats/min

I	A	B	C
II	A	B	C
III	A	B	C

Ventricular Tachycardia
- With sustained or nonsustained ventricular tachycardia:

  This recommendation applies whether the patient is untreated or treated with either drugs or catheter of surgical ablation

None

For at least 6 months after the last episode of ventricular tachycardia

- If there have been no clinical recurrences and:
  - ventricular fibrillation is not inducible by exercise
  - the athlete has no structural disease
- If the patient is asymptomatic and has:
  - no structural heart disease
  - brief episodes (<8–10 consecutive ventricular beats) of nonsustained monomorphic ventricular tachycardia, rates of < 150 beats/min

I	A	B	C
II	A	B	C
III	A	B	C

- -

- If the patient has structural heart disease and ventricular tachycardia

  This recommendation applies even if ventricular tachycardia is suppressed
- If the patient has an implantable defibrillators or antitachycardia device

I	A	B	C
II	A	B	C
III	A	B	C

Low intensity sports

SYSTEMIC HYPERTENSION

Hypertension
- With mild-to-moderate hypertension in the absence of target organ damage or concomitant heart disease

I	A	B	C
II	A	B	C
III	A	B	C

- With severe hypertension

I	A	B	C
II	A	B	C
III	A	B	C

- With other coexisting cardiovascular diseases

Follow recommendations for associated heart conditions

ACQUIRED VALVULAR HEART DISEASE

Aortic Regurgitation

- **With mild or moderate aortic regurgitation *and*:**
  - left ventricular size that is normal or only mildly increased above that expected to result solely from athletic training

	A	B	C
I	A	B	C
II	A	B	C
III	A	B	C

  - moderate left ventricular enlargement

	A	B	C
I	A	B	C
II	A	B	C
III	A	B	C

  - progressive left ventricular enlargement on serial studies

None

- **With mild or moderate aortic regurgitation and ventricular arrhythmia at rest or with exertion**

	A	B	C
I	A	B	C
II	A	B	C
III	A	B	C

- **With mild or moderate aortic regurgitation and symptoms**
- **With severe aortic regurgitation**

None

- **With associated Marfan's syndrome**

See section on Marfan's syndrome

Aortic Stenosis

Severity determined by mean aortic valve pressure gradient with continuous Doppler echocardiography

- **With mild aortic stenosis (< 20 mm Hg):**
  - with no history of syncope or arrhythmias with exercise

	A	B	C
I	A	B	C
II	A	B	C
III	A	B	C

- **With mild to moderate aortic stenosis (21–39 mm Hg):**

	A	B	C
I	A	B	C
II	A	B	C
III	A	B	C

  - For selected athletes in which the exercise capacity, the development of ST-segment depression, blood pressure response, and arrhythmias are evaluated at exercise tolerance testing at least at the level of activity achieved in competition

	A	B	C
I	A	B	C
II	A	B	C
III	A	B	C

- **With mild to moderate aortic stenosis and either:**
  - supraventricular tachycardia
  - multiple or complex ventricular arrhythmias at rest

	A	B	C
I	A	B	C
II	A	B	C
III	A	B	C

- **With severe aortic stenosis (> 40 mm Hg)**
- **Symptomatic patients with moderate aortic stenosis**

None

Mitral Regurgitation

Note: If on anticoagulants, avoid sports with danger of collision

- **With sinus rhythm and with normal left ventricular size and function**

	A	B	C
I	A	B	C
II	A	B	C
III	A	B	C

- **With sinus rhythm or atrial fibrillation with mild left ventricular enlargement and normal left ventricular function at rest**

	A	B	C
I	A	B	C
II	A	B	C
III	A	B	C

  - Selected athletes can engage in these sports

	A	B	C
I	A	B	C
II	A	B	C
III	A	B	C

• With definite ventricular enlargement or any degree of resting left ventricular dysfunction			None

Mitral Stenosis

• With sinus rhythm with mild mitral stenosis (mitral valve are > 1.5 cm^2 or exercise pulmonary wedge pressure < 20 mm Hg)

I	A	B	C
II	A	B	C
III	A	B	C

• Mild mitral stenosis and atrial fibrillation *or*
• Moderate mitral stenosis (mitral valve area 1.1–1.4 cm^2, or exercise pulmonary wedge pressure ≤ 25 mm Hg, or resting pulmonary artery systolic pressure ≤ 50 mm Hg

I	A	B	C
II	A	B	C
III	A	B	C

• With atrial fibrillation or normal sinus rhythm with mild mitral stenosis and
  • a peak pulmonary artery pressure of 50–80 mm Hg

I	A	B	C
II	A	B	C
III	A	B	C

• With either sinus rhythm or atrial fibrillation with severe mitral stenosis
• With pulmonary artery pressure > 80 mm Hg during exercise

	None

Mitral Valve Prolapse

• Structurally normal valve
• Abnormal valve with no cardiac complications

I	A	B	C
II	A	B	C
III	A	B	C

• Abnormal valve and have any of the following:
  • family history of sudden death associated with mitral valve prolapse
  • history of syncope of an arrhythmogenic origin
  • repetitive forms of sustained and nonsustained supraventricular tachycardia
  • moderate-to-marked mitral regurgitation
  • prior embolism

I	A	B	C
II	A	B	C
III	A	B	C

Multivalvular Disease

In general, patients with multivalvular disease should not participate in any competitive sports

	None

Specific recommendations should be based on the most hemodynamically severe lesion

Postoperative Patients with Bioprosthetic Valves

With prosthetic *mitral valve:*
• Are not taking anticoagulant therapy
• Have normal or near-normal left ventricular function
If anticoagulant agents are used, patients should not participate in sports with risk of bodily collision

I	A	B	C
II	A	B	C
III	A	B	C

With prosthetic *aortic valve:*
• Normal LV function
• Are not taking anticoagulant therapy
• Are without valvular dysfunction
Note: If anticoagulant agents are used, patients should not participate in sports with risk of bodily collision

I	A	B	C
II	A	B	C
III	A	B	C

• Selected athletes may be appropriate for the following activities

I	A	B	C
II	A	B	C
III	A	B	C

Postoperative Patients with Valvoplasty

- **With mitral stenosis (or occasionally mitral regurgitation)** *without* **left ventricular dysfunction**
  capacity to engage in physical exercise should be evaluated with an exercise tolerance test at least to the level of anticipated activity

Recommendations should be based on severity of residual mitral stenosis or mitral regurgitation

---

- **With mitral stenosis (or occasionally mitral regurgitation)** *with* **left ventricular dysfunction**

Consider as without operation

- **With mitral valve prolapse**

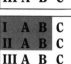

- In selected patients

Should not engage in sports with danger of collision

Tricuspid Regurgitation

- **Regardless of severity:**
  - in the absence of right atrial pressure > 20 mm Hg *and*
  - in the absence of elevation of right ventricular systolic pressure with normal right ventricular function

I	A	B	C
II	A	B	C
III	A	B	C

Tricuspid Stenosis

- **With associated mitral stenosis**

Follow recommendations according to the severity of the mitral stenosis

- **When isolated tricuspid stenosis**
  - if asymptomatic after exercise testing

I	A	B	C
II	A	B	C
III	A	B	C

Index

In this index, *italic* pages numbers refer to figures; the letter "t" refers to tables; *see also* refers to related topics and/or more detailed topic breakdowns.